D1404692

SCHOOL HEALTH INSTRUCTION

The Elementary & Middle School Years

SCHOOL HEALTH INSTRUCTION

The Elementary & Middle School Years

MARION B. POLLOCK, EdD

Professor Emeritus
Department of Health Science
California State University
Long Beach, California

KATHLEEN MIDDLETON, MS

Editor-in-Chief
ETR Associates
Santa Cruz, California

Third Edition

with 220 illustrations

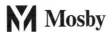 Mosby

St. Louis Baltimore Boston Chicago London Madrid Philadelphia Sydney Toronto

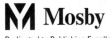

Mosby

Dedicated to Publishing Excellence

Publisher: Alison Miller
Acquisitions Editor: Vicki Malinee
Project Manager: Carol Sullivan Wiseman
Designer: Jeanne Wolfgeher
Design Manager: Betty Schulz
Cover Photo: Cathy Lander-Goldberg
Cover Design: GW Graphics & Publishing
Manufacturing Supervisor: Kathy Grone

THIRD EDITION
Copyright © 1994 by Mosby–Year Book, Inc.
Previous editions copyrighted 1984, 1989.

Printed in the United States of America
Composition by The Clarinda Company
Printing/binding by Maple-Vail Book Manufacturing Group

Mosby–Year Book, Inc.
11830 Westline Industrial Drive
St. Louis, Missouri 63146

Library of Congress Cataloging in Publication Data
Pollock, Marion B.
    School health instruction : the elementary and middle school years
  Marion B. Pollock, Kathleen Middleton. —3rd ed.
     p.   cm.
  Rev. ed. of: Elementary school health instruction. 1989.
  Includes bibliographical references and index.
  ISBN 0-8016-6745-3
    1. Health education (Elementary) I. Middleton, Kathleen.
  II. Pollock, Marion B. Elementary school health instruction.
  III. Title.
  LB1587.A3P64   1994
  372.3'7—c20   93-36645
                                      CIP

93 94 95 96 97 / 9 8 7 6 5 4 3 2 1

This book is dedicated

to the healthy growth and development of all school children,

and to their teachers, whose efforts and commitment contribute

so greatly to its protection and promotion

MBP

To Kirby

who brings new meaning to the importance of health and love;

may he, his teachers, and classmates

benefit from this work

KM

Preface

Health instruction during early school years can have a powerful influence on the quality of the lifestyle each youngster develops. These are the years during which most health-affecting habits and attitudes are being learned and can be shaped or reinforced most easily. Whatever other forces impact childrens' and adolescents' beliefs and actions, the schools are potentially among the most influential. What an effective teacher does to foster development of a healthy lifestyle among school children can be crucial not just to their present well-being but also to that of their families, friends, and their communities.

Health instruction is not an educational frill, it is a necessity. It is far too important to be delayed, as it often is, until the ninth or tenth grade. Children don't wait until they are in their teens to establish their values and health habits. Values and habits begin almost at birth.

AUDIENCE

This third edition, now titled *School Health Instruction: The Elementary and Middle School Years*, remains a textbook designed to help prospective elementary and middle school teachers teach children what they want and need to know about their health. At a minimum these teachers must have a sound background of up-to-date information about personal health and health behavior. Teachers need to have a clear understanding of the interrelationships among school health services, the quality of the school's environment (physical, social, and emotional), and the scope of the health instruction to be provided. Particularly, they need to know how to plan learning opportunities that encourage thinking, decision

making, and wise selection of health information sources when choosing among alternative health-affecting behaviors.

Although this book is primarily intended for use in college classrooms to guide the study of the school health program, it can also be used by health-concerned professionals as a medium for independent study. Everyone involved in making decisions affecting the quality of school health programs will find it a valuable resource, including elementary school teachers (grades K through 6) and middle school teachers (often grades 7 and 8) who have not had prior professional preparation for health teaching, school nurses, school principals, school physicians, and community health educators.

The overall intent is to provide the reader with the concepts and basic skills needed to understand, plan, and carry out a curriculum that reflects the very best of what is known about effective health teaching today. Although the book focuses primarily on instruction, the role of health services and provisions in protecting the safety and sanitation of the school's environment is emphasized throughout. A secondary intent is to provide the reader a general overview of health content as it is commonly covered in health education coursework.

"THE WAY IT WAS" IN HEALTH EDUCATION

Most adults, whether parents, administrators, or teachers, think of health instruction as *Hygiene*. In schools where some health education has been provided at primary and intermediate levels, the subject matter has tended to focus on grooming standards of personal care and watered down study of the anatomy and physiology of selected body systems. Often, lessons have been limited to the practice of tooth brushing or meal planning based on model meals that may or may not reflect realities of economics or cultural eating patterns. At best, this is not enough. Even our children know that there must be more than that to health education.

Moreover, teaching activities have tended to emphasize the acquisition of health-related facts as ends in themselves rather than a foundation for the ability to choose sensibly among alternative actions affecting well-being. The emphasis has been almost entirely given to provision of bits of information *about* health, rather than ways to promote and protect health. Today, there is a shift to experiential learning activities that are based on clearly specified and measurable objectives as guides to successful teaching and learning. Telling children what to do and believe about their health and equating ability to recite those *givens* with successful health instruction is being abandoned. Instead, the concepts and skills children are learning now promote acceptance of responsibility for their own actions and choices as these affect their health and safety. They are participating effectively and competently in self-care procedures appropriate to their age-group's abilities and understandings. Self-reliance and thinking skills are fostered in vital classroom health instruction today. Tested ways to plan and implement lessons of that kind are the focus of this textbook.

Historically, whenever new health problems have seemed uncontrollable through medical means, health education begins to be appreciated for its potential in solving the seemingly unsolvable. The current HIV/AIDS epidemic gives health education star status and boosts public recognition of its value as a weapon for disease control. Problems of drug use, including tobacco and alcohol use by children and adolescents, have created a surging market for related, packaged teaching programs. Which ones should you choose for yourself or your school? Studying the chapters of this book should equip any teacher at the very least to ask the right questions before purchasing computerized programs or learning guides focused on these problems.

THE THIRD EDITION

A wide range of ideas and findings gleaned from exhaustive search of current educational publications has been employed in the preparation of each chapter. Each chapter is headed by a set of measurable objectives specifying what the reader should know and be able to do when its study has been completed. Boxed information, propositions, case illustrations, summaries, updated lists of all references, and suggested readings are featured. In Part One, sets of questions, problems, and exercises at the close of each chapter have been completely revised or replaced with new items. Each set is intended to require the student to apply the just acquired concepts and information in new situations, not simply to repeat the material in words exactly as provided. These pedagogical activities will also encourage dialogue and cooperation among the class members.

NEW TO THIS EDITION

Changes to this edition are based on second edition reviews elicited from health education professors at schools offering courses in health instruction for elementary and middle school teachers. Instructors, whether users or nonusers of the second edition, were surveyed. Students enrolled in health instruction courses also submitted reviews suggesting changes. A synthesis of all these comments formed the basis for the design of this new edition.

As before, the third edition is divided into two distinct but interrelated sections. Part One covers theoretical aspects of health curriculum development, including instruction and evaluation. Part Two provides content supportive of the objectives proposed in Part One as appropriate for students at specified age levels. Part Two also gives valuable background information for the ten health-content areas.

Part One:

Theoretical Foundations

Part One has been totally updated where appropriate and revised extensively throughout. The sequence of its chapters has been reordered. Chapter 6, *Managing Categorical and Controversial Issues*, has been revised and now follows the first 5 chapters that deal with curriculum development procedures. This new position recognizes the role of the health educator in the community. The opportunity to work with individuals from communities with diverse standards and the need to use effective strategies for dealing with sensitive issues, such as HIV and human sexuality, are essential for a comprehensive health education curriculum. Chapter 7, *Health Education Evaluation*, and Chapter 8, *Designing Classroom Tests and Evaluation Activities*, focus on ways to measure and appraise the results of instruction. This presentation is more comprehensive than that in other health education texts. To facilitate its use, the Scope and Sequence chart has been totally revised and placed in Chapter 3 *Planning and Organizing the Curriculum*. Chapter 5, *Developing Effective Teaching and Learning Plans*, has been enriched by the addition of new material dealing with recent innovative and technological instructional advances, such as computer-assisted instruction and cooperative learning strategies.

Part Two:

Content and Practice

Part Two has now been extensively reorganized to facilitate its use. The chapters cover the ten generally accepted content areas: personal health, mental/emotional health, nutrition, family life education, disease prevention and control, injury prevention, drug use prevention, consumer education, environmental health and community health. Following the chapter on disease prevention and control, a new chapter on sexually transmitted diseases and HIV has been added.

Each of these health content chapters is organized by objectives for the reader, introduction to the content area, presentation of content, summary of the content, and listing of appropriate student objectives for that content area from the example Scope and Sequence chart developed by the authors. Also included are at least three examples of *fully* developed learning opportunities for primary, upper elementary, and middle school students, *fully* developed worksheets or teacher pages where appropriate, reduced versions of worksheets with answer keys in the margins of learning opportunities, and a listing of references and resources for each content area.

To improve the use of this text as a resource, our reviewers told us that the grade level presentation of the activities in the previous editions did not correspond to the way the course is being taught. We listened and reorganized! Now the information is easy to locate according to content area. Thus activities are all grouped together in primary, intermediate, and middle school order at the end of content chapters.

Content

Each chapter has a revised and expanded content section. This information is valuable to those students entering the course with limited knowledge of personal health content. Many of our colleagues indicated that this course might be the only one where important health information was presented. This presented us a with unique problem—should the health content presented be based on the needs and interests of college students or those of the elementary and middle school students they will be teaching? You will notice that we have taken a very different approach in the third edition. This new text highlights more current health information than earlier editions or competitive texts. Therefore, in using this text, students obtain practical information for themselves and the content background for their future role as a teacher.

School Health Instruction: The Elementary and Middle School Years is designed for educators charged with teaching content to children and adolescents. Therefore we have added the feature "What about my students?" to the content sections of chapters. This feature is designed to assist the teacher in determining the appropriateness and emphasis of content for elementary and middle school students. Often, we have chosen to present material in boxes to simplify complicated information or to highlight specific information.

Activities

We have retained the popular, effective activities and worksheets. For this edition, several new learning opportunities were developed based on the suggestions from reviewers that certain learning opportunities were weak. In *all* cases, learning opportunities were updated as necessary.

New Features

Terminology: New and important terminology changes were incorporated into both content and learning opportunity sections. For example, the term "accident" is no longer an appropriate term or concept. It is replaced by "injury prevention." The content section for Chapter 15 reflects the most current thinking in this area conceptually linking both intentional and unintentional injury.

New Chapter: Chapter 14, *Preventing STD and HIV: A Special Concern* is the only one of the eleven chapters in Part Two that is not a traditionally recognized content area. Since this topic has special significance to college students for their own health and needs sensitive treatment in elementary and middle school classrooms, a separate chapter on STDs, including HIV infection, was designated. This chapter largely follows similar organization as the content area chapters. Emphasis is placed on prevention of infection, ranging from choosing abstinence to making decisions about safer sex. Sections that indicate considerations for teaching about STD and HIV are featured in this chapter. The list of possible student objectives shows how this sensitive topic fits into planned health instruction. One example of a learning opportunity enables readers to see how sensitive and complicated content can be presented to upper elementary students.

Marion B. Pollock
Kathleen Middleton

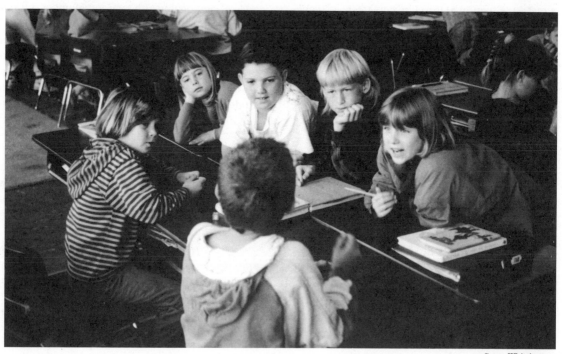

Scott Whittington

Acknowledgments

We wish to acknowledge the contributions of the following people whose thoughtful reviews of the second edition were valued aids in making revisions. These were:

Jacqueline R. Benedik
    University of Southwestern Louisiana
Donald L. Calitri
    Eastern Kentucky University
Sig Fagerberg
    University of Florida
Steven R. Furney
    Southwest Texas State University
Susan Giarratano
    California State University Long Beach
Onie Grosshans
    University of Utah
Sherman Sowby
    California State University Fresno

Many others whose contributions merit special thanks include our good friend and colleague, Don A. Beegle, MS, MPH, Professor of Health Science at California State University, Long Beach, who identified and obtained all of the references cited in Part One. Evalyn Gendel, MD, whose spe-cial expertise and advice were invaluable in the development of Chapter 6. We are indebted to teachers Angela Loya, Matt Fischer, Robin Gray Ballard, and the Computer Class teachers at the Arroyo Vista Elementary School in South Pasa-dena for their willingness to use their students as models for many of the new pictures featured in this edition. Beverly Bradley, PhD, was gener-ous in providing copies of some of the health record forms, including those that use the many languages necessary in the multicultural schools throughout the country. Nora Krantzler, PhD, MPH, brilliantly assisted in compiling content for Part Two. Many thanks also to the friends who assisted in this and previous editions, including Ric Loya, MS, Judy Scheer, EdS, and Betty Hub-bard, EdD.

Finally, with deeply felt gratitude we ac-knowledge the patient and painstaking attention to the numerous details by the editorial staff at Mosby as we worked together to prepare the fi-nal version of the text. Most particularly, we wish to thank Vicki Malinee, Wendy Schiff, and the many members of the editorial staff whose con-tributions were so significant, although we may never know their names or roles in the task.

Contents in Brief

Contents

CHAPTER 4

Defining Goals and Objectives for Health Teaching 96

CHAPTER 5

Developing Effective Teaching and Learning Plans 115

CHAPTER 6

Managing Categorical and Controversial Issues 148

CHAPTER 7

Health Education Evaluation   166

CHAPTER 8

Designing Classroom Tests and Evaluation Activities   189

CHAPTER 9

Personal Health and Fitness   215

CHAPTER 18

Environmental Health 440

CHAPTER 19

Community Health 464

Appendixes 485

Glossary 503

PART ONE

Theoretical Foundations

1 Health Instruction: Promoting Positive Lifestyles

When you finish this chapter, you should be able to:

- Define the meanings of key terms concerned with health promotion through health instruction.
- Describe the basic components of the total school health program.
- Explain the relevance of Piagetian and health belief model theories to the development of age-appropriate health teaching plans.
- Evaluate the influence of social, legislative, economic, educational, and other community influences in determining the quality of a school health program.
- Describe the unique role of the teacher in promoting the health of children and ultimately the community.

During the last hundred years, life expectancy for Americans has increased by more than 25 years. Advances in medicine and technology account for some of that. Yet what you can do for yourself every day of your life is twice as effective as medicine can do for you once you are ill. Improved lifestyles make the difference in longevity. The challenge for health education is to educate people not after but *before* they have made themselves ill. William Foege, distinguished scientist, medical practitioner, and educator says "each person is twice as powerful as twentieth century medicine . . . in public health we're going to have to realize that the educators are twice as powerful as all physicians" (16).

Think about that. As a teacher, you can be the most effective health educator a child will ever encounter during his or her entire school experi-ence. Childhood years are those during which most health practices and attitudes are being learned and established. Lewis and Lewis conclude that the principal determinants of health status in adulthood are formed very early and can be influenced for the better by those who care about the health of children (32).

Health behaviors begin to be shaped almost at birth. From then on, virtually everything we do affects health—and not just our own. Health information and a child do not wait to be introduced by a teacher, however. Long before children start school they have learned a great many aspects of health behavior. They have learned food likes and dislikes and ways of getting along with family and friends. They have well-established attitudes and value systems, based on a host of health-related experiences at home and

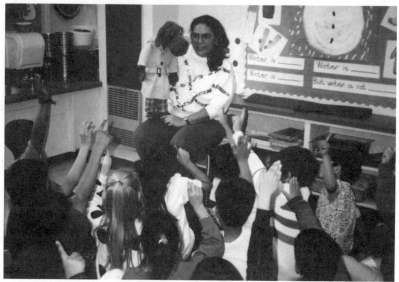

Angela Loya

The teacher can be a child's most effective health educator.

in the neighborhood. They have already accumulated a growing number of beliefs about health and the causes of illness.

The aim of health instruction is to help youngsters learn how to satisfy health related urges and needs in ways that are constructive and responsible. Those are the more immediate, everyday actions that typically are taken without conscious thought. The important decisions (and few do not affect health in some way) require problem-solving skills, which must be practiced and learned if we are not to be limited to choices based on trial and error, advertisements, or hearsay.

Health education is not accomplished through memorization and recitation of descriptions of the diseases to which children are vulnerable, body functions, or anatomy. Nor is it the outcome of single units of teaching focused on health problems of the moment or year. In short, health instruction is not learning to say "no" to potentially life-threatening behaviors. It is learning to say "yes" to choices marked by the abundant wellness, energy, and zest for the good life that are their reward.

The primary source of health training has always been one's parents. It still is, but today another "parent"—television—has become the favored babysitter and largest source of information about everything in life, including health. The average child between the ages of 6 and 11 spends 25 hours per week, roughly one third of nonschool hours, watching TV. By high school graduation, a student has been exposed to some 350,000 commercials (6). An example of the efficacy of this bombardment of sales pitches is illustrated by the following. Over a period of 5 years a study of viewers aged 6 to 17 found that TV viewing is the most powerful predictor of whether a child becomes obese. The more hours spent watching TV, the more apt it is that a child will be overweight. This is attributed to the fact that foods are the most heavily advertised product on television.

The fact that children learn by imitation is well established, and television shows offer many examples of behaviors that no one would describe as ideal. The implications of promoting eventual alcohol abuse, violence and aggressive behaviors, premature sexual activities, teenage pregnancy, use of tobacco products, and other harmful habits should be obvious (24).

Educational programs such as Sesame Street, although fun to watch, do teach fundamental concepts and cognitive skills. However, Postman believes what children learn to love is not education or schooling but television. Commercial television programs, which are those most often watched because there are so many more of them, are meant to sell a product (42). Often such programs seem to be advertisements interrupted by a bit of entertainment rather than the other way around, and the product being promoted is almost always something that affects health.

In short, education in school about health, even if it begins in kindergarten, must be carefully planned if it is to reinforce or counteract what children have already learned that affects their healthy growth and development. Direct health teaching cannot be safely postponed as it sometimes is until grade 7 or 10 without being too late, as well as too little.

What should be taught about health during elementary and middle school years? What does a child need to know about health after completing each of the grades? Clearly, there are no specific bits of information however true today that can be prescribed as adequate for solving health problems common among youngsters of any given age. Even if there were, their usefulness can only be judged according to today's best sources. By the time a child reaches adulthood, there will be new information making a lot of what has been learned already obsolete.

Lewis Thomas observes: "We ought to be developing a much better system for general education about human health with more curricular time for acknowledging, and even some celebration, of the absolute marvel of good health that is the real lot of most of us, most of the time" (48).

What can a very young child comprehend according to Piagetian theory? What methods are most appropriate based on what is known about levels of learning in terms of readiness? What skills and knowledge have the greatest potential for transfer?

If schools are to be effective in helping today's child survive in the twenty-first century, health teaching limited to study of the structure and functioning of the body systems won't help. The study of *hygiene* (i.e., focus on care of the body and grooming standards and practices) as conducted in the past is much less relevant to the solution of space-age health problems than it was even 20 years ago.

Health instruction that begins and continues throughout elementary and middle school years has the advantage of timeliness. Decisions and actions that affect an individual's health do not wait for physical, social, or legal maturity. They are needed and happen during early childhood. What a teacher does to foster the development of a healthful lifestyle among students can be crucial not only to their well-being today but also to that of their families and even the total community tomorrow.

THE LANGUAGE OF HEALTH EDUCATION

Notice how many words or word combinations related to health have already been used in the preceding pages. Rather than assume that certain key terms will be interpreted as intended, brief explanations and discussion are presented to help clarify some of these terms.

Health

Everybody knows what health is, but defining it is a different matter. Health is a concept, an abstraction. It's easier to describe than define. Concepts are generalizations based on a myriad of perceptions. We describe health on the basis of diagnostic tests, one's own perceptions, and the observations of others, professional or otherwise. Many definitions of health have been proposed over the years. Today, the one with widest official acceptance is "a state of complete physical, mental, and social well-being and not merely the absence of disease or infirmity" (52). This view represents a significant shift toward a holistic view of health as a quality of life having several dimensions, even though such a condition

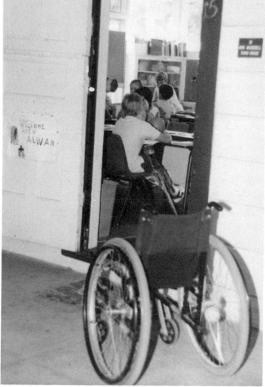

Armi Lizardi

Health is an optimal state of wellness for each individual, not just physical fitness.

admittedly is impossible to achieve. No one is ever entirely well in all three dimensions at once. Nevertheless, it was a landmark definition and remains the official definition for most of the world. More recent definitions include the following:

- Health is a state of well-being sufficient to perform at adequate levels of physical, mental, and social activity, taking age into account (31).
- Health is a relational concept . . . not an entity that can be directly promoted but a relationship between capacities and demands (5).
- Health can be regarded as a state of fitness to the environment, as a state of adaptation (13).

- Health is a quality of life involving dynamic interaction and interdependence among the individual's physical well-being, his mental and emotional reactions, and the social complex in which he exists (46).
- Health is what enables a person to be what he wants to be and do what he wants to do (27).

However defined, health is spoken about as being active rather than passive, as adapting, coping, and successful; as optimal functioning; and as indicating a strongly positive position on a continuum of well-being. The interdependence of the social, physical, mental, and emotional aspects of health makes it a dynamic that can only be understood as a constantly changing quality of life. One cannot be physically ill without an effect on mental and emotional well-being. Mental or emotional stress often causes physical illness, e.g., stomach ulcers or skin eruptions. Orphaned infants cared for in nurseries where the cuddling ordinarily given by loving parents is lacking do not thrive and sometimes die. In short, health is never attained wholly in a single dimension.

Health as a state of being can range from very good to very poor. On that continuum, whatever the challenges of illness, injury, or intolerable stress, how well one is able to cope depends on the choices typical of one's lifestyle. A positive lifestyle is the best preventive medicine available.

It is a reality of life, however, that perfect health does not exist. Even the healthy cannot escape illness or injuries entirely, but few people would consciously choose to be ill or limited in some way. There are some very simple ways one can avoid such problems if we know what they are and take advantage of them. There are immunizations available for some infectious diseases, e.g., hepatitis B, certain influenza strains, children's diseases such as polio, measles, pertussis, tetanus, and more. Diet choices affect the development of antibodies against bacterial infections. Adequate and balanced levels of exercise and rest reduce stress and promote strength. Avoidance of cigarette smoking or use of other harmful substances prevents damaging effects on the lungs or cardiovascular system. In short, one's lifestyle, which represents the sum of choices and actions taken by an individual, is the most powerful determinant of health, good or poor. It is the fundamental assumption of health education that most people will choose wellness over illness when they have learned how much their own actions can do to promote one or prevent the other.

The wellness continuum is illustrated here as a graph; the vertical axis refers to levels of wellness ranging from low, normal, and high. The horizontal axis represents a time factor, which is a theoretical life time that begins at birth and ends in death. The normal level is shown at center as a straight line moving along the normal level to the end of life. If the World Health Organization's definition of health could be realized, that straight line would depict "complete physical, social, and mental well-being." The jagged lines, identified as individuals *A*, *B*, and *C*, depict either positive or negative departures from normal. Which of them seems most normal? What would you conclude about the lifestyle of the remaining two individuals?

As a teacher you will be in an enviable position. First, you will be working with young people who are healthy, energetic, curious about their health, and eager to learn. They have few, if any, strongly developed poor health habits. You will not have to change their behavior so much as help them develop a pattern of positive beliefs and health practices. Don't fall into the habit of teaching them what *you* think they ought *not* to do, but teach them what they want to know about ways to grow to be the people they want to be.

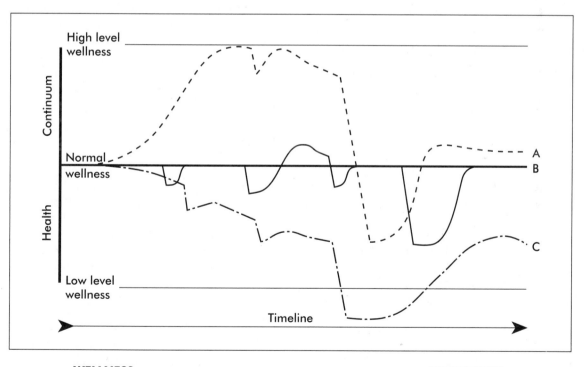

WELLNESS   **CONTINUUM**

FIGURE I-I
Wellness continuum graph.

Healthy/Healthful

There are few people who do not value health, although actual behavior is often inconsistent with that fact. In the United States, the consumer is constantly being urged to buy products or services because it is "healthy" or "healthful" to use them. Most often, the former term is used to describe anything that is supposed to be good for you. Is there any difference in the meaning of those two words? Healthy refers to an optimum state or quality. Healthful refers to some thing or action that promotes well-being. For example, a healthy rattlesnake can be very unhealthful for the victim of its bite. The more healthy the growth of pathogenic bacteria, the less healthful is the effect on the host. Vigorous exercise is healthful only if the individual is healthy enough to tolerate its physical expenditures. Viewed in this way, should a bowl of bran flakes be referred to as "healthy" or "healthful" food? (The latter is correct.) Watch for the use of these two words in advertising claims. How often are they misused? Resultant misconceptions may be the basis of decisions that can adversely affect health.

Health Behavior

McAlister defines health behavior as "any action that influences the probability of immediate and long-term physical and physiological consequences affecting physical well-being and longevity" (34). It may also be defined as the pattern of choices and actions representative of all of the decisions that affect one's total health.

Gochman proposed that "health behavior be considered substantively to denote personal attributes such as beliefs, expectations, motives, values, and other cognitive elements; personality characteristics, including affective and emotional states and traits; and overt behavior patterns, actions, and habits that relate to health maintenance and wellness, to health restoration, and to health improvement" (17).

Health Promotion

Health promotion is often used interchangeably with disease prevention, although the former has many other interpretations. The logic seems to be that whatever prevents disease is also health promoting. Carlyon says that the key element that distinguishes wellness (i.e., health) promotion from disease prevention is that it is not the purpose of wellness promotion to reduce or prevent risk factors for particular diseases; it is to help people develop lifestyles that can maintain or enhance health (9). Green and Kreuter define health promotion as "the combination of educational and environmental supports for actions and conditions of living conducive to health" (22). Duncan and Gold simply define the term as "all of the means by which healthy behavior may be encouraged" (14).

Disease Prevention

Disease prevention requires anticipatory action based on knowledge of disease causation and progression. Related actions may be primary, secondary, or tertiary in nature. Primary prevention is practiced before the disease occurs by taking measures to maintain health and taking specific actions to protect against disease (e.g., routine physical examinations, good nutrition, immunizations, use of seat belts, etc.). Secondary prevention depends on early diagnosis and treatment of disease, for example, prompt attention to and reporting warning symptoms of cancer, diabetes, unexplained and persistent changes in bodily functions, etc. Tertiary prevention has to do with rehabilitation, i.e., helping people disabled or handicapped by disease, accident, stroke, or other health problems to adjust as well as possible so as to resume normal life activities or employment (19).

The Joint Committee on Health Education terminology defines health promotion and disease prevention together as ". . . the aggregate of all purposeful activities designed to improve personal and public health through a combination of strategies, including the component implementation of behavioral change strategies, health education, health protection measures, risk factor detection, health enhancement and health maintenance (43). See also Appendix A.

Lifestyle

The concept of lifestyle covers the decisions made and actions taken by individuals that affect their health. Lalonde was one of the first to identify lifestyle as a major cause of illness and early death. He described it as "the aggregate of decisions by individuals which affect their health, and over which they more or less have control." He noted that personal decisions and habits that are bad from a health point of view create self-imposed risks (31). When these risks result in illness or death, the victim's lifestyle can be said to have contributed to or caused his or her own illness or death. Among such self-imposed risks, Lalonde listed destructive habits associated with drug use, faulty dietary choices, lack of appropriate exercise, careless driving, failure to wear seat belts, and promiscuity and carelessness leading to syphilis and gonorrhea.

Green and Anderson categorize four kinds of behavior, or health-related habits, as potentially harmful (20). These are alcohol abuse, smoking, eating patterns, and drug use. Those four patterns of behavior, together with physical activity or exercise, stress management or recreation, and safety practices, constitute the set of personal actions that are termed *lifestyle*. All of them are amenable to prevention as an outcome of comprehensive school health education programs. Although they are health related, they are not necessarily health directed. In 1992, unprotected sexual activity is perceived as a critical lifestyle behavior placing the individual at risk of contracting HIV.

Lifestyle is responsible for over half of the years prematurely lost in the more developed nations of the world. The children in your classes will not yet have built the set of habits that will constitute their lifestyle as an adult. However, the lifestyles of those they are observing and beginning to copy may be harmful or healthful. What you teach and how you teach it can make a difference.

Risk Factors

Risk factors are the characteristics or behavioral patterns that increase a person's risk of disease or disorders (in particular, heart disease, stroke, and cancer). Risk factors can be divided into those that cannot be modified (e.g., age, sex, family history, personality type) and those that can be modified (e.g., blood serum cholesterol level, high blood pressure, and cigarette smoking).

Self-Care

The active involvement of ordinary lay persons on their own behalf in health promotion, decision making, and disease detection and treatment is called *self-care* or *medical self-care*. It is not a substitute for professional care, but a partnership with it (29). Even small children can participate effectively in self-care activities. Experimental programs carried out by Lewis and Lewis led them to conclude that children are far more competent than adults believe them to be and that given the opportunity to practice self-care skills they might grow up to do "that which we as adults do very poorly"—that is, take care of themselves (32). Ferguson successfully taught medical skills (e.g., use of the stethoscope, thermometer, pressure cuff, pulse recording, etc.) to a group of first and second graders (15). The

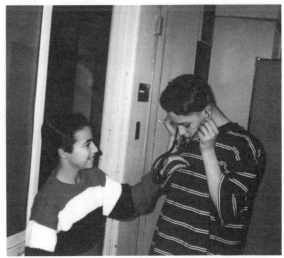

Matt Fischer

Children can learn basic medical skills.

teaching focused on things that the children said they would like to know about. It was discovered that one of the most important self-care skills was the ability to ask good questions and then figure out how to find the answers.

Before conducting a similar experimental course, Sehnert asked a group of sixth-grade children to indicate the person most responsible for maintaining their health among the following: mother, doctor, teacher, or myself (47). Only 21% chose "myself" before completing the course. Asked the same question after the course, the figure had increased to 85%. Clearly, as a corollary to learning self-care skills, these youngsters had also learned *self-reliance*. Brown argues that instead of trying to stuff as much knowledge, skills, and values into their heads as possible, we need to motivate children to manage their own lives (7). They need to learn self-reliance, not dependence, which is what teachers tend to do when they do things *for* children, telling them what to do and exerting control over them for their own good. He suggests that the rule should be "Do not do for children what they can do for themselves." The following three methods effective for making children self-reliant, independent thinkers are proposed:

1. Behavioral patterning—Arrange for children to behave in appropriate ways and they will become what they do. Children who act responsibly become responsible.
2. Expectation—Expect children to think, feel, and behave as self-reliant people do, and they will.
3. Modeling—The most powerful way children learn self-reliant behavior is by seeing that kind of behavior exhibited by parents, teachers, and other adults significant in their lives.

Admittedly, children cannot be completely independent of their families. The issue is whether we can find ways to help them grow into self-reliant individuals. Comprehensive school health education is the discipline whose subject matter and goals are most closely allied with and conducive to developing self-reliance.

WHAT IS HEALTH EDUCATION?

Generally speaking, health education refers to any health-related educational activities, whether in schools, community, clinical, or work settings. The same term is applied as descriptive of the discipline itself, the profession of its specialists, the outcome of its successful activities, any program designed to change health behaviors in some desirable way, and the special processes employed in effecting favorable changes in knowledge, attitudes, or practices.

Green et al define health education, whatever the setting, as "any designed combinations of methods to facilitate voluntary adaptations of behavior conducive to health" (23). That certainly fits all the settings and is probably the most often cited definition in the literature. But schools are in some ways different from those other settings. The fundamental assumption of the definition is that changing behavior is the primary goal, if not the only goal, of health education. Whether all of the health behaviors a child has learned need to be changed is debatable and certainly a question of importance for health instruction in schools.

Carlyon and Cook define health education as "any activity with clear goals planned for the purpose of improving health-related knowledge, attitudes, or behavior" (10). They say that "the prevalent notion that the sole purpose of health education is to change behavior is erroneous. It may be used to prevent, initiate, and sustain behavior as well." This would seem more appropriate as description of health education in schools.

Since this textbook focuses almost exclusively on health education in elementary and middle schools, the term will be used to refer to the total school health program, its purposes, procedures, and strategies. The school health program has three interrelated components: (1) health services, (2) environmental health (the provisions taken to ensure students a safe and sanitary place in which to study and play), and (3) health instruction. The overall purposes of the school health program are to protect, maintain, and promote the health of the children and adults who live and work together every day of the school year.

Although planned and sometimes unplanned teaching and learning experiences occur as an outcome of the first two program components, only those people involved in health instruction are directly concerned and responsible for planning the health education curriculum and providing the instruction designed to fulfill its goals.

Health education, or health, as it is sometimes termed, is seldom if ever listed among the courses school-aged students are required to study every year, but it is there. Goodlad's nationwide survey identified specific health education topics included in the curricula of science (nutrition and drugs/alcohol), social studies (themes of understanding self, family, and friends), and physical education (typically "wet days" emphasis on health and safety topics including nutrition) during both primary and upper-elementary school years (18).

WHAT HEALTH EDUCATION IS NOT

Sometimes it helps to define a term or activity by describing what it is not. Too often what is offered students in schools is best described as one of those things that it is not. Health education is not simply a minor aspect of physical education nor is it hygiene with another name. It is not a program focused on promoting physical fitness, although fitness is surely a parallel goal of health education. It is not simplified information about the anatomy and physiology of the body and its systems. It is not biology as it applies to human functioning. It is not sex education. It is not one or two short units specific to current health concerns, such as AIDS and drug abuse, temporarily hosted by another course as a means of meeting state requirements or satisfying community pressure. It most certainly is not simply an assembly lecture topic, a physical education rainy day activity or incidental teaching in response to momentary health-related problems or happenings. Most emphatically it is not a dreary

set of "do's" and "don'ts" applied to food selection, sexuality, or the satisfaction or denial of any other human need. It is education for healthful living—individual, family, and community.

SOURCES OF MISPERCEPTIONS OF HEALTH EDUCATION

If that is the case, why is health instruction often misinterpreted or confused with other related courses or disciplines, as we have just shown? There are several reasons. First, the professional preparation of school administrators, who make most of the decisions regarding what will be taught and how much time will be allotted, seldom includes study of either the content or the methodology of health education. Second, many of the teachers, parents, and other adults involved in curriculum planning have confused impressions of health education based on their own school experiences. As Kolbe and Gilbert point out, "Perceptions of health education are usually drawn from remembrances of relatively unsophisticated school lectures about 'personal hygiene' that administrators, parents, and influential community members experienced during their own schooling" (30). Third, health seems logically linked to physical education inasmuch as the purposes of both focus on the maintenance and promotion of health. Fourth, health teaching historically had its genesis in early state legislation mandating the teaching of "health and physical education"; the title has stuck despite the firmly established independence of health education as its own discipline. Although there are few today that attempt to provide a joint major, many colleges and universities still title the department or division as before, although offering separate majors in health education, physical education, and sports. The result is that the media and authorities in education outside the field of health education continue to speak of "health and physical education" as if they were one discipline rather than two. For example, the Paideia Proposal recommends that 12 years of physical education, sports, and athletic exercises be accompanied by instruction about health as part of the general education of all students in public schools* (1).

In Bennett's report on elementary education, "Health and Physical Education" is listed among the disciplines essential to the education of all elementary-age school children (6). Most of the related discussion focuses on the need for exercise, the ability to do a desirable number of pull-ups, and participation in sports and fitness. Later, it is specified that health and nutrition education should be included as part of this aspect of the elementary curriculum.

So, if you are confused by the fact that health is so often linked with physical education, remember that what you are seeing is what we call the "missing comma syndrome." Think "health" (comma) and "physical education" because that is what it's supposed to mean (51).

WHY HEALTH TEACHING IN ELEMENTARY SCHOOLS?

The early years of a child's life are those during which important health-related attitudes and practices are established. A lifestyle begins to take shape virtually at birth; health education begins just as early, as soon as an infant begins to react to the environment, both human and physical. Within the limits of their experience and understanding, even preschool children have already accumulated a set of attitudes and habits that will be the basis of their lifestyle as adults. Adult lifestyles do not suddenly emerge sometime after one's twenties to direct future behavior that may lead to chronic illnesses or early death. A lifestyle is learned, every bit of it, and it happens day by day.

For these reasons and many others, health teaching cannot be neglected until the seventh or tenth grade, as is the case in some school districts. Education for health is so universally ac-

cepted as a primary objective of education that its place among the basic subjects is virtually unquestioned. Nearly every statement of the goals of education since the 1917 "Cardinal Principles of Education" has placed health high on the list of its priorities. The National Education Association (NEA) Project on Instruction reaffirmed this commitment to the value of and need for health education in these words: "The school, as the only social institution that reaches all children and youth, has responsibility for teaching the basic information, and for helping young people develop the habits and attitudes essential for healthful living" (39).

Children at every grade are highly interested in information about their body and its parts, about safe living/first aid, and prevention of health problems. Asked whether they thought studying about health is important, 88% percent of those queried in a survey of over 5,000 Washington State students in grades 4 through 12 agreed that it is (49).

According to a survey published in 1989 (3), in 43 states a legal basis for health education was established through education codes or other state legislation either mandating, encouraging, or supporting the provision of health instruction in schools. In 38 of the states, health is specifically mandated. In 36 of these states, health education was mandated by law. Furthermore, in 40 states the boards of education had enacted policy statements, regulations, guidelines, and accreditation standards to address health education.

For example, the New Mexico State Board of Education has established 11 goals that all school systems are to pursue, including the following related to school health (2): "Districts are to design and implement programs which will ensure that students: (1) maintain a positive self image, and (2) practice good health habits and develop an awareness of environmental conditions for the maintenance of mental, physical, and emotional well being." Nineteen states require a specific number of health instruction hours during the K thru 6 school years.

Although compulsory immunizations have

---

*Paideia signifies the general learning that should be the possession of all human beings.

nearly eliminated the incidence of certain communicable childhood diseases, children do suffer colds and the flu, infestations of head lice, and other acute conditions that can be prevented or controlled by the services and instruction provided through the school health programs.

Today, specific health-related behavioral problems have become worrisome. For example, some youngsters are experimenting with alcohol. It is reported that the average age of first use of alcohol is 13, although pressure to begin use starts at even younger ages. Moreover 26% of fourth graders and 40% of sixth graders report than many of their peers had tried beer, wine, distilled spirits, or wine coolers (26). Obviously the best time to start teaching children to say "no" to alcohol or other drugs is in the preteen years.

About 25% to 30% of 10-year-olds have tried smoking cigarettes. Many children claim first use as young as age 5 or 6. While development of the habit usually does not occur until late childhood or adolescence, it is recommended that tobacco education programs be initiated while children are in elementary school, preferably during kindergarten or first grade (50).

Use of smokeless tobacco is growing rapidly, helped along by advertising promoting its use as an alternative to smoking and showing famous professional athletes spitting what is obviously tobacco juice. At present, the largest population of smokeless tobacco users are young adult males. However, a recent survey of Oklahoma school children indicated that about 13% of third-grade boys and 22% of fifth-grade boys were already users (11).

Hypertension is being found among children and adolescents in numbers large enough to suggest that intervention in the form of comprehensive health instruction will be necessary so those children will be less likely to develop hypertension as adults. The condition is associated with obesity, which is linked to poor nutrition and excessive TV watching, overconsumption of foods high in fats and sodium, cigarette smoking, and lack of exercise. The implications of all of this for health instruction should be clear as it relates to the development of a lifestyle that will help children make choices during their lives that may prevent coronary heart disease or other complications that could develop from hypertension (25).

Figure 1-2 lists the 22 national health problem priority areas (26). Of the 300 national health objectives developed as targets for success in alleviating these problems more than one-third could be attained directly or indirectly by schools or can be influenced in important ways by schools' health services, through procedures taken to ensure a healthful school environment, through health instruction, and through physical

Health Promotion
1. Physical activity and fitness
2. Nutrition
3. Tobacco
4. Alcohol and other drugs
5. Family planning
6. Mental health and mental disorders
7. Violent and abusive behavior
8. Educational and community-based programs

Health Protection
9. Unintentional injuries
10. Occupational safety and health
11. Environmental health
12. Food and drug safety
13. Oral health

Preventive Services
14. Maternal and infant health
15. Heart disease and stroke
16. Cancer
17. Diabetes and chronic disabling conditions
18. HIV infection
19. Sexually transmitted diseases
20. Immunization and infectious diseases
21. Clinical preventive services
22. Surveillance and data systems

FIGURE 1-2
Healthy people 2000.

education programs that promote cardiovascular and physical fitness.

During the critical elementary school years, the elementary teachers in our nation can have a tremendous influence on the health of the adults these children will some day be. Curricula designed to promote positive lifestyles need to be offered to children before they have developed patterns of behavior that need to be changed. It may be too optimistic to think that in the few hours available to teach about health (estimated average of 40 hours per year) much could be done to counter the persuasions of advertisers, the pressures of peers, and misconceptions derived from the conventional wisdom. But good teaching can make a difference, particularly if the instruction is mindful of the fact that lifestyles are learned, not born, and that many health problems can be prevented or controlled if you know how.

As evidence, there are the results of a recent 3-year study of several different health instruction programs recently conducted under the aegis of the Centers for Disease Control and the Office of Disease Prevention and Health Promotion. In general, it showed that health education does work, that it works better when there is more of it, and that it works best when it is carried out with broad administrative support and teacher training programs and when continuity across grades is planned for and implemented. Furthermore, it works best when there is attention to the building of foundations of basic health knowledge rather than starting with categorical health problems at secondary levels of education and beyond (44). School health instruction needs to provide that sound foundation of basic health knowledge but always as a means of promoting positive health behaviors.

WHO TEACHES HEALTH?

The answer to this question is everybody. Although responsibility for health education of the young is shared by the home, school, and community, there is no one who does not in some way influence the health of children. In that sense everybody is a health teacher, although often not in the positive sense.

Home

Primary responsibility for health education rests with the family, which usually includes more than the parents and a child. Often there are brothers and sisters, aunts and uncles, cousins, grandparents, and sometimes sets of step relatives, in-laws, and other family. Every family member with whom a child has contact is teaching that child something about health. Whether this instruction is done consciously or unconsciously, children's health beliefs, attitudes, and practices are most powerfully derived from those communicated by word or behavior by family members. It is not solely the outcome of specific training nor just the result of observing and adopting family practices. A family's religious beliefs and ceremonies, the emotional climate of the home (whether serene and pleasant or the reverse), the quality of family relationships (based on mutual respect and love versus dominated by fear or neglect), and many other social factors have a tremendous influence on the health and health behavior of small children. When they enter kindergarten, children bring with them an already well-established system of beliefs, attitudes, values, and habits associated with health.

School

Children are required to attend school for 5 or 6 hours a day, 5 days a week, over 30 weeks a year for up to 13 years. The school is the social institution legally responsible for educating the children and youth of this country, and health has long ranked high among the primary goals of education. But health instruction is only one part of the school health program. **Health services** (e.g., health counseling and guidance, communicable disease control, and emergency care) and a **healthful school environment** (e.g., regulated, healthful temperature levels; ventilation; sanitary food services; and provision of safety devices and procedures) are just as important.

(These two program elements are described in more detail in Chapter 2.)

Every member of the faculty and staff of a school in some way adds to whatever formal health teaching is provided at any one grade. This is because every adult in the school serves as a model for the children by virtue of his or her role. The harmful health habits that adults exhibit or whose effects are evident, e.g., poor grooming, tobacco breath and nicotine-stained fingers, or obesity, do not go unnoticed by children. It is difficult to persuade youngsters that smoking is harmful when they know that their parents and teachers are smokers. Because personal beliefs and attitudes underlie almost everything that adults say and do, children cannot fail to be influenced by teachers' statements and observed actions in and outside the teaching situation.

Community

Health teaching is as communitywide as it is schoolwide. Commercial organizations spend billions of dollars annually in the attempt to influence the health habits and choices of children. Sometimes this is done directly and constructively, as in the production and dissemination of useful instructional materials. More often it is done less directly through sponsorship of television shows whose advertisements are designed to convince the viewer to buy a product. That product is nearly always health related, whether for good or for bad, but the motive for promoting its use is profit, not health.

Individuals in the community, whom children hold in awe or admire, powerfully influence their beliefs and practices. Police officers, firefighters, physicians, musicians (particularly popular singers), television and film stars, and athletes are role models whether or not they wish to be. What is taught by their examples can be beneficial or harmful. Campaigns against drug abuse, cigarette smoking, sexually transmitted diseases (STDs), and other lifestyle risk factors often feature messages delivered by well-known community figures for this reason. Celebrities, professional athletic stars, and authority figures need to be aware

that their personal health habits are copied by children, who try to act like those whom they admire.

Not least among community influences are those exerted by a child's peers and older children. Children teach children, sometimes more effectively than adults can. Health concerns are high on the list of topics about which youngsters want to know. They tend to seek information from other young people more readily than from parents, teachers, or any other adults. The problem is that when peers do not know the answers, rather than lose face by admitting that they don't know, they often provide misconceptions or misinformation. Yet, if effective health instruction were a part of general education at every grade, the reliance of younger children on older ones might result in desirable reinforcement for the instruction provided by elementary teachers.

ANALYSES OF CHILDREN'S BELIEFS ABOUT HEALTH AND ILLNESS

We know that what children and adults believe about health and illness influences their day-to-day actions and the choices they make, which together constitute a lifestyle. Children have not yet formulated the fixed pattern of behaviors typical of adults, hence they are more responsive to instruction and accepting of change. The effectiveness of health instruction during elementary and middle school years is critical to the quality and perhaps even to the length of life those children will later enjoy as adults.

Effective health teaching in schools cannot be based solely on adult views of the value of healthful behavior or on assumptions about children's health beliefs and attitudes. What is needed is health instruction that is age-appropriate in content and in stage of cognitive development at every grade.

Most of the research devoted to investigating the origin and development of the health beliefs and attitudes held by children has employed three theoretical models: (1) the Health Belief Model (HBM), an expectancy theory derived from social psychology; (2) Piaget's cognitive development theory (35); and (3) the Children's Health Locus of Control Scale (CHLC). It is not possible to discuss these theories adequately here, but the basic concepts will be briefly sketched.

The Health Belief Model

The HBM provides information about what children believe about illness and what they think they can do to avoid it. This model theorizes that when you know what a youngster believes about a specific illness or specific hazardous activity, e.g., how unpleasant or life threatening it might be, what could be done to prevent its happening, or reasons why anyone might find the wise choice difficult or less tempting, health teaching can begin. Stated more formally, the HBM provides information about what people believe relative to (1) their personal susceptibility to particular illnesses, (2) how serious the related health risks seem to them, (3) the probable benefits of an action taken to reduce that susceptibility and seriousness, and (4) the barriers to undertaking or continuing actions recommended to reduce the possibility of contracting the illness or diminishing the seriousness of such an illness (expense, fear, pain, embarassment, etc.). Susceptibility and seriousness have strong cognitive components and are partially dependent on knowledge. The model is sensitive to the individual's value system as well (45). We probably all do some things that we know are harmful to our health or are risky or even dangerous, but we do it anyway because it's fun, we want to do what everybody else is doing, or any number of things may seem more important than the possible outcomes that threaten health or well-being.

Piaget's Cognitive Development Theory

Application of Piaget's theory bridges the gap between *what* children believe and *why* they believe what they do. Four major stages of cognitive development are identified, each of which is characterized by qualitatively different schemes and all of which are experienced in order by every child. These four invariant stages include: (1) the sensori-motor stage (birth to age 2); (2) the preoperational stage (age 2 to age 7); (3) the concrete operational stage (age 7 to age 11); and (4) the formal operational stage (age 11 to adulthood).

Preoperational children tend to view illness as punishment for some transgression and to confuse cause and effects of illness. They perceive health and illness as two separate happenings rather than as opposite ends of a continuum. Circular reasoning is prominent, and they lack the ability to generalize between similar experiences (35). Their definition of health is general and undifferentiated (28). They reason egocentrically, relating each health-related experience to themselves (21).

Children at the concrete operational level tend to see health as the ability to perform desired activities. In third or fourth grade they blame germs for disease and begin to grasp the concept of causal sequencing. This age group only gradually becomes future-oriented as they mature, hence behaviors promising rewards of future health are not relevant to them (36).

Children at the formal operational stage consider mental health as integral to global health status. They understand linkages between behavior and health outcomes and recognize individual susceptibility in the onset of disease (35). Only these oldest children, with a good grasp of reversibility in their judgments, can see health and sickness as reciprocal components of the larger aspect of "health."

It will be easy to find out what the children in your own class believe about health and illness. Just ask them. Their answers should not be too different from those given by most youngsters in American schools. For example, as part of the Connecticut study, Byler et al. (8) asked students in grades K through 6 "What is health?" Their answers are as delightful to read as they are informative. Some answers from grades K through 2 include "You brush the dirt off your teeth" and "You don't have measles or mumps." In grades 3 and 4, comments made included

"Smells clean" and "Eats only a cup of sugar." When students in grade 5 were asked "What is a healthy person?" some said, "He eats right and drinks milk" and "He doesn't smoke or drink." Sixth graders said, "Health is germs." "Health is whether you are alive." and "Health is not getting bored which brings on bad health."

All these children viewed health as a state arising from regular observance of certain practices or rules related to exercising, eating good food, not being sick, and keeping clean.

Social Learning Theory: Children's Health Locus of Control

Recently, measures of children's health locus of control have yielded fresh insights into the source of children's health beliefs and behavior (40,41).

Based on social learning theory, data generated by the CHLC (a carefully validated measurement instrument) show that children with an internal locus of control, meaning self-directed or responsible, believe that they have some control over the status of their own health. Children with external locus of control, meaning dependent on more powerful others, believe that they are helpless and that good or bad health is simply a matter of luck.

Conclusions drawn from Parcel and Meyer's findings have important implications for health teaching. First, if an internal locus of control is necessary for children to be able to assume responsibility for certain types of health behavior, then it is essential that health teaching provide learning activities that reinforce an internal locus of control. Second, as children reach age 7 and older, their instruction should shift from external sources of reinforcement to internal locus of control reinforcing activities. Third, focusing on health content, as is often the case in schools, should change to teaching strategies that help children experience success in making decisions about health. If children learn to apply reasoned decision making to health behavior and to practice these skills successfully and at increasing levels of responsibility, then the chances of their

being responsible decision makers as an adult are far more likely.

Selected Generalizations and Recommendations

Some observations and recommendations made by researchers who have studied children's beliefs about health include:

- Young children commonly view health as a long-term state and illness as a short-term condition.
- Across all grades, health was attributed to "foods I eat," and the causes of illness were attributed to germs and bad weather.
- Younger children differ more among themselves in their beliefs about health than do older children (12).
- School health educators and health-care professionals run the risk of confusing and frightening children if their messages are too sophisticated. Conversely, information that is too simplistic for a given cognitive developmental stage may bore or insult the child and may be ignored (35).
- Hispanic children overwhelmingly view health (100%) as the ability to carry out activities, compared with white children (2%) and black children (8%) (37).
- Teaching young children principles of health maintenance to prevent illness is meaningless to them (36).
- Health as a motive for acting wisely does not play a prominent part in most children's cognitive worlds, nor do they often perceive themselves as vulnerable to health problems (12).
- The differences between the adult at 35 and the adult at 40 are insignificant in comparison to the tremendous differences between a child of 5 and a child of 10 in the ability to understand causal relationships (35).
- Both handicapped and able-bodied children ages 6 to 14 define health in much the same way (37).
- Educational interventions designed to develop or modify health beliefs will have

greater success if they are introduced to 6-through 8-year-olds rather than to older groups (12).

- Very young children tend to believe that health is a matter of luck and that illness just happens (41).
- Children of middle-school age believe that they have some control over their own health (48).
- Health education that centers on a young child's desires and current goals will be more effective than programs that emphasize future health. The more health teaching is related to everyday activities, the more effective it will be (36).
- Children's concepts of health and illness change qualitatively with cognitive development that affects the progression from pre-operational to concrete to formal thought as proposed by Piaget (28).
- Health-oriented educational programs that are consistent with the child's ability to process information may be more effective than traditional disease-oriented programs (36).

THE GOALS OF HEALTH EDUCATION

The goals of health education support those of general education. The first goal is to help each child develop a pattern of health behavior that tends to maintain or enhance rather than to diminish wellness; second, to look beyond personal wants to the general well-being of the community, family, and friends when taking actions that can affect the health of others; and third, to consider not only the needs of those alive today but those of the generations to come. To achieve these ends, health teaching seeks to equip children with fundamental health concepts and problem-solving skills that will be as basic to sound decision making in the future as they are today. Perhaps the ultimate goal is the development of an individual who is self-reliant, comfortable with her or his weaknesses and strengths,

and humane and sensitive to the rights and needs of others. This requires building a meaningful and worthy system of values to serve as personal behavioral guidelines. Admittedly, such ideal development is not easily attained if it must depend on formal education alone. Nonetheless, it is the goal of the total school health program and of health teaching in particular.

THE SPECIAL ROLE OF THE SCHOOL TEACHER

The school's responsibility for the total school health program is based on four fundamental beliefs: (1) the school must help maintain the health of the students in its charge as a means of ensuring their continued fitness to learn; (2) the school should maintain an environment that contributes to rather than detracts in any way from social, emotional, mental, or physical health; (3) the school should do its best to ensure the optimum health of each child through appropriate health services designed to appraise, protect, and promote well-being; and (4) the school should educate young people to make sound decisions about matters affecting their health and that of their family and friends. All school personnel contribute to these goals, but the role of the elementary teacher is unique.

Although comprehensive school health education is increasingly recognized as a national priority by major health and education organizations, the professional preparation of elementary teachers for health teaching has often been minimal or even totally lacking. There were no established standards for such preparation, thus no way the lack could be identified or remedied. This problem has been addressed by a joint committee of the Association for the Advancement of Health Education and the American School Health Association. In 1990, five areas of responsibilities and related competencies for elementary classroom teachers were identified and accepted as guidelines for the development of programs adequate to the need (Figure 1-3). Whether equipped by any special coursework or not, the teacher is the key person in every school's health program.

Although some school district's health education is assigned to "floating" health specialists or school nurses, most commonly the classroom teacher is responsible for all health teaching, along with teaching the other basic subjects. In most elementary schools a teacher works with the same group of boys and girls throughout the school year. All the health instruction a child receives, as well as the daily monitoring and adjusting of the classroom environment, is the primary responsibility of that one teacher. Even though school health services are provided by health-care professionals, the teacher's observations and prompt referrals provide the link between each child and any health care that may be needed during the school day. Mayshark et al acknowledged the significance of the elementary school teacher's contribution to the health of the school child in these words (33):

> If we were told that only one category of school personnel would be permitted to work for student health and that we had the authority to select this category, it would have to be the elementary teachers. Such a choice does not depreciate the important contributions of other school personnel, but it does recognize the immense responsibility that falls to this dedicated group.

Only the elementary school teacher works every school day, all day, with the same children. As a consequence, each child's total performance is well known, not only in terms of that youngster's usual appearance and behavior but also compared with the others in the room of the same age and level of development. Even small changes from the usual or expected behaviors are more quickly apparent to the classroom teacher than to any other observer. In fact the elementary school's first line of defense against an epidemic of communicable disease is the alert teacher's ability to spot signs of illness and to see to it that a sick child is quickly separated from the others and sent home. In addition to visual perceptions, teacher observation includes the sense of smell in detecting the use of substances, such as smokeless tobacco, cigarettes, alcohol, marijuana, or any other mind-altering substance. Touch may be important, as in the case of noting possible fever. Hearing also could be a source of information about a child's well-being (sounds of hoarseness, coughing, sniffling, or wheezing).

A more subtle but no less profound influence on health can be traced to the daily close relationship between teacher and students. Teachers are role models for impressionable young children. In the primary grades, but also during the intermediate school years, youngsters tend to love, admire, and emulate their teachers' behaviors. Brown suggests that "adults can promote self-reliance by showing an awareness of their own identity and autonomy, by defining for themselves appropriate values and behavior standards, by acting responsibly, and by providing children with experiences that help them grow into self-reliant adults" (7).

Classroom teachers shape a child's concept of health and health education as powerfully by what they do as by what they say. Thus a teacher's personal health behavior can enhance or counteract the message intended by health instruction. The very *way* a teacher presents health information, even the topics selected and the method employed, can reveal her or his attitude toward the importance or worth of that material and thus influence students' acceptance and use of it in their daily lives.

Comprehensive health education in schools has the potential to promote and protect the health of children, not just while they are in school but also during adolescence and adulthood. However important the contributions of other school personnel, family, and community, the classroom teacher's role is special and often pivotal in shaping children's attitudes and beliefs about self-reliance and the value of self-care in promoting their own health. Health teaching is not *telling* children about health and illness. It is giving them the concepts and intellectual tools they need in order to build and maintain a healthful lifestyle.

Responsibility I — Communicating the concepts and purposes of health education.
 Competency A: Describe the discipline of health education within the school setting.
  Sub-Competencies:
  1. Describe the interdependence of health education and the other components of a comprehensive school health program.
  2. Describe comprehensive school health instruction, including the most common content areas.
 Competency B: Provide a rationale for K-12 health education.
 Competency C: Explain the role of knowledge, skills, and attitudes in shaping patterns of health behavior.
 Competency D: Define the role of the elementary teacher within a comprehensive school health education program.
  Sub-competencies:
  1. Describe the importance of health education for elementary teachers.
  2. Summarize the kinds of support needed by the K-6 teacher from administrators and others to implement an elementary school health education program.
  3. Identify available quality continuing education programs in health education for elementary teachers.
  4. Describe the importance of modeling positive health behaviors.
Responsibility II — Assessing the health instruction needs and interests of elementary students.
 Competency A: Utilize information about health needs and interests of students.
 Competency B: List behaviors and how they promote or compromise health.
Responsibility III — Planning elementary school health instruction.
 Competency A: Select realistic program goals and objectives.
 Competency B: Identify a scope and sequence plan for elementary school health instruction.
 Competency C: Plan elementary school health education lessons which reflect the abilities, needs, interests, development levels, and cultural backgrounds of students.
 Competency D: Describe effective ways to promote cooperation with and feedback from administrators, parents, and other interested citizens.
 Competency E: Determine procedures which are compatible with school policy for implementing curricula containing sensitive health topics.
Responsibility IV — Implementing elementary school health instruction.
 Competency A: Employ a variety of strategies to facilitate implementation of an elementary school health education curriculum.
  Sub-Competencies:
  1. Provide a core health education curriculum.
  2. Integrate health and other content areas.
  3. Incorporate topics introduced by students into the health education curriculum.
  4. Utilize affective skill-building techniques to help students apply health knowledge to their daily lives.
  5. Involve parents in the teaching/learning process.
 Competency B: Incorporate appropriate resources and materials.
  Sub-Competencies:
  1. Select valid and reliable sources of information about health appropriate for K-6.
  2. Utilize school and community resources within a comprehensive program.
  3. Refer students to valid sources of health information and services.
 Competency C: Employ appropriate strategies for dealing with sensitive health issues.
 Competency D: Adapt existing health education curricular models to community and student needs and interests.
Responsibility V — Evaluating the effectiveness of elementary school health instruction.
 Competency A: Utilize appropriate criteria and methods unique to health education for evaluating students outcomes.
 Competency B: Interpret and apply student evaluation results to improve health instruction.

FIGURE 1-3
Health instruction responsibilities and competencies for elementary (K-6) classroom teachers.

SUMMARY

The purpose of health instruction is to foster the development of healthful lifestyles among children and youth during their public school education, K through 12. Elementary teachers have limited time available for health teaching and typically little background in health coursework. Nevertheless, they are potentially the most influential health instructors any child will ever encounter. Several advantages go with an elementary-level assignment to compensate for these limitations. First, there is the element of timeliness. These teachers are working with youngsters who are eager to learn about their bodies, how each part works, and what they can do to help themselves grow to be like grown-ups whom they admire. Second, elementary school children and their teachers live and work together all day, every day in the school year. Health teaching can be integrated throughout the curriculum as enrichment, rather than set apart as topics unrelated to the other studies. There is an opportunity to provide incidental teaching responsive to everyday, real-life health concerns and interests as they occur, rather than tied to the chapters in a textbook or topics in a curriculum guide. Third, young children tend to regard their teacher with admiration, affection, and respect; more than anything they want to please him or her. Thus they are far more readily motivated to change any behaviors that might need modification or to accept new ideas or practices presented to them. It takes more than that, of course. Because health education is a discipline as basic to the general education of children as are reading, writing, and arithmetic, there is a certain irreducible minimum of information about it that elementary teachers need to know. Most importantly, they need to be comfortable in their understanding of the language and the goals of health education. They must know what health education is, which means that they must also be clear about what it is not.

The term *comprehensive health education* as used in this text refers to the total school health program, which includes formal health instruc-

tion, required health services and procedures, and facilities designed to provide a safe and healthful environment for students and staff. Children are learning about healthful living as an outcome of the total program, and every member of the staff plays a part in that education. But planning and implementing health instruction is the responsibility of the teaching staff.

Elementary and middle school teachers need to have some experience with the stuff of health instruction, its content areas, supporting concepts and facts, and the experiential teaching strategies that bring it to life, whether gained in preservice or inservice study. They need to be able to apply what they have learned about learning theory and readiness to the selection of the health content and teaching activities appropriate for specified age groups of children. They must be able to identify children's existing health beliefs and attitudes and to infer what learning opportunities would effectively reinforce those that reflect good practice or could motivate new or improved health behaviors.

Most importantly, perhaps, they need to know that health instruction places less emphasis on personal hygiene and the prevention of common communicable diseases, and instead seeks to promote self-reliance, self-responsibility, and the development of a healthful lifestyle. The goal is never memorization of health-related facts or rules to live by; it is to give children the chance to discover how to find the answers to their own questions and health problems within the limits of their ability to think and act upon those answers.

QUESTIONS AND EXERCISES
Discussion questions

1. In what ways do the purposes of health promotion differ from those of disease prevention programs? How would those differences influence the focus of health instruction expected to promote health?

2. Interpret the meaning of the following statement: "Health teaching in the elementary school has the advantage of timeliness over that done at any other level of education."

3. Describe the unique role of the elementary or middle school teacher in preparing children to be effective health consumers and eventual self-reliant adults.

4. In what ways do the goals of health education support and overlap those of general education?

Problems and exercises

1. Differentiate between *healthy* and *healthful*. Which would you use to describe: (a) a daily regimen of exercise planned for a young office worker; (b) regular patterns of adequate rest and sleep for everyone; (c) a state of optimum physical fitness; (d) the ability to get along well with friends, family, and neighbors; and (e) flossing and brushing one's teeth as recommended by dental authorities.

2. Assume that you are invited to appear before a parent group to answer questions about the health curriculum in your school. One parent asks, "Aren't parents responsible for teaching their children to practice good health habits? Why do we need health teaching taking up important time in the elementary school curriculum?" How would you answer this query? How could you synthesize what you have learned here about community influences and possible negative health teaching to justify the importance of school health instruction? In a short paper, outline all of the principal reasons why school health programs are essential to maintain and protect the health of children while they are in school and to support and complement the goals of general education.

3. Consider these two definitions of health.
   1. Good health is a process of continuous adaptation to the many microbes, irritants, pressures, and problems that challenge humans daily.
   2. Health is a quality of life involving dynamic interaction and interdependence between the individual's physical well-being, mental and emotional reactions, and the social complex in which he or she exists.

   Which of them seems to be a better description of health? How might acceptance of either one over the other influence (a) the emphasis of health instruction given to support it, (b) the comprehensiveness of a resulting curriculum plan, and (c) the relevance of that health teaching to the stated goals of health education? Prepare a written set of answers to these questions for use in class discussions.

4. Make an informal survey of five or six young children in your immediate neighborhood. Having determined their age and grade in school, record their answers to the question, "What is health?" Analyze the answers you obtain relative to the age of the children surveyed and see if you can identify patterns of beliefs corresponding to Piaget's levels of cognition. If possible, compile the survey results of your entire class and draw some conclusions regarding the results.

5. From the moment you get up in the morning until you fall asleep at night, you are making decisions and taking actions based on those decisions. Of the actions common to those in our society, how many can you name that do not affect health in some way? Can decisions of this kind depend on conventional wisdom ("everybody knows that so and so is what one should do")? Should there be a planned curriculum for health teaching at every grade, K through 12? Be ready to support your point of view with specific reasons.

6. In your opinion, should the 22 priority areas upon which the Healthy People 2000 objectives for the nation have been based (see Figure 1-2) define the curriculum for health teaching for all school children? Name those that you would recommend for elementary and middle school level consideration, as well as any you would add that are not among those listed. Write a short paragraph justifying your selection of topics based on what you have learned about children's beliefs and abilities.

7. Looking ahead to your first job as a teacher, what other courses might you elect now to help you fulfill your future responsibilities for health teaching? Would you look for health content courses? If so, which ones and for what reasons?

REFERENCES

1. Adler M: *The Paideia proposal,* New York, 1982, Macmillan.
2. American School Health Association: *School health in America,* ed 4, Kent, Ohio, 1987, The Association.
3. American School Health Association: *School health in America,* ed 5, Kent, Ohio, 1989, The Association.
4. Bandura A: *Social learning theory,* Englewood Cliffs, NJ, Prentice Hall, 1977.
5. Baranowski T: Toward the definition of concepts

of health and disease, wellness and illness, *Health Values* 5:6, Nov/Dec 1981.

6. Bennett W: *First lessons: a report on elementary education in America*, Washington, DC, 1986, US Department of Education.

7. Brown B: We can help children to be self-reliant, *Children Today* 15:1, Jan/Feb 1986.

8. Byler R et al: *Teach us what we want to know*, 1968, Connecticut State Board of Education.

9. Carlyon W: Disease prevention/health promotion: bridging the gap to wellness, *Health Values* 8:3, May/June 1984.

10. Carlyon W, Cook D: Science education and health instruction, *BSCS* 4:1, 1981.

11. Christen A, Glover E: History of smokeless tobacco use in the United States, *Health Educ* 18:3, June/July 1987.

12. Dielman TE et al: Dimensions of children's health beliefs, *Health Educ Q* 7:3, 1980.

13. Dubos R: *Man adapting*, New Haven, Conn, 1965, Yale University Press.

14. Duncan D, Gold R: Health promotion—what is it? *Health Values* 10:3, May/June 1986.

15. Ferguson T: *Teaching medicine to kids: medical self-care*, New York, 1980, Summit Books.

16. Foege W: Closing the gaps: ensuring the application of available knowledge in the promotion of health and prevention of disease, *J Sch Health*, 60:4, 1990.

17. Gochman D: Labels, systems and motives: some perspectives for future research and programs, children's health beliefs and health behaviors, *Health Educ Q* 9:2, 3, Summer/Fall 1982.

18. Goodlad J: *A place called school*, New York, 1984, McGraw-Hill.

19. Green K: Health promotion: its terminology, concepts, and modes of practice, *Health Values* 9:3, May/June 1985.

20. Green L, Anderson C: *Community Health*, ed 6, St. Louis, 1986, Mosby.

21. Green K, Bird J: The structure of children's beliefs about health and illness, *J Sch Health* 56(8):325-328, 1986.

22. Green L, Kreuter M: Health promotion planning: an educational and environmental approach, Mountain View, Calif, 1991, Mayfield.

23. Green L, Kreuter M, Deeds S, Patridge K: Health education planning—a diagnostic approach, Palo Alto, Calif, 1980, Mayfield.

24. Grzelka C: Children and television, *Health Links* 3:(2), July 1987.

25. Harris J: High blood pressure in children and adolescents, *Health Educ* 18:3, June/July 1987.

26. *Healthy people 2000*, Washington, DC, 1990, Public Health Service.

27. Hochbaum G: An alternative approach to health education, *Health Values* 3:4, July/August 1979.

28. Kalnins I, Love R: Children's concepts of health and illness: implications for health education: an overview, *Health Educ Q* 9:2,3, Summer/Fall 1982.

29. Keever B, Lelm K: Introducing medical self-care in the curriculum, *Health Educ* 15:3, May/June 1984.

30. Kolbe L, Gilbert G: *Involving the schools in the national strategy to improve the health of Americans, Prospects for a healthier America: achieving the nation's health promotion objectives*, Washington, DC, 1984, Department of Health and Human Services.

31. Lalonde M: *A new perspective on the health of Canadians*, Ottawa, 1974, Information Canada.

32. Lewis C, Lewis M: Child-initiated health care, *Sch Health* 50:3, March 1980.

33. Mayshark C et al: *Administration of school health programs*, St Louis, 1977, Mosby.

34. McAlister A: Social and environmental influences on health behavior, *Health Educ Q* 8:1, Spring 1981.

35. Mickalide A: Children's understanding of health and illness: implications for health promotion, *Health Values* 10:3, May/June 1986.

36. Natapoff J: A developmental analysis of children's ideas of health, *Health Educ Q* 9:2, 3, Summer/Fall 1982.

37. Natapoff J, Essoka G: Handicapped and able-bodied children's ideas of health, *J School Health* 59:10, December 1989.

38. National Education Association: Committee on the reorganization of secondary education: Cardinal principles of secondary education, US Bureau of Educ Bulletin 35:32, 1918. In Vredevoe, LE: *An introduction and outline of secondary education*, Ann Arbor, 1957, Edwards Bros.

39. National Education Association: *Project on instruction: schools for the sixties*, New York, 1963, McGraw-Hill.

40. O'Brien R, Bush P, Parcel G: Stability in a measure of children's health locus of control, *J School Health* 59(4):161, April 1989.

41. Parcel GS, Meyer MP: Development of an instrument to measure children's locus of control. *Health Education Monographs* 149-159, Spring 1978.

42. Postman N: *Amusing ourselves to death*, New York, 1985, Viking Penguin.

43. Report of the 1990 Joint Committee on Health Education terminology, *J School Health* 61(6):237, August 1991.

44. Results of the school health education evaluation, *J Sch Health* 55:8, October 1985, entire issue.

45. Rosenstock I: Historical origins of the health belief model. In Becker, M (ed): The health belief model and personal health behavior, *Health Education Monographs* 2(4):328, Winter 1974.

46. School Health Education Study: *Health education: a conceptual approach to curriculum design*, St Paul, 1967, 3M Education Press.

47. Sehnert K: On teaching self-care to children. In *Medical self-care*, New York, 1980, Summit Books.

48. Thomas L: *Lives of a cell*, New York, 1974 Viking Press.

49. Trucano L: *Students speak*, Seattle, 1984, Comprehensive Health Education Foundation.

50. Tucker A: Elementary school children and cigarette smoking, a review of the literature, *Health Educ* 18:3, June/July 1987.

51. Vitello E: *Personal communication*, 1988.

52. World Health Organization: *Chronicle of the WHO*, New York, 1947, The Organization.

SUGGESTED READINGS

Anspaugh D, Hunter S: Building a sense of community through friendship training in the classroom, Journal of *J Health Education* 23(5):304, July/August 1992.

Bush P, Iannati R: A Children's Health Belief Model, *Medical Care* 28(1):69, 1990.

Fisher R: An empirical investigation of health teacher credibility, *J Health Education* 423-428, November/December 1992.

Green L, Kreuter M: Applications in school settings. In *Health promotion planning: an educational and environmental approach*, Mountain View, Calif, 1991, Mayfield.

Hearne J, Klockars A: Applicability of the Parcel-Meyer children's locus of control scale, *J School Health* 59(4):161, January 1988.

Lavin A, Shapiro G, Weill K: Creating an agenda for school-based health promotion: a review of 25 selected reports, *J School Health* 62(6):212, August 1992.

O'Brien R, Bush P, Parcel G: "Stability in a measure of children's locus of control, *J School Health* 59(4):161, April 1989.

2 The Comprehensive School Health Program

When you finish this chapter, you should be able to:

- Explain the purposes and functions of a comprehensive school health program.
- Analyze the interrelationships among the basic components of such a program.
- Appraise the quality of an existing school health program.
- Interpret student cumulative health records.
- Develop a feasible system for the orderly emergency care of injured or ill school children.
- Identify available community resources appropriate for use in solving school health problems.
- Describe appearances and behaviors symptomatic of hearing and vision problems as well as common illnesses of children.
- Distinguish among mandatory, permissive, and tort laws affecting the school health program.

What is a comprehensive school health program? Although health instruction is intended to be the primary focus of this textbook, it is neither the sole purpose of a school health program nor the only source of activities designed to teach and learn positive health concepts and practices. Generally speaking, a school health program is a composite of activities, procedures, facilities, and services provided by a school, in collaboration with parents and community organizations, to protect the safety and promote the well-being of its students and personnel. Such programs usually encompass three interdependent components of equal importance:

health instruction, health services, and provisions for a healthful school environment. Each of these program elements complement and are complemented by the planned or implicit teaching and learning activity procedures and activities involved in administering the total program.

A health program of some kind can be found in every school in the nation; however, not all of these programs can be described as comprehensive if the term is intended to reflect the best practice possible. Usually health instruction is the least well-developed aspect of a program. Education in this country has always been subject to local control, hence the quality and quan-

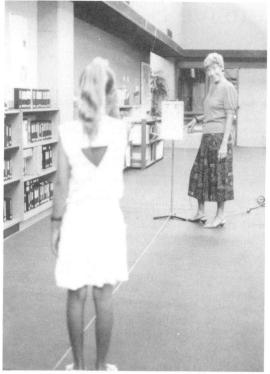

Beverly Bradley

Visual acuity testing is an important procedure often carried out by teachers.

tity of health instruction vary widely among districts and even among schools within a district. Particularly at the elementary level, health education is seldom given top priority except in the case of topics temporarily viewed as crucial by the community. Although teachers' attention to planned health teaching may often be minimal, legally and professionally they are responsible for certain activities associated with health services and the quality of the school environment. A complete description of the many aspects of these two important components of the total program is not possible in a book focused primarily on health instruction; however, it is the intention of this chapter to give you an overview of the potential for health teaching and learning implicit in those other areas.

No child should be admitted to a public school unless his or her health has been certified by medical examination and all required immunizations have been completed or formally waived. Once admitted, it is the school's responsibility to maintain, protect, and promote the health of that well child. That is the purpose of every school health program.

Figure 2-1 depicts the three major components and illustrates their interrelationships. At the center is the student surrounded by the school, the family, and the community. The word "community" in this instance refers to the contributions made by individuals, organizations, and agencies outside the school for the purpose of promoting school health programs. Below that central focus, all of the elements shown are school based. Above it, all of the elements are community based. Two special kinds of organizations (youth groups and parent-teacher organizations) are set to the sides because they are uniquely both school and community based. Liaison bodies, a community health council and a school health committee, facilitate effective coordination and cooperation between school and community. As the concerns and principal activities of the individuals, groups, or primary divisions are explained in the following pages, refer to the chart and note how each fits into and contributes to the total program (25).

Building on the model in Figure 2-1, others propose that expanded versions better fit the needs of students in the 1990s and beyond. Allensworth and Kolbe suggest an eight-element plan that adds five elements to the original three:

1. The integrated efforts of school and community agencies to improve the health of students
2. The school physical education program
3. School food service
4. School counseling and psychology programs
5. School programs to protect and improve the health of faculty and staff (1).

Other recent models include the Nader triangle (26) and ACCESS (an acronym taken from

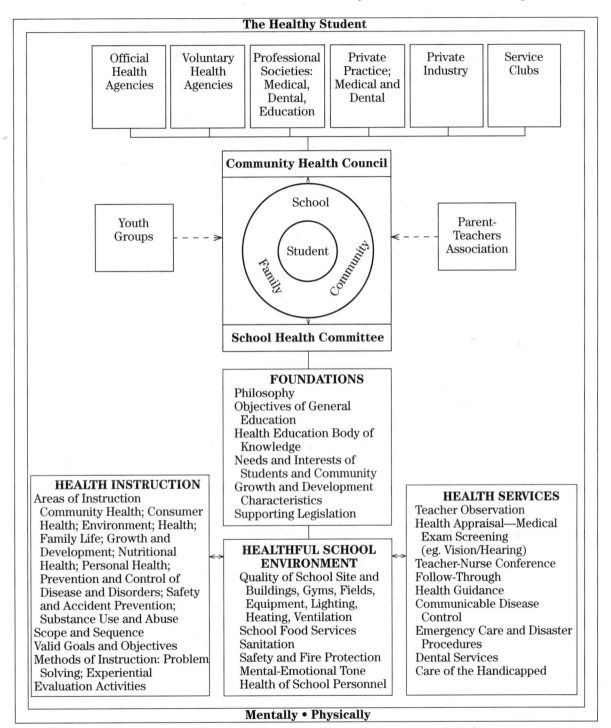

FIGURE 2-1
A concept of a comprehensive school health program.

its five keystone components, *A*dministration, *C*ommunity, *C*urriculum, *E*nvironment, *S*chool, and *S*ervices) shown in Figure 2-2 (36).

The difference between these newer models and the long-established Johns' concept is more a matter of changed placement and emphasis on the parts than of innovation. For example, in the case of the eight-element model, four of those added have simply been separated out and given equal status with the originals. Physical education, although admittedly health promoting in purpose, is no longer the discipline once so closely identified with health education. At the elementary school level, physical education is usually expected to be the responsibility of the classroom teacher. Middle schools may have health and physical education faculty with credentials. But even at this level the notion of the expanded comprehensive school health program is more effectively addressed at the district rather than individual school levels.

LEGAL ASPECTS OF THE SCHOOL HEALTH PROGRAM

Because every aspect of public school education is regulated by the individual states, legislation affecting the school health program varies among states as well. In general, the laws governing health services and the school environment are far more restrictive and comprehensive than those concerning health instruction. Public health laws usually are enforced more rigorously than those of state education codes. Most schools are inspected regularly (especially food-service areas) to see that they are complying with state laws governing sanitation and safe maintenance of buildings and grounds. In addition, state health and safety codes spell out requirements for the design of school facilities for fire protection, disaster control, asbestos removal, and other environmental safety provisions. Currently 36 (71%) of the states have laws mandating comprehensive school health education (23). However, this does not mean that implementation is always monitored or enforced. Essentially the

kind and amount of health instruction a child receives depends on decisions made at the local level (28). It is largely state law, however, as expressed in its health and safety codes, that accounts for the fact that basic health services and provisions for a safe and sanitary school environment are universally provided by schools. Variations in the number and quality of those afforded students in a school can be attributed to the difference between mandated and permissive legislation. Cost and budget are also factors.

Mandated Versus Permissive Legislation

The difference between **mandated** and **permissive** legislation is that the first says that something shall be done, and the second usually says that something may be done. In the latter case, the school is not required to do what is specified, but it can if it wishes. With mandated procedures, those who are charged with implementing the law can be held accountable if its provisions are not carried out. Ignorance of the law does not protect the individual from blame if for that reason alone it was not obeyed. Are there mandates currently defining the scope of health instruction in the schools in your state? If so, what are these requirements?

Legislation Affecting Teachers Directly: Tort Law

The laws discussed above are concerned with the total school health program. Other laws concern specific responsibilities of teachers and other school personnel with respect to the health and safety of students. Every teacher needs to be aware of these tort (civil liability) laws. A tort is an act, or absence of an act, by which someone either directly or indirectly causes an injury to a person, property, or reputation. In every state, the teacher is liable for his or her own tort. A few states, such as California, New York, and Washington, have enacted laws making the district liable also; however, in other states, under common law, the district can do no wrong. Thus in most states, the teachers is the only one who can be sued for damages when a student is injured

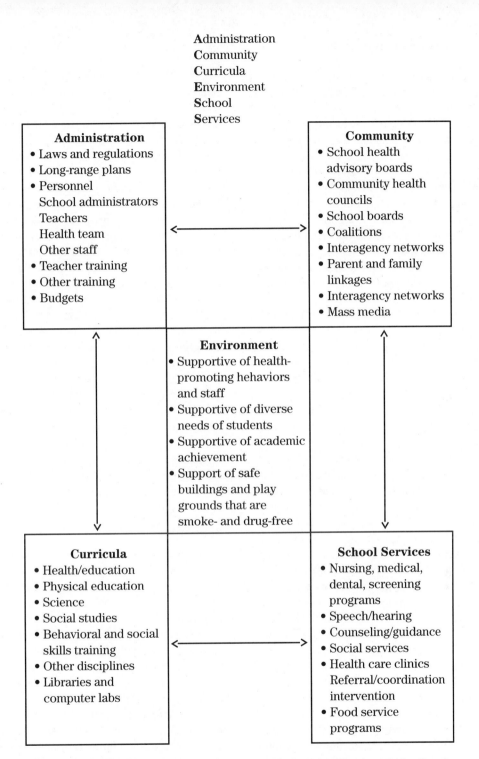

Administration
Community
Curricula
Environment
School
Services

Administration
- Laws and regulations
- Long-range plans
- Personnel
  School administrators
  Teachers
  Health team
  Other staff
- Teacher training
- Other training
- Budgets

Community
- School health advisory boards
- Community health councils
- School boards
- Coalitions
- Interagency networks
- Parent and family linkages
- Interagency networks
- Mass media

Environment
- Supportive of health-promoting hehaviors and staff
- Supportive of diverse needs of students
- Supportive of academic achievement
- Support of safe buildings and play grounds that are smoke- and drug-free

Curricula
- Health/education
- Physical education
- Science
- Social studies
- Behavioral and social skills training
- Other disciplines
- Libraries and computer labs

School Services
- Nursing, medical, dental, screening programs
- Speech/hearing
- Counseling/guidance
- Social services
- Health care clinics
  Referral/coordination intervention
- Food service programs

The ACCESS model has 5 major building blocks that provide an organizational structure for planning, implementing, and or evaluating a school health promotion program

FIGURE 2-2
School health promotion program—ACCESS model.

or a reputation is damaged. In general, a tort is considered to be the result of negligence. **Negligence** is defined as either *failure* to do something that a reasonable person would do, or *doing* something that a reasonable or prudent person would *not* do. So negligence can be an act either of omission or commission. For instance, California law mandates that a first-aid kit be taken along whenever students are to be away from school on a field trip. If an injury occurred and no first-aid equipment was available, the teacher would be liable to a suit for negligence. Find out what your state laws specify as essential equipment to be taken along or procedures to be followed on field trips.

It is not uncommon for parents or guardians of children injured in school to bring suit for damages against school personnel. (About 60% of the injuries to children of school age occur on school grounds, in the building, or between school and home.) Teachers are responsible for the children in the classroom and on the playground. Whether they can be held liable for damages in case of an injury occurring on school grounds depends on the circumstances. The difference between responsibility and liability is significant. **Responsibility** is established by school and community policy. **Liability** is established by law and is decided by the courts. Liability can be established only if the teacher or other school personnel being sued can be proven either negligent in the performance of duties ordinarily associated with the position or imprudent in the discharge of those responsibilities. In the event of an injury, a teacher may be held liable if she or he has (1) failed to warn children of danger or to provide adequate supervision, (2) knowingly conducted a class under unsafe conditions, or (3) committed any other imprudent act. Failure to provide first-aid treatment or provision of the wrong kind of first aid can be interpreted as negligence and therefore grounds for a liability judgment. All schools should have a clearly stated first-aid policy, and all teachers should be required to obtain and maintain certification in first-aid procedures.

Mandatory Reporting Law: Child Abuse

Nearly all states require that suspected child abuse be reported, although definitions of that crime differ somewhat. Most states require that a report be made immediately. A teacher or school worker is not obligated to investigate the matter, but suspected child abuse must be reported. Failure to do so is deemed negligence. Those required by law to report suspected abuse include teachers, principals, school superintendents, physicians, nurses, dentists, and other professionals concerned with the health care of children. These persons are not liable for either civil damage or criminal prosecution as a result of a report, even if it turns out to be unfounded, unless it is proved that the report was made falsely and with malice. One or more of the following categories of injury is included in the definitions of child abuse in all states: (1) physical injury, (2) emotional assault or deprivation, (3) physical neglect, and (4) sexual exploitation.

Every educator should know her or his state's mandatory reporting statute, how child abuse is defined in that state, and what the indications are for possible abuse. This information can be obtained from several sources, including a district attorney's office, a state attorney general's office, or a local superintendent's office.

School Health Policy

Policy statements should specify how far school personnel may and should go in providing first aid, how and under what circumstances parents (or their designees) will be notified in the event of illness or other emergency, and how and under what circumstances injured children will be removed from school for treatment. A signed statement establishing parental responsibility for the expense of any such treatment should be obtained and kept on file.

As a teacher you will be responsible for protecting the health and safety of the children while in your classroom and on the school grounds. Be certain that you know what your responsibilities are and that you take appropriate action to fulfill them at all times. For example, most elemen-

IDENTIFYING CHILD ABUSE OR NEGLECT

Physical Injury

Unexplained or poorly explained injury(ies); burns, bruises, cuts, red marks, broken bones, clumps of hair missing

Injuries occur over a period of time.

Complains about or discloses experience of abuse.

Wears clothing inappropriate for the season to conceal injuries on arms or legs

Emotional Assault or Deprivation

Withdrawn or depressed

Excessive absenteeism, tardiness, or dropped off at school too early and/or retrieved too late

Nervous, aggressive, disruptive, or destructive behavior

Overly compliant or uncommunicative

Uncomfortable around adults or other children

Antisocial behavior, such as drug abuse

Physical Neglect

Dressed inappropriately for the season

Appears unclean, smelly or has rotten teeth

Wears unclean clothes, clothing that is too small or in poor condition

Shows signs of malnutrition; thin, weak, poor skin color, hunger, frequent illnesses

Sleeps in class

Shows evidence of drug abuse

Experiences repeated lice infestations

Left alone and unsupervised for long periods

Unsanitary home

Sexual Exploitation

Expresses knowledge about sexual behavior that is inappropriate for grade level

Complains about an older family friend, acquaintance, or relative touching them in "private" places

Complains of genital or anal irritation; discomfort when urinating or defecating

Diagnosis of a sexually transmitted disease

Evidence of incest, seduction, or forced sexual contact

---

tary teachers are assigned specific play yard supervision times. If for any reason an assigned teacher was late in getting to the playground and in the interim a child was injured, that teacher would be guilty of negligence and liable for damages.

If you plan any out-of-the-ordinary school activities, be certain that state laws and school policy permit their being carried out and that you know what safety procedures will be required. Be ready to implement them if necessary.

HEALTH SERVICES

Health services include the procedures carried out by members of the school health team (physicians, nurses, dentists, psychologists, counselors, teachers, custodians, dietitians, pupil personnel specialists, and others) to appraise, promote, and protect the health of every child in the school. The total well-being of the child—physical, social, emotional, and intellectual—is the primary concern (18). Certain activities usually provided to accomplish this goal include the following.

Continuous Observation

Observation must be carried out by every teacher almost without conscious effort. Although a simple form of appraisal, observation is extremely important as a means of detecting any deviation from expected patterns of growth and development. Comparisons are based on established norms and also on past observations of a particular child's body build, health status, and behavior. These observations depend on the experi-

CHARACTERISTICS OF ABUSIVE/NEGLECTFUL PARENT(S)

Does not return calls to teacher; does not respond to other efforts to communicate

Shows lack of concern for child's welfare or problems

Projects blame for injuries on others or provides inconsistent explanations concerning the cause of the injury

Cannot be located; child is left in the care of others

Abuses alcohol or other drugs

Reports lack of social support network that could provide assistance during crises

Displays unrealistic expectations concerning child's abilities

Uses overly strict or cruel methods of punishment

Becomes hostile, angry, or evasive when discussing child's health

Fails to provide information about child when asked

Was victim of abuse or neglect as a child

---

enced eye and perceptions of the teacher during each year of a child's grade-school experience. The teacher is the only one who sees the child every day in the company of numbers of other children who are of the same age and who are required to fulfill the same educational assignments. For this reason a teacher is in some ways better able than parents to observe small but significant changes in appearance or behavior.

Observation can enable a teacher to detect signs and symptoms of common childhood diseases and of physical and emotional problems that if left uncorrected could interfere with learning. Every teacher must be alert to signs of ill health or disability linked to alterations in a student's appearance or performance. Obvious signs such as a pale or flushed face, noticeable weight loss or gain, or physical or emotional distress signal problems. More subtle signs such as inattention or straining to see or hear should not be overlooked. Sudden negative personality changes or changes in standards of work provide clues to health status problems as well. Some of the conditions that can easily be noted by a classroom teacher include the following:*

- General appearance—very thin or obese; sudden change in weight; unusually pale or flushed; poor posture; unkempt hair; change in gait; lethargic or hyperactive.
- Eyes—crossed, inflamed, or watery; squinting to see; frowning or scowling; holding book very close or unusually far away from the eyes; frequent sties; unnecessary wearing of dark glasses.
- Ears—noticeable discharge; turning head to one side when listening; failure to hear well revealed by irrelevant replies to questions or lack of response.
- Nose and throat—persistent mouth breathing; enlarged glands in neck; frequent colds; persistent runny nose or sniffling; odor from mouth or nose.
- Skin or scalp—rash on face or body; sores on face or body; numerous pimples; excessively dry skin; nits on hair or visible lice; scratching; bald spots.
- Teeth and mouth—irregular teeth; stained or eroded teeth; cracking of lips; pale or blue lips; puffy or bleeding gums.
- Behavior when playing—tiring easily; shortness of breath after moderate exercise; lack of interest in games or activities; unusual clumsiness; poor coordination; unusual excitability.
- General behavior—docile and withdrawn; drowsy; aggressiveness; depression; day dreaming excessively; inability to work well with other children; excessive thirst; frequent need to use the toilet; unusual tenseness.

In addition, watch for behaviors such as inat-

---

*Adapted from Dukelow DA, editor: *Health appraisal of school children,* Washington, DC, 1969, Joint Committee on Health Problems in Education, National Education Association, and American Medical Association.

tention in class, irritability, acting out, stammering or other speech abnormality, or too frequent absences, especially when any of these is unusual for a child.

Depending on the criticality of a problem and its persistence, a teacher should make a note of symptoms needing further investigation or make an immediate referral to the school nurse or other designated person. For example, inattention displayed by a normally eager student might be remarkable but would not be a cause for concern unless noted for more than a few days. On the other hand, a child who is watery eyed and feverish and complains of a sore throat or stomach ache should be referred at once. Immediate action in the latter situation protects not just the health of the sick child but also that of the other children.

Always pay close attention to a pupil's complaints about pain or illness. Even when not accompanied by other signs of illness, the child should be referred to the appropriate school person for further diagnosis and action.

Child Abuse Prevention.   Teacher observation has been described as the first line of defense against child abuse because the teacher is in such close and continuing contact with children older than five years (11). Child abuse is not limited to physical acts of aggression against a child; it includes any act of either omission or commission that endangers or hinders a child's physical or emotional growth and development. Child abuse is more readily apparent when physical injury rather than emotional deprivation is the source. Fortunately, a teacher has the child's health record and the cooperation of the school nurse for evidence of past incidents that may provide further clues to the problem.

Health Appraisals

Medical Examinations.   At least four physical examinations during the school life of a child are recommended by every professional group concerned with the well-being of children. All fifty states require such examinations as a condition of admission to kindergarten (23). Examination by the family physician with the parents present is the best procedure for the small child about to enter school. If a problem is detected, its solution can begin at once. Most school districts have an established health history form that is sent to parents for appropriate notations by the physician and returned to the school files. Frequently physicians are employed by school districts or assigned to schools by the public health department to provide at least minimum examinations in cases where parents are unable or unwilling to pay for private health care.

Screening.   Screening tests are preliminary appraisal techniques used by teachers, nurses, or trained volunteers to identify children who appear to need diagnosis by health-care specialists. Of those performed in schools, the most common are the vision and hearing tests.

Vision Screening Tests.   Teacher observation of symptoms of eye disease is a reliable kind of vision screening. In fact, it may be more meaningful than the results of a rapid screening procedure (5). Swollen eyelids, sties, redness, discharges, squinting, and the need to hold a book close to or unusually far from the eyes when reading are clues to a need for a professional eye examination.

The Snellen test is frequently used in schools to test visual acuity (sharpness of vision). Eye specialists use this method in their offices almost universally. It is inexpensive, easily administered, and needs no particular electrical equipment, although the chart must be well lighted. No special training is needed for its use other than familiarity with the procedures, and only about one minute per child is needed for its completion. Elementary teachers frequently are expected to administer the test, but if there is a school nurse, it is the latter's responsibility (Figure 2-3). A teacher does need to know how to interpret the results, however.

The test involves the correct identification of simple objects or letters, often the "tumbling E," of progressively smaller sizes. Each letter size is numbered according to the standard distance at which a person with average vision should be

COMMUNICATING HEALTH SERVICES NEEDS TO BE MULTI-CULTURAL

Dear Parent/Guardian:

Your child _____ has an appointment at the School Health Center for _____. At that time we will collect a health history from you and do a physical exam. There will be no charge to you, but if your child has Medi-Cal please bring your stickers. If you do not speak English, it would be very helpful if you bring a translator with you. You also need to bring your child's immunization record.

Spanish

Queridos Padres o Acudientes:

Su niño(a) _____ tiene una cita en el Centro de Salud Escolar el día _____. En ese momento colectaremos de usted la informatión para la historia médica y haremos un examen físico. No habrá costo por esto, pero si su niño(a) tiene MediCal, por favor traiga las etiquetas. Si usted no habla inglés, será muy útil que traiga un traductor. También necesita traer los expedientes de las vacunas de su niño(a).

Chinese

敬愛的家長，監護人：

　　貴子女 _____ 在學校保健中心經已安排一約見時間，作 _____，以便登記貴子女的健康紀錄並作體格檢驗，全部免費，若貴子女有政府醫藥補助者，則請帶同醫藥補助標紙，若貴家長不懂英語，若能帶同一傳譯人員則更方便。請不要忘記，必須帶備貴子女的防疫注射紀錄。

Vietnamese

　　Kính gởi Phụ huynh/Giám hộ:

　　Em _____, con/em của ông/bà, có hẹn với Trung Tâm Y Tế Học Đường để _____. Khi đưa em đến trung tâm, chúng tôi sẽ phỏng vấn ông/bà để có được quá trình sức khỏe của em và sẽ khám thể chất cho em. Ông/bà sẽ không phải trả phí tổn nhưng nếu em có Medi-Cal xin ông/bà nhớ mang theo stickers. Nếu ông/bà không nói tiếng Anh mà mang theo được thông dịch viên thì thật là hữu ích. Ông/bà còn cần phải mang theo hồ sơ chích ngừa của con/em.

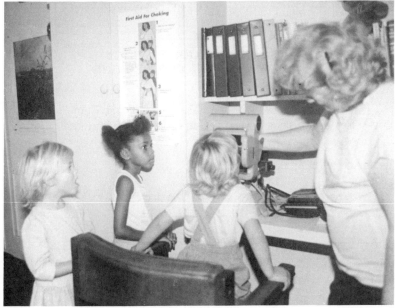

Armi Lizardi

FIGURE 2-3
Visual testing

able to read easily. The numerator represents the distance from the student to the chart, so it is always the same (usually 20 feet). The denominator represents the lowest line in the chart that the child can read (i.e., the smallest symbols that were identified correctly). Average visual acuity is recorded as 20/20, meaning that at a distance of 20 feet, the eye reads the 20-foot line on the chart. A test score of 20/30 means that the child reads at 20 feet the line that should be readable at a distance of 30 feet. What would a score of 20/40 mean? Interpret a score of 20/10.

All children who consistently show any signs of visual difficulty, regardless of their visual acuity scores, should be referred for further examination (Figure 2-4). In addition, children 4 years old through grade 3 with 20/40 or less visual acuity (i.e., 20/50, 20/60, etc.) and all children in grade 4 and above with visual acuity of 20/30 or less, should be referred for complete professional examination. Scores are interpreted differ-

ently for younger children because as they mature, the shape of the eyeball changes, and visual acuity usually increases as a result. In every case, however, when test scores indicate below-average vision (i.e., the second number is greater than 20), those individuals are retested at a later time to be certain that the findings are not just a result of a temporary reaction to an unusual circumstance.

The importance of periodic screening is also justified by many studies that show that the incidence of visual defects increases with age and that visual acuity can never be assumed to be constant (4), which is illustrated by an actual case. A school nurse, whose responsibility it was to check the eyesight of children in an elementary school district periodically, discovered that her own child's visual acuity had gone from 20/30 to 20/200 in 1 year. Ordinarily her child would not have been reexamined for another 2 years. Because she never saw her child at work in his

Date _____

UNIFIED SCHOOL DISTRICT
REPORT OF VISION SCREENING

Name _____ School _____ Grade _____

The above student has received a routine vision screening test during which the following observations were made:

Visual Acuity on Snellen Chart   R.E. _____   L.E. _____   Both _____

Appearance

Frowns to see	_____	Headache	_____
Eyelids crusted, swollen	_____	Dizziness	_____
Sensitive to light	_____	Blurring Vision	_____
Watery eyes	_____	Burning eyes	_____
Discharge	_____	Trouble reading	_____
Eye wanders	_____	Other	_____
Frequent styes	_____		

It is urged that you consult an eye specialist in regard to these observations to see what action, if any, should be taken. (C.A.C., Title V, Section 594, defines test failure.)

Please have the examiner complete the bottom portion of this form and return the entire form to the principal, teacher or nurse of this school.

_____   _____   _____
Principal or Nurse   Address   City

Eye Examiner's Report to the School

Visual acuity: without lenses   R.E. _____   L.E. _____   Both _____
                        with lenses   R.E. _____   L.E. _____   Both _____

Diagnosis: _____

Prognosis: _____

Recommendations:
　　Glasses prescribed: Yes _____   No _____
　　Glasses to be worn constantly _____ for class only _____ reading _____ other _____
　　Preferential seating _____ Child should return for further care _____
　　　　　　　　　　　　　　　　　　　　　　　　　　　　　　　　　　　　(when)
　　Other recommendations _____

Signed _____ Date _____

Address _____ City _____ Phone_____

FIGURE 2-4
Report of visual screening.

classroom but only at home, his reading problems were not apparent. It was his teacher who noticed that he was having a great deal of difficulty and sent word to his parents. With professional diagnosis and appropriate eyeglasses, the boy's reading and schoolwork were soon back to normal. What might have been the outcome had there been no other observation of the child's problem in reading?

Hearing Screening Tests.   Again, the classroom teacher can note behaviors indicative of hearing loss even before it can be verified by screening tests. Inattention or failure to carry out assignments sometimes can be traced to the fact that the child simply does not hear well. Cocking the head to one side, faulty pronunciation of certain words, and frequent requests for repetition or directions or words are additional symptoms. When a child seems slow to understand, a hearing problem may be the cause.

In such a case, consult the child's health re-cord to see if a hearing problem has already been identified and check with the school nurse. Just moving such a youngster to a seat nearer the teacher might do a lot to solve the problem.

Hearing screening is the task of a trained audiometrist, although school nurses often hold credentials for this work (Figure 2-5). In most school districts, hearing screening is conducted at intervals of 2 to 3 years. Referral to a physician normally depends on the results of a pure-tone audiometry threshold test showing some amount of hearing loss or any significant teacher observation or history of hearing disorders (Figure 2-6).

The kind of hearing loss most common among elementary school children is called *conductive* loss, which can be caused by impacted ear wax, foreign objects in the ear, otitis media (inflammation of the middle ear), or severe ear infections.

The need for instruction about hearing and its

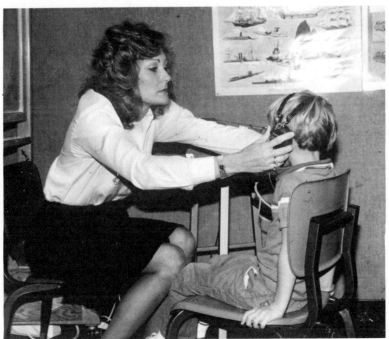

Armi Lizardi

FIGURE 2-5
Audiometry. School nurses are often trained audiometrists as well.

UNIFIED SCHOOL DISTRICT

HEARING SCREENING REPORT

Student's Name _Robert Olson_   Age _6_ Date _5/10/87_

School _____ School Address _____

Dear Parents: A series of hearing tests have been completed on your child. The results indicate a possible hearing problem in the

Right Ear [   ]   Left Ear [   ]   Both Ears [X]

This audiogram is enclosed for your doctor's interpretation. It is suggested that you ask your physician to complete this form and return it to the school named above.

_____
School Nurse

Right Ear   Left Ear

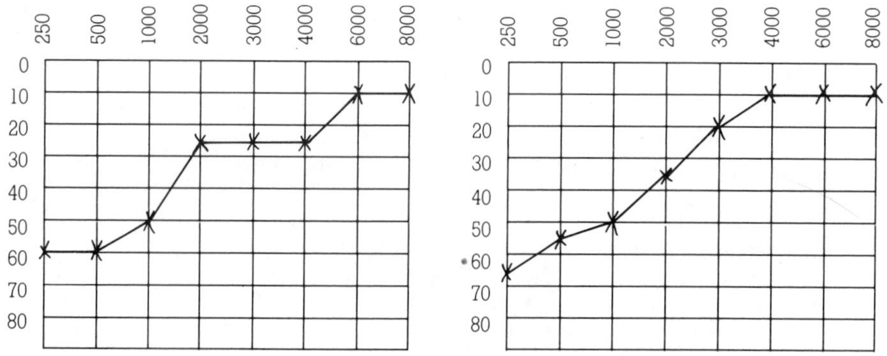

ISO 1964 Standard
Date of Test _5/10_

Dear Doctor: The school seeks the advice and cooperation of parents and physicians in maintaining the student's health and making the best plans for his school program.

Physician's Report to the School

Audiometric Findings

Right Ear

250	500	1000	2000	3000	4000	6000	8000
60	60	50	25	25	25	10	10

Left Ear

250	500	1000	2000	3000	4000	6000	8000
65	55	50	35	20	10	10	10

Results of other hearing tests: Date: _5/25_

Otitis media – acute

Date of examination: _5/25/87_

[X] Child is under medical treatment   ☐ No further medical treatment is needed

Joseph Otto, M.D.   _____
Signature of Physician   Date

FIGURE 2-6
Sample hearing screening report.

protection is attested to by the high incidence of hearing loss in our society. Noise pollution is a major problem in industry and the community. Studies show that although elementary school teachers report that they teach about hearing health, most of that instruction is based on show and tell. Frager urges that more time be given to providing hands-on activities to help youngsters understand why and how noise threatens hearing (10). For example, students could be allowed to examine sound measurement devices and to use them in actual noisy environments. Experiments with a marble dropped from a given distance onto surfaces, such as wood, tile, foam, and carpet, could be arranged to help them understand the role of sound insulation in protecting hearing.

Scoliosis Screening. Scoliosis is an abnormal curvature of the spine that causes a slow, steady change in the back or chest and resultant pressure on the heart or lungs. It can be deforming and painful and may even shorten life if not recognized or treated. In some states it is state law that middle-school boys and girls be screened to facilitate early diagnosis. (The condition seldom appears among younger children.) The best way to find out if a child has scoliosis is to have the back examined by a school nurse or someone in the family. If there is an unequal waistline or if the ribs in the back are higher on one side when the child bends forward, you must assume that the child has scoliosis. As soon as possible the child should be examined by a physician, and x-rays of spine be ordered if necessary.

Teacher-Nurse Conference. A school nurse often is given responsibility for the health of the children in a number of schools. In small districts there may be just one nurse who visits all of the schools. In any case, the nurse sees a child infrequently except in unusual cases. A referral may be the first time a particular child visits the nurse's office. The child's teacher may know far better how atypical a child's behavior or appearance is. It is impossible for a nurse to know every child in even one school as well as a child's teacher does. Therefore the most impor-

tant link between school-provided health care and the individual child is the conference between the nurse and the teacher. Health records can only provide an index of status and history up to the last date of entry. The nurse depends on the teacher to refer a child who appears to have a health problem at present. Similarly, a teacher often can solve a child's learning problem through consultation with the nurse. The nurse has more experience in interpreting the medical history in a child's health folder and in evaluating present symptoms in light of that record. Consultations are sometimes scheduled annually so that both the teacher and the nurse can better understand the needs of the children whose health and education are their mutual concern.

A teacher-nurse collaboration is much more than just a team approach to the solution of a suspected student health problem. A case history vividly illustrates this point. An 8-year-old child, normally high-spirited, self-assured, and outgoing visibly changed between one day and the next. She coughed weakly from time to time and looked half frightened, half puzzled. She told the teacher that she had a funny feeling in her stomach. The nurse talked to her but could get no more information nor was there anything in the health record that might help to explain the problem. She sent the youngster back to class. The teacher, not satisfied, persisted and urged that the child's parents be contacted and advised. This was done, the family physician was consulted, and before the day was over the child was in surgery. An x-ray examination and other tests had revealed that a tumor pressing on the child's heart was the cause of her distress. This is an unusual case, but it demonstrates that you should never hesitate to refer a child a second time if you believe that there is a chance that something has been missed. Sometimes a child will feel better for a little while just because of the referral. Trust your wider experience with a student if you see changes that signal a possible problem.

Follow-Through Procedures. Follow-through procedures are intended to provide a check on what is done for a child once a condition needing treatment or correction has been called to the attention of parents. When there is no nurse assigned to a school, the teacher or school administrator must assume this responsibility. The essential aspect of the follow-through procedure is telling the person who made the original appraisal what has happened in the case. If a teacher requests that the nurse evaluate a child's hearing acuity, for example, and the test shows that more elaborate examinations are needed, the parents are notified. In follow-through procedures, the nurse would contact the parents after a week or so to find out what has been done about the problem. This information would be entered in the child's health record and also reported to the teacher. If nothing has been done about it, further referrals are made until some action is taken to remedy the problem. If you make a referral but never receive any report of its outcome, don't forget it. Follow through yourself. Contact the person to whom you made the referral and find out what, if anything, was done about it. If necessary, make another referral.

Health Records. Most school districts maintain cumulative health folders as a means of storing and organizing all the data accumulated for each child during school years. A health record typically contains information from every relevant health examination or treatment and all important information related to the health history of the individual: height and weight at specified intervals, dates and types of immunizations received, anecdotal records of significant teacher observations, dental records, parental information, records of illnesses, results of any psychometric procedures, and nurse's reports (see Figures 2-4 and 2-6).

Confidentiality. A health record should be started when the child enters school and added to as the child progresses from grade to grade. Ordinarily, if a child transfers to another school, whether in the same city or another, the record goes with him or her. It is an indispensable resource for understanding a child's special needs and thereby contributes to his or her optimum health and achievement.

Such a comprehensive record must be used with discretion. An important rule to be obeyed is maintenance of confidentiality. Only specified personnel should have access to these folders. Student office aides should *never* be allowed to file or retrieve data from these records. They should not be combined with academic records, disciplinary records, or any other data that may be open to individuals not directly concerned with health and medical matters. In addition, possible liability for libel and slander should be considered. Teachers and others must not make subjective statements in a health folder reflecting judgments about a child's character or personal habits. At best these can only be personal opinions or unconscious biases; at worst they could harm the child's future achievement and life (2).

Health Guidance. Some kind of planned health guidance must be included for a school health program to be fully effective. All teachers have a role in guidance. Elementary school teachers have both the responsibility and a unique opportunity to guide because they usually work closely with the same small group of children all day.

The major guidance problem areas include physical and emotional health, home and family relationships, and peer group or boy-girl relationships. One of the tools of guidance is **counseling**—the procedures by which nurses, teachers, physicians, and others interpret a problem for students and parents and help them to work out their own plan for its solution. Teachers and nurses must only assist them in the process.

Health counseling and follow-through activities do more to promote health than any other school activity. Sometimes parents, not aware or convinced of its seriousness, allow a health problem to go uncorrected. Health guidance is essential as a means of motivating appropriate action to treat any potentially handicapping conditions. In essence, the process is a problem-solving activity, and the steps are the same whatever the problem. The teacher or nurse helps the student and family understand the problem and identify ways to obtain information needed to solve it;

they discuss tentative solutions and help the student and family choose the one best suited to their circumstances. The final step in guidance, as in referrals, is follow-through action.

Communicable Disease Control. Control of communicable diseases is a responsibility shared by the home, school, and community. Primarily it is the responsibility of parents to keep a sick child at home. The practice of rewarding continuous attendance is not compatible with the best protection against disease or epidemic. Absences should be encouraged when children have even minor cold symptoms, since most childhood diseases have those same signs in the early stages. Table 2-1 lists some common communicable diseases and their signs and symptoms.

The teacher is responsible for detecting and excluding any child from the classroom who has symptoms of a communicable disease. Each day's first task must be to look at each arriving child for signs such as the flushed cheeks of fever, watery or red eyes, skin rash or eruptions, persistent coughing, sniffles, hoarseness, frequent head scratching, or unusual pallor. Children exhibiting such conditions should be taken at once to the nurse or person designated as the excluding authority in the event of a child's illness.

If it is decided that a child may have a communicable disease and should be sent home, the next step is the responsibility of the nurse or school administrator. Policies should be established in accordance with local public health regulations. They must be thoroughly understood and complied with by all those concerned. These policies usually contain provisions for follow-through procedures to ascertain the diagnosis, provisions for notifying the parents and safely transporting the child home, and specified means of verifying total recovery as a condition of readmission to school.

Procedures must be established to determine if it is safe for a child to return to class, not only for the sake of the affected youngster, but also to protect the health of every other person in the school. In the case of a minor illness, such as an upset stomach, a note from a parent and inspection by the school nurse are usually adequate. In case of a more severe illness such as chicken pox or mumps, a statement from a physician may be required. With certain diseases where isolation is mandated by public health law, a certificate from a health department is required. In any case, the person whose responsibility it is to admit a child after an illness should be competent by training to make such a judgment.

Control of communicable diseases in the community is legally the responsibility of the board of health, but there are basic rules concerning the control and prevention of these diseases that must be obeyed by parents and school personnel. No communicable disease control program can be fully effective without the cooperation of parents. Therefore, schools must make every effort to acquaint parents with their role in disease prevention and control. Children should also be aware of the necessity for strict adherence to public health rules.

Principals and superintendents must have accurate information concerning the legal status of immunization in their state. State laws vary, and they are revised often. Administrators can require that immunizations have been obtained, but they can only go as far as state law permits. If a school board wants to require immunization against specified diseases as a condition of entrance to school, the right to do so must be established by law.

Emergency Care and Disaster Procedures. The school has three responsibilities for emergency care and disaster control: (1) to prevent injuries from happening in school, (2) to provide safety education, and (3) to develop a plan for handling emergencies. The last of these is sometimes neglected because it is assumed either that injuries will not occur or that what should be done in such an event can be left to common sense. Yet injuries do happen in the classroom and on the playground, and they are not always handled wisely because of excitement, forgetfulness, lack of knowledge, or panic on the part of school personnel. The unexpected must always

TABLE 2-1

Teacher Resource: Communicable Diseases

Disease	Type of Pathogen	Source	Transmission
Head lice (pediculosis)	Louse	Humans	Use of borrowed combs, brushes; close contact with infected humans
Impetigo	Bacteria	Humans	Contact
Rubeola	Virus	Humans	Respiratory discharge
Scabies	Mites	Humans	Infected skin and clothing worn by infected person
Ringworm	Fungi	Humans, animals	Direct contact; indirect contact with clothing, hair
Influenza ("flu")*	Virus	Humans, some animals suspected	Direct contact; indirect contact through droplet spread; discharge from nose and throat, possibly airborne
Mumps*	Virus	Humans	Direct contact; indirect contact by droplet spread or articles freshly soiled with saliva
Chickenpox	Virus	Humans	Direct contact; indirect contact by droplet spread or articles freshly soiled by discharges
Conjunctivitis ("pink eye")	Bacteria	Humans	Contact with discharge from eyes or upper respiratory tract, usually through fingers or clothing
Pinworm disease (enterobiasis)	Intestinal roundworm	Infected humans, particularly children	Direct transfer of eggs (same host); indirect transfer of eggs through clothes or bedding
Hepatitis B* (HBV)	Virus	Humans	Person to person; contaminated needles and syringes; transfusions from an infected person
Common cold	Virus	Humans	Direct contact, indirect contact through droplet spread or soiled articles
German measles (rubella)*	Virus	Humans	Direct contact with secretions from an infected person; indirect contact through droplet spread

Modified from School health curriculum project, grade 7, San Bruno, Calif, 1981, US Center for Health Promotion and Education.
*Diseases best controlled through use of vaccine.

Entry	Period of Communicability	Prevention	Control
Hair or head	As long as lice and nits remain	Nonuse of borrowed combs, etc.; inspection	Applications of medications to hair and scalp; frequent inspection
Skin	2 to 7 days	Isolate any infected children	Medical attention and readmission only with medical advice
	1 to 2 weeks	Immunization	Isolation and treatment
	As long as skin is affected	Isolation of infected individuals; cleanliness of body and bedding	Medical treatment and personal hygiene
On skin	As long as lesions are present	No vaccine; avoid contact with infected person	Cleanse infected areas daily; disinfect articles in contact with infected area; apply antibacterial agent topically
Mouth, nose	3 days from onset of symptoms	Vaccination dependent on viral strain; avoid enclosed, crowded places during epidemic	Isolate infected person; disinfect bedding or clothing in contact with discharges
Mouth, nose	48 hours before swelling occurs to 9 days after	Vaccination lasts about 4 years; life-long immunity after infection	Isolate infected person during period of communicability
Mouth, nose	5 days before eruptions first occur to 6 days after	Long immunity after infection; immune globulin may lessen severity of attack	Isolate infected person for 1 week after eruptions occur; disinfect contact articles
Eyes	During the course of active infection	Good personal hygiene	Infected person should not attend school during acute stage; disinfect soiled articles
Mouth	2 to 8 weeks if untreated	Frequent bathing; good personal hygiene; daily bedding and clothing changes	Disinfect soiled articles (eggs killed at temperatures of 132° F or higher)
Mouth, skin puncture	Latter half of incubation period (30 to 35 days) to 3 to 5 days after onset of jaundice	Passive and active immunization by HBV vaccine, gamma globulin; good personal hygiene; sanitary disposal of feces; sterilization of needles and syringes; careful screening of blood donors	Isolate infected person first 2 weeks of illness and 1 week after onset of jaundice
Nose, mouth	First 24 hours of symptoms to 5 days	None known; however, adequate nutrition and rest may increase resistance	Rest; avoid contact with infected person; treat symptoms
Nose, mouth	2 to 4 days before rash until 2 to 5 days thereafter	Vaccination, natural immunity	Isolate infected person

Continued.

TABLE 2-1

Teacher Resource: Communicable Diseases—cont'd

Disease	Type of Pathogen	Source	Transmission
Scarlet fever	Bacteria (streptococci)	Humans	Direct contact; indirect contact
Tetanus*	Bacteria	Intestinal canal of animals and humans	Puncture wounds, scratches, burns
Diphtheria*	Bacteria	Humans	Direct contact; indirect contact with articles soiled with discharges from infected person; ingestion of infected raw milk
Pertussis (whooping cough)*	Bacteria	Humans	Direct contact with mucous membrane discharges; indirect contact through droplet spread or contact with articles freshly soiled with discharges
Tuberculosis	Mycobacteria Tuberculosis	Humans	Via air, and blood transfer by illegal drug use

Modified from School health curriculum project, grade 7, San Bruno Calif, 1981, US Center for Health Promotion & Education.
*Diseases best controlled through use of vaccine.

be expected; every contingency must be anticipated and a plan ready and practiced to meet it.

Several steps are necessary to develop effective plans for emergency situations. The faculty must be made aware of the possibility of injury and emergencies and must be willing to think through plans to cope with any eventuality in their classrooms. These individual plans should be correlated to form a written master plan, which should be thoroughly studied and understood by all school personnel.

Data files for every student and staff member should be quickly accessible to the main office. The file should include name, parents' names (or names of nearest relative) and their address and home and business telephone numbers, name and telephone of the family physician or physician of choice, hospital of choice, special directions for dealing with an injury involving that person, any known allergies or special conditions (e.g., hemophilia, epilepsy), and the person's religion. In case of an injury, the school is responsible for providing immediate care and should do so in accordance with previously agreed-to practices and instructions from the parents or stipulated relative.

Parents should be informed of every plan made by the school in anticipation of emergencies and given the opportunity to state the kind of care they want their children to receive. Informing parents of plans in advance gives them the chance to suggest modifications and helps prevent any criticism or litigation that might occur later if a parent did not approve of some action taken.

First-aid kits or cabinets must be provided and placed in strategic spots around the school. Their contents should be fresh and in accordance with accepted standards for first-aid needs. Every teacher should be qualified to administer first-aid procedures. A school nurse with first-aid expert status could make an important contribution to the school health program by giving instruction to new teachers.

Entry	Period of Communicability	Prevention	Control
Nose, mouth	Approximately 10 days from onset of infection	Some immunity from first infection	Isolate infected person; disinfect contaminated articles
Skin puncture	Not directly communicable among humans	Repeated vaccinations	Thoroughly clean all wounds; update immunization
Mouth, skin wounds	Usually 2 weeks or less	Vaccinations with booster	Isolate infected person; disinfect soiled articles; contacts immunized, antibiotics prescribed
Mouth, nose	7 days after exposure to 3 weeks after onset of cough	Vaccinations with booster	Isolate infected person; disinfect soiled articles; antibiotics prescribed
Respiratory tract; skin puncture in intravenous drug abuse	While sputum and/or blood contains TB bacilli	Treatment of sputum-positive persons. Case finding important; avoid overcrowding in housing, etc.	Chemotherapy with two or more drugs at same time; good nutrition, failure to properly treat disease may produce drug-resistant strains of the agent

At the first indication of an emergency, code signals should be sounded throughout the school, calling specified school personnel (as established by plan) or calling for a general exodus from the building, as in a fire drill.

Parents or relatives should be calmly notified as soon as possible, and every needed assistance should be given them in caring for their children.

The school medical adviser should prepare detailed instructions for the guidance of teachers and the school nurse with reference to the immediate treatment of common emergencies such as abdominal pain, menstrual problems, and headaches, as well as less frequent emergencies such as epileptic attacks or insulin shock. The school nurse is responsible for making certain that injury provisions and plans for immediate treatment are known by all school personnel. When no nurse is assigned to the school, the principal or other designee must be ready to fulfill this responsibility.

A report of each injury or other emergency should be prepared and kept on file. This report should include names of persons concerned, date, time, location, and nature of the event that caused injury, names of witnesses, and the manner in which the case was handled. Such records are frequently of great importance in later discussions of additional preventive measures or of liability. Frequently, forms for reporting serious injuries are supplied to schools by the liability insurance company with which they are insured.

Plans for transporting injured or ill children to home or hospital must be made. The school should provide private cars, school buses, ambulances, or other dependable means, as well as a method of summoning a driver and paying for such a trip. Nothing should be left for an after-the-injury argument. If private cars are used at times of injuries, the insurance covering those cars and their drivers should be adequate and up to date. It is advisable to establish in advance which exits to use in taking injured children from the building to a car. In short, every possible detail needs to be thought about and planned for.

Moreover, each teacher must be a part of the school health team. They should be informed, practiced, and ready to handle emergencies if they occur. The best-written plans are only words. You must be prepared to translate them into action if need be.

Dental Services.   Dental disease begins in childhood. Until very recently it was not uncommon to see nearly two thirds of the school population affected to some degree by dental caries. Now, as reported by the National Institute of Dental Research, about half of all children up to the age of 17 are free from any tooth decay (22). This dramatic change is attributed to the early training children are receiving in brushing and flossing techniques and to the increased use of fluorides as decay prevention. Nearly half the children have never seen a dentist, and 45% of the rest of the population has infrequent dental care (less than one visit per year), usually sought only for emergency conditions. Dental health is the responsibility of the individual, family, and community, in that order. The schools, as part of the community, are in a particularly strategic position to promote the dental health of children. As a part of its program, school health education should motivate children to practice good oral hygiene, especially correct use of dental floss, and seek dental consultation on a regular basis.

Undoubtedly the best place to teach children good oral health practices is in the home. Classroom teaching provides reinforcement and sometimes more effective instruction in specific dental hygiene techniques, particularly if it is pro-

---

DRY BRUSHING ANYTIME, ANYPLACE: DO IT RIGHT!

The "dry brushing" technique is a method of toothbrushing suggested for classroom use. No toothpaste is required; it is not necessary to spit; no sinks are needed. This method supplements the dental care practiced by the student at home.

The technique reduces the incidence of tooth decay and gum disease by removing plaque, a sticky layer of harmful bacteria that continually forms on teeth, and eliminates a major cause of bad breath. It should be remembered, however, that once dental problems are present, the technique cannot cure them. Therefore, it is important to see your dentist periodically to make sure that your mouth is free from disease.

The suggested technique for dry brushing is as follows:

1. Wipe all soft tissue in the mouth, including cheeks, roof, and inside the lips and gums, with a dry, soft and small toothbrush. Do not brush the tongue yet. This step will stimulate the flow of fresh saliva and help remove debris.
2. Work bristle tips now wet with saliva between the gum margin and the tooth and vibrate the brush with bristles in place. This technique will remove plaque, stimulate circulation and work saliva around the gums.
3. Direct the bristles between the teeth and toward the biting surfaces. Vibrate the bristles in place. Brush biting surfaces.
4. Polish and brush your teeth in your usual manner, but do not damage the tissues.
5. Now, brush your tongue as thoroughly as possible.
6. The use of dental floss is introduced as soon as properly supervised teaching and monitoring is available, and adequate manual dexterity is demonstrated. To use floss, work it gently between the teeth. Curve it around the tooth and under the gum line. Move floss up and down across the tooth to remove the plaque.
7. When water is available after brushing and flossing, thoroughly rinse your mouth.

Endorsed by the California Dental Association, State Department of Health, Dental Division.

vided over time. Studies show that a well-designed, ongoing curriculum based on specific cognitive and behavioral objectives of dental hygiene can result in better skill development, as well as increased knowledge about oral hygiene (16). Not only should information concerning nutrition and dental hygiene be provided, but arrangements should be made to allow students to practice basic dental care procedures in school.

Access to running water for toothbrushing practice for 25 or more students at a time is not likely to be possible in schools. However, students can be taught to clean their teeth by dry brushing. This method of toothbrushing requires neither toothpaste nor sinks. It involves the use of a dry, soft toothbrush to sweep and stimulate the oral cavity and tongue. Studies have demonstrated that the technique reduces the incidence of tooth decay and results in improved oral cleanliness even among children as young as kindergarten age (21).

Annual dental examinations and direct fluoride applications to the teeth, when needed, are recommended dental procedures. Those who urge provision of dental examinations at school believe that this supports dental health instruction, brings children's dental problems to the attention of school personnel, provides the children experience with a dentist in a familiar setting (thus relieving fears about dental treatment), and provides data for the assessment of the overall school dental health status (31). Others believe that examinations made in dental offices or clinics have the advantage of better equipment, the feeling of security provided by parental presence, and a better chance that needed dental treatment will be obtained. Either way, the educational value of the examination experience is more apt to motivate good dental hygiene than any amount of teacher talk. The provision of a lesson in advance of an actual examination prepares the students for what is to happen and enhances the total learning outcome (15).

Controls should be maintained over vending machines at school so that they are stocked with noncariogenic (noncaries-causing) snacks. It probably is nearly impossible to provide nutritious foods that are totally devoid of any sugars; however, there is evidence that it is the frequency with which snack foods are consumed that may be the greater hazard. The length of time they stay in the mouth and their physical form increase the potential for harm. Most hazardous to oral health are snacks such as confections, hard candies, and sticky dried fruit (14). The following are reasonable choices: milk, nuts, cheese, plain yogurt, popcorn, and unsugared gum (3). In general, eating between meals should be limited and followed by brushing the teeth as soon as possible.

There are many variations possible in developing a school dental health program. Whatever the plan, three basic forms of activity should be included: (1) dental health education, (2) preventive measures, and (3) referral with follow-through procedures in cases of discovered dental problems. Neglect of one of these aspects diminishes the effectiveness of the others.

Care of the Disabled: Special Education. Every child has the right to an education, and disabled children are no exception. For many years schools were allowed to exclude certain children who were judged ineducable because of some disability. Some of these children simply stayed home, others were sent to expensive private schools, some were admitted to state institutions, and a select few in some school districts were admitted to special schools such as those for children who are multiply disabled but educable. Today that picture has changed dramatically because of new strong federal laws and accompanying funds to assist in the education of physically, mentally, or emotionally disabled children. Special education has become a separate career choice for prospective teachers.

Disabling conditions include mental retardation, speech impairment, visual impairment, learning disability, emotional disturbance, orthopedic problems, deaf-blindness, or health impairments from other problems such as autism. To qualify for special education, a child must have one or more such disabilities and also have need of special teaching because that condition limits her or his mobility, strength, or well-being.

The Education for All Handicapped Children Act (Public Law 94-142) went into effect in September 1978. Five principles of special education summarize key provisions of this act:

1. *Zero reject:*
   No handicapped child may be excluded from free appropriate public education.
2. *Nondiscriminatory evaluation:*
   Every handicapped child must be fairly assessed so that he or she may be properly placed and served.
3. *Appropriate education:*
   Every handicapped child must be given an education that is meaningful to him or her, taking the handicap into account.
4. *Least restrictive placement:*
   A handicapped child may not be segregated inappropriately from his or her nonhandicapped peers.
5. *Procedural due process:*
   Each handicapped child has the right to protest a school's decision about his or her placement (33).

Additional provisions stipulate structural changes that must be made where necessary to ensure wheelchair access to buildings, free movement in the halls, and entrance to restrooms and classrooms. All buildings constructed after June 1977 are required to provide such access to restrooms and classrooms.

The schools have embraced the philosophy that every child has the right to learn to the fullest extent possible, to be prepared for useful employment, and to be as independent as possible. Programs have been set up in most schools for this purpose. In 1981 it was reported that fully 98% of those children requiring this sort of education appeared to be participating in some sort of special education program (7). As of 1984, the estimated number of children being educated in this way was over 4 million, or 11% of all those then in elementary and secondary schools in the United States (8).

HEALTHFUL SCHOOL ENVIRONMENT

Although the school health program is a composite of three interrelated areas of activity, obviously none of these exists in isolation from the others. Thus the activities of health services contribute to the quality of the school's environment, and health instruction is reinforced by learning gained through health services and participation in a safe and sanitary school environment (27). The key components of healthful school living include not only the physical aspects but also the social and emotional currents in which the school's inhabitants live and work.

School Site and Plant

Most states have carefully prescribed requirements defining the acreage needed for a school, the size of its rooms, the type of construction, the kind and number of sanitary facilities, the number and location of fire hoses, and other health and safety features. Although standards vary from state to state, usually 5 acres, plus an additional acre for every 100 students enrolled, is the minimum land allocation for an elementary school.

Playgrounds

Recommendations for the number of acres needed for schools are based on the need for playgrounds. Children, especially in the primary grades, need time to relax and play during school hours. Play not only enables the youngster to return to the classroom refreshed and ready to work, but it provides other kinds of learning experiences. Muscle coordination, teamwork, sportsmanship, and a host of game skills are practiced and learned during play.

Lighting

Most provisions for the quantity and quality of lighting are made by those responsible for designing and constructing the school building. The teacher's responsibility is to see that the lighting remains constant, with conditions, sources, and seating adjusted as necessary. Students should be allowed to arrange or change seats whenever this improves their ability to see their work. Activities involving close work such as reading should be alternated with other tasks for which vision is not as critical a factor. Failed lighting equipment should be reported at once. Observe the students as they read what is written on the chalkboard from their seats. Do they appear to read easily, or must they squint to see it? If they are having difficulty, check the light levels in the room with a light meter. The recommended illumination for chalkboard reading is 150 **footcandles** (a footcandle is the amount of light on a surface one foot from a standard lighted candle.)

Heating and Ventilation

Studies show that children react to temperature more directly and in some ways differently than do adults. Elementary school children have a higher metabolism rate than adults do. What will be comfortable for one age group may not be for the other. But anyone becomes sluggish when it is too warm, and temperatures that are too cold make people restless in the natural urge to get warm. The primary consideration must be the child's comfort. With more and more schools moving to year-around attendance patterns, extremes of temperature become more threatening to learning potential.

School Food Services

Food services have been an integral part of the school health program since the National School Lunch Act was signed by President Truman in 1946. Since then the Special Milk Program (1954) and School Breakfast Programs (1966, 1972) have been added. In 1980 it was reported that 26 million children in more than 94,000 schools were being provided free or low-cost lunches. Another 13 million were receiving nutritious breakfasts at school. Federal subsidies in support of these programs rose from the initial $100 million in 1946 to more than $2.7 billion in 1980.

The need for school food services is supported by studies revealing that not just the poor or neglected children but also those from well-to-do families come to school unfed or poorly fed. Good nutrition promotes health, builds energy, and enhances both the ability and desire to participate in the activities and demands of the day. Learning is hindered when the student is hungry.

However, lunches and other nourishment provided by the school are not intended solely to satisfy hunger and build energy; concurrently, children learn about the social and sanitary aspects of foods and eating patterns. Concepts of good nutrition are given practical application in the menus provided, thus reinforcing lessons experienced in health classes. The Dairy Council of California has developed a food guide for teachers to help them teach food classifications to children of seven Asian cultures in their own languages with phonetic translation in English (9). Lists of common foods translated into Spanish can also be obtained (13). It seems likely that whatever the extent of federal influence and subsidization of such programs, school food services will continue to be a priority of a good school health program.

Certain principles concerning the operation of school food services have been suggested as basic guidelines.

Balanced Meals.   Every lunch should be nutritionally balanced in accordance with the recommendations of nutrition authorities. Millions of children depend on the provision of school food services to meet their total nutrition requirements. A nutritious lunch at least five days a week is as important a school enterprise as special education for handicapped children.

School Lunch Menus.   To receive federal aid, schools must serve nutritious lunches that meet the requirements for a type-A lunch as established by the Secretary of Agriculture (6). These lunches must meet one third of the National Research Council's recommended daily nutritional allowance for school-age children. A type-A lunch consists of a meat or meat alternate, two or more vegetables or fruits, bread, and milk. A home-packed lunch can be well balanced, nutritious, and hot if thermos bottles are used.

Health instruction might focus on identifying the kinds and amounts of food that can be used to prepare such a meal at home (see Fig 12-1). Aspects of sanitary food preservation can be emphasized as well.

Sanitation.   Serving food in school requires perfect food-sanitation procedures: good refrigeration, nonporous and undamaged dishes, tables and counters without cracks that are scrubbed clean after every use, and effective sterilization equipment for all eating and cooking utensils. Cooking and serving personnel must be free of communicable diseases and must comply with state, county, and city sanitation codes governing the handling of food.

Personal Sanitation.   Handwashing and toilet facilities should be adequately supplied with soap and hot water and be convenient for users of the lunchroom.

Instruction.   The school lunch programs should go beyond the function of feeding hungry children. If those in charge consider the educational possibilities, not only the nutritional aspects of diet choices but also courtesy, table manners, and polite dining-room behavior can be learned or reinforced.

Administration.   Most school food service programs are controlled and administered by the school itself. In large school districts it is necessary to hire full-time food specialists. The educational authorities should be responsible for selecting the school lunch manager and other personnel. The manager is responsible for carrying out a program that is an integral part of the school health program, one that operates efficiently and provides an adequate and nutritious lunch under sanitary, attractive, and pleasant conditions. The training and supervision of the other food service workers is a parallel responsibility. Therefore the manager needs an understanding of nutrition, food buying, food preparation and care, and personnel management.

Enough time should be scheduled for lunch to allow food selection and eating at a leisurely pace. At least 20 minutes at the table should be allotted for elementary school children, with another 10 minutes for handwashing and passing from room to room. The earliest lunch hour should be 11:30 a.m. and the latest 12:30 p.m., with the youngest children served first.

Safety and Fire Prevention

More injuries affecting children occur on school grounds or between school and home than anywhere else in the community. Safety precautions should be spelled out carefully and responsibility assigned for each specified procedure (35).

A school safety program should involve the identification of hazards, development of measures to prevent unintended injuries, and regular inspection of such measures to check their continuing effectiveness and usage. Fire drills must be held regularly, and every member of the school staff must be thoroughly familiar with the location of fire exits and equipment, as well as being practiced in whatever responsibility has been assigned. A "buddy" system might be instituted and made an ongoing procedure practiced during fire drills or emergency situations of any kind. Each child, especially one who has a limitation of any kind (visual, hearing, wheel chair, crutches), should have an assigned buddy so that no child ever has to cope with the situation alone, and every child is responsibly involved in his or her buddy's safety during such crises.

General recommendations for the development of a school safety program include an all-school safety council composed of teachers, students, and administrators to continually examine the school for hazardous situations and devise ways of preventing injuries.

A thorough plan for traffic safety, both inside and outside the school, must be worked out. Cooperation of the police can be obtained easily for installing traffic lights, marking crosswalks, and even for discussing with the children how to cross streets safely. Traffic inside the school must be regulated to ensure efficient movement when children move from classroom to classroom (more frequently done in middle schools).

All school personnel should be required to study local laws and ordinances pertaining to school safety and fire prevention as well as those concerning liability for injuries. Subcommittees on safety might be appointed from among the students in upper elementary and middle-school grades. Such committees could help direct the orderly response to a fire drill and could be given responsibility for monitoring safe practices in classrooms as appropriate.

Mental and Emotional Tone

The school health program depends on the willing cooperation of everyone concerned. Unless all teachers, administrators, and members of the staff do their work responsibly, competently, and with enthusiasm, the total program is less effective. The mental and emotional tone or quality of the interpersonal environment, is crucial to every aspect of the program.

A good mental and emotional climate is one in which the morale of the teachers is high. They are relaxed and confident and enjoy their work, just as their students enjoy being in school. The classroom environment is conducive to learning. The room is orderly, and everyone cheerfully takes part in keeping it so. Pupils feel that they are accepted and respected as individuals by their teachers and by classmates. Both teachers and students are involved in setting standards for behavior and in finding solutions for school health problems. There is an active and welcome interest in the school on the part of the children's parents.

We've been describing the ideal environment. That some classrooms in some places fall short of that description does not mean that it should not be continually sought as the goal (24).

Health of School Personnel

The health of the men and women who carry out the school's program is a crucial aspect of a school's environment. The primary consideration is, as always, protection of the child's health. Only persons who are shown through medical and psychological tests to be free of emotional and physical disorders should be employed in a school.

A teacher's health affects a student in many ways. Emotional health, and especially lack of it, can have a profound effect on the happiness and achievement of the children. An unhappy, frustrated, or emotionally disturbed teacher can create an atmosphere so full of hostility and tension that children fear coming to school (32).

A teacher's personal health behavior can be a more powerful influence than any lesson. For example, a teacher who is obese may be uncomfortable about teaching good nutrition habits or figure control and either avoid it or give little time to the topic. A teacher who comes to school obviously suffering from a severe case of common cold is teaching irresponsible behavior, at least by example, and at the same time endangering the health of everyone in the room.

Providing facilities for rest, conferences, and sanitation promotes the health of faculty and staff. Work loads must be fair and equal. Arrangements for some free time each day are essential, particularly in the case of elementary school teachers, who in most schools work closely with the same students in one room for the entire day. The health of school personnel is not limited to the control of communicable diseases; it includes careful attention to the economic, social, and emotional well-being of teachers, as well as of every other school employee.

HEALTH INSTRUCTION

As health services are provided and the many aspects of a safe and sanitary school environment are experienced and enjoyed, learning something that relates to one's own health interests is an inevitable and concurrent happening. People learn by experience, and there is a wealth of health-related experiences in the two components of a school health program just described. Formal health instruction, involving curriculum development, lesson planning, classroom teaching techniques, and evaluation will be the focus of the remainder of this text. These elements of the teaching-learning tasks are common to all teaching, but health teaching is in many ways different, even unique. Its purposes are concerned with lifestyle choices, not health information as an end in itself.

COMMUNITY HEALTH RESOURCES

The community resources available to help the health teacher are plentiful and available for the asking. Generally, community resource groups are categorized as (1) official, (2) voluntary, (3) professional, (4) private physicians and dentists, (5) industrial, (6) service clubs, (7) youth groups, (8) parent-teacher groups. Whatever the agency, group, or organization, their interest in health makes them willing allies for health teaching. Find out what services and materials are easily available to you in your community. Pick those that complement the textbook you are using and use them in ways that can add to and broaden the scope of your students' health instruction.

Official health agencies are tax supported and responsible under law for the protection of the people within their jurisdiction. A public health agency may be local, state, or national in scope. A wide range of services, which vary to some degree depending on the budget, is available to all members of the community. A teacher might contact the health educator of a local public health office for a list of available films or other audiovisual aids or for consultation. A letter to the state health department asking for a catalogue of visual or written materials may open avenues to resources not available from the local office. At the national level the various health institutes, such as the National Cancer Institute, National Institute of Allergy and Infectious Diseases, and other branches of the U.S. Department of Health and Human Services, have large catalogues of pamphlets, booklets, and printed materials concerning health statistics and health problems in all age groups. Send a request for lists of available materials on school stationery because a copy of such publications is usually free to teach-

ers. You can also call one of the national clearinghouses for information (see Appendix B).

Voluntary health agencies typically are concerned with a specific health problem or disease. They are supported by donations and are organized and controlled by volunteers. A key purpose of such agencies is education about the health problem of their interest. Therefore certain amounts of their budgets are allocated to the development and dissemination of educational materials. The American Cancer Society, American Heart Association, and National Society for Crippled Children and Adults are some of those agencies that commonly have offices in major cities. Materials such as films, posters, pamphlets, charts, and student workbooks and worksheets often are printed in several languages. Speakers' bureaus are another frequently available service. All these aids are readily obtainable, often with no more effort than a telephone call to the nearest office. If a voluntary agency has no local listing, write to the national office and ask for the address nearest your home or school (see Appendix C).

Professional health organizations include local medical, dental, nursing, or educational associations and, at the National level, the American Medical Association (AMA), the National Education Association (NEA), the American Dental Association (ADA), and the American Nurse's Association (ANA). The AMA, with the NEA, for many years produced a host of significant references and resources for school health. *Health Services* (18) and *Healthful School Environment* (17) remain the classic references regarding these two aspects of the school health program.

Several national professional organizations, including the Association for the Advancement of Health Education (AAHE), the American School Health Association (ASHA), and the School Health Education and Services section of the American Public Health Association (SHES/APHA), specifically focus on health education in schools. The membership of these organizations includes health teachers, school physicians and nurses, and other individuals whose primary concern is the health and health education of children and youth. By affiliating with one or more of these groups, teachers can keep up to date through the articles in the journals, as well as through meetings with teachers with similar interests at regional and national meetings. In addition, position papers, curriculum guides, and other resource materials are regularly developed or updated and made available.

Locally, a teacher might obtain classroom subscriptions to health-related magazines and journals through the cooperation of the medical society. A teacher might interest a dental group in promoting a dental hygiene campaign by classroom demonstrations and examinations. Nursing groups might be persuaded to provide volunteers for schools in which such services are limited or to provide resource persons for the school health instruction program.

Private physicians and dentists and other local health advisers are a potential source of information, as well as service in special situations. Private practitioners who are parents of children in a school often are willing to serve as resource persons, to explain health problems to children, or to provide a field trip experience for a class. For instance, a dentist might allow a group of children to visit the office to view the dental equipment and to explain its function in the maintenance and promotion of oral health. Children would be far more likely to develop positive attitudes toward dentists and dental services after such an experience (34).

These are but a few of the ways community resources can be used in health teaching. The public library and reference librarian are also community resources. The familiar *Yellow Pages* directory supplies the addresses and telephone numbers of most health-related organizations. A classroom without walls can be a reality if a teacher will just open the door to the abundance of community resources available for use in the classroom and outside the school.

Industrial organizations, either individually or with others, have developed a great number of instructional aids specifically for use in schools. For example, the Metropolitan Life Insurance Company has materials for use at every level of health education, from K through 12. The National Dairy Council, representing the nation's milk industry, allocates a major portion of its budget to nutrition education. Their materials are not limited to the promotion of milk products but cover all aspects of nutrition. The teaching aids developed by this group are creative, dynamic, and educationally sound. National Dairy Council nutritionists frequently will assist with inservice education or even give demonstrations in some areas of the country. Other cooperative groups such as the Cereal Institute and the National Livestock and Meat Board also provide some teaching aids and student materials related to nutrition in general and their products in particular.

Most large industrial organizations are very concerned with safety, and many also are directing attention to alcoholism because of the impact this problem has on the performance of otherwise competent employees. It might be possible either to arrange a field trip to learn about their safety program or to persuade the safety or medical director to visit the school to describe such a program and its applications in a school or home. Toothpaste manufacturers often offer dental hygiene training kits or sound-assisted filmstrips designed to teach young children oral health-care techniques. Charts, booklets, and materials useful in teaching about menstruation are free to the teacher who requests them from companies, such as Kimberly-Clark and the Tambrand Corporation. The Kaiser Health Plan sponsors regional dramatic presentations titled "Professor Body-Wise" on health topics for elementary students.

In short, there is no limit to the kinds of free or inexpensive teaching aids that can be obtained from commercial organizations. The main thing to be guarded against is the possibility that some aspect of the material may not be acceptable in terms of district policy. It is prudent to preview any teaching aids obtained from resources out-side the school to be certain that no objection-able advertising copy is included and that it is ap-propriate for use with the age group for which you are responsible. Appendix C includes sources of free or low cost health instructional materials from various national organizations.

Service clubs such as the Elks, Lions, Kiwa-nis, Shriners, and Optimists, although primarily social in purpose, always include community ser-vice as an integral part of their programs, hence the name *service* is used to describe them. Usu-ally a specific health problem is chosen as the club's special interest. For example, tiny white canes are given by the Lions' Club to those who donate money for service to the blind. The Lions also sponsor antidrug abuse education. The Elks' club raises money to fight cerebral palsy. The Shriners' annual charity football games or pa-rades provide the money to support their hospi-tals for the care and treatment of burned or crippled children. Find out what local service clubs can be called on to assist in solving spe-cific health problems that hinders learning for any youngsters in your class.

Youth groups, although composed of children and youth, are administered by community-based organizations and personnel; these include the Boy Scouts, Girl Scouts, Campfire Girls, Y-Guides, 4H Clubs, and church clubs. The pro-grams of such groups are usually committed to the promotion of health in any way they can. A teacher might ask for their help in organizing fire prevention surveys, in participating or leading en-vironmental clean-up projects, in serving as crossing guards, and in teaching younger chil-dren safety procedures or other positive health behaviors. The possibilities are limited only by the imagination and interest of the teacher.

Parent-teacher groups, such as the National Congress of Parents and Teachers (NCPT) are an-other kind of organization whose members are derived from both community and school. The NCPT is dedicated to the health of school chil-dren. It has spearheaded the drive to secure na-tional legislation supporting and promotion of comprehensive school health education. On the local level, the chairperson of the health commit-tee in particular is ready to help in any way pos-sible and should be invited to serve as a regular member of the school health council. Parent members are often willing to assist with field trip arrangements and to help with individual prob-lems, such as lack of adequate shoes, clothing, or health services of some kind. Parent members can be called on to provide materials that can be used for health teaching, such as discarded maga-zines for clipping pictures or health-related ar-ticles or advertisements, to make costumes for school health dramatizations, or to raise money for needed teaching aids by selling fruit or other foods on school grounds as permitted by school policy and health laws.

School-Community Liaison Groups

Community Health Council. The eight kinds of community-based groups just discussed are possible sources of assistance for those ad-ministering a school health program. However, there are too many community-based organiza-tions in most areas for a school to approach one by one. In these cases a cooperative body such as a community health council may be the an-swer. It ensures representation, at least on a ro-tating basis, of all eight kinds of agencies, and it provides a mechanism for mobilizing community resources to assist the school with problems that threaten the health or safety of teachers or stu-dents. Added community representation can be obtained by including religious leaders, inter-ested and qualified civic leaders, and specialists from fields such as law enforcement, social work, and recreation. Whatever the problem or need brought to the council, each member can consult with the larger group that is represented and bring back suggestions or offers of assis-tance that are appropriate and feasible.

School Health Committee. Just as a com-munity health council is a representative body of agencies and individuals interested in promoting community health, so a school health committee is a representative group of individuals interested in promoting and protecting the well-being of the child while at school.

In a district where a school health committee is in operation, it functions as a coordinating body. It has no regulatory powers but can only make recommendations to the administration. Membership is drawn from the administration, faculty, staff, student body, and parents. It may include the principal or a designee of the administration, school nurse, custodian, dietician, or food service manager, and teachers who have expressed interest in health education. Possibly the most important aspect is the student representation. All people, including children, are better able to understand and accept new rules or requirements if they have a voice in their development.

A school health committee functions as a data-gathering, problem-solving body. The problems are brought to it by administrators, teachers, crossing guards, bus drivers, parents, or staff. Its function is to analyze the problems and determine possible solutions. The kinds of problems that a school health committee might be asked to study are as varied as human behavior and may include prevention of drug abuse among students, prevention of spray-can graffiti on school walls, control of a school-wide epidemic of the flu, coping with vandalism of school property or facilities, and even establishment of a school dress code. Whatever the problem, a school health committee can be an effective mechanism for dealing with it.

A school health committee can be organized informally so that a member is allowed to solve the problem individually but must follow agreed upon channels of communication when doing so. It can be an *ad hoc* committee that is disbanded once the problem has been solved. The third and best organization is as a formal, continuing committee that functions as a problem-solving, recommending body when necessary and works to smooth any conflict that arises between school policy and shifts in community needs.

The development and implementation of a school health program can never be a unilateral task; it is a shared responsibility of the home, school, and community. Each has a role in the education of children, in promoting and protecting their health, and in shaping and protecting the environment in which they must live and learn.

SUMMARY

The comprehensiveness of a school health program is defined by the quality and quantity of the activities, procedures, and facilities and services provided by its three basic program components (i.e., health instruction, health services, and a healthful environment). Every school in the nation has some kind of a school health program; however, not all of them can be described as comprehensive. There are several reasons for the differences that exist: legal considerations, local school policies, budgetary constraints, community needs and concerns, and the philosophy of local decision makers regarding the value or need for a given aspect of the program. Often more than one of these has influenced the nature of an existing program.

State and sometimes federal legislation have an impact on school health programs. For example, in order to receive federal financing for the school health program, the menus must include specified amounts and kinds of foods representative of all food groups. Federal law and supporting funds are responsible for the establishment of nationwide special education programs for handicapped children. Health education curriculum projects have been funded and disseminated with the help of federal funds and the supervision of federal agencies.

State requirements as spelled out in an education code and a health and safety code affect school health programs significantly, depending on whether they specify health services, environmental protection or controls, or health instruction. Of the three, legislation regarding health instruction is typically least restrictive; even when instructional programs are mandated, their implementation is not often monitored or enforced. At the elementary level, recommendations for health instruction tend to be ambiguous and global. Recommendations may include teaching "health habits" and promoting "good moral character." However, state health and safety codes are usually specific, and many of them are universally required among the states because they deal with health problems that might either endanger the health and safety of students and school personnel or in some way hinder a child's potential for learning.

School policies, whether established at the district level or a particular school, have far more impact on health instruction than on health services and environmental aspects of the program. Education in this country has always been subject to local control; hence the quality and quantity of health instruction vary widely among districts and sometimes even among schools in the same district. Mandated health services and environmental standards usually are provided at least at required minimum levels. As a rule how much beyond those minimums a school goes in building its program depends on local school policy.

Budgetary constraints affect the quality of a program. However desirable it may be to employ enough qualified school nurses to carry out appraisal procedures, to be quickly available to meet emergency needs, to provide student counseling, and to supplement instructional services, many school districts have severely cut the number of such specialists. There is seldom enough money to support a nursing staff of that size. Similarly, purchase of materials and resources for health instruction or even the employment of health teaching specialists as district health coordinators or teachers is more often tied to cost considerations than to need or value.

Community needs and pressures can be a positive or a negative force when a school health program is being planned. When the incidence of some health problem becomes critical, typically a public clamor arises for education designed to alleviate that problem. If it is a new problem, then the schools try to respond to the public's concern by fitting the new topic into the existing curriculum. On the other hand, sometimes the public outcry focuses on removing some health topic from consideration by the schools. More often the vote is divided. Usually the fewer who urge a change, the louder their voices will be.

The schools are required to meet community needs and interests. School administrators have the problem of deciding whose wishes should have priority. No matter whose wishes are satisfied, the change will have been wrought by the community. Sex education is a perennial case in point. Whether or not education concerned with human sexuality should be provided to young people by the schools has been controversial even at the secondary level. But now HIV-AIDS is so terrifying a problem that there is considerable support for curricula providing information on the mode of transmission and methods of prevention, starting as early as the third grade. Many adults will support this recommendation; many will not. It is likely that the decisions that will be made will vary from one community to another.

Community health agencies interested in a specific health disorder or disability often devote considerable time and money to devising educational materials concerned with teaching children what it is believed they need to know about the problem. Understandably, such agencies want to see those materials being used, so they put pressure on school authorities to include them in a curriculum, usually health education.

It is appropriate that a school health program be based on knowledge of student and community needs and, to the extent possible, represent the activities needed to meet them. But it takes a balance between what is possible and what is beyond the purview of the schools as the instrument of so great a responsibility.

The Johns' chart depected in Figure 2-1 graphically illustrates a model school health program. If a school provides those services competently, maintains the safety, sanitation and comfort of the children and adults who live and work in its environment, provides health instruction appropriate to the needs and interests of its students, cooperates effectively with interested community agencies, and maintains positive relationships with parents and community leaders, then it can be described as a comprehensive school health program. As a prospective teacher you should be able to describe a quality program and anticipate the very real contribution that you will be able to make in your future role.

QUESTIONS AND EXERCISES

Discussion questions

1. Teachers are expected to teach a full curriculum specified for any given grade level. Why should they also be concerned with health services or the quality of the school's environment? What is the relevance of attention to these aspects of the school program to instruction?

2. Why is teacher observation so crucial a factor in the maintenance and promotion of student learning and health?

3. The principal purposes of the total school health program are to maintain, protect, and promote the health of the child. For each of the components of that program (health services, healthful environment, and health instruction) describe at least four specific functions with which teachers are directly involved or responsible.

4. If you suspected that a student was in need of protection from what appeared to be child abuse, the symptoms of which were more behavioral than physical, what would be the best thing to do, both professionally and legally?

5. Which is the more important service to students and their parents that a classroom teacher can provide—guidance or counseling? How might the nature of the problem affect your answer to that question?

6. Should the same nutritional standards required of a federally sponsored school lunch menu be applied to the selection of snack foods supplied by vending machines on school grounds? Why or why not? Defend your point of view with specific arguments.

7. If you were asked to recommend the ten most essential members of a school-community liaison group, whom would you list? What would be your rationale for those choices?

Exercises and problems

1. Prepare a bibliography of at least six key references on school health that could be used when setting up a functional school health program. Explain your choices on the basis of their authorship, subject matter, and potential long-term validity as resources.

2. Visit an elementary school and arrange to interview the principal or other school administrator on school policy relative to emergency care and disaster control. Is safety education provided? If so, what is the nature of that instruction and how is it carried out? Is there an established plan of action? Is every school worker familiar with his or her responsibilities in the event of an emergency? If possible, obtain a copy of the plan and check to see if it satisfies the suggestions made in this text or others dealing with safety in schools.

3. Familiarize yourself with the dry brushing technique for classroom practice. Write or call your nearest dental association for suggestions regarding sources of classroom sets of free brushes, disclosing tablets, or educational pamphlets. Then offer to instruct one or more elementary school classes in the procedure and write a short report of the entire experience. What did you learn about teaching children how to do something as opposed to teaching them facts? Would you do anything differently another time?

4. Inspect a school building or at least the building in which your education class is being held. Are public telephones, drinking fountains, toilets and wash basins, aisles between desks, cafeteria counters, or other facilities reachable by a person in a wheel chair? In a short paper, describe any problems you identify and list possible solutions.

5. As a second-grade teacher you have observed that one of your students often squints when looking at the chalkboard and soon loses interest when required to read at that distance. His health record shows that last year his eyes were tested and recorded as 20/40, but the most recent test showed visual acuity of 20/20. Should the child be referred for a more comprehensive examination at this time? Why or why not?

6. Consider the following health problems often encountered by a teacher of elementary school children and name a community group who might assist in solving each:

a. You have been asked to serve as the school co-ordinator of health instruction, and you want to obtain relevant and up-to-date films or other resource materials for use in setting up an inservice program.

b. A school nurse is asked to present instruction regarding menstruation to fifth-grade girls and wants some pamphlets and charts appropriate for this purpose.

c. A school wishes to set up a peer group-conducted street-crossing safety program.

d. A class wishes to take a field trip and needs help with local transportation and supervision during the trip.

e. The school nurse discovers that many of the children in a school have a great need for dental care. Many factors are involved in the problem, such as economics, ignorance, and malnutrition.

f. In order to comply with community pressure to begin some instruction in schools relative to the prevention of HIV infection, a middle-school principal wishes to arrange appropriate instruction for all of the faculty as a first step in such an endeavor.

7. You are asked by your principal to serve as the convening chairperson of a new school health committee. Because there are no specialists on the school faculty, presumably every teacher is equally competent to serve. What criteria might you consider for use in choosing among the school teachers, and which members of the total staff would you select as most representative of the total school program?

REFERENCES

1. Allensworth D, Kolbe L: The comprehensive school health program: exploring an expanded concept, *J Sch Health* 57(10):409-412, 1987.

2. American Academy of Pediatrics, Committee on School Health: *School health: a guide for health professionals*, Elk Grove Village, Ill, 1987, AAP.

3. American Dental Association: *Diet and dental health*, Chicago, 1986, ADA.

4. Appleboom T: A history of vision screening, *J Sch Health* 55(4):138-41, 1985.

5. California Association of Ophthalmology: *The vision screening committee.* Cited by Orange County Department of Education, California, 1985.

6. California State Education Administration Code (CFR) Title 5-15558, 1987.

7. *Condition of education, statistical report*, Washington, DC, 1981, National Center for Statistics, US Department of Education.

8. *Condition of education, statistical report*, Washington, DC, 1987, National Center for Statistics, US Department of Education.

9. Dairy Council of California: *Asian foods guide for teachers*, Fall 1981.

10. Frager A: Toward improved instruction in hearing health at the elementary level, *J Sch Health* 56(5):166-169, 1986.

11. Fraser B: *The educator and child abuse*, Chicago, 1979, National Committee for Prevention of Child Abuse.

12. Healthy People 2000: National Health Promotion and Disease Prevention Objectives and Healthy

Schools. *J Sch Health* 61:7, Sept. 1991 (entire issue).

13. Hernandez M et al: *Valor nutritivo de les alimentes Mexicanos*, Mexico City, DF, 1972, Instituto Nacional de la Nutricion.

14. Hinkle M: A mixed message: the school vending machine, *J Sch Health* 52:1, 1982.

15. Horowitz L et al: Self-care motivation: a model for primary preventive oral health behavior change, *J Sch Health* 57(3):114-118, 1987.

16. Houle B: The impact of long-term dental health education on oral hygiene behavior, *J Sch Health* 52(4):256-261, 1982.

17. Joint Committee on Health Problems in Education: *Healthful school environment*, Washington, DC, 1969, NEA-AMA.

18. Joint Committee on Health Problems in Education: *School health services*, Washington, DC, 1964, NEA-AMA.

19. Kolbe L et al: School health in America, ed 4, Kent, Ohio, 1987, ASHA.

20. Lammers J: *I don't feel good*, Santa Cruz, Calif, 1991, Network Publishers.

21. Lee J: Daily dry toothbrushing in kindergarten, *J Sch Health* 50(9):506-509, 1980.

22. Los Angeles Times: *Where the ouch went*, part II, p 8, June 25, 1988.

23. Lovato C, Allensworth D, Chan F: *School health in America*, ed 5, Kent, Ohio, 1989, ASHA.

24. Mills M: *Classrooms in Compton cited as "horrible" by NEA chief*, Los Angeles Times, part CC, p 1, May 28, 1987.

25. Nader P: The concept of comprehensiveness in the design and implementation of school health programs, *J of Sch Health*, 60(4):133-137, April, 1990.

26. National Professional School Health Education Organizations: Comprehensive school health education: a definition, *J Sch Health* 54(8):312-315, 1984.

27. Newman I: Integrating health services and health education: seeking a balance, *J Sch Health* 52(8):490-501, 1982.

28. Noak M: *State policy support for health education*, Denver, 1982, Education Commission of the States.

29. Oda D: Is school nursing really the invisible practice? *J Sch Health* 62(3):112, March 1992.

30. Oda D et al: The resolution of health problems in school children, *J Sch Health* 55(3):96-98, March, 1985.

31. Rabich T et al: The need for dental health screening and referral programs, *J Sch Health* 52(1):50-52, 1982.

32. Sauls C, Fuller A: School phobia: a paralyzing fear in a child's life, *Early Years* 17(1):88-90, 1986.

33. Scheiber B: Parents campaign for handicapped children and youth, *Closer Look*, Washington, DC, 1981.

34. Smardo F: Dental health of young children: how can we help them cope? *Health Values* 9:3, May/June 1985.

35. Sorenson E: Plan to prevent accidents, *A Sch Board J* 72:6, June 1985.

36. Stone E: ACCESS: Keystones for School Health Promotion, *J Sch Health*, Sept 1990, 60(7):30.

37. Tower C: *Child abuse and neglect*, Washington, DC, 1984, NEA.

SUGGESTED READINGS

Floyd J, Lawson J: Look before you leap: guidelines and caveats for school-site health promotion, *J Health Education* 23(2):74-80, March, 1992.

Kirst M: Improving children's services: overcoming barriers, creating new opportunities, *Phi Delta Kappan* 72(8):615-618, April 1991.

Kobokovich L, Bonovich L: Adolescent pregnancy prevention strategies used by school nurses, *J Sch Health* 62(1):11-14, January 1992.

Kozlak L: Comprehensive school health programs: the challenge for school nurses, *J Sch Health* 62(10):475-76, December 1992.

Nader, P: The concept of comprehensiveness in the design and implementation of school health programs, *J Sch Health* 60(4):133-137, April 1990.

O'Rourke, T: Reflections on directions in health education: implications for policy and practice, *Health Education* 20(6):4-14, Oct/Nov 1989.

3 Planning and Organizing the Health Curriculum

When you finish this chapter, you should be able to:

- Define the meanings of planning and organizing as they refer to curriculum development.

- Interpret the role of a school's philosophy of health education in determining scope.

- Compare advantages and disadvantages of using any particular curriculum design.

- Explain the teacher's special role in planning and organizing a curriculum for teaching.

- Describe ways to investigate each of the primary sources of the curriculum.

- Predict changes in children's health needs and interests as they grow and develop during the school years.

- Differentiate between horizontal and vertical organization of the scope of a discipline.

- Develop a feasible cycle plan for a selected level of school health instruction.

Planning and organizing are inextricably interrelated functions in curriculum development. Both are involved when decisions affecting when and what will be taught must be made. Generally, **planning** is concerned with determining the long-range goals and instructional objectives of teaching and with designing effective means of attaining them. **Organizing** involves decisions defining the scope and sequence of the plans for teaching and learning.

Effective planning for health teaching depends on the worth and feasibility of proposed goals. Worthwhile goals must be synthesized from data gathered through careful investigation of the following three principal sources: (1) the needs, interests, abilities, and concerns of the learners; (2) the culture and the community in which they must learn to live and to participate effectively as citizens; and (3) the body of knowledge believed to be essential to the development of a person who is health educated (35). These are the sources fundamental to curriculum decision making in any discipline. Yet in no field are the data generated through study of these sources more crucial than in health education because we are basing teaching plans on the needs and concerns of real people, on human behaviors, and often on solvable or preventable community problems. The more current the curriculum, the more meaningful and the more transferable the learning.

By definition, goals are long-range plans; no one lesson or single course can assure their attainment. As a result, goals provide stability to a program so that instructional objectives expressed at course- or lesson-planning levels can be responsive to what is relevant to a particular group of students yet at the same time contribute to achievement of the broader aims. But no matter how unique or entertaining the lessons might be, if thoughtfully derived goals are lacking, it is like taking a trip without any destination in mind. It should not be surprising, in that case, if the teaching ends up nowhere and the students cannot tell you what they have learned or even what the purpose of the activity was. Have you ever had a course that disorganized?

THE AIMS OF HEALTH INSTRUCTION

Before planning for effective teaching and learning, a clear statement of aims is an essential first step. The principal aim of school health instruction is to promote favorable health behavior, to help children learn how to choose actions that enhance and protect health rather than the reverse. To achieve that goal, acquisition of knowledge and the development of positive attitudes and beliefs about health and health behavior are critical. To impart information is easy, but whether that information will have much influence on a child's lifestyle choices depends in part on the way it was acquired and in part upon a variety of other factors over which no teacher has control. For example, knowledge of the 5 food groups will have to vie with peer group pressures, cultural and family preferences, budgetary constraints, eating habits, and other forces affecting a youngster's dietary choices.

Attitudes and beliefs about health and the effects of unhealthful behaviors also determine what a person does in a given situation. Children come to school with a great many attitudes already firmly established; however, these can be modified by vital new information. Knowledge that seems important to a child because it fits into his or her own concerns and interests is more apt to promote changes in behavior or attitudes than information having no apparent significance in real life.

The aims of health education might be expressed as follows:

1. To promote health behavior (choices, actions, habits) that is favorable to the development of a positive lifestyle.
2. To foster development of a well-balanced personality, based on a realistic acceptance of one's limitations as well as capacities.
3. To clarify misconceptions, remove superstitions, and provide accurate information about personal and public health matters.
4. To contribute to the health of the community through the development of health-educated citizens who will support future health measures intended to protect and promote the common good.
5. To develop ability in students to see causes and effects on health, to take preventive or remedial steps when possible, and thus to lengthen and improve the quality of life.

THE SOURCES OF THE HEALTH CURRICULUM

Planning a curriculum that is likely to help students achieve personally satisfying goals is difficult, and so is devising learning opportunities relevant to their present needs and concerns. Added to these problems is the teacher's perennial challenge—that is, how to create an educational program that can help their students prepare to live effectively in a society that changes so rapidly. The kind of education that can facilitate the development of human capabilities must be directly related to the world outside the school. The questions that need to be asked are: Who is to be educated? What does that person *need* and *want* to know about health? What are the important ideas that health education specialists believe are representative of their body of knowledge? How can these ideas become a functional part of the learner's personal framework of knowledge? What health-related skills are needed by and what health and social behaviors are expected of members of our society?

Needs of the Learners

The primary source of data from which educational goals can be inferred is the learner—the needs, interests, concerns, stage of maturation, skills, and abilities of the student.

Needs can be looked at in several ways. One view of **need** is the degree to which the present condition of the individual differs from some acceptable norm. An educational objective based on this notion of a need would focus on a plan to provide learning opportunities designed to fill this gap—that is, to teach what the student needs to know. Measurement of knowledge or its lack is probably the easiest aspect of needs assessment (see Chapters 7 and 8 for a detailed discussion of measurement techniques).

Another kind of need is reflected in the natural urge to maintain a balance between internal human drives and external conditions. These are the physiological needs such as food, water, and warmth; psychological needs such as affection, status, and belongingness; and integrative needs such as feelings of identity, self-fulfillment, and self-respect.

A third kind of need is revealed by the learner's interests and concerns. *Felt* needs are more readily identified, and it is easier to plan lessons that meet them. Planning lessons focused on needs that are not felt at all is more difficult. Children may need to know which people help keep them healthy and what they do to help, but studies show that this is a topic of little or no interest to children at any grade level (34).

Ways to Identify Needs. Considerable research has shown that similar needs are likely to be shared by children of the same age, develop-

mental level, or sex living anywhere in the United States. The **Denver study,** a classic study conducted in Colorado from 1948 to 1954, surveyed children, parents, and teachers about the health interests of 3,600 schoolchildren, representative of a total school population of about 50,000. Analysis of the responses obtained showed that there was a consistent pattern of shifting interests that paralleled expected and actual physical and social development in these children (12).

In 1969 the **Connecticut study,** a study of student health interests, asked some 5,000 schoolchildren what they wanted to know about health (8). The findings were categorized by topics and in relation to age groups. Three main age groups at the elementary level and another at the middle-school level will be of interest to the elementary teacher.

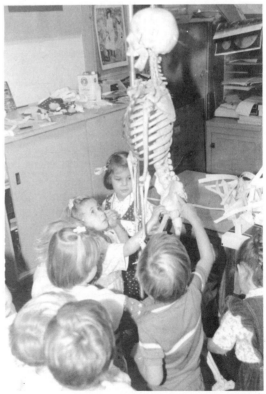

Armi Lizardi

Children have a great interest in the function of bones.

As expected, the interests of very young children (K through 2) are found to be concrete and concerned with the here and now. Their questions tend to focus on "how" and "what." Many questions are directly related to their own health, growth, and development (e.g., "How does my heart beat?" "What makes the bones?" "How do you get colds?"). By grades 3 and 4, interest in the details of the entire body rises steadily. These youngsters want to know "how many" and "why" (e.g., "How many gallons of blood are there in my body?" "Why do we lose baby teeth?"). They want to know how the body works.

Children in grades 5 and 6 continue to have great interest in the body, especially the organs, asking questions such as "How does the mind work?" and "What is inside the body?" Questions about puberty begin during grade 5 as boys and girls are maturing physically. These include "Why does a girl menstruate?" and "Why was I born male instead of female?" Their questions also reveal rising curiosity about drug abuse and its effects. Many ask, "Why do people use drugs?" "What do they do to you?" or "Why do people want to smoke?" Children in both grades express a growing need to understand themselves, their peers, and their families.

Middle school youngsters are keenly interested in learning the full story of their own development. They are concerned with their appearance and how they are accepted by the opposite sex. It was discovered that the major health interest areas are common to all children of every age level, no matter where they lived or what their economic status was. However, the survey team urged that their findings not be regarded as universal, saying that "teachers or curriculum workers still need to answer questions such as 'What are the priorities in *my* class?'" (8).

In the early 1980s, over 5,000 school children, representative of a population of 750,000 in grades K through 12, were surveyed in Washington state. This study, referred to as Students Speak (34), was a replication of the Connecticut study; however, the intention was not to make comparisons but to ascertain health interests and concerns in the eighties.

Data were gathered by means of (1) questionnaires written for and applied at four levels (grades K through 3, 4 through 5, 6 through 8, and 9 through 12), (2) classroom observations noted by teachers and aides, (3) open classroom discussions with students in grades K through 5, and (4) voluntary responses made by individual students during the procedures. All of the data were tabulated and reported by grades. Many of the health topics evoked questions and responses not dissimilar from those reported in the 1969 study. However, certain health topics were selected for additional discussion either because they were mentioned often, mentioned at every grade level, or seemed to be of special concern in the 1980s. These topics included handicapping conditions/birth defects; genetics; child and sexual abuse; fears and worries (about divorce of parents, death, not being loved or losing love, suicide, and stress); self-concept enhancement; understanding human behavior; effects of drugs and drug abuse; nutrition (including weight control from grade 4 on); aging; first aid/accident prevention; and sexuality/family/babies/pregnancy.

It was noted that although some health topics or areas appeared to be of high interest at all grade levels, different aspects of these topics became priorities at different age levels. It was speculated that part of this continued similarity of interests could be traced to the fact that students had not received enough health education along the way to answer their questions; hence, they continued to have questions. Moreover, these findings shed light not only on health interests of students but on the growth and development patterns of students at these ages as well.

It is not fully possible to convey the richness of the data reported in the Washington study. It would be well worth your while to obtain a copy and use it as a reference when planning for teaching and learning at any level of school (10).

How can you determine the special concerns and interests of the students in your own class? There are several ways to do this. The most informed person about student interests is the student, and a very good way to learn about

THE WASHINGTON STATE STUDY: STUDENT HEALTH CONCERNS

At all grade levels there was high interest in handicapping conditions.

Child and sexual abuse questions appeared at every level, including the primary grades.

Fears and worries were expressed at all grade levels.

Almost every grade level mentioned divorce, why it occurs, how to cope with it. There was fear of not being loved. "How can you tell if your family loves you?"

Fears about death, how to avoid being trapped in a fire, how to get over the death of a loved one, why death occurs, were issues of concern.

From the seventh grade on, questions about stress, suicide, how to help a friend who may be thinking about suicide, and why people commit suicide were common.

There were concerns about being liked by others, being a good friend, and getting along with people.

Interest in drugs was very high in all students, increasing as the individual progressed from third to eighth grade.

Weight control was a concern from fourth grade on.

First aid/accident prevention was a big interest at all grades. Students wanted to know how to prevent accidents and what to do if a brother or sister had taken poison or pills.

Interest in babies was shown in primary grades; students asked how babies develop, how they are made, how they grow inside the mother, how twins and handicapped babies happen.

In general, the highest interest for primary level children was in human body/growth and development and mental health; for children at fourth grade to eighth it was in mental health and drugs. Whatever the grade, however, the least interesting topic was health care systems.

From Trucano L: *Students speak*, Seattle, 1984, Comprehensive Health Education Foundation.

---

students' interests is to let them tell you what these are.

Student Questions. Given the chance, children will ask questions in abundance, and for the most part these are reliable indicators of need. There are several ways in which such questions can be gathered and organized so they can be used in lesson planning.

1. Ask your students to hand in written lists of questions that they would like answers to. With *sixth grade or older* students this is better done anonymously so they do not feel pressured and so they can ask questions that otherwise might embarrass them. Younger children's questions may need to be recorded for them by the teacher or an aide for later analysis.

2. Take note of significant questions asked during class and file them for future reference under a classification system corresponding to the health topics or content areas specified in your district's curriculum plan. This will serve to identify those asked most frequently, thus reflecting common needs or interests of children of that age in your school.

3. Solicit the cooperation of other teachers, the school nurse, or other school personnel in recording on index cards any significant health-related questions the children ask them. Such questions provide a different perspective on health interests because they were motivated by situations outside the health class.

4. Develop a list of perhaps 50 common words related to health actions or concepts. Ask the students to react to each word if it in any way suggests a question to them. Each child has had unique life experiences in connection with one or more

of those words, so the potential for new and unusual questions is great.

5. Prepare a health problem or interest checklist. This can be put together easily by using particularly interesting questions asked by earlier students. Yarber described such an instrument to be used with students in grades 3, 5, and 6 to ascertain their desire for much more, a little more, or no more information about specified health content areas (39). With younger children, such surveys can be read aloud by the teacher or an older child and their responses recorded by checking whichever answer best reflects their wish. Older children can read and check their own list and even participate in tabulating the results.

6. Arrange conferences, interviews, or informal discussions with individuals or groups of students to focus on their health concerns. When these shared concerns result in related learning opportunities, both interest and motivation to participate will be high.

Evaluation of School Life. Consider what health problems may have had their origins in the school itself. Going to school is not always a totally healthful experience. Some children, as a direct consequence of being in school, become nervous and emotionally disturbed or develop such a strong sense of failure that they quit trying. Some suffer a series of communicable diseases contracted from other children and fall so far behind in their school work that they never quite catch up.

The emotional climate of the classroom needs careful analysis as a source of health problems. A child who frequently complains of being sick in the stomach may actually have severe stomach cramps or nausea, but the symptoms may be an emotional reaction to an unhappy teacher-student relationship or to peer group rejection. School experiences leave many marks. Most of these experiences enhance a child's well-being and growth, but others leave very real

scars. The teacher who hopes to make health instruction vital and effective should arrange a social and emotional environment that helps a child cope with stress and learn at his or her own pace.

Analysis of Health Records. Because knowledge of health problems of individual students provides valuable data useful not only for lesson planning but also in preparing for any needed health care arrangements, you should be familiar with the information recorded in each student's cumulative health folder. Health needs and problems may also be identified through children's self-reports about personal health problems. Patterns of illness or disorders that frequently interrupt school attendance or hinder performance indicate the need for specific health instruction or a conference with the school nurse or parent.

Growth and Developmental Characteristics. Knowledge of expected physical, social, mental, and emotional development makes it possible to predict what a child should be able to do at a particular age and, just as importantly, what a child should *not* be expected to do. This means that growth and development have more to do with readiness (i.e., *when* children can handle learning opportunities competently) than with *what* they should be taught at any age.

Consideration of the several dimensions of growth and development—physical, social, emotional, and intellectual—is not limited to decisions affecting cognitive development but needs to be included in making classroom arrangements that facilitate affective and social growth (25). However, readiness to learn will be the focus here.

It is assumed that prospective elementary teachers will have recently completed courses on growth and development of children and will be familiar with related learning and developmental theories, including Piaget's cognitive development (13), Erikson's psychosocial development, and Kohlberg's moral reasoning development (20) theories. Charts listing physical, mental-emotional, and social characteristics of children of successive ages show that specific changes in those dimensions are consistent over time. Examples of those sure to appear in most such charts include the information in Table 3-1. All of this information has obvious applications for health teaching and learning. However, for the purposes of this book, discussion of cognitive growth and development characteristics will be limited to a brief application of Piaget's theories as they relate to planning curriculum sequence.

Children enter school during Piaget's preoperational period (ages 2 to 7) and progress to the period of concrete operations during elementary school grades. The pre-operational child cannot consider the whole and the part simultaneously. Health and health behavior are viewed as a series of unrelated practices and ideas. Somewhere around age 7 or 8 a child begins to conserve ideas and to reverse thinking processes (the concrete operational stage); yet cause and effect are not well understood, and the future is too abstract to contemplate. Health education that focuses on a child's immediate goals and desires will be more effective than education that promises future health benefits. The more health teaching is related to everyday actions, the more effective it will be.

Research shows that at age 8 or 9 children can begin to be active health consumers and make many of their own health decisions. It is recommended that health education be started before this age, but it should remain present-oriented despite the change in cognitive ability. Future-oriented teaching, stressing the value of health as a lifetime quality, is feasible only when children begin to understand abstractions and can formulate hypotheses based on reality testing (the formal operational stage) (23).

Kolbe and others maintain that children do not possess the cognitive skills needed to make sound health-related decisions during the concrete operational stage of development (21). Instead, they argue that either *training* or *indoctrinating* must be the process employed:

> When children are young, we need to train them to *do* so and so . . . and to teach them that so and so

is the case (i.e., to believe something). . . . Thus as children mature developmentally we need to move away from training and indoctrinating them . . . and toward educating them (21).

Studies of the moral development of children have shown that they tend to reason egocentrically because they are concerned mainly with consequences to themselves; yet when they are allowed to answer "why" questions and are then encouraged to examine consequences of an act on themselves and others—to develop reasons for behavior on their own—they are capable of higher reasoning with regard to concern for others (11).

Health concerns or problems of children, wherever they are found, should be identified, analyzed for their relevance and cruciality, and used in developing teaching-learning plans as much as possible. These may reflect persistent situations faced by all children in their daily life, as related to nutritional needs, safety rules, family disruptions, or worries about peer group acceptance.

In today's pluralistic society, children need to understand that all people have the right to contribute and participate without giving up their own language, ethnicity, or culture. They need to learn that differences exist, differences are good, that unjust treatment of differences exists, and that unjust treatment of differences is wrong. Health education in elementary school years can be a powerful factor in building an environment where self esteem is nurtured and children take pride in their own uniqueness (24).

Other problems may involve health behavior standards such as personal health-care habits, certain social behaviors and manners, and acceptance of one's gender role. Of course, none of the aforementioned aspects of the learner are mutually exclusive. An interest exists because it is a concern. A concern or problem may be traced to a growth and developmental characteristic that occurs too early, too rapidly, or too late compared to the individual's peers, and so on.

Everything that can be learned about the chil-

TABLE 3-1

Growth and Development Characteristics

Grades K-3 (Ages 5-8)

Physical Characteristics

Growth relatively slow.

Increase in large muscle coordination, beginning of development of small muscle control.

Bones growing.

Nose grows larger.

Permanent teeth appearing or replacing primary teeth; lower part of face more prominent.

Hungry at short intervals; may overeat and become overweight.

Enjoys active play-climbing, jumping, running.

Susceptible to fatigue and limits self.

Visual acuity reaches normal.

Susceptible to respiratory & communicable diseases.

Suggested activities: vigorous games emphasizing outdoor play with basic movement patterns and skills as well as singing games and rhythms.

Needs

To develop large muscle control through motor skills.

To have play space and materials.

To use instructional tools and equipment geared to stage of development.

To establish basic health habits: toileting, eating, covering nose and mouth with cough, etc.

To have snack time and opportunity to develop social graces.

To have plenty of sleep, and exercise interspersed with rest.

To have health examinations and follow-up.

To have visual and auditory checks.

To have dental attention.

Emotional Characteristics

Self-centered, desires immediate attention to his/her problem—wants to be first.

Sensitive about being left out.

Sensitive about ridicule, criticism, or loss of prestige.

Easily aroused emotionally.

Can take responsibility but needs adult supervision.

Parent image strong; also identifies with teacher.

Expresses likes and dislikes readily.

Questioning attitude about sex differences.

Needs

To receive encouragement, recognition, ample praise, patience, adult support.

To express inner feelings, anxieties and fears.

To feel secure, loved, wanted, accepted (at home and at school).

To be free from pressure to achieve beyond capabilities.

To have a consistent, cooperatively planned program of classroom control. Must have guidance.

To develop self-confidence.

To have some immediate desirable satisfactions.

To know limitations within which to operate effectively.

To develop realistic expectations of self.

Social Characteristics

Lack of interest in personal grooming.

Engages in imitative play.

Friendly, frank, sometimes aggressive, "bossy," assertive.

Generally tolerant of race, economic status, etc.

Gradually more socially oriented and adjusted.

Boys and girls play together as sex equals, but aware of sex differences.

Needs

To have satisfactory peer relationships, receive group approval.

To learn the importance of sharing, planning, working and playing together—both boys and girls.

To have help in developing socially acceptable behavior.

To learn to assume some responsibility, to have opportunities to initiate activities, to lead.

To work independently and in groups.

To accept sex role.

To develop an appreciation of social values, such as honesty, sportsmanship, etc.

Intellectual Characteristics

Varied intellectual growth and ability

Interested in things that move, bright colors, dramatizations, rhythmics, making collections.

Interested in the present, not the future.

Learns best through active participation in concrete, meaningful situations.

Can abide by safety rules.

Wants to know "why."

Attention span short.

Needs

To experience frequent success and learn to accept failure when it occurs.

To have concrete learning experiences and direct participation.

To be in a rich, stable challenging environment.

To have time to adjust to new experiences and new situations.

To learn to follow through to completion.

To develop a love for learning.

To learn without developing feelings of hostility.

To communicate effectively.

From *A pocket guide to health and health problems in school,* Kent, Ohio, 1981, American School Health Association.

Grades 4-6 (Ages 8-11)

Physical Characteristics

Growth slow and steady.
Girls begin to forge ahead of boys in height and weight.
Extremities begin to lengthen toward end of this period.
Muscle coordination improving.
Continued small muscle development.
Bones growing, vulnerable to injury.
Permanent dentition continues.
Malocclusion may be a problem.
Appetite good, increasing interest in food.
Boundless energy.
Tires easily.
Visual acuity normal.
Menarche possible toward end of this period.

Suggested activities: more formal games with emphasis on body mechanics.

Needs

To develop and improve coordination of both large and small muscles.
To have plenty of activities and games that develop body control, strength, endurance, and skills-stunts (throwing, catching, running, biking, skating).
To have careful supervision of games appropriate to strength and developmental needs; protective equipment.
To have competitive activity with children of comparable size.
To have sleep, rest, well-balanced meals.
To have health examinations and follow-up.
To have visual and auditory checks.
To have dental attention.

Emotional Characteristics

Seeks approval of peer group.
Desire to succeed.
Enthusiastic, noisy, imaginative, desire to explore.
Negativistic (early part of period).
Begins to accept responsibility for clothing and behavior.
Increasingly anxious about family & possible tragedy.
Increasing self-consciousness.
Sex hostility.
Becomes "modest" but not too interested in details of sex.

Needs

To begin seriously to gain a realistic image of self and appreciate uniqueness of personality.
To be recognized for individual worth; to feel self-assurance and self-esteem.
To receive encouragement and affection; to be understood and appreciated.
To exercise self-control.
To talk about problems and receive reasonable explanations. To have questions answered.

Social Characteristics

Learns to cooperate better in group planning and group play and abides by group decisions.
Interested in competitive activities and prestige.
Competition keen.
Begins to show qualities of leadership.
Developing interest in appearance.
Strong sense of fair play.
Belongs to a gang or secret club; loyal to group.
Close friendships with members of own sex.
Separate play for boys and girls.

Needs

To be recognized and accepted by peer groups; receive social approval.
To have relationships with adults which give feelings of security and acceptance.
To assume responsibilities, have increased opportunities for independent actions and decisions.
To develop appreciation for others and their rights.
To learn to get along with others and accept those different from self.

Intellectual Characteristics

Likes to talk and express ideas.
High potential of learning in science, adventure, the world.
Eager to acquire skills.
Wide range of interests; curious, wants to experiment.
Goals are immediate.
Demands consistency.
Generally reliable about following instructions.
Attention span short.

Needs

To experiment, explore, solve problems, challenges; use initiative, select, plan, evaluate.
To receive individual help in skill areas without harmful or undue pressure.
To have opportunities for creative self-expression.
To have a rich environment of materials and the opportunity to explore it.
To participate in concrete, real-life situations.
To be able to accept one's self with strengths and weaknesses.

dren for whom a curriculum is to be planned should be considered when making decisions about what they need to know, what they want to know, and when it should be presented to them. This information cannot be used as the only basis for planning curricula, but it provides important clues that cannot be ignored if health teaching is to be meaningful to its audience.

Needs of the Community

The second source of data essential to sound curriculum development is the society in which we live. What does the student need to know about wise use of community health-care systems, and what concepts, skills, and abilities are needed to be an effective health consumer and a responsible neighbor, family member, and citizen? Some answers to these questions can be ascertained by studying the social, economic, and political communities in which we work and live. National health concerns must be considered, as well as more immediate and local health issues and problems. If you are going to teach about health, it is necessary to look beyond school walls for clues to a curriculum that deals with life.

National Health and Education Goals. There is an abundance of data on national health and education goals. The surgeon general's report on health promotion and disease prevention, *Healthy People*, emphasized four major factors that affect the nation's health: (1) unhealthy life styles, (2) inadequacies in the existing health-care system, (3) environmental hazards, and (4) human biological factors. Fifteen priority areas among preventable threats to health were named: high-blood pressure control, family planning, pregnancy and infant health, immunization, sexually transmitted diseases, toxic agent control, occupational health and safety, accident prevention and injury control, fluoridation and dental health, surveillance and control of infectious diseases, smoking and health, misuse of alcohol and drugs, nutrition, physical fitness and exercise, and control of stress and violent behavior (36).

Among that early report's many recommendations, one specifically linked national health goals with school health education:

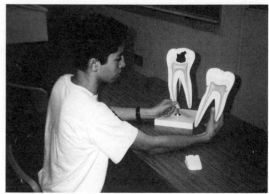

Ric Loya

Dental health education is important for all children.

The schools may be the richest source of potential behavior change. Comprehensive school health education should include promoting health knowledge, the causes of disease, and the influence on health by personal decisions related to smoking, alcohol, and drug abuse, exercise, and sexual activity (36).

During the following year, *Objectives for the Nation* were proposed for each of the priority areas, along with related health implications, specific objectives to be attained by 1990 or earlier, and other data (37). Later, a 2-day conference, *Prospects for a Healthier America: Achieving the Nation's Health Promotion Objectives* was held in Washington, D.C. to study and discuss the objectives and make recommendations (38). Members of more than 50 national organizations representing health-care settings, health professions, business and industry, voluntary organizations, and schools were involved. The schools' workgroup was made up of 10 members of major professional educational associations representing school administrators, teachers, and others. The group quickly agreed that schools could best contribute to the achievement of the 1980 *Objectives for the Nation* to be attained by 1990 by offering quality health programs. All of this information is relevant in developing a curriculum for tomorrow's health classes (38).

Most recently, *Healthy People 2000: National Health Promotion and Disease Prevention Ob-*

jectives, 1990 introduced a set of 300 national health objectives, which evolved from the foregoing *Prospects* report (19). An expanded list of 22 priority areas was introduced, categorized as concerned with health promotion, health protection, preventive services or surveillance and data systems. (See Figure 1-2 for the complete listing of the areas.) The related objectives are proposed as guides to health promotion and disease prevention policy and programs at federal, state, and local levels throughout the 90s. Each of the priority categories is addressed by three sets of objectives: *health status objectives*, e.g., "Reduce deaths caused by unintentional injuries to no more than 29.3 per 100,000 people," *risk reduction objectives*, e.g., "Increase use of occupant protection systems such as safety belts, inflatable safety restraints, and child safety seats, to at least 85 percent of motor vehicle occupants"; and, *services and protection objectives*, e.g., "Extend to 50 states laws requiring safety belt and motorcycle helmets use for all ages" (19).

The following are examples of some of the objectives directly or indirectly attainable by schools:

8.2 Increase to at least 75 percent the proportion of the nation's elementary and secondary schools that provide planned and sequential kindergarten through 12th grade quality school health education.

9.18 Increase to at least 95 percent the proportion of schools that have age-appropriate HIV education for students in the 4th through 12th grade, preferably as part of quality school health education.

All of this information is relevant in developing a curriculum for tomorrow's health classes.

Local Community Health Needs and Concerns. Local community needs assessment often is overlooked entirely in school health curriculum planning. Yet to base the goals and objectives for health education solely on national needs and objectives would be foolish and philosophically unsound. Knowledge of local health needs, especially those specific to a given school, neighborhood, or community is essential when planning a health education curriculum. Such needs are not difficult to identify. Look in any journal or newspaper, and you discover a wealth of social issues, problems, and trends with implications for health teaching. Various ethnic or socioeconomic factors may justify curriculum emphases in one community that are not as imperative in other communities. For example, poor nutrition may be a problem in a high-socioeconomic area, but it may exist for different reasons and be of a different nature than the same problem in an inner-city area. Health-related choices often are dictated by necessity or by ethnic or cultural forces rather than by willful neglect or ignorance. That is why the kinds of teaching strategies that succeed with children in one school may be totally ineffective in another for a number of reasons.

Community Influences on Curriculum Planning. Although the community is a source of the kinds of data just listed, the curriculum is in many ways the *product* of the community as well. For example, local morbidity statistics may show that the incidence of sexually transmitted diseases has increased alarmingly among school-aged children; nevertheless, certain parent groups may be so opposed to education planned to counter this problem that they fight against any proposal to offer related instruction.

Legislative and political factors have a powerful impact on curriculum decisions. State legislatures decide what the requirements for teacher credentials will be. Whether elementary school teachers receive specific preparation for their health teaching responsibilities depends to a great extent on state laws. A current investigation of teacher certification requirements revealed that only one state required teachers to be certified in health education in order to teach the subject in elementary schools. However, 26 (51%) required prospective elementary school teachers to take course work in health education to qualify for elementary certification (6). Furthermore, lawmakers, not educators, decide whether health education will be provided and, if so, how comprehensive it will be. Local and state boards of education are elected bodies, and no public school can carry out a program contrary to board policy, regardless of how urgent a community need may be judged to be by school personnel.

Other external influences on decisions about the health curriculum are the values or philosophy of the community regarding the need for or the worth of health education. It is not likely that a teacher would propose an educational goal that was inconsistent with her or his own value system. However, an educator's values may conflict with those of some other members of the community. This kind of conflict is exemplified by the disagreements about sensitive health topics such as human sexuality or family planning. Somehow such curriculum issues must be resolved, with the needs of the learner as the primary consideration.

Scales has said, "Regardless of the areas of difference that surface among us, responsible adults on all sides know that sexuality education is neither panacea nor poison, but that it is part of an effective response to the challenge of promoting the healthy growth and development of young people" (31). He suggests that schools focus more on the unifying forces in our communities—our shared values and concerns—"that in our basic beliefs there is more that unites us than divides us."

Where there is established community support of and parental participation in the total school health program, including the curriculum, the chance of controversy is minimal. Chapter 6 discusses the role of policy statements regulating selection of both materials and subject matter for use in health instruction. Common sense guidelines, ways of managing controversy should it develop, and principles crucial to developing new programs are key elements of the chapter.

The health curriculum for the 1990s probably will continue to reflect the increasing national concern with drug abuse among children and youth and with the crucial problems of HIV-AIDS prevention, environmental pollution, teenage pregnancies, and stress and violence control. These priorities will change if other health problems are later perceived as having greater urgency. That urgency will come from the community in most cases.

Crisis–generated community pressures are more often the cause of curriculum priority-setting changes in health education than in most subjects commonly taught in the public schools. Unfortunately, such a bandwagon approach is categorical and reactive, whereas health education, to be effective, must be comprehensive and proactive. If health education is to be effective, it must consider the whole person, not merely the diseases and disorders to which humans are prey. Children need and want to know about wellness rather than how to cope with next year's expected diseases. A set of lessons designed to keep one jump ahead of specified health problems year after year would be not just dull but dreary. Another problem is that, as we have already suggested, young children do not relate to future problems or benefits. They want to know about what is happening now. Health education for the 1990s and beyond seeks to emphasize promotion far more than prevention or control, as has previously been the case. The goal is a healthy lifestyle and abundant wellness—now and tomorrow.

The Body of Knowledge

Seffrin said, "Respecting differences between and among various school districts, a core body of knowledge exists which should be included within all curricula which are truly comprehensive" (32). This core body is recommended by the national professional school health education organizations (27). The body of knowledge, the third source of information affecting curriculum planning, is defined by consensus of its subject matter specialists. Every subject area lays claim to some broad but definite range of principles, concepts, and generalizations. But information, however well it may be structured and organized, is not by itself the content of a discipline. There is also process, the constellation of intellectual skills employed in acquiring and using that knowledge. Neither content nor process can exist or be taught or learned in the absence of the other. Parker and Rubin argue that process is in fact the life blood of content. In classrooms where transmission of information is primary, learners play a passive role (29). Where the emphasis is instead placed on process (e.g., analyzing, decision making, problem solving), the learners are actively involved. Transmission or assimilation of information is not less important, but subject matter becomes the vehicle for learning rather than merely a destination selected for the learners by the teacher. This outcome has been aptly described as representing the difference between knowing something, and knowing what it is good for.

Students need to learn how to search out what is known about a problem and how to analyze, compare, and sensibly choose the best among alternative solutions. Use of problem-solving and decision-making skills is stimulating in elementary school years, and it may be more important to begin using them then than at later levels of education. Thinking should not be a process deferred until secondary school levels, nor should its happening be left to assumption. Bruner said that "Intellectual activity anywhere is the same, whether at the frontier of knowledge or in a third grade classroom . . . the difference is in degree, not in kind" (7). The subject matter used in investigating health topics arises from the problem being worked on and should never be viewed as the primary goal of instruction. The teacher must be a facilitator of learning, not a communicator of information.

Health information doesn't long stay the same, and even if it did, no system for presenting that information could equip children with enough of it to deal sensibly with every manner of health-related problem or decision over a lifetime. Learning *how* to learn is imperative in education today because it has lifelong utility and application. Information can become obsolete or irrelevant, but the ability to discover fresh facts when they are needed increases each time it is used. The person who has mastered problem solving and informed decision making has the

versatility needed to cope with new challenges, technologies, and health problems whenever they occur.

However, there must be a system for selecting the principal topics to be used to structure the subject matter of concern, so it follows that content and values will be inseparable. The questions that must be addressed to the subject specialists in a field are these: What knowledge is of most worth in today's world? What knowledge does an educated person need to function effectively as an individual and as a worthwhile member of our society? The answers will always be somewhat different over time because the essential knowledge about health and health behavior is changing more rapidly than can be communicated to the public. So much is being learned about life and health at so fast a pace that teachers are hard pressed to keep up to date. However, unless they do and adjust their teaching plans accordingly, their students may have to cope with tomorrow's problems using yesterday's information.

The trend in every discipline has been to abandon any attempt to describe its total body of knowledge, for this is impossible. Faced with this reality, scholars have sought to identify the most powerful concepts and generalizations in their fields to structure and define the scope of their discipline—the most logical and economical way to organize a field's content matter. As Bruner said, "To focus on structure is to learn how things are related" (7). Once a student has grasped the fundamentals of healthful living, each new idea fits in neatly and is quickly understood because it belongs. Even young children can learn how things affect and are connected to each other.

A Philosophy Statement: Curriculum Guidelines

Curriculum planning waits upon data gathering, needs assessments, and synthesis of the resulting data. An important first step must now be taken. The beginning point in planning an instructional program is the development of an effective statement of the set of basic beliefs upon which subsequent curriculum decisions will be based. In effect, this is the function of the United States Constitution. Without the guidance and justification of such a document, planning curricula is similar to starting a difficult journey in the absence of a dependable map. Given the existence of an effective statement of philosophy, schools can resist pressures to add or delete studies according to every passing fad. Teachers are able to plan instruction consonant with the purposes spelled out in the statement. In short, every curriculum decision is provided with focused direction if the document is a good one.

Perrin argues that many statements purporting to be "philosophies" are instead descriptions of methods of operation, personal thoughts about educational methods and programs, or prescriptive lists of "shoulds" relative to administration, organization or curriculum (30).

Tyler believes that a philosophy statement should define the nature of a good life and a good society (35). Perrin agrees, saying, "A philosophy should describe the ideal 'educated' person whom the public schools seek to produce, and the conditions of society which demand an individual with that kind of education" (30). He suggests that the 1961 Educational Policies Commission produced one of the best examples of philosophy stated properly. A section relevant to health education follows:

> The traditionally accepted obligation of the school to teach the *fundamental processes*—an obligation stressed in the 1918 and 1938 statements of educational purposes—is obviously directed toward the development of the ability to think. Each of the schools' other traditional objectives can be better achieved as pupils develop this ability and learn to apply it to all the problems that face them.
>
> Health, for example, depends upon a reasoned awareness of the value of mental and physical fitness and of the means by which it may be developed and maintained. Fitness is not merely a function of living and acting; it requires that the individual understand the connection among health, nutrition, activity, and environment, and that he take action to improve his mental and physical condition" (30).

Currently a point of view approved by the AAHE Board of Directors presents such a statement totally concerned with health education (3). Portions of that paper may serve to illustrate its appropriateness as an illustration of beliefs basic to health teaching and program development:

> Health is a personal and societal matter. Health education, therefore, must become a part of the experience of each learner and extend itself into the surrounding society. For health education to indeed take place, health must eventually become a directing factor in one's ever-present lifestyle. The subject matter of health education must be established and taught within the context of students' lives, not treated as something to be transmitted simply because it is available. Knowledge about the structure and physiology of the human body, for instance, is of value in teaching solutions only when it contributes to the understanding or solution of individual or solution of individual and group human problems and thus fosters the enrichment of human development and learning (30).

Whatever curriculum design selected for a program, there should be a philosophical statement justifying its selection as an effective means of developing the kind of health-educated person needed today.

DEFINING THE SCOPE OF HEALTH EDUCATION

The term **scope** in health education refers to the total range of subject areas or health topics selected to represent the body of knowledge of the discipline. It is usually categorized and ordered by means of a series of units referred to as its "organizing elements." To use a simple analogy, if we were to speak of an ordinary ruler as a scope having 12 units, then we might say that its organizing elements were inches and the plan was the "inches system." The way any scope is described depends on the point of view of those given responsibility for determining how it is to be organized. Although in essence it is always the same material, the form in which it is presented differs somewhat. Whatever the plan chosen, the subject matter considered by all of its organizing elements taken together is its scope.

The organizing elements most commonly employed in health education are the major body systems, current health problems, traditional content areas, health topics, or health concepts. For example, those viewing the appropriate focus of health instruction as being physiological-anatomical would probably use body systems as their organizing elements. Each plan has certain strengths and weaknesses. Whichever structure is chosen for a school curriculum, there will unavoidably be some effect on the way the body of knowledge titled "Health Education" will be perceived and taught.

Which of the following plans fits your own beliefs concerning the best possible presentation of health instruction? In your opinion, which one seems most oriented to the promotion of wellness?

Body Systems Design

Obviously the body systems design focuses on an anatomical and physiological study of the body and its functions. The strength of this plan, particularly at the elementary level is that young children have great interest in learning about their bodies and how they work. The weakness in using body systems as a curriculum framework is that the focus tends to be more on physiology than on health education. Also, there is no logical reason for including health content, other than that implicit in the area of optimum physical growth and development. Consumer health, prevention and control of diseases, community health, and environmental health must be tacked on if they are to be considered at all. Teachers who lack preparation in health teaching cannot be blamed if they mistake the systems for the total body of knowledge. Moreover, because some communities object to any mention of the reproductive system, especially at the elementary level, the teacher is in the awkward position of having to avoid discussion of the system about which student interest is apt to be greatest.

The body systems design was used in the Primary Grades Health Curriculum Project and the School Health Curriculum Project. Each grade's study focused on a body system, part, or sense. However, attention was later given to the need for comprehensiveness during the revision of the original units between 1979 and 1982. At that time the organization plan was changed from the body system design and expanded to encompass ten more or less traditional content areas into which the earlier objectives and activities were interwoven as appropriate. Retitled, *Growing Healthy*, the curriculum today reportedly reaches more than 1,000,000 students in grades K through 7 in 41 states (26). It was the first curriculum design to be recommended by the Department of Education, although it seems likely that the School Health Education Study curriculum would have earned that accolade had the award been in existence earlier.

Health Problems Design

A scope employing the health problems design reflects the conviction that effective use of the limited time and resources available for health instruction is possible only if the curriculum focuses on the crucial health problems of the day. An early example of this rationale was the development of a guide to instruction by a Commission of the American Alliance for Health, Physical Education, and Recreation (2). Their first step was to identify the most crucial health problems for the 1960s and 1970s. This judgment was determined by a process of reaching consensus among the commission members. By inference, those not specified did not meet the criterion of cruciality. The problem areas selected were accident prevention, aging, alcohol, disaster preparedness, disease and disease control, economics of health care, environmental conditions, ionizing radiation, evaluation of health information, family health, international health, mental health, nutrition, and smoking. The list was not intended to be representative of the total scope of health education, but the exclusion of drug abuse and misuse as a major health problem area is surprising.

During the late 1970s, 15 priority areas were identified in the Surgeon General's report

Healthy People (36). (In fact, these were also *problem areas*, so the title could as aptly have been *Unhealthy People*).

The advantage of using health problems to structure health teaching and curricula is that the greatest emphasis can be given to the prevention or control of threats to health that are most likely to be encountered by the learner. As such, the material is both current and meaningful. The disadvantage is that related health instruction is limited to the selected problems, which may or may not be crucial by the time the instruction occurs. Moreover, what seems crucial to adults may be far less threatening to healthy youngsters.

There are other disadvantages. For example, a problem-focused curriculum is based on the assumption that students need know nothing more about healthful behaviors than how to cope with those problems. Learning how to prevent or solve common health problems is not the same as learning how to make wise everyday choices that affect wellness in important ways. The approach also ignores the pressures that motivate unhealthful actions. As Neubauer and Pratt point out:

> In very concrete ways the health of individuals is a reflection of the social, economic, and political patterns of the community, and is in fact simply a symptom of those patterns. To talk about "health" as if it were disconnected from dominant institutions and community life is to fall into the trap that tells us that isolating events gives us control over them (28).

To focus on disease as though knowledge about symptoms, causes, and prevention or risk reduction were the primary or only requisite factor in health promotion is the very opposite of what health education should be.

Health Content Area Design

The use of content areas as the organizing elements for curriculum development is the traditional and most familiar form by which the scope of health instruction is defined. There are many strengths associated with this plan, one of which is that when fully developed and implemented, it provides a comprehensive survey of the body of knowledge. The format is so well accepted that a wealth of resource materials (e.g., books, textbooks, pamphlets, articles, films, filmstrips, and tapes) keyed to those areas is easily obtainable and frequently updated. For the same reasons, school health educators anywhere in the country will interpret and teach the subject matter in much the same way. The content area titles are consistent with the actual subject matter and serve to define the boundaries of the information contained in each.

Content areas are often used as the organizing elements in official curriculum documents such as those formulated by state boards of education, state departments of education, and national health organizations, both voluntary and professional. Two such lists of recommended content areas illustrate how nearly universal their titles are:

California State Board of Education (1993)
1. Personal health.
2. Family living
3. Nutrition education
4. Tobacco, alcohol and other drugs
5. Communicable and chronic diseases
6. Environmental health
7. Individual growth and development
8. Injury prevention and safety
9. Consumer and community health

National Comprehensive School Health Guidelines Committee (1984)
1. Community health
2. Consumer health
3. Environmental health
4. Family life
5. Growth and development
6. Nutritional health
7. Personal health
8. Prevention and control of diseases and disorders
9. Safety and accident prevention
10. Substance use and abuse

The latter list was endorsed and accepted by all of the school health-interested national professional groups (ASHA, AAHE, SHES/APHA, and the Society for State Directors of HPER). The seeming omission of mental-emotional health as an area is based upon the belief that these dimensions of health are always a part of each of the ten content areas.

A weakness associated with use of content areas is that the very compactness and neatness of those titles leads to division and compartmentalization of instruction. Unless care is taken to plan meaningful and logical transitions between the areas, the result can be a series of short courses with little to link them other than their concern with health or its absence. Also, because the cue for instruction is taken from the content area titles, what is taught or learned tends to be subject matter, not processes, with the focus on *knowing* rather than *doing* or thinking. Finally, when there is not enough time allocated for full study of all the areas, those left until last are given little attention or are omitted entirely. This diminishes the effectiveness and comprehensiveness of the program as it was intended to be taught.

Topic Design

A topic differs from a content area in that it is usually a subordinate area or a theme related to a content area. A subordinate area might be oral health, stress reduction, or rest, sleep, and relaxation. Stated as a theme, it might be "eating for energy and health," living safely at school and at home," or "protecting the world we live in." An advantage of using a topic design is its flexibility in planning health instruction according to student interests and curriculum time constraints. Topics meaningful to a given grade level can be studied in ways that contribute to learning in other basic studies.

Topics tend to be built around lifestyles or day-to-day health decisions so that they relate well to specific needs and concerns of the learner. However, they seldom encompass the total scope of health instruction, even added together following the entire elementary school experience. It also takes a very skilled teacher who knows the difference between health education and physiology or hygiene to plan and integrate

health topics into a day's teaching so that it has real impact. A busy elementary school teacher already burdened with teaching many subjects may not have time to do the special planning this requires. The topic design works best when it is promoted vigorously by the school administrator and coordinated by someone who is qualified and given the free time needed to do so.

Conceptual Approach

A conceptual approach to curriculum planning might be described as one that (1) employs powerful generalizations or concepts as a means of structuring a given area of subject matter, (2) derives its scope from those concepts, (3) stresses teaching strategies that provide practice in applying cognitive skills, and (4) uses factual data to facilitate conceptualization rather than as bits of information to be memorized (Figure 3-1).

Conceptual teaching takes advantage of the fact that conceptual learning is the way people learn naturally. It is centered on the learner, not the teacher. The classroom is not a scene typified by rows of passive students listening or filling out worksheets; instead it is characterized by the vital sounds and sights of active participation in the investigation of real problems and interests. The goal of conceptual teaching is the discovery of answers to questions that lead to meaningful conclusions. Conceptual learning goes on all the time, in and out of school. In the conceptual approach the teacher provides an accepting environment, arranges experiences facilitative of that kind of learning, and then simply allows it to happen.

Probably the best-known example of a conceptual framework defining the body of knowledge in health education is the SHES curriculum (2). Based on the results of a carefully designed and implemented research project, its ten concepts have had a lasting impact on health education curricula. For example, when the study was begun, more than 35 different subject areas were commonly listed in curricula across the country. Somehow, few curricula offered since those ten

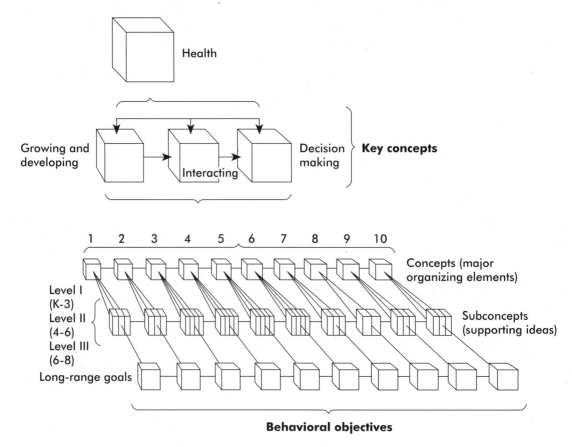

FIGURE 3-1
Conceptual model for the SHES curriculum.

concepts were devised to categorize the subject matter have either changed the number of organizing elements or departed very much from its basic categorization scheme. In fact, the project was very possibly too far ahead of the profession when it was introduced to be understood or well accepted. In a very real sense, the SHES curriculum was fated to succeed by osmosis rather than by acclamation, although a great many school districts adopted the full curriculum during the 1970s.

Since the concepts are stated as complete ideas, they provide far more guidance to their meaning than do other kinds of organizing elements. For example, the concept "Use of sub-

stances that modify mood and behavior arises from a variety of motivations" is a complete idea and probably has been understood as long as humans have known of substances that can do that. When one reduces the concept to a couple of words like "substance abuse," as in a content area designation, the real meaning of the concept is lost along with much of its power as an idea. In the first place, there are lots of substances that we eat or drink or ingest somehow. Which of them is intended by the word substance, even when linked with "abuse" is uncertain. Ice cream modifies one's mood, but if you eat too much of it, you tend to add unwanted pounds. And, ironically, because the word "substance" has been so

SHES CONCEPTS FOR DEFINING BODY OF KNOWLEDGE IMPORTANT IN HEALTH EDUCATION

1. Growth and development influences and is influenced by the structure and functioning of the individual.
2. Growing and developing follows a predictable sequence yet is unique for each individual.
3. Protection and promotion of health is an individual, community, and international responsibility.
4. The potential for hazards and accidents exists whatever the environment.
5. There are reciprocal relationships involving man, disease, and the environment.
6. The family serves to perpetuate man and to fulfill certain health needs.
7. Personal health practices are affected by a complexity of forces, often conflicting.
8. Utilization of health information, products, and services is guided by values and perceptions.
9. Use of substances that modify mood and behavior arises from a variety of motivations.
10. Food selection and eating patterns are determined by physical, social, economic, and cultural patterns.

widely and thoughtlessly accepted, for many it has come to mean only illegal or controlled chemicals as in cocaine, heroin, and marijuana. The real point of the concept is that whatever the substance may be, the motives for taking it can differ widely.

When the physical, social, mental, and emotional dimensions of these concepts (big ideas) are explored, the outcome is a holistic view of health and health behavior, not one limited to the physical alone. In addition, the conceptual approach provides a rationale for study at every grade level. Although specific enabling objectives must be designed for every level of teaching, the concepts keep them on target. Kreuter observed, "The SHES approach remains the most conceptually and philosophically sound guide to the development of school health education curriculum" (22).

The weakness of the conceptual approach probably lies in the fact that it takes more skill and planning to teach concepts instead of facts. Green and Kreuter opined that "Paradoxically, the philosophical and conceptual strength of the SHES curriculum may have been its major weakness. Many health educators apparently found it hard to understand and apply in the classroom situation" (17). The problem is not in arranging for children to conceptualize; the challenge lies

in arranging the kinds of perceptual experiences (lessons) that will lead to the formulation of the concept wanted. Elementary teachers do not always possess the background in health sciences needed to plan meaningful and valid learning opportunities. It is often desirable and necessary to arrange inservice training in health teaching, whatever the curriculum plan chosen for a school. The provision of at least a part-time consultant to advise and suggest ways to enrich the program would be a valuable addition to a curriculum committee's roster.

DETERMINING THE SEQUENCE OF HEALTH INSTRUCTION

Sequence, the ordering of the content areas, is a problem that must be dealt with once the scope is defined. **Vertical sequence** is the ordering of organizing elements from year to year, grades K through 12, and is usually established at the administrative or district level. **Horizontal sequence** involves a plan for ordering the elements within the time allotted for teaching, whether as a semester course or as a single grade's curriculum plan. Specific decisions concerning horizontal sequence are best made by school curriculum committees and teachers (18). Figure 3-2 illustrates the complex interrelationships among vari-

ORGANIZATION

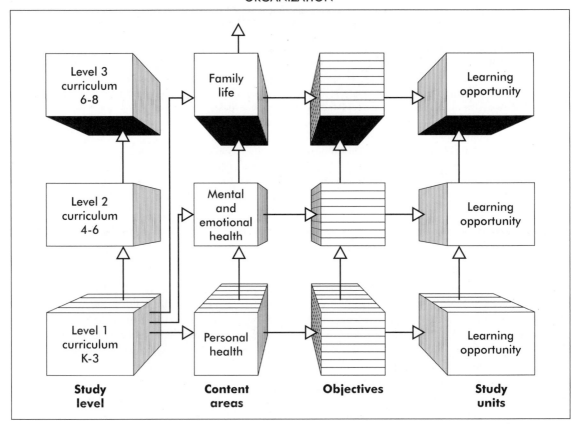

FIGURE 3-2
Vertical and horizontal organizational chart.

ous curriculum elements using a vertical and horizontal diagram.

Determining when study of any particular organizing element (concept, topic, content area, health problem, or body system) should be scheduled is a complex problem. There must be a reason for the position assigned in every case. There is no one right sequence, but there must be logic connecting one element to the next. The sequence represented by the chapters in the textbook you may be expected to use provides a sequence, but it is somebody else's sequence. Ask yourself, "Based on what I have learned about children of this age (their concerns, what they

need to know, their cognitive abilities, etc.), what would get their interest on the very first day of school, and what would they feel most confident and comfortable about discussing in a new situation like that?" When that has been decided, look at the other elements of the scope that you are asked to teach and choose the one that seems appropriate as a next step. For example, suppose you decide that because second grade students typically are very interested in having friends and being a friend, you plan a way that helps them get to know each other during the health lesson. Growth and development in ability to make friends is important to children. Learning to do

TABLE 3-2

Proposed Organization of Cycle Plan Health Curriculum

Content Areas	Horizontal Sequence								
	Levels								
	I				II			III	
	K	1	2	3	4	5	6	7	8
Personal health and fitness	X	X	—	—	X	—	—	X	—
Mental health	—	—	X	—	—	X	—	—	X
Family life	—	—	—	X	—	—	X	—	X
Nutrition	X	X	—	—	X	—	—	X	—
Disease prevention and control	—	—	X	—	—	X	—	—	X
Injury prevention and safety	X	X	—	—	X	—	—	X	—
Consumer health	—	—	X	—	—	X	—	X	—
Avoiding drug misuse	—	—	—	X	—	X	—	X	—
Environmental health	—	—	—	X	—	—	X	—	X
Community health	—	—	—	X	—	—	X	—	X

so helps them to recognize that growth is good and happens in many ways. Ask them to suggest other ways we help each other grow.

Once growth and development have been studied in all dimensions, what might reasonably be considered next? Whatever the sequence you adopt, whether your own or one recommended, the important thing is that there *is* a plan and the children can see what it is. A little time spent during the first day or even the first week of school might profitably be spent asking them to tell you what they would like to know and what they would like to learn first. The more you can involve them in making these kinds of decisions the more likely it is that the health lesson will be their favorite time of the day.

It is not always possible to schedule the total scope of health instruction during any one grade or course of study. This means that the task of planning horizontal sequence involves a sort of vertical aspect. In general, two scheduling schemes, the **cycle plan** and the **spiral plan,** are employed in order to accommodate all of the subject matter within a period of time encompassing two or more school grades.

In the cycle plan, placement of each of the content areas in the grades where indicated has been based on known needs, interests, and the physical, social, mental, and emotional growth and development characteristics of each age or grade level (Table 3-2). Notice that all of the content areas are emphasized at least three times during grades K through 8, although more of them are covered in some years than in others. Such a plan does not preclude natural overlaps into unscheduled content areas as a consequence of interest generated by planned study or an unexpected community problem or issue. Don't get so locked into your plan that you can't take advantage of student interest of the moment if it is worthwhile.

The advantage of the cycle plan is that every teacher knows the minimum that each student in his or her class is expected to learn in that year. The disadvantage is that it rests upon the interest and competence of each teacher to accomplish the goals of the total curriculum if later grades are to progress as intended. Unless there is careful coordination of these units and commitment to the goals of the total health curriculum, the minimum is apt also to be the maximum.

A spiral *horizontal* scheme is illustrated in the plan here proposed for elementary and middle-school health instruction and will be developed in considerable detail in Part II of this textbook. Table 3-3 outlines both the scope and suggested sequence of the content areas selected for study. Illustrative instructional objectives are listed relative to each content area and for all three levels of schooling; however, these are not intended to comprise all of the objectives that need to be addressed. They typify a range of objectives feasible for students at the indicated level. In addition, because objectives serve as cornerstones for the development of teaching plans, several have been selected at every level and for every content area as the focus for fully developed learning opportunities that describe several ways to achieve those designated. The selected objectives are identified by an asterisk. Notice the overlap in the case of grade 6, which is shown in both the intermediate and middle-school groupings. This is because grade 6 can be found in either setting, depending on a particular district's preference.

As you can see, the depth and breadth of health information covered during these years is considerable. To complicate matters, "facts" can change rapidly as research continues in health science. What is believed to be true one day may appear to be wrong or different the next. It is unlikely that any one text can include all of the pertinent health information that an elementary or middle-school teacher might need to know. Because specific facts and other data are changing so quickly, a school, college, or local librarian could be of help in locating the most current information on a specific topic before preparing lesson plans. In today's computerized filling systems, research of that kind is easier and more quickly achieved than teachers could have imagined only a few years ago.

Scope and vertical sequence development is a more critical problem in elementary and middle-school grades because it considers about nine years of a child's school life. Children's needs, interests, and their growth and development levels change far more dramatically during these years than during high school. In addition, it is usual to offer health education only once during high school years, ordinarily in 9th or 10th grade.

Notice that each column of objectives presents curriculum level objectives at three succeeding stages of children's education. Each provides a clue to the intended content and is appropriate to the abilities that can be expected of youngsters of that age. All are general objectives that are broadly designed to give teachers flexibility in lesson planning, while serving as a stabilizing frame of reference and means of maintaining consistency among the strategies used to implement them.

The behaviors (expressed as verbs) specified in the objectives progress from simple to more complex, and the subject matter from factual and concrete to more abstract. Yet remember that achievement of the most abstract content to be mastered and dealt with by means of higher level cognitive skills during high school or college rests upon successful learnings experienced as an result of the elementary school plans.

Although this scope and sequence plan is but one of many possible arrangements, it is consistent with current recommendations relative to comprehensive school health education at the elementary and middle-school levels. The advantage of the spiral plan is its greater flexibility and adaptability to the needs of the learners. Actually, the curriculum objectives proposed here could be used to plan instruction for any age group, assuming only that those being taught had the necessary background information and skills to cope with the objectives selected for them. The disadvantage is that teachers must be able to design learning opportunities that match the objectives as proposed or must be able to devise new enabling objectives as needed or more appropriate objectives that would lead toward achievement of the general objectives for a given group of students.

During the lower two levels of elementary

TABLE 3-3

A Scope and Sequence Plan for Elementary and Middle School Health Instruction

Personal Health and Fitness

Primary Level K-3 Student:

1. Names health habits that protect self and others.*
2. Identifies physical, mental, and social benefits of good health.
3. Explains why daily dental care is essential for the growth and development of sound teeth and gums.
4. Describes ways decision making affects personal health practices.

Intermediate Level 4-5/6 Student:

1. Explains ways personal health behavior is influenced by friends and family members.*
2. Describes the relationship of personal health behavior to the optimum structure and function of the body.
3. Explains the relationship of physical fitness to sound body function.

Middle-School Level 6/7-8 Student:

1. Analyzes the relationship between diet choices and fitness
2. Designs personal health care and fitness programs to meet individual needs and interests.*
3. Describes both immediate and long-range effects of personal health care choices.

Mental and Emotional Health

Primary Level K-3 Student:

1. Classifies social behaviors as acceptable and unacceptable.
2. Differentiates between pleasant and unpleasant emotions.
3. Illustrates ways to show friendship.*

Intermediate Level 4-5/6 Student:

1. Explains the difference between physical well-being and mental and emotional health.
2. Identifies positive and negative effects of stress.
3. Proposes acceptable ways to deal with strong negative emotions.*

Middle-School Level 6/7-8 Student:

1. Identifies constructive ways to manage stress.*
2. Analyzes the influence of peer pressure health-related choices.
3. Describes the importance of setting realistic goals.
4. Explains the interrelationships among physical, mental, emotional, and social well-being.

Family Life

Primary Level K-3 Student:

1. Defines the meaning of family.
2. Identifies responsibilities and privileges of various family members.
3. Describes ways family membership changes*
4. Explains that all living things come from other living things.

Intermediate Level 4-5/6 Student:

1. Proposes constructive ways to solve conflicts with friends and family.
2. Interprets changes in social activities as family members mature.
3. Describes the progression of the individual through the life cycle from birth to death.
4. Identifies growth and developmental characteristics common in puberty*

---

*These objectives are illustrated by sample learning opportunities in Chapters 9 through 19.   *Continued.*

TABLE 3-3

A Scope and Sequence Plan for Elementary and Middle School Health Instruction—cont'd

Middle-School Level 6/7-8 Student:
1. Predicts physical, mental and emotional, and social changes that occur during adolescence.
2. Explains why growth and development is individual, although predictable.
3. Describes the reproductive processes.*
4. Identifies social and cultural factors in the development of responsible health behavior.

Nutrition

Primary Level K-3 Student:
1. Lists distinctive characteristics of foods.*
2. Explains the importance of eating a variety of foods.
3. Describes food combinations that provide a balanced diet.
4. Identifies snack foods that are nutritious.

Intermediate Level 4-5/6 Student
1. Identifies factors that influence personal food choices.
2. Classifies foods according to their major nutrients.
3. Analyzes the nutritional value of food choices for meals and snacks.*
4. Explains reasons for differences in nutritional requirement between individuals.

Middle-School Level 6/7-8 Student:
1. Evaluates diets appropriate for individual needs.
2. Explains the relationship between calorie intake, level of activity, and body weight.*
3. Analyzes nutritional value of food in fad diets.
4. Predicts long-range outcomes of poor diet choices.

Disease Prevention and Control

Primary Level K-3 Student:
1. Explains differences between illness and wellness.*
2. Differentiates between infectious and other diseases.
3. Identifies ways to prevent the spread of disease.
4. Explains the importance of health checkups and immunization to health maintenance.

Intermediate Level 4/5-6 Student:
1. Identifies factors that may cause diseases and disorders.
2. Differentiates between control of infectious and other diseases.*
3. Explains the contribution of science to the detection, prevention, and control of disease.

Middle-School Level (6/7-8) Student:
1. Analyzes the relationship of personal life-style choices to disease prevention*
2. Identifies symptoms of diseases common among young people.
3. Explains the effects of disease on individuals, families, and communities.
4. Describes appropriate courses of action when a disease is suspected.

Injury Prevention and Safety

Primary Level (K-3) Student:
1. Explains the relationship between observing safety rules and preventing injuries.
2. Identifies potential hazards at home, school, and community.
3. Explains how to obtain help in an emergency.

*These objectives are illustrated by sample learning opportunities in Chapters 9 through 19.

TABLE 3-3

A Scope and Sequence Plan for Elementary and Middle School Health Instruction—cont'd

Intermediate Level 4/5-6 Student:

1. Evaluates actions of bicycle riders for safety.
2. Demonstrates basic first aid procedures for stopped breathing.*
3. Identifies individual responsibilities for reducing hazards and preventing injuries.

Middle-School Level 6/7-8 Student:

1. Develops a home safety program.*
2. Demonstrates standard first aid procedures appropriate in life-threatening situations.
3. Explains how properly used protective equipment increases enjoyment and diminishes the possibility of injury when engaging in potentially risky activities.

Consumer Health

Primary Level K-3 Student:

1. Differentiates between health products and services.
2. Names people who help promote and protect health.*
3. Explains the influence of advertising in promoting sale of health products.

Intermediate Level 4-5/6 Student:

1. Interprets information provided on health product labels.
2. Lists sources of reliable health information and services.
3. Describes advertising appeal of foods and medications used by children.*
4. Differentiates between health quackery and licensed health care.

Middle-School Level 6/7-8 Student

1. Analyzes methods used to promote health products and services.
2. Compares scientific and faddish bases for choices among health products.
3. Describes the function of consumer-protection agencies.
4. Identifies criteria for the selection of a qualified health adviser.

Avoiding Drug Misuse

Primary Level K-3 Student:

1. Explains reasons for avoiding use of controlled drugs or unknown substances.
2. Explains reasons why many people avoid using any drugs including tobacco and alcohol.
3. Demonstrates effective ways of refusing offers of drugs.*

Intermediate Level 4-5/6 Student:

1. Analyzes reasons why some people abuse drugs.
2. Explains why we have laws controlling use of drugs.*
3. Evaluates the effectiveness of problem-solving skills in choosing alternatives to drug use.

Middle-School Level 6/7-8 Student:

1. Predicts effects of drugs on physical, mental and social functioning.
2. Analyzes factors motivating individuals to avoid or abuse drugs.
3. Interprets the significance of peer pressure on decisions regarding drug use*

*These objectives are illustrated by sample learning opportunities in Chapters 9 through 19.

Continued.

TABLE 3-3

A Scope and Sequence Plan for Elementary and Middle School Health Instruction—cont'd

Environmental Health

Primary Level K-3 Student:
1. Identifies the sources of environmental (air, land, and water) pollution.*
2. Names actions that conserve natural resources.
3. Describes ways to work with others to help provide a healthful environment.

Intermediate Level 4-5/6 Student:
1. Explains how improving the environment can enhance physical, social, and mental health.
2. Identifies causes and preventives against environmental pollution.

Middle-School Level 6/7-8 Student:
1. Analyzes ways individuals and communities can promote a healthful and safe environment.
2. Evaluates the effects of community groups and agencies in improving and protecting the environment.*

Community Health

Primary Level K-3 Student:
1. Identifies familiar community health workers (health helpers)
2. Explains the function of various health workers in the community.
3. Lists services provided by community health agencies and organizations*

Intermediate Level 4-5/6 Student:
1. Describes ways community members work together to solve health problems.
2. Identifies functions of interesting career opportunities in the health field*

Middle-School Level 6/7-8 Student:
1. Describes community efforts to prevent and control disease.
2. Concludes that individual participation is essential if community health activities are to be successful.*

*These objectives are illustrated by sample learning opportunities in Chapters 9 through 19.

school, a supplementary cycle plan might need to be worked out if time allocations are too few or too short. Some ways that the objectives develop as the framework is sequenced to fit both the subject matter and the students' existing abilities are explained in Chapter 5, along with discussion of criteria to be applied to the evaluation of the quality of proposed objectives.

CHOOSING CURRICULUM PATTERNS FOR HEALTH TEACHING

If those responsible for the administration of a school or school system believe that comprehensive school health education should be provided, or if it is mandated and supported by state fund-

ing, then health education will be included in the school's curriculum plan. How it will be implemented depends again on decisions made at the administrative level. Patterns of organization at the elementary level may be integration (infusion) or direct teaching. The latter pattern is more typical of upper elementary and middle-school organization.

Integration

To integrate or infuse is to relate the parts of something within the whole. To employ integration in planning for teaching and learning is to focus on relationships, generalizations, or concepts that tie experiences or facts together. As a curriculum plan, **integration** refers to the means by which a subject area is introduced and treated in a given educational setting. In traditional educational patterns from elementary school onward, learning is often compartmentalized and specialized. Each subject area is dealt with in turn as a separate entity. The relevance of what is learned in one subject area to that learned in others may be less than clear if students are not helped to see significant relationships among them.

As a process, integration or, as it is currently sometimes termed, *infusion* functions as a part of *any* effective teaching and learning program, whether it be elementary, secondary, or higher education. At the elementary level, often what is considered a core curriculum based on a broad theme or concept is in fact an integration model. In learning about issues or problems associated with a broad theme such as transportation, the students begin to examine the implications for health that are inescapably involved. They begin to identify questions concerning ways transportation is related to availability of foods, preservation of perishable foods, safety of passengers, rapid transmission of disease agents, accessibility of health care, air and noise pollution and more. At the same time they are learning related science, geography, history, climate, mathematics and supporting skills such as reading and writing—not as separate, unconnected bits of information, nor as ends in themselves but as contributions to the study of transportation. Moreover, they are learning and applying lifelong cognitive skills such as problem solving, thinking and reasoning with transfer to all learning. Students actively participate in investigations dealing with their own needs and those of the community. They learn about living, and at the same time they learn ways of processing the flood of data that pours in daily. These are the kinds of lessons that children must have if they are to live in the twenty-first century as effective family members and citizens.

Health instruction in elementary schools is often infused with social studies and science. Goodlad concluded that development of truly in-tegrated programs of study (those that involve a wide number of disciplines in a program focused on larger themes) is something that no level of school does well (16). His investigation revealed that many first and second grade classes put together the theme of understanding self and others, with discussion of the family and community as part of social studies. By third grade, children were frequently studying community needs such as health care. As a part of science studies, grades 1 through 3 were focusing on personal orientation to the natural world, and fourth graders were learning about nutrition and drugs/alcohol problems. In general, Goodlad found that it was the science curriculum at the elementary level that appeared to be linked with health.

The strength of an infused curriculum pattern is that students are active participants in their own learning. As they investigate real community needs and problems, they learn about living healthfully and productively. They learn ways of processing new information as it is offered to them. They learn how to identify reliable sources of information and how to access it as needed to solve their own health problems and that of family members. They learn that personal behaviors and choices give them some control over their own well-being. They are not passive listeners but active learners of the skills required for the development of responsible lifestyles.

A weakness of the infused or integrated model is that its success depends so heavily on the interest, motivation, and skill of the classroom teacher. Few are given much, if any, preparation for the health instruction for which they are the primary source during the vital first years of school. In the absence of a qualified health coordinator and planned in-service programs to promote the quality and quantity of health teaching across the grades, what results is apt to be fragmented at best. Elementary teachers (K-6) are generalists, and they do a remarkable job of teaching the many basic subjects for which they are responsible. Some become interested enough as undergraduates to take electives that help them fulfill their responsibility for effective health teaching. Many states employ health-teaching specialists as coordinators or instructors in junior high or middle schools. These are individuals whose preparation has been in health education and who are credentialed as health-teaching specialists. But the preponderance of elementary teachers need all the help they can get. Inservice training and careful use of prepared health-instruction programs can help bridge the gap between the responsibilities elementary teachers face and the scanty preparation for the task most receive in teacher-preparation studies.

Direct Teaching

The most successful pattern for health instruction is **direct teaching,** with a regular, daily class period allotted to health instruction. How much time is scheduled is ordinarily an administrative decision. What is covered in direct teaching, its scope, often depends on the content of the textbook or the curriculum plan adopted by the school. Hence, the scope and sequence of health education in elementary schools are often determined less by schools than by authors and publishers.

When direct teaching will be provided is an administrative decision and varies with the philosophy of the school or its principal. There is no standard practice in elementary schools regarding the content or grades in which health instruction is provided. Some health instruction usually is given each year, based on recognized health problems and the growth and developmental characteristics of the age group of concern. The quality and quantity of that instruction depends to a great extent on the interest of individual teachers or the nature of their credential during the first six years of school. Middle-school health teachers are often specialists and teach only health education, although they may and often do have split assignments, teaching other subjects in the curriculum as necessary.

Many health-concerned organizations, professional groups, and experts in health education recommend that elementary school children be given a minimum of 20 minutes of health instruc-

tion each day. Students in grades 7 and 8 should have *at least* a full class period once a week for a year and preferably a full semester of daily health instruction. Specified health topics usually are emphasized in some years and not in others according to a determined plan (see Table 3-1). For example, injury prevention and safety may be stressed every year from K through 6. Another topic often included in the primary grades is dental health. Topics such as drug misuse and abuse and boy-girl relationships often are not approached until grade 7 or 8. What do you already know about the health needs and interests and the growth and development of children that affects decisions regarding the sequence of health topics at any particular grade level? Look at the growth and development characteristics in Table 3-1 with reference to a grade level that interests you. Do those topics appear logical based on the facts listed in the table?

When the administrative commitment is to direct teaching, the program must be of high quality and should be coordinated by qualified health-education specialists. The subject must be given time, space, and material support equal to those provided other basic subjects. Unfortunately, there is not enough time, even with daily health lessons, to teach children all they want and need to know.

There are many advantages to direct teaching. It is the traditional pattern, so teachers are most familiar and comfortable with it. Health textbooks are written with direct teaching in mind. The teachers' editions or supplements include suggestions for lessons designed to be used in a separate course. The packaged curriculum programs widely used in schools are similarly designed to be implemented by direct teaching. And with the set amount of regularly scheduled class time typical of direct teaching patterns, a teacher can be more responsive to current needs and concerns. Interest and motivation are naturally sustained when a daily program is possible; health can be considered in all of its dimensions.

A disadvantage of direct teaching is that where it exists, there is a tendency to view health education as having been given complete coverage. Potential enrichment by means of integrating experiences in other subject areas is forgotten. When health instruction is assigned to unqualified or uninterested teachers, instruction may be limited to reading the book. Although "health is more than hygiene," the student in such a class may be lucky to learn even that much. As a result of dependence on the textbook, the sequence may be a lockstep march through the chapters with no attempt to give priority or emphasis to those topics most relevant to a given group of learners. Finally, where teaching is confused with "telling," lecture becomes the sole technique used. Health instruction becomes a series of "no-no's," health rules, and warnings instead of stimulating learning opportunities that offer ideas and strategies for self-care and maintenance of wellness.

Nevertheless, direct teaching has been shown to be the most effective single pattern for organizing the health curriculum. School health education at its best develops a student who has learned to generalize and has formulated a set of useful concepts and skills that will remain long after specific facts have been forgotten. Direct teaching provided by a competent instructor is, potentially at least, health education at its best.

THE TEACHER'S ROLE IN CURRICULUM DECISIONS

Because of its complexities, curriculum development has emerged as a major field in education. Curriculum specialists have to be knowledgeable about current and past research findings related to curriculum problems and must be skilled in conducting and interpreting research. They must have the ability to design and carry out valid program evaluation procedures. They must be thoroughly grounded in curriculum theory and methodology. Extraordinary skill in writing and creating curriculum materials is a must. Fortunately, although teachers need to be able to speak the language of curriculum developers, it is not necessary that they be curriculum specialists. Teach-

ers should not be expected to add curriculum designing to all the responsibilities already given them.

Sliepcevich differentiated between two levels of curriculum planning, one no more essential than the other, but each essential to the effectiveness of the other (33). The broader, more general view of curriculum development entails careful research leading to a product applicable in any community because it is based upon universal needs and concerns. She termed this level the *macroscopic* view of curriculum organization. The more specific curriculum problems encountered at the classroom level are termed the *microscopic* view of curriculum organization. This is the teacher's special area of decision making and curriculum planning.

A teacher brings unique competencies, skills, insights, and practical experience to the tasks of adapting, modifying, and implementing programs proposed by the specialists. Where this division of labor exists, the teacher and curriculum specialist complement each other's skills. The result of such a dynamic partnership is increased efficiency, economy of effort, and effectiveness of the total school health program. Sliepcevich concluded that teachers are not *less* involved as a consequence, but *more* involved, and at a more sophisticated and meaningful level. (33)

Developing packaged curriculum materials for schools requires the macroscopic view of the problems and goals of health education. A set of broadly described objectives forms the framework of such materials. Each of these general objectives specifies a measurable skill as well as some significant subject matter with which it is to be employed. However, instead of listing a series of lesson ideas, **learning opportunities** are described that could be used in achieving that objective. The principal difference between a learning opportunity and a lesson is that a learning opportunity focuses on a curriculum-level objective, is described in general terms, and requires several lessons for its accomplishment. A lesson plan focuses on enabling objectives subordinate to a general objective and describes an activity that usually can be accomplished within the limits of a day's class, yet contributes to the achievement of the learning opportunities.

The words "packaged curriculum program" may suggest a mechanistic approach to health instruction, reducing the teacher's role to that of the tool used to activate the plan. Nothing could be further from the truth; in fact, it is quite the other way around. In the absence of skilled teachers who can interpret and adapt such materials to fit their students' needs and abilities, the finest and most innovative curriculum package is just a lot of words and paper. When you think of it, a textbook is a packaged learning system, especially the teacher's edition, but it is how the teacher uses that textbook that makes it as effective as it is intended to be. If nobody reads it, a book is just a lot of paper and words. And if teachers do nothing more with a textbook than use it for quiet work, those words cannot make much of an impact on the reader. In the case of packaged curriculum programs, the emphasis is on *how*, not merely *what*. It cannot be handed to the students; it is a teacher's aid.

The real testing and adaptation of a curriculum program takes place in the classroom, and the responsibility will be yours. You have to know what it ought to include and how to judge the quality and validity of its goals and objectives. Remember that the use you make of it must be appropriate to the needs and interests of *your* students, not students in general. Base your plans on the information you have gathered about your own students and the communities of which they and your school are a part. Then if the choice is yours, examine the most widely used programs to see which of them best fits your students' needs as well as your system of beliefs about health education as an educational purpose.

Packaged curriculum plans, though expensive, are popular with schools, especially at elementary and middle-school levels. Because prospective elementary teachers receive little or no preparation for health teaching, a strong, well-organized health education program is a welcome addition to their kit of teaching tools. Such programs come in all shapes and sizes. Some are developed by or in cooperation with state boards of education; many are prepared by publishers of educational materials in general. Voluntary health organizations such as the American Cancer Society, American Heart Association, the American Lung Society, and others have prepared curriculum plans for teaching what students need to know about a particular health problem. (See Appendix B for the names and addresses of voluntary and non-profit agencies that provide educational materials.) Private industry-related organizations such as the Metropolitan Life Insurance Company, the National Dairy Council, and the National Lifestock and Meat Institute are valuable sources of free or inexpensive health-related teaching materials.

Some programs are concerned with a single topic only. Many programs require the purchase of a wide range of teaching aids; others mandate teacher training in the use of the materials, while some can be used by the teacher just as received and read. Some require that the total program be purchased, but others can be obtained on a single unit basis depending on a school's need. Most of them are designed for use with students from grades K through 6, in some cases there are also middle-school components available. A few of the most popular programs follow:

The Great Body Shop is a comprehensive health education program developed by the Children's Health Market, Inc. (9). Obviously employing the body system approach, the scope of the curriculum includes functions of the body, nutrition, physical fitness, safety, AIDS and illness prevention, substance abuse, self-worth and emotional health, growth and development, and consumer and community health. At every grade, the three learning goals for each of these 10 topics are a knowledge or understanding, a value, and a skill. The scope and sequence chart developed for the user lists the 3 goals for every topic. These are not instructional objectives usually found in scope and sequence presentations but ambiguously stated goals. For example, the goals in connection with breathing are (1) "To understand how the lungs function" and "To understand asthma, the common cold etc," (2) "To value clean lungs and recognize how pollution, smoking, etc. can hurt them," and (3) "To practice healthy behavior to protect the lungs." A teacher's guide promises activities that span all 6 cognitive levels of learning and considers interwoven themes such as self-worth, responsibility, and values throughout.

Growing Healthy evolved from an original body system format (The School Health Curriculum Project) now encompassed within a comprehensive health education curriculum for children in grades K through 6 as developed by the National Center for Health Education (26). Reputedly the most widely adopted curriculum of any supported by the National Diffusion Network (NDN), which recognizes exemplary educational programs and promotes their adoption by the nation's schools. Growing Healthy covers the recommended 10 major content areas, combining community and environmental health management into one area and including mental/emotional health as a separate area. Lifestyle goals are spelled out for each of the content areas, and instructional objectives are defined for each goal at every grade. Teachers selected from schools intending to implement the Growing Healthy program attend organized workshops for training, and these teachers in turn train others in their schools. Detailed teaching guides are provided for use by teachers at each grade. Children participate actively in small groups at successive learning centers that provide hands-on activities relevant to the objectives. A wide range of multimedia materials are included as part of the program.

The Michigan Model is a comprehensive school health curriculum for grades K through 8, adapted from the original Growing Healthy curriculum. The program covers the same 10 content areas. Each grade level's instructional materials are provided to the teacher in "phase" boxes, I to VI, which contain a variety of related, multimedia, hands-on learning aids. Special booklets have been developed to acquaint parents with the program and to promote their involvement in the project. Teacher training is available and urged. Skills addressed in the program include self esteem, emotions, stress coping, relaxation, and other resiliency skills. AIDS is discussed at the eighth grade level. The program is basically a body system approach and is popular with teachers whose training has been science oriented.

Actions for Health is a comprehensive health education curriculum designed for students in grades K through 6 (15). Its scope encompasses growth and development, mental and emotional health, family life and health, nutrition, substance use prevention, personal health and hygiene, disease prevention and control (special attention given to HIV/AIDS at every grade level), injury prevention and safety, consumer health, and community and environmental health. Skill development is the organizing element and emphasis in this innovative program. Every grade focuses on a specified skill with the related knowledge aspect of study serving as vehicle rather than end of instruction. Grade K's skill is self-esteem, grade one's skill is self-esteem and rewarding healthy behavior; grade two's skill is communication, grade three's is decision making; grade four's is health assertiveness, grade five's is managing stress, and grade six's is setting and achieving goals. Classroom tested materials are featured instead of a textbook. For each grade level there is a theme animal, student booklets that illustrate health themes in fun-to-read stories, activity posters, a proposed culminating special event, and take-home letters involving family and community in the program.

For example, grade one includes seven units of study: Unit 1, *Me, myself, and I;* Unit 2, *I am part of a family;* Unit 3, *Taking care of myself every day;* Unit 4, *Everybody gets sick sometimes;* Unit 5, *Keeping myself safe;* Unit 6, *No drugs for me;* and Unit 7, *Health helpers in the community.* The special event, which is titled "A Healthy Behavior Celebration," details writing invitations, arranging the room, making healthful snacks, arranging student work displays, preparing role plays or demonstrations, and filling out certificates attesting students' healthy behaviors. Unarguably user friendly, the program satisfies every criterion of sound curriculum design from measurable objectives to evaluation plan.

The American Heart Association School Site Program, *Getting to Know Your Heart,* is comprised of 2 packages: one for lower elementary grades 1-3 and one for upper elementary grades 4-6 (4). The middle-school program is called **Heart Decisions** (5). The two elementary packages cover three modules: physiology of the heart, effects of smoking, and nutrition and exercise. The middle-school package covers the same three modules plus emergency cardiac care. Each package includes a comprehensive teacher's guide that leads teachers step by step through the activities within each module and provides objectives, key concepts, activities-at-a-glance, background information, kickoff activities and follow-up activities and more. Support materials include a videotape, 21 reproducible masters, 6 brightly colored posters, a songbook, rubber tubing to illustrate blood vessel concepts, 2 stethoscopes and *"What Every Teacher Should Know about the Heart,"* a booklet that provides teachers with additional background information.

Here's Looking at You, 2000 is a complete drug education curriculum for students in grades K through 12 (10). Each grade level unit comes with a teacher's guide and a kit including audiotapes, books, videotapes, puppets and games. Teacher-training sessions (3 or 5 day) are offered at various locations around the country. Although the program is totally concerned with drug- and alcohol-abuse prevention, it does deal with topics such as sexuality, making friends, and decision making but only as they relate to drug use and abuse.

Know Your Body is a multicomponent, teacher-delivered health promotion program for grades K through 7 (3). First developed in 1975 by the American Health Foundation (AHF), it has been approved by the U.S. Department of Education's Program Effectiveness Panel and is supported by the National Diffusion Network. The Foundation has developed teacher and coordinator training programs that are conducted over 1, 2, or 3 days. Teachers may be trained either by AHF personnel or by local project coordinators who have been trained by the Foundation. The materials have been updated to reflect current health concerns (3).

The program has been extensively evaluated for effectiveness. Children participating in studies of its application have demonstrated increased health knowledge as well as decreased serum cholesterol levels, blood pressure, and use of cigarettes. Questionaires for each grade level are available to teachers, administrators, and funding agencies to assess changes in students' health-related knowledge, attitudes and behavior. Classroom materials consist of teacher manuals and student activity books for each grade level. In all grades, Know Your Body utilizes a combination of developmentally appropriate health instruction as well as cognitive and behavioral skills relevant to substance use, smoking, exercise, nutrition, dental health, self management, first aid, accident prevention, risk factor reduction, and environmental and consumer awareness.

What has been discussed in this chapter should be helpful to you if you are asked to evaluate programs for your students. Look for the answers to these: Who are the authors of the curriculum, and what is their professional background? Is the program staff-developed, or written by practicing health educators? Have measurable objectives been stated, and are they employed as the organizing centers for the suggested activities? Is the content of the learning activities part of the lessons or simply an assumption? Do any suggested evaluation activities specify *ways* to measure achievement or only *what* to look for? Does the program fit with your beliefs about the nature of meaningful health education for the year 2000? More suggestions for evaluation of written materials will be presented in Chapter 7.

SUMMARY

There are but three basic sources of information to be analyzed in curriculum development: the learners, their needs, interests, problems, maturity, and abilities; the demands and problems of the society in which they live; and the valued subject matter. There was a time when the only consideration when planning for instruction was the named subject matter. That might have worked 50 years ago, but it is no longer possible for anyone to know everything there is to know about anything. So the problem is to decide what knowledge is of the most worth today, and that depends on many other things (e.g., the nature of the students, where they live, and what they need to know to live in that environment and society).

In recent years, the study of curriculum has become a discipline in its own right, having a special vocabulary and distinctive modes of procedure. Teachers need not be experts in curriculum design, but they do need to be comfortable in their grasp of its language and relevant data sources, first, because they are responsible for the interpretation and application of curriculum plans where it counts most, at the classroom level; second, because they are so often asked to participate in the development or updating of school or district level curricula; and third, because the processes employed and the information needed for curriculum planning applicable and essential to the development of study units, learning opportunities, and lessons.

Any vocabulary that might seem strange or new is just a matter of using another word or words to mean what is already familiar language for teachers. What curriculum specialists call organizing elements, teachers often refer to as "units." In health education, units are ordinarily titled according to the design selected for a particular curriculum, i.e., as health content areas, topics, health problems, body systems, or concepts. A scope lists the number and kind of organizing elements chosen for a curriculum plan. Sequence is the word used to describe the plan for ordering the organizing elements from K

through 12 so that one learning experience builds on another by reasoned intention. Horizontal sequence is the planned arrangement of elements side by side so that they buttress each other in effect and logic. When curriculum specialists refer to organizing centers, they are talking about the suggested learning opportunities as proposed in a curriculum guide.

However thorough the investigation of the sources of a curriculum may be, an essential preliminary statement must be prepared. This is the philosophy or set of basic beliefs about health education held by those who will plan the curriculum. Such a document specifies the nature and skills of the health educated person the schools seek to develop and justifies this goal on the basis of demonstrated needs. Subsequent decisions that set goals, objectives, content focus, and learning activities are based on and guided by that philosophy. The result is a plan that is consistent with the avowed purpose of the program, whatever the level of instruction.

How the scope of the curriculum is taught requires another set of decisions, similarly based upon what we know about the learners, the community and the body of knowledge. Health teaching at the elementary and middle-school levels may be integrated with other subjects such as social studies, science, or physical education. Or it may be accorded equal treatment with other basic subjects and allotted single subject status, including adequate amounts of time, resources, and facilities. Ideally, a combination of both patterns is provided, which requires careful coordination of activities and objectives and inservice training for all of the teachers who will be doing the teaching.

QUESTIONS AND EXERCISES
Discussion questions

1. What would be the advantages and disadvantages of basing curriculum decisions solely on the interests of the learner?

2. Differentiate between needs and interests and the developmental characteristics of children. Which set of data do you see as having the greater influ-

ence on *what* is taught and which one on *how* it is taught?

3. What is the relationship between general education and health education?

4. Which plan for organizing the scope of health instruction seems best suited to a focus on wellness? Which plan might present the greatest problem if health promotion were to be the goal of instruction? Why would it be difficult? `

5. If health is viewed as a concept with interacting physical, social, mental, and emotional dimensions, can mental health be dealt with as a distinct and separate area? If so, explain your rationale for such a separation. If not, explain why not.

6. In what ways do community values influence health curriculum planning? Give examples of some ways you perceive to be significant.

7. What do you see as the major differences between integrated or infused and direct teaching of health science? What would be the best way to offset the weaknesses of each?

Problems and exercises

1a. For an elementary school grade of your choice, find out as much as you can about the needs and interests of elementary students as reported in the literature: the levels of physical, social, mental and emotional development to be expected of these children; the scope of health instruction recommended or mandated in your state or school district; and a listing of the local health needs and problems relevant to a health curriculum for children of that age.

1b. Based on careful consideration of all these data, (1) define the scope of health instruction by means of the organizing elements that you believe to be most suitable, and (2) order these elements according to a stated logic for a horizontal sequence for one year. Present your plan to the class and be prepared to support your decisions by reference to the data from which they were inferred.

2. Make a scrapbook of current news clippings collected from local, state, or national publications that have implications for health curriculum planning. Organize them according to their relevance to the organizing elements you have chosen, whether these are content areas, topics, or other. Note which elements are most often a community

concern and which are mentioned least. How could this information affect your plans concerning sequence?

3. Interview at least five children of either primary, upper elementary or middle-school age and ask them to tell you what they want to know about health or health problems. Encourage them to think about health as a means of enjoying life and growing up to be what they would like to be. Record every question that they ask. Share your list with others in your group and draw some conclusions, based on the accumulation of questions, about the interests and the needs revealed, as well as about the frequency with which each of these is expressed. Which kinds of questions were asked most frequently? Were there questions you expected but did not get? Speculate about the reasons that this might have been the case.

4. Obtain a copy of a local school health curriculum guide (or one prepared by a community health agency or professional health organization) and analyze its components. What are the organizing elements used to structure the subject matter? What is the scope of the curriculum? Is there a plan for horizontal sequence? If so, what is suggested for first consideration? Is there a plan for vertical sequence? Does the scope reflect a comprehensive view of health education, or is it limited in any way? If it is limited, what is missing? What would you add if it were in your power to amend the plan? Write a report of your analysis.

REFERENCES

1. American Alliance for Health Education: Point of View, *J Health Educ* 23:1, 1992.

2. American Alliance for Health, Physical Education, and Recreation: *Health concepts: guides for instruction*, Washington, DC, 1967, AAHPER.

3. American Health Foundation: *Know your body*, New York, 1988. The Foundation.

4. American Heart Association: *Getting to know your heart*, Dallas, 1988, The Association

5. American Heart Association: *Heart decisions*, Dallas, 1990, The Association.

6. American School Health Association: *School health in America*, ed 5, Kent, Ohio, 1989, The Association.

7. Bruner J: *The process of education*, Cambridge, Mass, 1963, Harvard University Press.

8. Byler L, Totman R: *Teach us what we want to know*, New York, 1969. Mental health materials center, Inc., Connecticut State Board of Education.

9. Children's Health Market, Inc: *The great body shop*, Wilton, Conn, 1992.

10. Comprehensive Health Education Foundation: *Here's looking at you 2000*, Seattle, 1991.

11. Dapice A, et al: Teaching and learning values, *Educ Horizons* 66(3):107-109, Spring 1988.

12. Denver Public Schools: *The health interests of children*, Denver, 1954.

13. Droz R: *Understanding Piaget*, New York, 1976, International Press.

14. Educational Policies Commission: *The central purpose of education*, Washington, DC, 1961, National Education Association.

15. ETR Associates: *Actions for health*, Santa Cruz, Calif, 1993/1994.

16. Goodlad J: *A place called school*, New York, 1984, McGraw-Hill.

17. Green LW, Kreuter M: *Health promotion planning: an educational and environmental approach*, Mountain View, Calif, 1980, Mayfield.

18. Hartoonian H, Laughlin M: Designing a scope and sequence, *Social Educ* 50:7, Nov/Dec 1986.

19. *Healthy people:* national health promotion and disease prevention objectives, Washington, D.C., 1990, US Department of Health and Human Services.

20. Kohlberg L. *The philosophy of moral judgment*, New York, 1981, Harper & Row.

21. Kolbe L et al: Propositions for an alternate and complementary health education paradigm, *Health Educ* 12:3, May/June 1981.

22. Kreuter MW: *Considering realistic outcomes for school health education.* Unpublished paper presented at Promoting Health through Schools Conference, Denver, 1980.

23. Lowrey G: *Growth and development of children*, Chicago, 1986, Year Book Medical Publishers.

24. Matiella C: *Positively different. Creating a bias-free environment for young children*, Santa Cruz, Calif, 1991, Network Publications.

25. Moyer J: Child development as a base for decision making, *Child Educ* 62(5):325-329, 1986.

26. National Center for Health Education: *Growing healthy*, vol 3, New York, 1984.

27. National Comprehensive School Health Education Guidelines Committee: Comprehensive school health education, *J Sch Health*, 54(8):312-315, 1984.

28. Newbauer D, Pratt R: The second public health revolution: a critical appraisal, *J Health Politics, Policy Law*, 6:205, Summer 1981.

29. Parker J, Rubin L: *Process as content*, Chicago, 1966, Rand McNally.

30. Perrin K: Instructional leadership: a statement of philosophy is the first step, *NASSP Bulletin*, 70(494):65-73, 1986.

31. Scales, P. Sexuality education in school: let's focus on what unites us. *Health Educ* 24(2):121, March/April 1993.

32. Seffrin J: The comprehensive curriculum: closing the gap between state-of-the-art and state of the practice, *Sch Health*, 60(4):151, April 1990.

33. Sliepcevich E: Curriculum development: a macroscopic or microscopic view, *National Elem Principal*, 48:2, 1969.

34. Trucano L: *Students speak*, Seattle, 1984, Comprehensive Health Education Foundation.

35. Tyler R: *Basic principles of curriculum and instruction*, Chicago, 1963, University of Chicago Press. (Originally published in 1949.)

36. US Department of Health and Human Services: *Healthy people.* Washington, D.C., 1979.

37. US Department of Health and Human Services, Public Health Services: *Objectives for the Nation*, Washington, D.C., 1980.

38. US Department of Health and Human Services, Public Health Services: *Prospects for healthier America*, Washington, D.C., 1984.

39. Yarber W. *Accounting for health instruction*, *Health Educ* 8:4, July/Aug 1977.

SUGGESTED READINGS

A point of view for health education, *J Health Educ* 23(1):4-6, Jan/Feb 1992.

Nielsen, M: Integrative learning for young children: a thematic approach, *Educational Horizons* 68(1):19-24, Fall 1989.

Perry C, Murray D, Griffin G: Evaluating the state-wide dissemination of smoking prevention curricula: factors in teacher compliance, *J Sch Health* 60(10):501-504, December 1990.

Smith D, Robinson K, Olsen, L: The longevity of "growing healthy": an analysis of the eight original sites implementing the school health curriculum project, *J Sch Health* Vol 62(3):83-87 March 1992.

White D, Ballard D: The status of AIDS/HIV education in the professional preparation of preservice elementary teachers, *J Sch Health* 24(2):69-72, March/April, 1993.

4 Defining Goals and Objectives for Health Teaching

When you finish this chapter, you should be able to:

- Differentiate between the structure and functions of educational goals and instructional objectives.
- Analyze the advantages of using measurable objectives as the framework for planning health teaching.
- Evaluate the worth and functionality of goals and objectives proposed for health teaching in elementary schools.
- Apply the criteria for preparing clearly stated objectives to the development of a set of classroom-level objectives.

Since it is your intention to become an elementary school teacher, you may already have had some experience in writing goals and objectives. Is there anything about writing goals and objectives for health teaching that is different? We think so. The other basics of the elementary school curriculum focus on communication and computation skills (i.e., reading, writing, and arithmetic). What is to be learned is clearly defined, and what is taught is much the same anywhere in the country. Health teaching has to do with helping children learn and apply problem-solving skills for making the realistic choices that characterize a healthful life style. Its subject matter is far more complex and dynamic, and its objectives must elicit activities involving active participation, not passive listening or desk work. The goals of health teaching do not propose ends without real-life utility, nor can its instructional objectives be effective in attaining those ends in the absence of clearly drawn relevance to the learners.

Can you write an objective that describes an educational outcome with potential use in solving an actual health problem? Can you differentiate between a goal statement and a measurable objective? The following 10 statements labeled *objectives* are taken from current elementary school curriculum guides published by major, health-concerned organizations. The student will be able to:

1. Understand some of the reciprocal relationships involving man, disease, and environment.
2. Be able to state that the heart is a muscle that never stops working.
3. Explain why certain foods have limited nutritional value.

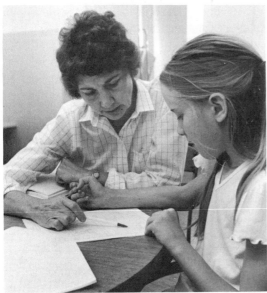

Armi Lizardi

Effective problem-solving requires careful thinking.

4. The student will be able to discuss three major differences between active and passive immunity.

5. Students will have opportunities to identify the characteristics of human blood.

6. Children will recognize what they can do to maintain and protect the environment.

7. After listening to, completing, and discussing several riddles and poems, the pupil will be able to identify the function of several body parts by completing the given worksheet with 80% accuracy

8. Recall why individual, community, and international health problems prevail on the local, state, national, and international scenes.

9. The students will help make a model breathing apparatus and participate in three tests to determine the adequacy of their lung power.

10. Cite the difference between a vaccine and a serum.

Do you see any differences among these ten statements? How many of them would you ac-cept as being meaningful and achievable objec-tives for health teaching in elementary schools? If they all look good to you now, we hope you will read on before you decide.

FUNCTION OF GOAL STATEMENTS IN CURRICULUM DESIGN

Goal statements describe the *ends* or purposes of a curriculum plan. Whatever their level of specificity, **objectives** always describe ways and means of attaining those ends. Differences be-tween goals and objectives also depend on their intended function in curriculum development and on their distance from the students them-selves. Krathwohl divides these distances into three levels (8). At the most remote level—far-thest from the classroom and the student—are the **goals,** the broad, abstract, and most general statements describing the educational goals for a total program for grades K through 12. At the next level are the **general** objectives used to structure plans for a semester course or curricu-lum unit. Such an objective is broad enough in its content to require many learning opportuni-ties for its achievement. The third level—that closest in impact to the learner—is composed of the most specific, or **enabling** objectives, used to structure a single lesson, or part of a lesson.

The broadest statements, the cognitive por-tion of which is often ambiguous, may be re-ferred to as aims, as well as goals. The subordi-nate and more measurable general objectives and instructional objectives allow teachers flexibility in choosing among them and in selecting the strategies and techniques to be used in carrying them out.

Goodlad agrees that the term *objectives* should be used only when referring to purposes stated in terms of learner activities; the terms *goals* or *aims* are used to define purposes to be carried out by schools (4). He also defines three educational decision-making levels of remote-ness from the classroom, but they differ from those of Krathwohl. Most remote, says Goodlad, is the *societal* level, which includes the educational goals set by school boards, legislators, and federal agencies. Closer are the institutional goals—those set by school administrators and teachers when making curriculum plans intended for an entire school or school district. Closest to the students is the instructional level. Only these purposes, he says, should be termed behavioral or instructional objectives (4).

Notice that in this chapter we are concerned with writing and implementing educational goals and instructional objectives. In Chapter 3, when we cited national health and educational goals as one of the sources of the school curriculum, we described the national report *"Healthy People 2000"* subtitled *"National Health Promotion and Disease Prevention Objectives"* (7). The same terms, goals and objectives, have been used in that report, but they are not the same thing in that context either in substance or form.

Briefly, *"Healthy People"* lists the three major goals intended to give structure and define the challenge for health planners, health policy makers, and health providers. The goals are brief and narrowly specific to public health concerns:

1. To increase the span of healthy life for Americans.
2. To reduce health disparities among Americans.
3. To achieve access to preventive services for all Americans.

The hundreds of "objectives" described as means to those ends are more exactly subgoals because they are not intended to provide direction to those expected to implement them. Instead they describe hoped-for outcomes along with specific desired percentages of total achievement. Examples of these so-called objectives are: "18.2 By the year 2000 to confine HIV infection to no more than 800 per 100,000 people" and "3.4 To reduce cigarette smoking prevalence to no more than 15% of adults."

FORMULATING LONG-RANGE HEALTH EDUCATION GOALS

Every statement of educational purposes, whatever its level of generality, includes the same two dimensions: (1) a behavior and (2) some amount of subject matter. The differences between goals and objectives are most apparent in the behaviors used in each case and the relative abstractiveness of the specified content. The behavior, or verb, used to state long range goals is often ambiguous, such as "knows", "understands," or "believes." This is acceptable for goal statements because, in effect, the meaning of that ambiguous behavior will be defined by the objectives proposed as effective means to its achievement.

In health teaching, long range goals represent target outcomes and remain the same throughout the entire curriculum plan. Thus they provide stability and give direction for every teacher responsible for fulfilling them at every grade level. Typically goals are stated in terms of what is hoped the students will learn, believe and do about health-related practices and problems. Accordingly, the goals are categorized as belonging to the cognitive, affective, or action domains of behaviors. The cognitive domain includes those objectives that deal with recalling or recognizing information and those requiring higher cognitive intellectual skills and abilities, such as comprehension, application, analysis, synthesis, and evaluation. The affective domain includes those objectives that describe desired changes in interests, attitudes, and values. There is a third domain, the psychomotor, which includes manipulation or motor skills and performance components. These have primary relevance to physical education goals (6).

There are health education objectives with psychomotor components. They include objectives that can be practiced and evaluated overtly, such as the ability to carry out cardiopulmonary resuscitation (CPR), use dental floss or a toothbrush effectively, carry out certain basic first-aid procedures, or demonstrate recommended personal health care practices such as those involving care of the skin, hair, and nails.

Instead of using the psychomotor domain as its third category of long range goals, the School Health Education Study writing team selected a new term, *action*, as more descriptive of the hoped-for outcome of its curriculum. The action domain was defined as "those aspects of health behaviors in which one applies health knowledge, attitudes, and problem solving skills to an actual life situation" (13). Since its introduction in this role, the action domain has been employed by many health educators to categorize the third group of health education goals. Examples of goals categorized according to these three domains include:

Cognitive: knows that body parts, systems, and functions grow and develop at varying rates both among and within individuals.

Affective: believes that the potential for growth and development can be fostered or hindered by an individual's own choices and actions.

Action: exhibits health behaviors that promote or maintain optimum growth and development.

COMPETENCIES AS GOALS

Instead of long-range goals, many states and school districts have proposed competency statements as descriptors of desired learning outcomes. The notion of competency as a goal has been widely adopted, and sets of competencies have been recommended for every level of instruction from kindergarten through graduate school.

Competencies written in regard to health education are usually stated at two levels of abstraction. The high-level competencies are virtually indistinguishable from statements otherwise termed goals, and the specific competency statements, inferred from the broader statements, are in no way different from behavioral objectives.

The principal difference between the two levels appears to depend on whether the behavior is ambiguous (e.g., *knows, appreciates, behaves*) or specific (e.g., *identifies, names, lists*) and whether the statement describes an outcome that corresponds to one of the previously mentioned domains of learning.

A general competency and its supporting objectives, adapted from those specified for a high school in California, follow:

Competency: Students will understand the effects of nutrition on their immediate and long-term personal well-being.

Objectives: Names the essential nutrients and their functions.

Identifies beneficial effects of foods commonly consumed by children and adults.

Describes long term effects of poor nutrition.

The following long-range goal is almost identical to the above competency statement. "The student comprehends that the choice of foods determines the nutrient balance vital to effective functioning of the body." The form has not been altered; only the label is different. Nevertheless, the use of competencies as desired outcomes of instruction has brought much greater attention to the quality of the instructional objectives designed to attain them. Goal statements are apt to be forgotten by those who write instructional objectives. Perhaps the word "competency" makes the difference? Competency statements seem to be more provocative targets; hence, the objectives that are subsumed tend to be more relevant and interesting than they otherwise might be. In fact, the greatest contribution of the competency movement may have been this emphasis on measurement of student learning in terms of predetermined abilities and the consequent sharpening of the objectives.

RELATIONSHIP OF GENERAL TO SPECIFIC OBJECTIVES

Curriculum-level, or general, objectives are implied by the long-range goals. Instructional objectives, in turn, are inferred from the general objectives. At each level, these statements attempt to answer the question "What are the skills and knowledge an educated person needs in order to maintain a positive lifestyle and to solve health-related problems effectively when they arise?"

Objectives designed to implement goals should be stated at the classroom level. Whether they are broadly or narrowly defined depends on their intended function. A few broadly stated general objectives can be used to structure a unit or

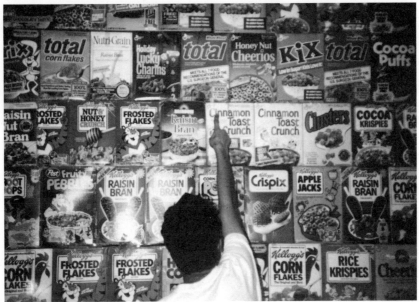

Ric Loya

Comparing similar foods for nutritional value requires analytical skills.

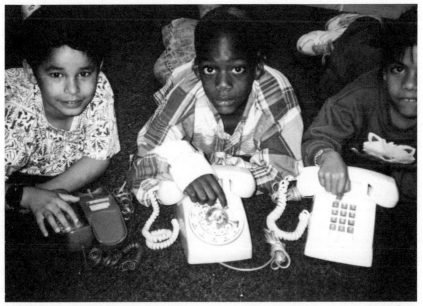

Angela Loya

Dialing the emergency number requires specific skills and knowledge.

course of study with considerable economy of detail and no loss of clarity. All of the illustrative objectives in the scope and sequence chart (see Table 3-3) are general objectives. The most specific objectives subordinate to these general statements are best left for the classroom teacher to prepare because different groups of students have different interests, past experiences, and abilities. Only their own teacher can effectively tailor the specific objectives designed to fulfill the purposes expressed in a general objective. As long as the specific objectives collectively result in the achievement of the general objectives, small differences in the enabling (specific) objectives have little, if any, importance. For example, if a proposed general objective were "Develops criteria for choosing among commonly used personal health products," some enabling objectives that a teacher might use as a means to that end might include:

1. Defines the meaning of the term "health product"
2. Names health products commonly used at home
3. Identifies reasons why certain health products were chosen
4. Lists criteria used by parents and friends when choosing health products
5. Describes key factors involved in determining each criterion

Although general objectives do not differ in form from the specific objectives, they *are* different, either in the breadth of the subject matter they encompass or in the complexity of the behavior they elicit. The more complex the behavior, the more experience and skill the learner needs to carry it out. The broader the content, the more elaborate the learner's system of previously learned concepts must be. These two major components, behavior and content, can be manipulated to suit a given level of student readiness. Figure 4-1 illustrates four possible patterns for combining the two dimensions to adjust for the needs and abilities of individual groups of students.

Examples of each of the four possible combinations, from the simplest to the most complex objectives, include:

A. Lists ways to avoid exposure to germs.
B. Describes characteristics common to all living things.
C. Classifies foods according to the major food groups.
D. Evaluates social, cultural, and economic influences on health behavior.

It is essential that the objectives you devise be attainable by your students. Also within any set of general *or* instructional objectives, each objective must be consistent with the others at that level of generality. That is, in a given set, all ob-

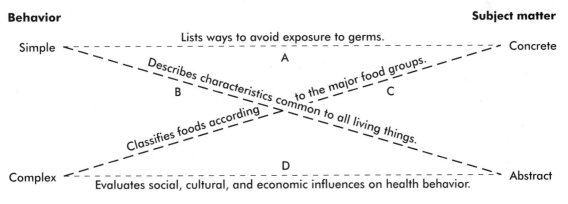

FIGURE 4-1
General objectives.

jectives must have the same combination of the two dimensions which you decide is best suited to the abilities and needs of your students (the A, B, C, or D combination) (see Figure 4-1). For students at elementary levels, a mixture of two or more of these patterns confuses both the purposes and the results.

BEHAVIORAL AS MEASURABLE OBJECTIVES

Most educators are willing to admit that anyone planning to teach needs to decide what the objectives are to be. The principal issue seems to center on the degree of measurability such statements should possess. This point has been debated for some time without much resolution, probably because the two sides are not all that far apart in their approaches. The curious thing is that despite all the debate, few instructors find it easy to write objectives and fewer still bother to write them at all. Nevertheless, whether or not you believe that precision and measurability are essential elements of an instructional objective, you should know how to write one and how to use it to facilitate lesson planning. Objectives that are measurable should describe *what the learner will be able to do following instruction that she or he could not do before.*

Perhaps the problem is not that educators believe that there is no need to write objectives that describe actions or behaviors that can be seen and measured but that the word *behavioral* is not clear in meaning. Often behavioral objectives are descriptive of lesson-specific activities, for instance, "Given a diagram of a particular part of the body (e.g., the eye) the student will be able to correctly label that diagram" (3). Some see "behavioral" as referring only to cognitive skills which have been sharpened and increased as a result of the activity called for in the objective, for example, "Describes the structure and function of the eye and ear" (12). Others reject the word in this sense because the resulting objectives seem to them either trivial or mechanistic (and therefore dehumanizing) or as part of a plan to mold or control the minds and behaviors of children. Still others see "behavioral" as referring to changes effected in actual health practices, for example, the learner no longer exhibits a harmful behavior or adopts a healthful behavior as a result of the learning experience provided. This connotation is more apt to be an expectation of community health educators whose objectives and activities are focused on existing health-related behaviors that need to be changed, (e.g., smoking, overeating, alcoholism, etc.)

For the purposes of this textbook, when the word *measurable* is used, it will mean that the objective describes an activity, mastery of which can be assessed now, in the classroom. Whatever you call it, an instructional objective for health education in schools specifies a measurable cognitive or affective behavior associated with some amount of meaningful and useful health content. It is a tool for planning teaching strategies.

COGNITIVE BEHAVIORS

Certain behaviors descriptive of cognitive processes are more useful in stating measurable objectives than others. Some verbs have wide acceptance because their meaning is specific enough to be interpreted in much the same way by most educators. However, even slight differences in interpretation can alter both the approach selected and the outcome of the instruction. It is wise to specify the meaning of the behaviors to be used rather than assume that each will be perceived by everyone else exactly as intended by its developer. Whenever you set out to design a series of instructional objectives, define the terms you are going to use before you begin; it simplifies the task of choosing behaviors that are feasible for your students, promotes consistency in form, and facilitates the development of lessons that provide appropriate practice. The following are examples of definitions that might help establish what the learners should be doing as they carry out the objective. Each of these has been tentatively categorized according to the hierarchy proposed by the Bloom Taxonomy of

Educational Objectives (2). Remember that these are not *the* definitions—only possible examples.

1. **Knowledge**
   a. Naming: using the correct word to designate a given person, object, or idea.
   b. Defining: stating the exact meaning of a word or sense of a word.
   c. Listing: making an ordered record of persons or objects, usually of the same nature.
   d. Identifying: ascertaining the nature or definitive characteristics of a thing or person.

2. **Comprehension**
   a. Explaining: verbally making the nature or meaning of something clear; giving reasons for a condition or happening.
   b. Describing: telling about something in detail; picturing with words.
   c. Interpreting: translating complex ideas or situations into simpler terms that mean the same thing.

3. **Application**
   a. Illustrating: clarifying by using examples and comparisons with words, pictures, or actions.
   b. Predicting: stating what might happen in a given situation on the basis of prior or newly obtained information.
   c. Discriminating: distinguishing relationships or differences among elements of a communication or problem.
   d. Applying: transferring learned concepts and skills, as needed, to solve new problems.

4. **Analysis**
   a. Analyzing: separating a communication, problem, or concept into its component parts as a means of clarifying the meaning of the whole.
   b. Categorizing: determining the placement of an idea or object in a specific division of a classification system.
   c. Classifying: arranging or sorting items according to a set of shared characteristics.

   d. Differentiating: noting or showing specific variations in or between objects.

5. **Synthesis**
   a. Concluding: making a reasoned judgment or inference based on all the data available.
   b. Proposing: suggesting a novel plan or solution to a problem for consideration and adoption.
   c. Synthesizing: combining separate substances, elements or ideas to form a whole new product.

6. **Evaluation**
   a. Contrasting (with): showing or emphasizing differences between or among objects, persons, or ideas.
   b. Comparing (with): examining objects, persons, or ideas to note similarities between or among them.
   c. Evaluating: appraising the quality of a product or plan according to a set of predetermined standards.

Stating Measurable Objectives

Authorities differ somewhat in their recommendations regarding the form of a well-stated objective. Most agree that it should propose a behavior that can be practiced and observed in the classroom (as opposed to the ambiguous long-range behaviors used in stating goals). Major differences in opinion, as we have said, center around the precision with which those behaviors must be stated and whether the criterion of achievement must be included in the objective itself. In general, three patterns of developing objectives seem to have evolved. One is the *programmed instruction model*, another is taxonomy, influenced by the Bloom *taxonomy* of educational objectives (2), and the third is termed the *operational model* in this discussion.

Programmed instruction model. Those who have adopted a programmed instruction would write an objective of this kind: "Given a list of ten common foodstuffs, the student will be able to identify each according to its food group with at least 80% accuracy." Use of this very specific, criterion-associated objective had its origin in Mager's little book *Preparing Objectives for Programmed Instruction* (10). At that time there was great interest in programmed instruction, and teachers were pressed to write objectives of that sort. Needing help, teachers created such a demand for Mager's book that the next year the title was changed to *Preparing Instructional Objectives.* Nothing else in the book was changed, but that new title led to the assumption that what had been intended as an aid in developing programmed instructional materials was appropriate for every kind of education. The programmed instruction era ended soon, but the model for objectives still lives. In an attempt to apply this model at all levels of instruction, lesson, course, school, and district, curriculum developers found themselves drowning in a sea of mini-objectives. Critics looked at the mass of minutia and decided that any objectives that attempted to specify learning outcomes were useless—or worse.

Popham an early advocate of behavioral objectives, commented:

> Certainly there are abuses of instructional objectives. These are usually perpetrated by administrators, who having read Mager's little volume on objectives feel themselves blessed with instant expertise and thus institute a free-wheeling circus in their schools (11).

A related problem was the fact that objectives so narrowly conceived and rigidly prescriptive tended to stifle teaching creativity and flexibility. Moreover, individualization of instruction in such a situation became difficult, if not impossible.

Taxonomy model. Bloom and his colleagues (2) identified cognitive skills at 6 levels, ranging from simple to most complex (i.e., knowledge, comprehension, application, analysis, synthesis, and evaluation). The rationale was that each level presupposes achievement of that preceding it. And if care is taken to give equal emphasis to all of the six categories of cognition, this model can be a useful framework for the design of health education objectives. However, studies show that the overwhelming majority of

objectives based on this approach focus on the lowest level of the hierarchy, *knowing.* At that level it is the *content* dimension on which the specificity depends, particularly in the case of objectives designed for the elementary school years. An example of such a fact-oriented statement is "Knows that a food which is derived from the flesh of animals belongs to the meat group." Use of the single behavior *knows* for so many objectives gives the teacher no guidance in selecting an activity but only in deciding *what* to teach. Yet the goal of health education is to develop the ability to think and use the information learned in making decisions, not the acquisition of a lot of facts about health.

A set of consumer health objectives, devised according to the entire taxonomy illustrates such a hierarchy of proposed cognitive skills:

Knowledge: Names people whose job it is to keep us well.

Comprehension: Explains ways advertising influences choices of foods and other health products.

Application: Interprets the meaning of information on food labels.

Analysis: Distinguishes between health quackery and reliable health advice.

Synthesis: Formulates a set of criteria for the selection of health products.

Evaluation: Evaluates the reliability of claims promoting the sale and use of health products.

Operational model. Instructional objectives intended to structure health teaching are most efficiently stated in operational terms. *Operational* means that the statement clearly describes what the student will be able to do *after* instruction and what she or he will be practicing *during* instruction. Furthermore, the criterion or test of its achievement can be inferred from the objective itself, exactly as stated. Objectives can be broadly stated as to the content, yet are measurable so long as the associated skill can be demonstrated by the student. Examples of operational objectives are "Explains the influence of peer pressure on one's health behavior" and "In-

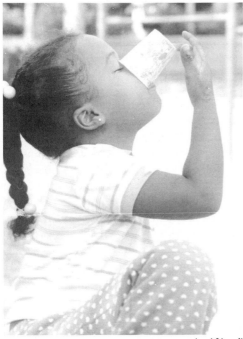

Armi Lizardi

Snack time can be a learning activity.

terprets advertising claims promoting the use of over-the-counter drugs."

Both teaching and evaluation can be based on such an objective by *any* means a teacher chooses as long as the students are (1) helped to learn how to accomplish the objective, and (2) ultimately asked to demonstrate their new ability. Operational objectives provide direction but do not restrict teachers in choosing how they will be implemented. They allow teachers freedom to vary techniques to suit their own style and the special needs of their own students.

Another problem that can be avoided by use of operational objectives is ambiguity. For example, consider this objective: "Identifies foods that are essential for a balanced diet." There is no single list of foods that are essential in a balanced and nutritious diet. In other words, health is not like mathematics. There is not always one right answer. The goals of health teaching are not to develop singular abilities. What might be a

good list in this country for a person of a certain age and sex could be totally inapplicable in another situation. What needs to be learned is the ability to choose a diet that fulfills one's current nutritional needs from the total range of available foodstuffs. And that is undeniably a worthwhile skill.

CHARACTERISTICS OF FUNCTIONAL INSTRUCTIONAL OBJECTIVES

Before the functions of an objective or sequence of objectives are discussed, some guidelines for the development of objectives that work well must be considered. As Mager has said, "If you don't know where you are going, you might wind up somewhere else"(10). Whether specific or general, a well-stated objective fits the following description:

1. It is stated in terms of a learner's behavior, not in terms of a teacher's intentions.
2. It specifies both a behavior and the content matter of interest.
3. It describes just one behavior and one content component.
4. It is operational, meaning that the learner can practice the skill and work with the subject matter in the classroom setting.
5. It specifies a behavior that is explicit, not ambiguous, hence is measurable.
6. It describes a cognitive or affective outcome rather than an activity that is an end in itself.
7. It describes an outcome with apparent lifelong application and worth.
8. It is feasible for the students for whom it is designed.

Characteristic 1

An operational objective is stated in terms of a proposed learner activity, not as descriptive of something the teacher plans to do, for example, "To teach reasons why so many people continue to smoke despite official warnings of possible ill effects." Learning happens in the learner. The stated objective could be carried out by the teacher in an empty room, speaking for the benefit of an admiring tape recorder. A better objective is, "The student explains why people begin and continue to smoke cigarettes." This statement says exactly what the student is expected to be doing during the learning opportunity, yet the teacher has considerable latitude in planning because there are many ways that practice in explaining the reasons involved could be provided.

Characteristic 2

An operational objective has two basic components: a measurable behavior and some clearly defined subject matter. "The effects of drug abuse" is a topic, not an objective, because it merely states generally *what* will be covered. On the other hand, "To analyze critically" is a behavior without any subject matter. A complete objective would be "The student describes hazards associated with abuse of any harmful substance." Both components, the behavior and the subject matter, are included, and achievement of the objective can be demonstrated several ways.

Characteristic 3

An operational objective specifies just one behavior and one element of content. The statement, "Names methods of disease control and explains how each method is most appropriately applied" combines two objectives. Separately stated, they are easier to carry out, and, in sum, the outcome is at least the same and probably better. "Identifies and describes methods of disease control" is an objective with two behaviors but only one element of subject matter. These behaviors will have to be practiced one at a time. A better statement might simply ask the student to "describe," since "identify" would be a necessary first step in doing any describing of those methods. "Describes methods of disease control and how each control is applied" has two content elements. The student will have to deal with these one at a time, so there is no avoiding the fact that there are two objectives to be reached. A better behavior might have been suggested for

the second content element if two objectives had instead been proposed, for example, "Describes methods of disease control" and "Explains how different methods of disease control are applied."

Characteristic 4

An operational objective elicits a teaching strategy that allows the student appropriate practice and permits its achievement to be immediately demonstrated in the classroom. "Refrains from using substances that are harmful to health" is a goal, not an objective. The teacher would have to monitor the student's behavior for the rest of his or her life in order to evaluate its success. A better objective is "Differentiates between uses of mind-altering substances that may be helpful and those that are harmful." A number of hypothetical problems or simulated situations can be devised to evaluate achievement of that objective, and the student either can or cannot make that differentiation. Whether that ability leads to wise decisions in later life is not something that the teacher can or should attempt to test.

Characteristic 5

An operational objective specifies a behavior that is clearly measurable rather than ambiguous. Certain action words or verbs are more descriptive of skills and therefore communicate their meaning more universally than others. Cognitive behaviors commonly used in objectives and accepted as being measurable include *identify, describe, compare, analyze, explain,* and *evaluate.* Although individual teachers may interpret these behaviors somewhat differently, most would generally agree about what is happening when a student is describing, or listing, or comparing things.

Verbs that are too ambiguous (open to many equally plausible interpretations) to dependably communicate the intended behavior include *know, understand, comprehend, appreciate, learn, recognize,* and *realize.* What would you ask a student to do to show that she or he appreciates, or knows, or comprehends? The teacher who bases learning opportunities on these kinds of fuzzy behaviors may not decide what the student will be asked to do until the examinations are being written. However, whatever the examination asks the student to do, the task will not be ambiguous but specific. If the teacher does not know what will be asked while the lesson is going on, who can blame the hapless students who have no way of knowing what they will be asked about the lesson later? For example, "Appreciates the value of good health" is nice but ambiguous. Everybody appreciates good health (although those who appreciate it most are those who have it least). But how would you measure how much a person's appreciation had increased as a result of your instruction? And how would that objective help you plan a lesson that would contribute to your students' appreciation? "Explains the relationship between good health and enjoyment of work and play" might get at the same thing. Even small children can carry out a lesson giving them appropriate practice in doing that and later explain the relationship to others.

Characteristic 6

An operational objective specifies a cognitive or affective skill or behavior that transfers to other times and other problems rather than a word that simply describes a means of exhibiting or expressing such a skill. Words such as *discuss*, *write*, *state*, and *tell* verbally express what is happening cognitively or emotionally. But is it possible to discuss something without explaining, describing, or comparing, for example? Try it.

Discuss, which is the most overworked word in the lexicon of curriculum developers, actually describes a means of verbalizing cognitive skills. Other words such as *observe*, *participate*, or *demonstrate* usually describe an activity, or assignment. The real objective, which should tell us why this would be done, is unstated. *Do not confuse a description of an assignment with a statement of an instructional objective.*

An objective such as "Discuss the correct use of dental floss" poses several questions. Who is to discuss it? Is it to be the teacher? What does "discussing" mean in that event—lecturing or telling? If it is to be the students who are doing the discussing, won't they actually be describing the way to use dental floss? If so, why not say so? And how would you devise a means of evaluating a discussion? A measurable behavior is all that it takes, hence "Describes the correct use of dental floss" is acceptable and workable.

"Demonstrates ability to take a pulse rate" is another activity. It is not an objective, but rather the outcome of an unspecified objective. What happens once the student can demonstrate the skill? How does that relate to health behavior? Do the children learn the relevance of this activity to their own health or later learnings? Or more likely, is it simply an end in itself?

Characteristic 7

An educational objective should describe an outcome with potential life-long utility and value. Thus, a worthwhile objective involves problem solving and deals with content that can be generalized to solve similar problems at other times and places. Only rarely are decisions made that do not in some way affect health, both our own and that of others. Not only should an objective be measurable in the classroom, but what has been learned should also be useful in the future. At the very least, an objective ought to contribute to the ultimate achievement of another objective that does have that potential. For instance, study of the physiology of the heart might be justified as a part of health education if it were integrated with learning how diet choices are a factor in preventing coronary heart disease.

"Names the principal bones of the human skeleton" is not an objective clearly relevant to health behavior. How does ability to name bones help the student of health education? Can it help a person to walk better, run faster, or stand straighter? Unless it is deemed an asset to be able to pass a test on the names of bones, achievement of such an objective is simply an end in itself. On the other hand, "Explains how adequate fluoride levels in drinking water can affect the development of teeth and bones" has both physical and social uses beyond the immediate learning situation. The learner discovers the implications of fluoride use for the skeletal growth of children and in the maintenance of healthy bone tissue in the elderly. As a potential voter, the learner is better prepared to make a reasoned decision about the addition of fluorides to public water supplies if this becomes an issue.

Characteristic 8

An instructional objective must be feasible. An objective might exhibit all the foregoing characteristics and yet lack this one. The abilities and comprehension of the subject matter specified in the objective must be within the range of possibility for the students for whom it is intended. For example, "Analyzes the impact of environmental pollution on the quality of urban living" might be feasible for high school students but not for those in the third grade. The appropriateness of an objective must be justified on the basis of studies of the learners, as recommended previously, so that the objective reasonably matches expected skill development and builds on past content learnings. Third grade students probably will not be able to demonstrate the ability to analyze or to deal with the concept of quality as it relates to urban living. "Identifies physical characteristics that are inherited" is a relatively simple behavior, and the content element is factual rather than abstract. The Trucano Study revealed that interest in genetics was high at all grade levels (15). Such an objective should be interesting and feasible for elementary and middle-school students, given appropriate enabling objectives developed for each grade.

Another aspect of feasibility has to do with the available time, money, and facilities. It is pointless to develop objectives that cannot possibly be achieved. Cost, time requirements, and the availability of qualified staff and supplies, which can have a significant influence on implementation, must also be considered when defining teaching objectives. Thus the objective "Develops a videotaped survey of sources of water, air, and noise pollution" could result in a dramatic production and give great satisfaction to both students and their parents. However, it probably involves more sophisticated and expensive equipment, technical expertise, and more time than schools are able to devote to health education at any level of schooling. A substitute objective needs to be devised that describes something that *can* be done and is just as satisfying but is also feasible.

Now that you have examined the eight characteristics of a well-stated and operational objective, let's look at them again. Consider that each of them can be categorized as either a characteristic of an objective's *structure* or its *function*. Here is a quick-check chart for use in screening proposed objectives for use in teaching. A well-stated objective will receive checkmarks for all items in both screens.

Affective Objectives

Although all the objectives discussed so far have been drawn from the cognitive domain, this does not mean that affective objectives cannot be defined in a form that is measurable to some degree. Affective objectives are primarily con-

---

CHARACTERISTICS OF OBJECTIVES

Structural Screen	Yes	Functional Screen	Yes
1. Learner focused	☐	1. Measurability	☐
2. Two dimensional	☐	2. Feasibility	☐
3. Singularity	☐	3. Operationality	☐
4. Outcome oriented	☐	4. Future applicability	☐

cerned with the development of positive attitudes, values, and interests. Krathwohl, Bloom, and Masia, who devised a taxonomy of affective educational objectives, believe that the term *internalization*, used to describe these kinds of learnings, refers to the inner growth that occurs as one becomes aware of and then adopts attitudes, codes of behavior, and values that make up the personal system of beliefs that influences health-related decisions (9). The five categories

RATING SCALE FOR INSTRUCTIONAL OBJECTIVES

Objective	Acceptable	Unacceptable	Number of characteristics lacking
The pupil can indicate the number of primary teeth.			
Learns to say no.			
The student will demonstrate an increase in cognitive knowledge by taking a test.			
The pupil can name the three basic functions of teeth and tell why teeth are important.			
Keep the fingernails clean.			
Students will list their five favorite foods and their five least-liked foods.			
Understands the major factors that influence healthful living.			
Describes the structure of the eye and ear and explains the functions of each.			
The principal causes of premature death and disability.			
Cooperates with others to promote a healthful environment at school, in the home, and in the community.			
To teach the techniques of CPR			
To use problem-solving skills correctly.			
Discusses the benefits of wellness versus illness.			
Analyzes the cost effectiveness of preventive medical treatment as a means of controlling health care expenditures.			
Recognizes qualities of a good friend.			
Knows the relationship between food choices and dental health.			

of objectives in the affective domain range from the lowest and nearly cognitive level of learning, termed *awareness*, followed by *responding*, *valuing*, and *organization*, to the highest level of the taxonomy, *characterization by a value or value concept*.

Achievement of an affective objective may be as difficult to measure as it is to define. For this reason, some educators neither try to write such objectives nor consider one that seeks to modify an attitude as feasible or necessary; yet the goals of health education are inextricably linked to the promotion and maintenance of attitudes favorable to their attainment.

Learning activities can be planned to help students analyze their existing beliefs and make a reasoned interpretation of the impact those beliefs have on their daily choices among behaviors. Objectives for this purpose can be stated nearly as operationally as those for cognitive purposes (14). Affective objectives such as the following have been proposed by health educators: "Volunteers to participate in a campaign to promote a neighborhood cleanup program", "Seeks to persuade family members to improve poor health practices when these are noted", or "Evidences willingness to comply with school safety procedures." Admittedly, these are more exactly descriptions of desired outcomes of instruction based upon meaningful cognitive objectives, whether stated or not.

Meaningful cognitive objectives have much to contribute to affective outcomes. For example, in one classroom, two students, whose existing negative attitude toward fluoridation of drinking water made them reject any information that supported its worth, were permitted to argue their point of view as a class project. It was agreed that they would first study both sides of the issue as carefully and thoroughly as they could. To their surprise, they found themselves persuaded that fluoridation of drinking water supplies does in fact have a positive effect on the development of strong teeth and bones. Their prior convictions and attitudes had been entirely

reversed as a result of what could have been perceived as a cognitive objective such as, "Describes the effect of fluoridated water on growth and development of teeth and bones." Had a measurable affective objective also been defined, it might have been, "Believes that fluoridation of water supplies promotes optimum bone and teeth development."

ADVANTAGES OF USING MEASURABLE OBJECTIVES

Although it cannot be argued that good teaching is impossible in the absence of guidelines in the form of measurable objectives, it cannot be denied that their use makes good teaching more likely. There is no one set of health instructional objectives whose mastery is essential to the achievement of the goals of every elementary school. Even if there were, it would be necessary to evaluate and revise it continually in order to adjust for changes in needs, conditions, health problems, and health information. Nevertheless, there are some very concrete advantages to using objectives as tools for planning and implementing effective health instruction.

First, specifying educational objectives in terms of the cognitive processes to be practiced is the most meaningful and powerful way to begin the task of planning learning activities that are relevant to curriculum goals whatever the discipline involved. The teacher must decide on the purpose of a lesson before deciding how to teach it. Process-focused objectives make teaching a professional, decision-making function instead of an accumulation of fuzzy plans to "discuss how body parts grow," "talk about the chapter that was assigned," "draw a picture that describes one's family," "show a film about drug abuse," or "invite a dentist to talk to the class about dental hygiene." Such plans are formulated day by day as coping strategies based not on skill development but on subject matter alone. With specific objectives, skill and subject matter are not two things, but one. Guided by these kinds of statements, teaching is a reasoned process rather than a haphazard mixture of activities and textbook reading.

A teacher who knows exactly what a student needs to be able to do and know when the lesson has been completed is more effective in planning matching learning opportunities. That is what an operational objective describes. On the other hand, a teacher who is guided by ambiguous objectives such as, "To help the students understand and appreciate the role of the family," understandably confuses teaching with telling.

Second, an operational objective facilitates teaching because it contains clues to the four basic teaching tasks. (1) The cognitive skill to be practiced in a lesson or lessons is explicit in the specified behavior. (2) The technique or strategy appropriate to that behavior is implicit in the statement as well. Certain techniques are suited to practicing a given behavior, whereas others are not. Panel discussions, debates, or preparation and presentation of a report would allow the student practice in synthesizing. But if the behavior were "describe" or "explain," a lecture or film could not be the sole technique employed because only watching or listening are required. (Whether the students actually see and hear what is being presented is another problem.) So the operational objective suggests which techniques you can use as well as which ones are unsuitable. (3) The objective sets the boundaries of the subject matter to be studied. If the content specified is the effects of drug abuse," any other information, such as their chemical components, slang names, laws concerning their use, or historical highlights of usage is completely irrelevant. If any of that seems essential to the goals of the unit being studied, then you need to develop additional enabling objectives that deal with that information. A measurable objective tells you what subject needs to be included as well as what ought not to be covered. (4) A measurable objective is the best guide to its own evaluation. Evaluation is not just facilitated, but its validity is assured when it is based on a measurable ob-

jective because it matches what the student presumably has been helped to learn.

Often classroom tests bear little relationship to what actually has been taught and learned; this is especially the case when the objectives of the teaching have never been clearly defined and employed as guidelines to the teaching. When the expressed intention is unclear, as in, "The student will really appreciate the potential harmfulness of misusing or abusing drugs," how would you arrange for practice or evaluation of that behavior? What is a student doing when appreciation is being practiced or really exhibited? The ability to recall facts about the subject matter is usually what is assessed, the assumption apparently being that the more facts students know, the greater their appreciation.

Third, evaluation of the teacher's success and of the feasibility of the objective itself is facilitated when a measurable objective is used. If students cannot yet demonstrate mastery of the specified subject matter and skill, new or different learning opportunities can be devised to give added practice or broadened study of the subject matter. If it seems likely that failure to achieve the objective is not an indication of inadequate teaching but instead due to the fact that the objective simply was not feasible for these students, the statement can be discarded or rewritten, as the teacher decides.

Fourth, use of measurable objectives as a framework for curriculum development at any level of implementation minimizes the risk of irrelevance to student needs or educational goals, with a waste of time and materials as a consequence. The clarity of such statements, as derived from careful analysis of the sources described in Chapter 3, makes it easier to assess both the worth and potential contribution of each to the overall plan.

Fifth, supervision and in-service education are facilitated when what the teacher expects to accomplish has been clearly specified in advance of instruction. The degree of success or failure can be assessed and the strengths and weaknesses diagnosed based on the criteria implicit in the objectives.

Sixth, communication is facilitated, especially between teacher and student, but also between teacher and supervisor, and between one teacher and another who are teaching the same material. Carefully planned and clearly defined objectives, developed at levels of increasing complexity and comprehension from K through 8 and beyond, allow successive teachers to build on and reinforce desired competencies. Each teacher can see what the student needs to have learned at any particular level in order to participate effectively in the objective proposed for the next. When objectives are stated clearly and unambiguously enough to convey a similar meaning to any teacher, then the final outcome should be much the same whatever the means chosen to carry them out.

Finally, and perhaps most importantly, students who are involved actively in the learning process (and measurable objectives are far more apt to motivate choices for these kinds of teaching strategies than are the "knows" and "appreciates" kinds of statements) are more likely to adopt and value the behaviors basic to positive health attitudes than students who are merely passive recipients of health information or health rules (1).

As we began this chapter you evaluated the 10 objectives offered to you as a sort of pre-test. Now examine those listed in a rating scale on p. 109. How many of these would you accept as well-stated *operational* objectives at this point?

SUMMARY

Education holds no patent on the terms "goals" and "objectives" nor on the manner in which they are stated and employed. *Healthy People 2000* and its objectives illustrate this point quite well (7). This is to say again that the models and characteristics of well-stated objectives we have recommended for use in planning and organizing health teaching should be perceived as tailored

to the purposes of teachers and curriculum developers. Even in education you will find "goals" that are not really goals and "objectives" that do not satisfy some of the standards proposed in these pages. Some statements labeled objectives may not satisfy any of the standards, in fact.

Goodlad's study of the nation's schools found that, while state education guides were a "conceptual swamp," district guides were usually more directly oriented to the classroom, proposing more and better goal statements; yet even district guides listed a jumble of desired behaviors in students, purposes for teachers, and admonitions to schools under the title of goals (5). He concluded that those working at all levels of the educational system must be accountable for the quality of the education planned for and offered children in our schools, which means that every educator, not just curriculum specialists, needs to know how to construct and use well-stated goals and objectives.

Teachers may not think of themselves as sharing in the responsibility for establishing or fulfilling the long-range goals for health education. In reality, they have the key role in fulfilling the hopes and plans implicit in those goals. At the bottom line, it is the classroom teacher who brings them to life. Teachers need to know what the goals and general objectives proposed for district schools at all levels are and how to infer from them a set of instructional objectives capable of contributing to their achievement.

Whatever grade you teach, you also need to know what objectives your students will have already completed and what they will need to know and be able to do at the level that follows your own teaching. Only when successive elementary teachers know how to define meaningful and measurable objectives with full knowledge of what has preceded them and what is to follow will children be afforded the firm foundation of health-related information basic to the effective problem-solving and decision-making skills essential in building a healthful lifestyle for themselves.

QUESTIONS AND EXERCISES

Discussion questions

1. What difficulties do you see in planning a health education curriculum in the absence of stated long-range goals?

2. Explain the advantages of basing health instruction plans on clearly stated operational objectives.

3. Which of the characteristics of well-stated objectives would not apply to goal statements?

4. What would be the disadvantage of specifying performance standards as part of an instructional objective?

5. Why is it nearly impossible to write an instructional objective that is totally cognitive or affective in its intent and outcome?

6. Which element of an instructional objective would you identify as the most apt to be the cause of complaints that "behavioral objectives" focus on trivialities? What could you do to avoid that problem?

7. Based on examples provided in the literature, how would you explain the difference between a competency statement and a measurable objective?

8. Why is it important that an instructional objective be demonstrable in a classroom setting?

9. Explain the notion of feasibility as it applies to objectives of health teaching in particular.

Problems and Exercises

1. Using the categories described by Krathwohl, Bloom, and Masia (9), (see p. 110) develop a set of affective behaviors for each. Formulate a definition for each behavior to serve as a guide for planning a lesson so the students can practice that skill.

2. Develop a general objective that would require a number of enabling, or subordinate, objectives for its achievement. Then define a list of such enabling objectives to allow for as many different levels of ability and knowledge as might be expected among children of a given age. Which of those you propose would be essential for all children, and which ones would probably be needed by only a few?

3. The box on p. 109 contains a list of "objectives" taken from many kinds of publications for health education in elementary schools. Read each one, and decide whether it has all the characteristics of a measurable objective. If it does not, enter the number (1 through 8) that identifies any of the characteristics it lacks in the appropriate space.

4. Rewrite each of the objectives you judged unacceptable in the previous question to make it acceptable. Which characteristic was most often the problem? What is your conclusion about objectives and the problems involved in writing operational statements?

5. Select a health content area or concept that interests you and develop a long-range goal for each of the cognitive, affective, and action domains. Next define a curriculum (general) level objective for each of the first two goals. Finally, prepare an instructional, or enabling, objective for each of those two curriculum objectives. Study the progression that you have established. Do the statements at each level exhibit the essential characteristics of an operational objective? Does each logically depend on those below it for its achievement? Does the behavior become more explicit and the subject matter more narrow as the concern of the statements moves closer to the classroom? If not, how could you correct that?

6. Choose one of the content areas listed in the scope and sequence chart (see Table 3-3). From one of the general objectives proposed at a level of instruction that interests you develop a set of enabling objectives that should help students of that age group to achieve the general objective. Does each of them pass the structure and function screens?

REFERENCES

1. Black JL, Newton J: Should health behavior change be an objective of school health personnel? *J Sch Health* 51(3):189-190, 1981.

2. Bloom BS et al: *Taxonomy of educational objectives, handbook I, cognitive domain*, New York, 1956, David McKay.

3. Feuerstein P, Galli N: Linking health screening to health education learning modules for elementary school student: a feasibility study, *J Sch Health* 53(1):10-13, Jan 1983.

4. Goodlad JI: *Planning and organizing for teaching, project on the instructional program of the public schools*, Washington DC, 1963, Rand McNally.

5. Goodlad JI: *A place called school: prospects for the future*, New York, 1984, McGraw-Hill.

6. Harrow AJ: *A taxonomy of the psychomotor domain*, New York, 1972, David McKay.

7. *Healthy People 2000.* Washington, DC, 1990, Department of Health and Human Services, Public Health Services.

8. Krathwohl DR: Stating objectives appropriately for programs, for curriculums, and for instructional materials development, *J Teach Educ* 83, March 1965.

9. Krathwohl DR, Bloom BS, Masia BB: *Taxonomy of educational objectives. Handbook II: Affective domain*, New York, 1964, David McKay.

10. Mager RF: *Preparing instructional objectives*, Palo Alto, Calif, 1961, Fearon Publishers.

11. Popham WJ: Objectives '72, *Phi Delta Kappan* 53:433, 1972.

12. School Health Education Project (SHEP): *Health education curricular progression chart*, New York City, 1981, National Center for Health Education.

13. School Health Education Study (SHES): *Health education: a conceptual approach to curriculum design*, St Paul, 1967, 3M Education Press.

14. Thayer L, Beeler K: *Activities and exercises for affective education*, Washington, DC, 1975, American Educational Research Association.

15. Trucano L: *Students speak*, Seattle, 1984, Comprehensive Health Education Foundation.

SUGGESTED READINGS

Fodor J, Dalis G: Formulating goals and objectives for health instruction. In: Health instruction, theory and application, ed 4, Philadelphia, 1989, Lea and Febiger.

5 Developing Effective Teaching and Learning Plans

When you finish this chapter, you should be able to:

- Analyze the interdependence of process and content in the promotion of problem solving and thinking abilities.
- Synthesize cognitive and social learning theories in the design of lessons.
- Describe the procedures and purposes of commonly employed, active teaching techniques.
- Explain the problem-solving method.
- Design experiential health teaching strategies appropriate to the needs and abilities of specified students.
- Interpret the influence of values on an individual's health-related actions.
- Develop adequately detailed lesson plans based upon instructional objectives attainable by selected students.

However worthwhile and carefully crafted the stated goals and objectives of a curriculum for health teaching, without the enthusiasm and skillful planning of a classroom teacher, they are just words. Typically, the broadest objectives have been agreed upon by consensus of state or district curriculum committees composed of school administrators, curriculum specialists, and content consultants (who may be teachers). Objectives may also be supplied as components of commercially developed curriculum packages complete with proposed lesson plans and coordinated resource materials.

This chapter will consider the basic questions that teachers must continually ask themselves as they infer enabling objectives from the general objectives they are expected to implement. The content and behaviors specified in their own objectives should guide the choices from among techniques that are appropriate for their lessons. Remember that achievement of the objectives you develop must be (1) feasible for your students in terms of their readiness, experience, and the time and resources you have; (2) a legitimate concern of the schools; and (3) consistent with school and district curriculum goals and policies.

Given that goals represent overall target competencies, remember that every class is different. These differences must be kept in mind when lessons are being planned because they must direct the choice of both teaching techniques and content.

Madeline Hunter, probably the best known and most influential authority on elementary school teaching today, says,

> Regardless of any particular method or program, the planning of the teacher is probably the most critical element in generating the transfer which yields student productivity and creativity. This planning makes the difference between "hoping that it will happen" and "seeing that it does" (14).

When to teach the content and skills explicit in your objectives is a problem of horizontal sequence. The chapters in the textbook provided for your students may or may not present a logical sequence of subject matter that matches your class needs. If you like the way the textbook is organized, it can be used as is. If you like the book, but not the sequence, you can change the order of the chapters to be studied to fit your own plan.

What content would you choose as the focus of your first lesson in health education for a group of second grade children? Think about that for a moment before you read on. Why would you

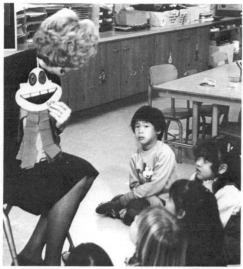

Don Merwin

Adequate teaching planning generates the transfer of information.

choose to introduce that subject matter over any other for the introductory lesson? Are there any health content areas that you would *not* schedule first? Why? How could knowledge of the needs and interests of 7-year-old children help you to make sensible choices among content areas and teaching strategies for their health lessons? It is generally agreed that decisions affecting curriculum need to be based on knowledge of all aspects of child growth and development—physical, social, emotional, and intellectual (23). Think about what you have learned about Piaget's stages of cognitive development. What implications for sequence for either subject matter or skills do you find in that information?

To plan a sequence of instruction that fits every aspect of student readiness is not easy, nor is it easy to distinguish between unnecessary repetition and desirable reinforcement. It depends, to a great degree, on your students; you will have to be sensitive to their special needs as you make your plans. Some revisiting of subject matter is needed every year for most students. What they need to know about nutrition, for example, cannot be mastered in a few lessons even if a few were provided every year. As students grow older they have more control over food choices. Lessons have to shift from learning about basic facts, such as the nutrients categorized within the five food groups, to understanding some of the many forces that motivate diet choices.

Health problems keep recurring but in different forms and with different degrees of severity. The social and emotional needs of children in grade 6 are very different from those typical of children in first grade or eighth grade. Although Bruner proposed that any subject can be taught effectively in some intellectually honest form at any stage of development, cognitive and moral developmental abilities are higher among children in upper elementary grades (6). This means that during early school years more emphasis has to be given to *training* children to practice desirable health behaviors. Only as abilities increase can health-teaching activities begin to focus on decision-making skills (19).

These are some of the things we talked about in Chapter 3 that must be considered before you can decide how to teach and what techniques are best suited to the implementation of any particular objective. It might be worth your time to quickly review those aspects of growth and development as they affect teaching and learning.

PROCESS-FOCUSED INSTRUCTION

Health instruction is not limited to the communication of health-related information. It is as concerned with the development of cognitive skills as with providing the learner with information.

Because we have spoken of the two dimensions of an instructional objective as being content and a measurable cognitive skill, it might seem that the two are separate elements of a teaching-learning plan. What do we mean by *process* in this context? The term is used in education to describe all the operations of which the human mind is capable, encompassing theorizing, conceptualizing, analyzing, decision-making, thinking, and generalizing, to name just a few of the cognitive skills employed in active learning. Like any other skill, intellectual skills must be practiced to be mastered. Learning opportunities must be planned as much for their potential contribution to the development of mental processes as for the accumulation of health information. Whether the health problems or behaviors of interest to children are real or hypothetical, the processes employed in investigating them are the same. Problem solving is perhaps *the* method of health education and the way humans decide on any particular health behavior.

But first, what do we mean when we speak of problems in connection with health behavior? The word sounds negative, implying that something is wrong or needs fixing. A better definition might be "a question proposed for solution." Most of our health problems are so routinely solved through habit that we are not aware of them at all. Health habits are, in essence, learned solutions to long forgotten health-related needs.

When we are hungry that's a problem, but for most of us it is solved so easily that we don't think of it as being a problem. Thirsty? The solution is not so much *how* as *what* to use to fix that. But if you were left by accident in an arid plain, you'd discover in a hurry that you had a big problem. Behaviors that we call "etiquette" are learned solutions to social problems. Which fork? Can I eat this with my fingers? It might be said that problems are situations in which familiar solutions do not work, or do not work well, so that creative thinking is required. And that is when problem-solving skills are so useful in coping with the dilemma, whatever it may be.

> . . . Our public education system has not successfully made the shift from a system that focuses on memorizing facts to one that has achieved the learning of critical thinking skills (26).

Health behavior is the result of decision making, which must be based on a reasoned examination of possible alternatives. The belief that the purpose of education is to develop intellectual skills is not new, but sometimes it has been assumed that stuffing students' minds with facts is the most effective way to do this; yet encyclopedias and computers are filled with facts, none of which are of any use without the ability of a human being to retrieve and apply those facts productively.

Content, as we use the word in health teaching, refers to the fund of accurate information with which the discipline is concerned. That information consists of the set of concepts, principles, and generalizations that, by agreement of its scholars, represents its body of knowledge. These are categorized under general headings such as content areas, subject matter, topics, or problems. Content is static. It becomes dynamic only as we use it in employing the processes with which humans carry on their work and do their thinking (25). Paradoxically, cognitive skills, once mastered, have life-long utility and transferability, whereas content can only be considered as a tentative quantity of information. Content needs to be tested frequently for its dependability because its application is essential in solving a problem.

I would suggest that problem solving be given the leading position among learner goals, from the primary years on and for all children. By this, I mean schools should create conditions under which students are motivated to solve problems and thus become eager to learn both problem solving strategies and relevant factual content and communication skills in order to succeed (9).

Emphasis on reasoning rather than information is essential for health teaching. Combs supports this view when he describes problem solving as a creative process that is useful whatever the subject or whenever the need (7). Use of this method as appropriate during elementary school years seems implicit in these remarks:

The student's own personal problems seem like a logical place to begin. In problem solving, process takes precedence over subject matter. Moreover, personal problems have the distinct advantage of built-in motivation. A review of research on motivation suggests that students are most likely to be motivated when problems are real and personally relevant, when students feel solutions are reasonably within their capabilities, and when results are immediately discernible.

The use of cognitive skills or creative thinking goes on all the time, whenever people need something or want to do something they don't know how to do—in short, whenever a problem occurs. This is true at every age. It is the schools' responsibility to help students from kindergarten on up to learn and use those skills effectively so that they can live better both now and in the future.

Other disciplines recognize their obligation to teach thinking and decision making. For example, here is a statement taken from social science literature:

The emphasis of elementary social studies should be on process, not content, specifically the process of gathering, categorizing, and analyzing information, and then making generalizations based on this analysis (26).

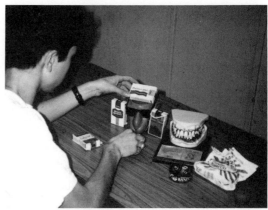

Ric Loya

Health education teaches thinking and decision-making skills.

Measurable objectives provide direction in selecting teaching strategies that require learners to practice cognitive skills.

LEARNING AS CONCEPTUALIZING

Conceptual learning is the way people learn naturally, without (and sometimes in spite of) formal teaching, yet it depends entirely on the senses as receivers of information. Interpretation of that information is heavily influenced by the individual's past perceptions. Communication between the teacher and the learner is bounded by two realities: *(1) the five senses are our only avenues of communication, and (2) what is perceived will always be affected by related past experiences.*

In order to plan how to teach, you have to understand how a person learns. Learning is a very personal thing, *first, because no two people have had exactly the same experience in life, and second because every one of us has different abilities, interests, learning styles, and motivations.*

An infant begins to sense almost at once that certain things or experiences belong to a family of like things or experiences. One of the first generalizations a human being formulates is from a

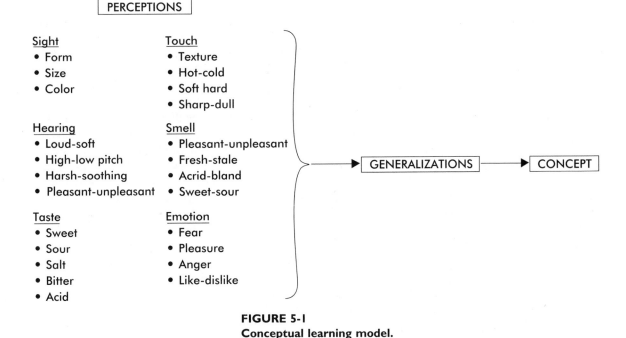

FIGURE 5-1
Conceptual learning model.

myriad of perceptions about food. At first the infant reacts with pleasure when hunger has been satisfied and begins to associate that contented state with the touch of familiar food on the lips and in the mouth. Then more senses—taste, smell, and sight—are stimulated, and the infant adds those perceptions to the first ones. As time goes by, colors, sounds, odors, even textures of food begin to be added to the "things that bring relief of hunger" pleasure. All the while, the senses are also yielding information about things that can be put in the mouth but are *not* food. Very soon, long before he or she has learned a word for it, the concept of food is well established in the baby's mind. Anyone who has tried to persuade an infant to eat something new or disliked knows this very well. In short, generalizing is a natural process, and generalizations based on our perceptions are the milestones of learning (Figure 5-1).

A teacher who depends on nothing but *telling* could be successfully replaced by a tape re-corder. Lecturing limits the number of senses that are stimulated and thus the range of perceptual experiences afforded the audience. *The more senses involved in a learning experience, the more effective the lesson will be.* Think about your own experiences as a student. What kinds of learning activities have you found to be the most rewarding and interesting? What kinds have seemed least absorbing and memorable? How many senses have been involved in each category of those teaching strategies?

LEARNING AS BEHAVIORAL CHANGE

School health education isn't just hygiene any more, nor is it limited to ways to avoid addictions, illness or chronic diseases. In the case of AIDS, a problem that at this writing appears to have no medical solution, behavioral change effected through health education currently offers the only hope for any sort of control.

It is a long-held belief of health educators that health-informed people are more likely to behave in ways that are beneficial to their physical and emotional health. Alas, it isn't that simple. Behavior is the result of decisions, whether conscious or subconscious, that may be either negative or positive in effect. Decisions affecting health behavior are not always good ones, nor are they always rational. They may be based on too little information or on misinformation, and they often reflect some miscalculation of the consequences of the chosen behavior. Even when they know what can happen, people don't always do what they know is best. Risky behavior is more fun— that's what makes roller coasters so popular. Because something is risky, it is a lot more exciting, whether the actual activity is fun or not. Clearly, cognitive learning is a necessary—but not sufficient—outcome of health education if the learner is to adopt a pattern of behaviors that adds up to a healthful lifestyle.

Owing to its significance in understanding the complexity of human behavior choices, many health educators and behavioral scientists view social learning theory (SLT) as paramount among the learning theories with application to health teaching. Briefly, SLT posits that every person exhibits a variety of behaviors, some of which are reinforced and will recur when the stimulus is the same. Reinforced means that the behavior being exhibited seems to work for that individual. Negative behaviors are reinforced just as easily as positive behaviors, of course. Those that are reinforced often enough eventually become the behavior of choice or habit. Bandura said:

> It is largely through their actions that people produce the environmental conditions that affect their behavior in a reciprocal manner. The experiences generated by behavior also partly determine what a person becomes or can do, which in turn affects subsequent behavior (2).

Behaviors can be learned or changed **directly** according to social learning theory by directly providing the reinforcement, as in an experiential lesson; **vicariously,** by arranging for the learner to observe someone else being rein-

forced for a behavior (social modeling); or by **self-management,** having learners monitor their own behaviors and provide their own rewards (by encouraging them to carry out a healthful behavior for a specified period of time, at the end of which they grant themselves a predetermined prize). All of this has great potential for the development of lessons that stimulate thinking, foster creativity, and generate positive behaviors among children and youth. Moreover it dramatically changes an erroneous concept of health education as simply being concerned with teaching good grooming, physiology, or the symptoms and avoidance of diseases or disorders.

Educational techniques based on social learning theory include **modeling, skill training, contracting,** and **self-control** (24). In the case of elementary school children, these concepts seem promising as sources of lesson plans designed to motivate development of decision-making skills and favorable health behaviors.

Modeling affords children an opportunity to observe others performing a desired behavior, which is an effective way of promoting that behavior's adoption. Content is communicated as students watch the action and listen to the dialogue. Concrete examples of how it is done are provided simultaneously as in real life. **Vicarious modeling** can be provided through films (in which the focus is on observed behaviors rather than information), video tapes, role playing, puppetry, and dramatizations. For example, children can be shown models that demonstrate how to resist peer pressure to try drugs, how to be a friend, how to select healthful snack foods, how to behave in social situations with poise, and so on.

Health behaviors are actions, and nobody learns to demonstrate an action solely through observation; there must also be skill training. An essential element in teaching desirable health behaviors is the provision of opportunities to practice the behavior, first in small steps separated out and practiced as means of learning its component skills, and finally as a whole, when these have been mastered. For example, in order to teach youngsters how to use dental floss and a toothbrush correctly, the following steps might be practiced as a preliminary motivating experience: self-application of disclosing tablets to reveal any existing plaque; learning how to measure off the amount of floss to be used, and the manner in which it is held between the fingers; then learning the technique to be employed in cleaning between the teeth and under the gum line; (2) learning the manner in which the brush is positioned depending on the shape and function of the teeth; and (3) learning the brushing motion most effective in removing plaque. At each of these steps, there should be immediate feedback to the student, reinforcing correct practice and correcting any errors as needed. These practices could be combined with techniques of **self-monitoring** and **self-rewarding,** in which students agree to follow these procedures as carefully and completely as possible for a specified period of time, at the end of which a test by application of disclosing dyes provide an indisputable measure of the results. The outcome would be a mouthful of very clean teeth and whatever reward the students might have stipulated as worthy of their efforts.

SPECIAL CHARACTERISTICS OF LEARNERS

Spend some time during the first weeks of school finding out as much as you can about the students in your class. Instruction has to begin "where they are" if it is to interest them. Do any or all of them have the necessary educational background for what you plan to teach? What are their cultural and socioeconomic characteristics? Assumptions about prior experience, whether in or out of school, must be avoided; for example, so called "middle-class values" will not be held by all children and, in some areas, not by any of them. Some youngsters learn less from what they hear than from what they can see or touch (indeed, this is probably true of all young children). More attention may have to be given to teaching listening skills to the child from an inner city environment, where the ability to shut out unwanted sound is an effective way of coping with

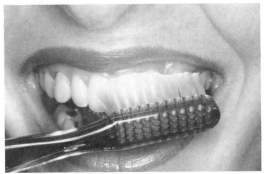

American Dental Association

Practicing skills for proper tooth brushing.

it. Children who are living in poverty may be less interested in learning activities that promise something as nebulous as "good health," or that have little to do with their real problems. For these children, teaching strategies that deal with the immediate and concrete may be more effective. Many children have feelings of low self-esteem or shyness that make them distrust their own judgment and conclusions. During the first weeks, task setting should be planned so that success is inevitable. Success is essential to self-esteem, and self-esteem breeds the confidence that allows its possessor to risk failure, suggest theories, propose tentative solutions to problems, and try new ways of doing things. Confidence flourishes in a classroom environment where failure is viewed as a learning experience and that kind of risk taking is viewed as fun.

The time needed to learn certain skills varies among people. Children learn and develop intellectually, as in all ways, at their own pace and in their own style. Teaching and learning methods should not be tied to a "one style fits all" criterion. Bloom's concept of mastery teaching is based on the conviction that, given enough time, all students can attain mastery of a learning task (5). He says:

Each student should be allowed the time he needs to learn a subject. And the time he needs is likely to be affected by his aptitudes and verbal ability, the quality of instruction he receives in class, and the quality of help he receives out of class. The task of a strategy for mastery learning is to find ways of altering the time individual students need for learning as well as finding ways of providing whatever time is needed by each (5).

The same teaching goals can be attained for most children. *The differences between children do not change the goals as much as the teaching strategies selected to achieve them.* The teacher's task is to provide an experience that will make a child's active participation both likely and productive. Assimilation of useful information is a logical outcome of that kind of activity.

Skill in diagnosing a student's special needs is basic to the selection of appropriate learning opportunities. It is not enough to know how to carry out teaching techniques or follow specific procedures. That's like confusing the cookbook with cooking. Choosing a technique must be based on analysis of needs rather than on whim or habit. The question to ask yourself is, "What has this plan to do with the needs of these students?" The answer to that question should be as clear to them as it is to you.

> It may be said that there is no use at all in teaching the structure and function of the body unless the learner can use the material to further his or her development and solve his or her problems (23).

RECITING VERSUS THINKING

The Bloom taxonomy of objectives identifies six categories of cognitive skills—**knowing, comprehending, applying, analyzing, synthesizing, and evaluating** (4). The first category is the simplest because the only process required is remembering. Knowledge is basic to all of the categories and essential in the practice of complex cognitive skills such as categorizing, interpreting, judging, organizing, and thinking.

The tendency to focus on simple recall as the desired outcome of learning persists at every level of education, up to and beyond the doctoral; yet information is useless without the cognitive skills needed to apply it appropriately. Cognitive processes are not fostered by means of lessons and curricula that emphasize memorization. Nev-

ertheless, this is the pattern of instruction predominantly found in schools. In his 1984 study, Goodlad said with regard to science teaching (which is typically the host area for health teaching in elementary grades), "The tests used emphasized heavily the recall of specific information rather than exercise of higher intellectual functions" (13).

Children will learn to think if lessons are planned to elicit thinking rather than reciting. Feldman says that although we are doing a good job of teaching the "basics," too many kids are not learning to think (11). She adds,

> We know for a fact that thinking can be taught and that it flourishes in a school environment that encourages initiative, independence, and originality, rather than obedience and docility. Encourage them to think of themselves as thinkers. Be a good role model. State the reasons for your actions, admit errors or lack of knowledge, and show them how you get back on track.

Wales et al. suggest a new paradigm for education to replace the long-standing focus on transmission of factual information (28). The new paradigm is "schooling based on decision making, the thinking skills that serve it, and the knowledge that supports it." Before this can happen, those thinking skills will have to be learned.

Focusing on higher cognitive skills does not change the subject matter used in teaching, only the way the learner handles it. The activity called for in a lesson changes, and in most cases learning becomes a lot more fun, without losing one iota of its worth and transferability.

The following tasks illustrate how thinking about and using subject matter can involve increasingly complex cognitive behaviors. The tasks represent different levels of cognition, arranged as nearly as possible according to Bloom's taxonomy *(see box)*. The subject matter remains the same (sources and functions of protein in human nutrition), and all tasks require the student to apply the basic knowledge. Only the first is limited to remembering; the others require thinking. Most importantly, the thinking tasks bring the facts to life.

EXAMPLES OF BLOOM'S TAXONOMY-TASKS ASSOCIATED WITH PROTEIN CONCEPTS

Knowing: Name the group of nutrients to which meat, poultry, fish, nuts, and peas belong.

Comprehending: Explain why protein is essential to good nutrition and human growth.

Applying: Predict what the outcome would be if an infant were given enough food but a diet nearly lacking in protein.

Analyzing: A 4-year-old child is given the following daily diet:

Breakfast: 1 cup of dry cereal, a half cup of skim milk, a slice of toast with jelly, and 1 pat of butter.

Lunch: 1 peanut butter sandwich, a cup of skim milk, 4 vanilla cookies.

Dinner: 1 small hamburger patty, 1 cup of french fries with catsup, 1 ear of corn, 1 glass of cola, 1 piece of apple pie.

What changes would you make in order to ensure adequate amounts of protein for a child of this age?

Synthesizing: Make up a day's diet that contains only one serving of meat yet supplies adequate amounts of protein for a student of your own age, sex, body build, and level of activity.

Evaluating: Protein can be obtained from a wide variety of foods derived from animal flesh, animal products (eggs, milk, and cheese), and vegetables. Which of these two sources, animal or vegetable, is the better source of protein? State the reasons why you think one is better than the other.

Measurable instructional objectives in which higher level behaviors are specified facilitate creative teaching. Ambiguous behaviors such as *knows*, *understands*, and *appreciates* lead to teacher-centered activities with memorizing and reciting as outcomes.

Yet even the most clearly stated objective is useless unless the teacher develops a lesson that matches its expressed intention. If the behavior is not elicited in the lesson, or if the objective serves only as a decoration, then it might as well have been ambiguous. Suppose that an objective called for a psychomotor skill rather than a cognitive skill, for example, "The student is able to demonstrate ability to perform CPR techniques." The teacher *tells* the students how CPR is done, asks them to read a pamphlet that describes the separate steps involved, shows them a film illustrating the procedures, and then arranges for an actual demonstration of CPR techniques. Satisfied that they should now know how, the instructor asks each student to demonstrate CPR resuscitation procedures. How well do you think the students would do that? Can you suggest anything that would have increased the quality of the performance of learners who had had all of these experiences? Right you are. Most importantly they needed to have had a chance to practice the techniques themselves.

Failure to implement the objective as stated is more obvious when it concerns a physical skill that can be evaluated on the basis of "can do" versus "can't do" Practicing the specified behavior is just as imperative when it is a cognitive skill and you can't see it happening.

Blackwood proposed the following criteria to appraise the worth of an elementary school science-learning activity (3). The criteria are equally applicable to health teaching plans and are as appropriate twenty years later as when first written. Ask yourself these questions as you review a lesson plan you have prepared or carried out.

Did the activity involve the children in describing or explaining the phenomenon?

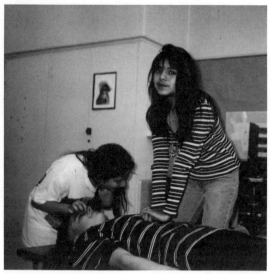

Matt Fischer

CPR training requires practice.

Did the children collect original data from which to draw conclusions?

Did the children organize and communicate about the data in useful ways?

Did the children have opportunities to speculate and predict?

Did the experience relate clearly to the development of a major science (health) concept?

Did some of the questions provide stimulation for further study?

If the answer to all of those questions is "No," then the chances are that you are teaching the facts as ends in themselves, not as vehicles for thinking.

METHODS AND TECHNIQUES OF TEACHING

Methods courses provided for prospective teachers usually stress ways of imparting information, rather than strategies for practicing creative thinking and decision making. We think that these specific ways are techniques, and the primary method of health education is problem solving. Activities such as field trips, lectures, debates, role-playing, panel discussions, and buzz-group discussions are techniques, and they, along with written materials, audiovisual equipment, and other teaching aids, constitute the set of tools from which a teacher can choose in designing teaching strategies.

Problem Solving: the Primary Method in Health Teaching

At the very heart of thinking processes is a problem of some sort. It may be something as ordinary as deciding whether to sleep another fifteen minutes and give up breakfast or deciding what to wear to a party, but the process is the same whenever a decision has to be made. Problems devised by teachers, for which there are neat, predetermined solutions, are no substitute for realistic, open-ended problems, for which there may be no pat answers or "correct" solutions. Children should be encouraged to formulate and solve their own problems—problems they care about.

A person's ability to do anything improves with practice. There is no better way to learn problem-solving processes than by solving problems. The method is always the same, consisting of a series of steps that move the thinker from the point where no solution exists, to the discovery of some new information that leads to a verifiable solution. These steps are generally described as follows.

Defining the Problem.   Health problems often are perceived by the individual as primarily physical (e.g., diabetes, obesity, or dental caries), social (e.g., shyness, overaggressiveness, or rejection), or emotional (e.g., feelings of loneliness, depression, or unworthiness). It is essential that activities focused on this step help the learner perceive the interacting influence of all three dimensions because all three are involved in every health problem. When the problem is clearly identified and is perceived as real and when a solution seems desirable and possible, the student is far more motivated to try to find a solution.

Theorizing   About   Solutions.   Some

thought must be given first to a reasonable theory as a means of limiting the search for relevant information. Even small children are capable of theorizing if they are encouraged to do so. Let them brainstorm in this step. Instruction may be necessary at this point to give them guidelines for identifying a theory as a logical starting point for their investigations, thereby avoiding blind-alley searches as much as possible.

Data Gathering. Depending on the problem and the individual, the basic information may already be available through past experience. Some information may have to be discovered, increased, or broadened. The teacher may act as adviser to help the students channel their search efficiently but should not serve as a source of ready-made answers. Whatever sources of information are used, they must be demonstrably sound and authoritative.

The process of collecting these data will be limited by the individual student's experience and ability. Children in grades 5 through 8 are capable of searching for information in popular and professional magazines and journals, as well as many other kinds of references. Younger children will have to be supplied with the needed data through carefully selected audiovisual materials or appropriate readings. Reading for problem solving must always be purposeful so that students read to find answers that they realize are necessary to fill in the gaps between what they know and what they need to know. In any case, the process of collecting data should be thorough and orderly, rather than incomplete and haphazard. Whatever sources are used, they must be objective and not slanted or biased.

Proposing Solutions. During this step, the student categorizes and analyzes the data she or he has gathered and tries to arrive at a good solution. A teacher may have to provide some guidance here to avoid wasting time on implausible solutions.

Verifying the Solution. This may be the final step if the student finds success on repeated testing of the tentative solution. If the first proposed solution does not solve the problem, then another promising approach is tried and another, if necessary, until the problem is solved.

Although these steps have been presented in a logical order, the process doesn't have to be developed exactly so. Instead of beginning by identifying a problem, the problem may suggest itself as an outcome of data gathering for an entirely different purpose. Some agile minds leap from the definition of a problem to a valid solution almost by intuition. Creative thinking is often unstructured rather than methodical, yet both approaches can produce solutions.

Theories are actually tentative solutions for which data gathering may be more of a verifying process than an investigation. Many cognitive skills are being developed in the total process of problem solving: analyzing, identifying, ordering, categorizing, evaluating, interpreting, concluding, and more—all of which are employed in thinking.

Solving problems builds competence in decision-making skills, and decision making determines health behavior. Good problem solvers are confident and persistent. They can live with uncertainty and do not jump to conclusions, but they make decisions when they must. They can risk being wrong or looking foolish. They act on hunches and change direction if it seems necessary, and they don't give up easily or look to others for their answers (11). Problem solving is a skill with total transferability.

A teacher can choose from a wide array of teaching techniques and instructional aids when planning lessons that help the student discover reliable information on which to base decisions affecting any aspect of human behavior.

Criteria for Selecting Teaching Techniques

The first step in selecting a technique to use with a particular instructional objective is to look at the proposed cognitive skill to be practiced. An objective, in effect, says "This is where the student should be." The lesson should answer the implicit question, "How can we best help him or her get there?" Whatever technique is chosen, it must give the learners an opportunity to practice the specified behavior. For example, suppose the objective calls for *evaluating*. You cannot simply tell the students or show them a film that tells them about the subject and be satisfied that you have provided practice in anything other than listening or observing. A student *may* be evaluating what was heard or seen, but that is an assumption at best and not an outcome on which you can depend or for which you can take any credit.

Thus the first two criteria in a plan for teaching are (1) the learner is given a chance to practice the behavior and to deal with the content described by the objective and (2) the lesson should be appropriate to the present abilities of the students for which it is intended. Lessons that promote the development of cognitive skills can be tailored to the needs of individual students according to their abilities or employed with the entire class, depending on grade level in general and individual abilities in particular. Some children may not be ready for the more advanced ways of thinking about a specific subject because they have not learned the facts needed; others who have learned the facts would be bored if they were forced to go over them again. Tasks can be varied to conform to individual readiness. The child who has learned enough to handle tasks at the lowest level of cognition—knowing—can succeed because what is required matches exactly what has been taught. At the same time, that child benefits from hearing how others have dealt with the same information in other ways.

There are other kinds of skills to be considered. For example, it is deceptively easy to plan a lesson that depends on the technique of discussion but disconcerting to discover that your students don't know how to discuss. Discussion skills have to be learned, and discussion leading is a skill too. "Discussion" often turns out to be teacher answers to student questions or vice versa. It may be more satisfying to the students when they are asking the questions (although these often stray from the intended topic), but the outcome is not discussion; it is telling or reciting.

A fourth test of an effective lesson is its worth as perceived by the students, based not on its entertainment value but on its relevance to their present needs and interests. The *worth* of a lesson is measured by the sense of satisfaction generated by having achieved the objective.

Because any number of different teaching techniques might be equally effective in satisfying the preceding four criteria, it is best to pick the one that can provide the greatest number of concurrent desirable outcomes. For example, while preparing for a group presentation on a health-related topic, the student improves library skills and learns to read with better comprehension and purpose, to organize data logically, to generalize, to make oral presentations, to work and plan cooperatively with others, and more.

However, not all concomitant learnings are positive in effect; the outcome of teaching can be negative, too. Even small children tire of "health" lessons that focus on the 5 food groups or the mechanics of toothbrushing year after year or that use scare tactics to prevent unwanted health behaviors. Health instruction for some luckless youngsters comes to mean, "Don't do anything that grown-ups seem to like to do; it's bad for your health." Unwanted negative outcomes are far more common when instruction focuses solely on facts, with no attention given to problem-solving processes. If the learner has helped to define a health problem, interest is nearly ensured, and discovering a solution to that problem can be very satisfying. Growth in knowledge is a desirable outcome, but the ability to obtain and apply needed information in similar situations is a primary goal of comprehensive health education.

ACTIVE TEACHING TECHNIQUES

The specific teaching strategies or techniques used in health teaching are the same as those in any other subject area. Those commonly used for health instruction may be categorized as either direct (the learner is directly involved intellectually, physically, and emotionally) or vicarious (the learner views activities recorded at another time and place). Both of these techniques can be carried out as group activities or as individual procedures. Group activities include buzz sessions, brainstorming, committee projects, panel discussions, forums, lecture-discussions, role playing, and field trips. Individual procedures, in which each student works independently, include textbook study, computer-assisted work, and individual projects. Overlaps are inevitable; for example, role playing or a field-trip assignment can be an individual or group activity. Vicarious teaching techniques involve audiovisual and other material resources, including television, overhead projection transparencies, films, slides, filmstrips, radio, videotapes, audiotapes, models, and mock-ups (simplified and clarified parts or working models of a real device, e.g., a working portion of an automobile used for driver training).

Direct Teaching Techniques

Lecture. In the past, lecturing has been the most commonly practiced technique. The rule used to be: "Tell them what you are going to tell them. Tell them. Then tell them what you told them." The notion of a lecture has strong negative overtones for many students because of past experiences. Admittedly there are dull lectures, but there are also absorbing lectures; the difference can be traced to the speaking skills of the lecturer. A lecture has its own uses and several advantages over any other techniques. It facilitates the quick communication of a common fund of information so that every student can start with the same background data. It functions as a stage-setting and focusing activity for discussions and other group procedures. It can also offer a welcome change of pace when it is not overused (which is true of all techniques).

Use demonstrations or visual aids (e.g., transparencies, pictures, models, posters, or puppets) to enliven your talks. Never simply read a prepared lecture. If your students fail to understand what you are trying to explain, you will know at once from their expressions if you watch, and you can't do that if you are reading to them. Don't continue until you have cleared up any misunderstanding or confusion. Urge them to ask questions. That takes skill, too. Often students prefer not to appear slow at understanding, so they wait until the class is finished and then ask each other what the teacher said. Sometimes if you pause after making a point instead of plunging ahead, after a second or two, someone will venture a question, and that will usually result in more questions. Maintain eye contact, move about the room, show enthusiasm about the topic you are explaining.

Don't be afraid to admit that you don't have all the answers. If a student's question is beyond your own expertise, and if it is relevant and of common interest, use it as a departure point for a class research project, a visiting speaker, a field trip or any other means of investigation that is feasible and appropriate. Once the lecture is completed, ask the students to summarize what they have learned, either verbally or in writing. What you learn about the effectiveness of the talk can be disappointing, but it is a very good way to find out how you need to modify your talk to make it a better communication technique.

Discussion. Judging by the frequency with which the word *discuss* appears in curriculum guides as a suggested activity, discussion must be the predominant technique used in health teaching. Because the suggestion is seldom accompanied by further advice, it is difficult to predict how it is interpreted or carried out. Feldman asserted that:

> True discussion, in which we join students in trying to resolve questions with unknown or indefinite answers, is rare. Our questions too often call for factual, one-word responses. In fact, it's been noted that most of us answer two thirds of our own questions (11).

Discussion is *supposed* to be a dynamic interchange of ideas that build, one on the other, until an issue is resolved or a conclusion is reached. This is difficult to do. Some teachers cannot seem to resist the urge to do most of the talking. Goodlad et al found that, on the average, about 75% of class time was spent on instruction and that nearly 70% of this was talk, usually teacher to students (11). "Teachers outtalked the entire class of students by a ratio of about three to one" (13). (Figure 5-2). Some teachers have difficulty tolerating the relatively unstructured classroom environment necessary for a pupil to pupil dialogue to build to vital discussion, so they limit discussion to teacher-pupil interactions. White says that teachers often act as if they "own" the knowledge, claiming the right to ask all the questions, as well as "owning" the right to decide if the answers supplied by students are correct or not (29). Even where pupil-to-pupil dialogue is encouraged, it is difficult to prevent "class talkers" from dominating the action. Generally, the larger the group, the more difficult it is to motivate and direct discussions without losing the spontaneity and freedom required.

A good way to facilitate productive discussions is to first provide the group with a common background of information about the issue or problem of interest. Any technique that results in the quick communication of the information needed can be used.

Often audiovisual materials are effective, but the students must be given cues to indicate the points for which they will be responsible in the discussion to follow. Once everyone has an established fund of information, the discussion can be initiated with a related, thought-provoking question for which there is no one right answer but which has meaning for the children. For example, "How many teeth are there in the full primary set?" may be relevant, but it leads to a factual answer not likely to lead to further comment. A better question might be "What are some foods that you like that you couldn't eat if you had no teeth?" The question, "What are the safety rules to follow when playing on school grounds?" is certainly relevant but is not as likely to motivate thinking and application of information as "What can *you* do every day to make play time safer and more fun for everyone?"

Each person's ideas must be given consideration and everyone's participation is essential to at least some degree. This balance is not easy to achieve. Be careful to avoid dominating the discussion so that in the end it is always your conclusions or solutions that are adopted. Let the students summarize and decide what they have learned.

Discussion is probably a part of *every* teaching and learning activity. However, there are a number of recognized forms by which a discussion may be organized. Four of these are discussed here, the first three of which can be used with any age group. The fourth is probably more effective with middle-school students. Before you plan any kind of discussion, find out whether your students know how to discuss. If they don't, spend some time introducing them to the joys of being free to offer ideas and to react to those of others just as they are accustomed to doing among their friends outside of school. Plan short sessions initially, setting some ground rules for speaking as the first step.

Lecture-Discussion. Teachers often describe their mode of teaching as a lecture-

THE CLASSROOM HOUR

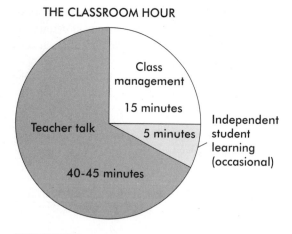

FIGURE 5-2

The classroom hour. (Adapted from Goodlad Jl: *A place called school,* New York, 1984, McGraw-Hill.)

discussion. This usually means that some new material is first introduced by the teacher in a direct lecture, after which the students are encouraged to ask questions, express any reactions, and talk about what has been offered. A lecture-discussion allows the teacher to set the stage for learning by providing a common base of information to the class in a short time, but there is typically more lecture than discussion. Its success depends primarily on the subject matter and the skill of the instructor in engaging the interest of the class during the lecture and in leading the subsequent discussion so that it is the students who are doing the thinking and talking.

Brainstorming. This activity can be led by the teacher for the whole class or employed in small groups as a quick means of obtaining a number of ideas for later analysis or evaluation. As an initiating procedure, the teacher or class identifies a problem or question such as, "How many ways can one person's actions affect his or her own health as well as that of others?" The teacher asks the children to think of as many physical, social, economic, environmental or other effects as they can. Every idea should be recorded without judging its worth until no more can be suggested. The tenor of the activity should be the free flow of ideas and complete acceptivity. When no more ideas can be elicited, each is then considered and classified as either positive or negative in its effect on personal or community health.

When the whole class is participating, the teacher acts as moderator and recorder. Use of the chalkboard or overhead transparency is an effective means of recording and summarizing any conclusions. Small groups can be led by an appointed or elected leader and notes taken by a group recorder. Each group brainstorms, considers the results, and categorizes the ideas as either positive or negative in effect.

As a culminating activity, the teacher might poll each group in turn for one effect that they identified as positive until all of them have been shared. Next, the negative effects are reported. Because the first group might have hit on most of the important effects, only one idea should be accepted from any one group at a time. Otherwise later groups are robbed of the satisfaction of contributing their work to the outcome.

Brainstorming is useful as a means of generating the ideas needed to define a problem of concern, to identify ways of locating needed data, and to theorize about possible solutions.

Buzz Sessions. This activity must be carried out in small groups of not more than five or six persons who are given a specified amount of time (usually 6 to 10 minutes) to talk over a problem or issue and to decide on a tentative solution. The buzz session gets its name from the sounds that result because the format promotes active participation by everyone. Each group may work with the same topic, or each may be assigned a different topic. In either case, the culminating activity involves communicating the groups' conclusions or recommendations to the total class. This can be done by means of individual reports given by the group leaders or by forming an impromptu panel of representatives from each group which would then share the groups' viewpoints. The remainder of the class forms the audience and should be encouraged to question or offer suggestions. Buzz sessions are useful in fostering creative thinking, building confidence in expressing new ideas, and promoting communication skills. They can be used effectively as preliminary planning activities for role playing, group projects, dramatizations, or any other procedure for which creativity is essential.

Panel Discussions. In the more formally organized panel discussions the panel members spend some time in advance preparation for the presentation. As a teaching and learning strategy, preparation for a panel discussion usually requires considerable time, spent both in and out of the classroom. This kind of discussion needs to be somewhat structured. Each group should be provided with a list of its responsibilities, along with suggestions for completing the assignment. Panel discussion projects may include more members than are required to participate in the final presentation. Time should be given in class for each group to elect a leader, prepare a tentative outline of their presentation, allocate the work to be done, and set a due date for each step involved. The leader should be given responsibility for submitting, before the presentation, an outline indicating what part each member will play in the total project. Planning the presentation, its theme, how it will be presented, and what visual or audio material, if any, will be required should be done by the total group. The specific tasks involved in preparation, such as doing research, producing the posters or other visual aids, writing the individual reports, and making the actual presentations, can be assigned by volunteering or drawing lots. Individual differences between students are best accommodated by allowing each person to choose the task that interests him or her most, when possible.

When the panel makes its presentation, usually as a conversational interaction among the group members, the leader is the discussion moderator and summarizer. The presentation also could be a series of brief descriptions of key aspects of the issue, after which the rest of the class is encouraged to join in the discussion. It is better to limit such panel discussions to no more than one a day, for when there are more, each successive group's work and conclusions are diminished in importance and effect. Too much of the same kind of activity can pall, even at the college level. Elementary school children need frequent changes of pace to keep their interest level high.

Panel discussions are particularly successful for considering issues or problems, such as boy-girl relationships, dress codes, environmental pollution, drug use or abuse, and any other topic that currently concerns the community or the school.

Whatever the form of discussion employed, help the class formulate summarizing conclusions or ideas for future action. These need not always be clear-cut but may be developed in the form of promising alternatives. Never let the outcome be lost because the bell rings and cuts off discussion. You know when the bell is going to ring and should anticipate it. If time is running out and there will not be enough time to reach any conclusions, propose a postponement of that part of the activity until another day. But the students should be left with some kind of summarizing thoughts and the clear expectation of further discussion on the topic. If the timing works out well, the class can make some decision or recommend a position to be taken. Most of all, it is essential that everyone sees the significance of what has been learned in relation to what is to come next.

Committee Projects.　The cooperative participation of a small group of students in exploring some designated topic is sometimes preliminary to other techniques. As already described, committee work is involved in preparations for panel discussions. It also precedes other forms of presentations, such as plays, skits, films, puppet shows, slide presentations accompanied by recorded narration, debates, or demonstrations. Committee work can help children learn how to discover answers to questions, work effectively as members of a team, and differentiate between fruitful and fruitless searches for valid information. A careful structure is essential to the success of this technique, however. It is not enough to simply make the assignment because the result may be a project to which only a few members contributed or a committee whose reports are largely derived from encyclopedias and are as boring to hear as they were meaningless to prepare. A good way to structure committee work is to prepare reporting forms that uniformly channel planning and reporting. The first form might ask the group to report the preliminary sources used to make plans, the second to specify what every committee member will do and when the work is due, and the last to indicate the title of the project, the format that will be employed (e.g., dramatization, debate, or media study), plans for involving the rest of the class in either the discussion or evaluation, and so on.

Committee projects can be a stimulating means to investigate health problems such as quackery, malnutrition, and local or school health needs. Whatever the issue, the important outcome is the development of valid conclusions by the students that tie the purpose of the project to those of the unit or course.

Role Playing. This technique appeals to all ages. It is an ad-lib, 3- to 5-minute informal acting out of a social situation in which the participants assume fictitious identities and then dramatize their parts. Role playing can be used to illustrate a concept or problem. Two or more persons may take part, and ordinarily a short amount of time is allowed for planning the action. Although informality and fun are associated with role playing, it should never be used simply for entertainment but always as a means of implementing a clearly evident instructional objective.

Role playing can be used to introduce a new area of study or to give students practice in applying what they have learned in another lesson. It can demonstrate the impact of tradition, values, attitudes, cultural beliefs, or social pressure on individual behaviors. Thus it can provide an outlet for feelings or convey ideas that, if approached more directly, might be awkward or uncomfortable for the students. For example, children may be too embarrassed to ask about some personal dilemma or health behavior, whereas role playing enables them to portray the unspoken query in the safe anonymity of the role being played. Understanding and empathy for the problems and responsibilities of others can be promoted by allowing a child to first play a role with one point of view and then switch to that of the other person in the situation. For example, a student might gain valuable insight into a parent's or teacher's problems by trying to play that role. When it is possible to present more than one dramatization without the players having seen the other version(s), the fact that differing perceptions can result in different behaviors can be demonstrated by giving the same problem to two or more groups.

In general, the teacher should first provide a well-structured explanation of the activity and its intent, either verbally or in writing, as on a transparency or prepared cards. Whatever the subject of the role playing, it should not have too personal a meaning for any one class member. The situation and resulting reactions should be those of people in general. It may be especially wise when the students have not had experience in this kind of activity, to call for volunteers rather than require everyone to take part.

Any nonparticipating class members should be given a feeling of belonging by being assigned something to do while the role players are planning their act. One way to ensure active participation of the audience is to allow the role players to choose and illustrate some principle, problem, or other health-related concept that the class members are challenged to interpret from the action. For example, teams of two or three persons might be given generalizations drawn from previous lessons such as, "Stress can be helpful or harmful in its effect on health." Each team should be given at least 5 minutes to plan a way of presenting this idea through role playing. Those who are shy or not ready to attempt this activity might be allowed to develop the generalizations or create the plan for portraying them. Role playing is an effective summarizing device, with the other students asking questions or commenting on how it was done. Used in this manner, it is employed only after lessons that have provided the students with the information needed to play the role.

Field Trips. A dynamic means of linking the course's purposes with individual concerns and responsibilities is a visit to a local community health agency or an on-the-spot exploration of a health hazard or problem. As with any teaching and learning strategy, this technique should be chosen for its potential contribution to a desired instructional objective and should offer evidence of being the best way of doing so. Although there is no reason why a field trip cannot be either an individual or small group activity, the term usually describes a total class movement to some place other than the classroom. The area can be on the school grounds or at a considerable distance from the school. Much preliminary planning is needed for a trip away from the school grounds. A class discussion might be used to identify the exact place to be visited, the information desired, and the relationship between this information and the health concepts being studied at the time. Depending on their age and ability, the class members may make some or all of the actual arrangements, such as arranging for the visit by telephone or interview, setting the date and time for the visit, providing the hosts with necessary information about the class and the purpose of the visit, and *always following up with a letter of appreciation signed by everyone.* In such a situation the teacher can act as a counselor but should stay in the background, allowing the students to practice the social skills and processes they need to develop.

The primary purpose of a field trip should not be to divert (although diversion it may be) but to provide the kinds of experiences that contribute to the acquisition of some powerful idea related to health protection or behavior. For example, on a field trip to a neighborhood health facility, rather than focusing on the services available simply by listing them, the students could find out what new services are being provided and what changing circumstances made them important (the idea being that community health programs must change as the community itself changes). The field trip should not be structured as a fact-finding endeavor but as a way to investigate and infer answers to questions such as, "Why are these services or facilities offered?" or "Why aren't some provided here that are offered elsewhere?"

All safety precautions for the students making the trip must be planned in accordance with school or district policy and state liability laws. Transportation, teacher aids, parental permission or assistance, and other logistical problems should be identified and solved well in advance of the scheduled travel.

After the field trip, it is essential to discuss what was observed. Cause and effect inferences should be examined and recommendations for change or improvement developed where appropriate. Another profitable field trip activity is to encourage interested students to take photographs, which can later be organized and a commentary dictated, taped, or written.

Public-opinion surveys concerning health issues or needs, searching for traffic or fire hazards that need to be corrected, or investigating prices and ingredients of over-the-counter medications are just a few examples of individual or small group projects that could be conducted outside the classroom.

Computer-Assisted Instruction (CAI)

Use of desk-top sized computers has escalated to the point that there may be more functioning computers in this country than there are people (12). Where once a typewriter was the primary instrument for written communication both at home and in business, today it is a microcomputer via word processing programs. Children in homes with computers come to school already familiar with keyboarding and are able to boot it

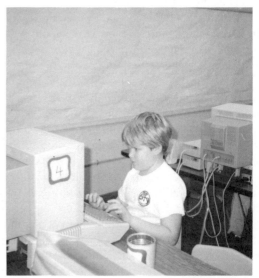

Marion Pollock

Computer software can be used to provide information and develop problem-solving skills.

up and play games or programs designed to fit their needs and interests. Virtually all children are given instruction in computer use beginning in kindergarten.

Instruction in operating the hardware is a necessary first step in using a computer. But it is the software that empowers a computer. **Software** is the term used to describe the instructions provided the hardware by a computer **program.** Software is widely available, but good software is not. More than 12,000 educational software programs are already available, and an estimated 2000 more are added every year. According to Dorman only about 5% of those programs can be rated as exemplary (10). Ninety-nine percent of all teaching material on the market, including educational software is not evaluated prior to distribution. "Only the Best", published by the Association for Supervision and Curriculum Development, lists just 136 software/multimedia programs offered among the thousands of programs available (1). Ratings are based upon data obtained from 31 evaluation services. Only 6 health education programs are listed for 1993 along with 3 others rated in 1992, with another two mentioned as prime candidates for inclusion among the best of 1994. Before purchasing any computer software, whether for school or home, find out as much as you can about its value for your own teaching needs. Information for evaluating computer software is provided in Chapter 7.

Microcomputer programs applicable as teaching strategies during elementary school years are commonly categorized as **drill and practice, tutorial, demonstration, simulation,** and **instructional games.** Although not directly concerned with instruction, **classroom management data storage** can be included among the uses of the microcomputer in schools. As an individual learning activity, the student works alone or with supervision at a computer in which an instructional program is installed. A laser disc player permits animated simulations or demonstrations for total classroom presentation. Interactive multimedia presentations can also be viewed individually, creating a more active learning situation.

Individual Computer Learning Activities

Drill and practice. Students are presented questions or problems, a response is elicited, and the computer scores the results and provides immediate knowledge of results. The student is given an opportunity to correct errors and to ask for review as needed until the material is mastered. In health teaching this is useful for quick learning or pretesting knowledge of terminology, definitions, or basic factual material.

Tutorial. New information is provided the student after which related questions are asked. Based upon the obtained responses, the computer either presents additional information or reviews the preceding lesson. Not all students progress at the same pace, but over time each learns the desired material. Tutorial programs usually provide the student with several options, e.g., he or she can request help or ask for examples, rules, or review. In school health classes such a program might be used to proceed from knowledge of the functions of the 5 food groups to the proposal of a nutritious diet for a specific individual.

Demonstration. The student views a functioning model or situation on the computer screen by means of a multimedia program. Graphic models of body systems, for example the heart or the circulatory system, illustrate their workings far more vividly than simple drawings supported by arrows showing blood flow direction can. CPR procedures or any such graphic situation can be demonstrated on screen when mannikins are not available or live demonstrations are not feasible.

Simulation. The student observes a model of a real or imaginary system or community health problem and then makes changes in some aspect of the model. The computer then tells the student whether the change made was positive or negative. Simulation allows hypothetical manipulations without threatening the system or the community. For example a situation is presented in which a community is threatened by dangerous levels of air pollution, and the student must consider banning the use of all gasoline-consuming vehicles older than 20 years. Analyzing the impact of such a change in terms of the economy, the transportation system, delivery of food stuffs, access to health care, the insurance industry, and every other aspect of community activity is possible without any threat to existing systems.

Instructional Games. The purpose of instructional games is entertainment, although a programmed game can result in instruction as well. The student must make decisions and then react to the results of those decisions. Games usually deal with fantasy, whereas simulations deal with reality. By definition games are fun, but they can also promote quick thinking and creativity.

Classroom management. Computers have many uses in the classroom that are not directly related to teaching activities. For example, a large pool of test items can be accumulated and stored in a computer's memory, categorized by kind of test (true-false, multiple choice, completion, essay, matching etc.) and by subject area. Tests can then be assembled in whatever combination desired and the results scored and analyzed for various kinds of statistics (mean scores, range, level of difficulty, reliability, functioning of responses etc.) Classroom attendance records, anecdotal reports for later entry in a student's health record, classroom evaluations, and other such data can be stored and retrieved as necessary.

The potential for the enrichment of children's education by computer applications is undeniably great. Perhaps the most dramatic effect is the reduced time required compared to the time needed for conventional teaching. Interest in learning is enhanced by the novelty of the game-like application. It's fun. There are difficulties, however. Effective software is hard to find, and it is usually expensive. Voluntary organizations in your community may be a source of free or relatively inexpensive computer programs.

Other problems include computer hardware purchase and maintenance expense. Preservice and inservice training of teachers in using computers as instructional aids is often lacking. Most software programs are designed to operate with specific computers. Computer hardware typically becomes obsolete within a short time, and that means that any associated software is useless as well. Nevertheless, computers are here to stay, and their potential in education is increasingly accepted. At this moment, the amount of data that can be stored in a disk no larger than a small match box is equivalent to the volume of words contained in nine very long novels. With a computer and a modem you can communicate by satellite with anyone anywhere in the world where there is another modem and computer. In short, anybody who intends to be working at any level of intellectual operations and who believes that computer literacy is not necessary for him/her had better think again.

Experiential Strategies. There is more than one concept of experiential education. It is commonly described as the outcome of activities that take place off-campus, most particularly as provided for college and university students. For example, Conrad and Hedin defined experiential programs as "educational programs offered as part of the general school curriculum but taking place outside of the conventional classroom" (7). James urged that students be provided opportunities for small group, community-based experiences and services. He said, "Cognitive learning and experiential learning need not be viewed as adversaries," which suggests that they usually are (16). Kierstead agreed that the two are not mutually exclusive but complementary in the hands of teachers who know how to synthesize them (18).

What seems to be the common denominator in any plan labeled *experiential* is not its setting but the use of techniques termed "hands-on." Hands-on learning activities are those that approximate reality as nearly as possible and provide the learner with an experience often having powerful physical, social, and emotional dimensions. For example, one health educator obtained the loan of a number of wheelchairs, and students had an opportunity to propel themselves around the school and carry out commonplace activities while chairbound. As a follow up, they shared the insights they had gained relative to the difficulties a paraplegic or other handicapped person has in satisfying what might have seemed to be simple personal needs otherwise. To learn how arthritis might make it difficult to use one's hands, children put on mittens and then tried to work the computer that they had learned to operate or tried to open a milk carton or soft drink can. They tried to use the telephone or, accompanied by a guide, cross the street with their eyes covered or their ears stopped up in some way. They examined animal lungs and watched them expand when air was blown through a straw into the principal airway. They took each other's pulse before and after running in place for a specified length of time and drew some conclusions about the effects of smoking on the efficiency of lungs in supplying the heart with oxygen during exercise.

The possibilities for experiential activities are limited only by the creativity and willingness of the teacher to spend the time and energy it takes to make these kinds of arrangements. A word of caution, however, must be given; be sure to check any plans for experiential activities with your school administrator in advance. There may be school policies or other problems of which you are not aware that would prevent your carrying them out. Should there be any complaint, you will be on safer ground if you have obtained approval beforehand.

The success of experiential teaching depends on the meaningfulness of the activity to the learners and the degree to which they are involved. Most simply, in experiential learning the students practice what the teacher used to preach. They learn by doing, and as many of the senses are involved as possible. Simulation games are experiential, as are many of the techniques commonly employed in health education—role playing, experimenting, demonstrations, dramatizations, and so on. In fact, effective health teaching is al-

ways experiential. Every lesson should have experiential elements.

Cooperative Learning Strategies

Cooperative learning, as it has been developed at The Johns Hopkins University and other centers over the past fifteen years, has been extensively studied and without exception has demonstrated its remarkable effectiveness in promoting the academic achievement of all students. Although cooperative learning models always include good instruction as a base, their activities supplement but do not replace direct teaching. What they *do* replace is individual seatwork.

In cooperative learning, students work together in teams to master material initially presented by the teacher in lecture-discussion, audio-visual, or other form. Yet it is not just group work with a new name. Asking students to work together without any group goal, to complete a single worksheet, or propose a group solution to a problem is not the same thing. A cooperative learning strategy must include the following two elements. First, the group must be rewarded for doing well *as a group*. Second, the group's success must depend on the *individual learning* of all of its members. There must be no way for individual students to ride on their teammates coattails. Each student's learning must be important to the team.

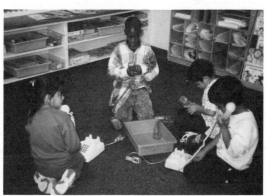

Angela Loya

Children can teach each other effectively.

The theory and practice of cooperative learning rest upon the following principles or beliefs.

Heterogeneous Grouping. The most effective student groups are those that are heterogeneous in membership. Ideally, cooperative learning groups are not randomly assembled but chosen as representative of the academic performance, sex, and race or ethnicity of the class. This means that those individuals selected must also satisfy the requirement for a high performer, a low performer, and two average performers in the team. Teams of four are ideal because they allow two sets of pairs, which doubles participation of each member in the learning activity and provides twice as much interaction as is possible with teams of fewer or more participants.

Simultaneous Interaction Among Students. The greater the participation, the greater the potential for learning and retention. In the traditional classroom, the teacher usually does all of the talking, and any student talk is limited to individual recitation or answers to teacher questions. In the whole-class question and answer format, only one student at a time answers. In a team-organized cooperative learning model, all of the students interact in answering a question or solving a problem. At any one time, half the class is talking, and the potential for active participation increases as a team is further separated into pairs.

Positive Interdependence. Students need to recognize and value their dependence on each other. Learning to work well with others and enjoy a feeling of mutual purpose and achievement builds ability to work cooperatively as opposed to competitively.

Individual Accountability. A group's achievement is greatest when every member of the team has contributed effectively to its goal. If evaluation is not based on individual products or tests, it is often the case that more able members of the group assigned a task find it easier to take over entirely, allowing others to coast yet receive a group grade. Students can be made individually accountable in several ways (grades given for a unique contribution, requirement that

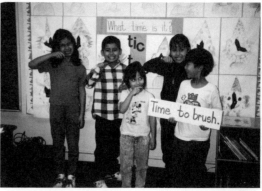
Angela Loya

A group's achievement gain is greatest when every member has contributed to the goal.

all members must complete a task before the team can progress, etc.). Whatever the contribution, the team is aware that it has been completed. When the group's success depends on the participation of all its members, activities necessarily focus on explaining, discussing, and assessing each other's understanding so that problems or weaknesses are revealed and corrected.

Social Skills Acquisition. Social skills are those interpersonal behaviors performed by all group members that help the group carry out a task and like each other when it is done. Social skill development should be integrated within the activities designed to sharpen the cognitive skills and learn the content specified in the objective. Active participation in cooperative learning activities fosters the development of these essentials for social success. At elementary school levels, development of even the simplest skills of this nature gives the student a head start on getting along in the world. For example, caring about others, sharing feelings, giving and responding to ideas, encouraging others, and following directions are social skills. Their use helps students feel better about the group and themselves. Without them, the learning task is empty of enjoyment, and students lack interest in going further with it.

Group autonomy. A fundamental belief of

cooperative learning is that the group must perform the task set for its members on its own. When students complete their task or work out their problems with a minimum of teacher input, they are learning to think and to be self-sufficient learners. Teachers can suggest or prompt if need be, but intervention and answer-giving robs group members of their chance to learn and grow.

Processing. Processing is a procedure by which individuals and groups examine their own behavior during a just completed lesson to ascertain whether or how well they practiced social skills. When processing is employed as the closing activity following every cooperative group lesson, use of positive group behaviors is increased, and the time required for their integration is less. The potential for transfer of the just-achieved knowledge is increased as well. Three types of processing can be used. *Analysis* considers the just completed activity, *application* asks the student to think about other situations in which the social skills just practiced could be used effectively as well, and *goal setting* gives the student an opportunity to identify a social skill to be practiced at the next lesson.

Monitoring. Group work, particularly when it is new to students, needs to be monitored so that the activities stay on track and its members behave responsibly and productively. It is the teacher's task to observe the groups in action and to record or note the application of the interpersonal behaviors that have been taught earlier. Until students have learned to work effectively in groups as expected, their progress needs to be checked and guidance provided as needed. Look for application of social skills such as listening, encouraging others, asking questions, praising, offering ideas, taking turns in speaking, and any other social skills that have been taught. Self-monitoring provides more insight into any behavioral problems that limit the effectiveness of the strategy. Ask students to write down or report answers to questions such as "What are two things that we did well in our group work and one thing that we need to work on next time?"

How does all of this fit into the established school curriculum? Kagan has said that there are just three basic structural patterns of instruction: individualistic, competitive, and cooperative (17). Most of us are used to the second pattern in which achievement is a matter of being among the best, usually judged by a system of grading. Competition for high grades and the recognition that goes with them is the norm. Students are not used to lessons that seek another goal entirely and asks them to help each other rather than beat as many as they can. Kagan recommends a structural approach which is based on the creation, analysis, and systematic application of *structures*, or content-free ways of organizing social interaction in the classroom. Structures in this sense usually involve a series of patterned steps. They can be applied in connection with any teaching goal and at any level of education. When a structure appropriate to a specific objective is combined with meaningful content Kagan terms the product a learning activity. Structures propose the *how* of a lesson, while the content with which the activity is to be concerned is the *what*.

How do you put all of this together when you start to teach? If it sounds complicated, that is because it is. Doing anything as a group takes more time than when the same task is given to an individual student. It takes more time to explain a task so clearly that every one understands perfectly what is expected. It takes time when each member of a team is to be given a turn at whatever is to be done, and the answers are compared, allowing group acceptance of the shared and checked answers. The reward is that everybody has learned what was proposed and at the same time has practiced social skills that may serve them in the future even more than at present.

Planning lessons requires 6 important decisions: (1) developing or selecting the objective that will be the focus of the learning experience, (2) deciding what information must be given the students prior to the lesson, (3) determining how much time it will take, (4) deciding how many members each group will include, (5) selecting the method you will use in choosing the members of the heterogeneous groups, and (6) anticipating and arranging for the shifting of desks or chairs necessary if the groups are to be accessible to you, yet comfortable for them. Only the last two steps are new or different from those involved in planning any lesson.

If cooperative learning is a concept or procedure new to you, and you want to incorporate it within your repertoire of teaching skills, you will find more than a few books and manuals on the subject. One in a particular that is comprehensive and easy to understand and apply is Spencer Kagan's *Cooperative Learning* (17).

Values-related Strategies. Inescapably, a person's values, or what seems important to her or him, shape the beliefs that underlie and give direction to every decision and resulting action that person takes. Like their first cousins, attitudes, values are essentially learned standards of behavior and products of the wide range of influences each person experiences from the moment of birth. What a person believes and does about his or her health perhaps is influenced more by values than by knowledge. The decision to begin smoking, stop smoking, eat sensibly, exercise appropriately, or do anything at all that affects health is inevitably based on values.

If you believe that health education needs to recognize this powerful influence, does consideration of values belong in the cognitive or the affective domain? Opinions on this issue are strong, and they differ. According to those who favor the affective approach, values cannot be dealt with as though they were facts to be memorized in the way that people learn that two times two is four. Because values involve feelings and beliefs, they can be approached only through activities that stir reactions. This includes the use of role-playing situations, thought-provoking visual materials, and devil's advocate discussions.

Those who favor the cognitive approach believe that values and moral judgments should be based on reasoning rather than on opinions or feelings. According to this view, affective education is perceived as manipulative rather than edu-

cational and is more aptly labelled *excitement education*. The primary purpose of role playing, in their view, should be to promote understanding. An affective impact will inevitably occur as a desirable secondary outcome of a meaningful experiential activity.

Tyler suggests that "clarifying values is an essential part of being an intelligent person. It is simply a sensible way of helping children as they go through life to find a way to think about the things they do and ask questions about the thinking involved in their actions." However, he suggests that the term "values clarification" be discarded because it is too often misunderstood (21).

Whatever strategies you choose as the means of promoting positive health attitudes, take care not to ask your students to discuss matters that could be interpreted as an invasion of personal or family privacy. Also, because some of the published values-clarifying activities are relatively unstructured and even fun, their purpose can get lost in the excitement. Be certain that you never lose sight of your objective and that the strategy you have chosen is best suited to its achievement. Above all, be certain that the students know *why* they have participated in that activity. Help them to interpret the meaning of what has happened and to relate their conclusions to future health-related decisions and actions.

Vicarious Teaching Techniques

Televised Instruction. Although the use of television in teaching is not universal, there is no question that it works as an educational tool. Students can learn from television as well as they can from teachers, textbooks, and other educational devices, as demonstrated by the success of *Sesame Street*. Where closed-circuit television equipment (a means of sending and receiving programs originated and received only within the school) is available, the potential for more effective use of demonstrations and experiments is obvious. Each student has a far better view than when everybody must crowd around a small area in order to see, and many classes can have a close look at a single show. Increasing use of videotapes makes it possible to record presentations by specialists or students themselves for future use. Taped demonstrations and presentations may even be better than live sessions for observation and study.

Many teachers use scheduled educational television broadcasts as supplementary instructional material. Very large school districts, such as that in Los Angeles, have their own educational television channel with programs available for public, as well as school, viewing. The weekly program schedules of both commercial and educational channels provide a means of identifying current shows with relevance to health education. Documentaries on topics such as environmental pollution, consumer issues, substance abuse problems, AIDS and other health-related concerns are frequent. Such programs usually are given advance publicity and can be announced and used as a homework assignment or recommended as voluntary viewing for extra points and subsequent class discussion. Effective use can be made of audiotape recorders for preserving the sound portions of televised materials where this does not affect its comprehensibility. For example, a taped series of commercials can be used to demonstrate kinds of sales appeals or to evaluate the student's ability to identify those appeals when they are heard and seen.

Overhead Projection Materials. Professionally prepared transparencies are available for use in connection with most aspects of health instruction. Drawings used for transparencies differ from photographs in that they are simplified line drawings, which are more effective in promoting understanding of structure and function. The transparencies enliven verbal descriptions and illustrate what is said. They can be used to introduce new topics, stimulate discussion, summarize, stress key points of a lesson, structure and explain assignments, or evaluate students. For example, instead of reproducing copies of tests, a transparency can be used to exhibit the questions and then store them for future use. The development of original transparencies

by students is a worthwhile and enjoyable project. Transparencies can be used to present the results of buzz sessions or to illustrate committee project or panel discussion points. A blank transparency is an effective substitute for the chalkboard because the writing is easier to read (if care is taken to print or write in inch-high letters) and the writer can face the class and thus be more audible and effective.

Films, Slides, and Filmstrips. Through the use of film media, a vicarious field trip, experiment, or demonstration can be arranged that otherwise might be difficult or impossible to do. Often a 15-minute film can cover an experience more effectively than an hour-long field trip or lecture. All students see and hear the same material, and certain details can be emphasized so that every part and its function are better described and observed than during an actual field trip. This is not to say that a film is always preferable to a field trip. There is undeniably greater impact and interest generated by seeing the real thing.

The effectiveness of filmed presentations depends as much on the way they are used as on the skill with which they were developed. Few films are of much value if they are shown without comment or discussion. The instructor must preview and note the key points that make up the message of the film. The entertainment quality of a film can be such that the educational purpose is overlooked. It is doubly important in such cases that the students be told in advance which points to look for while they are enjoying the story. As a means of further ensuring the students' close attention, it can be rewarding to ask for and use their evaluation of the film's worth as a learning activity. It is essential to establish in advance what objective the film is expected to fulfill. Although it may require more time than is available, research shows that learning is greatly enhanced when a film is shown, discussed, and then shown a second time.

The Metropolitan Life Foundation has developed a series of films for middle-school students (20). *Triggering Positive Health Choices* presents situations that young people may be or soon may be experiencing. A videocassette and detailed leader's guide are offered free of charge.

Slides and filmstrips do not have quite the dynamic realism of films, but they have the advantage of greater versatility. Individual frames can be viewed for as long as needed (Fig. 5-3), and the sequence can be altered as desired. Slide presentations are the most flexible of all. New pictures can be added, old ones deleted, and the sequence changed at any time. Slides can be created easily and inexpensively, even by young children. When combined with a taped commentary, a slide presentation rivals the dynamic quality of a motion picture. For example, a group of seventh grade students, invited to submit a color slide of themselves in a pose that illustrated their special view of "happiness," eagerly did so, and then each youngster read for audiotaping a line that explained the message intended by the picture. For example, a picture of a girl cuddling a kitten was accompanied by the voiced message,

"Happiness is having something to love that is your very own." The school glee club softly singing "Happiness Is" was recorded for background music. The resulting series of pictures and messages was featured at parents' night and other school meetings to great applause.

Teaching Aids

The use of teaching aids has increased enormously since the days when the slate was the only tool. In addition to the media already discussed, the teacher has radios, books, tape cassettes of visual and audio materials specific to health instruction, records, and a wealth of free or inexpensive teaching materials such as pamphlets, booklets, and article reprints. There are also visual aids such as scrapbooks, flannel boards, graphs, charts, posters, models, exhibits, and specimens, all of which can be used to actively involve the learner in many sensory experiences. Because learning is more likely to promote positive health behaviors when the teach-

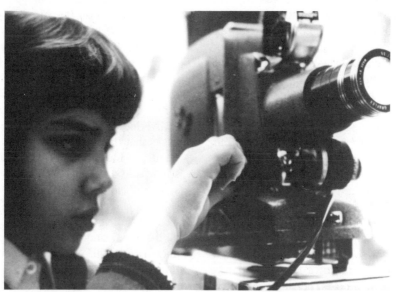

Ann Nolte and Philip Portlock

FIGURE 5-3
Using a filmstrip projector.   The filmstrip continues to be used as a common tool for health teaching.

ing activities engage the student emotionally and fully, teachers need to employ, as often as they can, techniques that are as close to real as possible. Models and mock-ups provide an artificial but realistic learning situation (e.g., the plastic head and torso for CPR practice). Drama forms such as sociodramas, skits, and plays also permit *action* on the part of the learner that reinforces desirable behaviors and attitudes. Exhibits of so-called health foods, quackish devices, or deceptive advertisements for "health" products can provide vital learning experiences for children.

A purely visual display using a pegboard, chalkboard, magnetic board, map, graph, cartoon, diagram, or other device may lack movement and auditory properties, but in many situations a simple display can bring a lecture or discussion point into focus better than more elaborate means. It cannot be said that any one medium is better than others; there are too many variables operating in the learning process. A teacher has to be competent in using them all and must choose the one best suited for the particular day, topic, and group of students. Each medium has advantages and disadvantages, but any one of them can be effective if used wisely and well. Some people learn more easily by hearing, some by reading, and others by watching or handling things. A wide variety of approaches and media should be provided so that each child experiences those which are most effective for him or her and also those which will reinforce what has been learned through their appeal to all the other senses.

LESSON PLANS THAT WORK

Hunter believes that there are three basic tasks in the teaching and learning process: (1) determining what is to be learned (2) determining what the learner will be doing to accomplish the desired learning, and (3) determining what the teacher will do to facilitate that accomplishment (14). These are tasks with which lesson planning is concerned. The lesson plan that evolves from and reflects the decisions relative to these three

tasks should communicate what will be taught and how it will be taught.

Only 20 years ago we were still operating on the notion that teachers are born, not made. I knew it was a myth because I had seen too many bumbling beginners—including me—turn into reasonably decent teachers. I'd also seen a lot of charismatic teachers, pied pipers who looked wonderful to the kids. The pied pipers managed to produce some of the happiest illiterates in the entire school. Charisma is great, but it's neither necessary nor sufficient to be a good teacher (3).

Lesson planning goes beyond the mere selection of subject matter, the teaching technique that will permit practice of the behavior specified in the objective, or how the lesson will be conducted. A lesson plan must be organized smoothly, logically, and concisely, clearly matching the intent of the proposed objective. Lesson plans submitted by a student teacher must be more explicit and detailed than those prepared by an experienced teacher. The latter has had the time to learn what works and knows how children of a given grade or age group react to the health concepts proposed. Student teachers usually are required to present detailed daily plans specifying what will be taught and how it will be done. The following suggestions are made with the assumption that the reader is a prospective rather than an experienced teacher. Ideally, a feasible and measurable objective, an outline of the key ideas, a brief plan of the activity, a list of resources that will be employed, and a culminating activity should be included. Student teachers should always consider the fact that whatever can go wrong may go wrong and should have a plan to cope with anything that might threaten successful achievement of the lesson.

Once the objective of the lesson has been determined, all the other decisions are directed accordingly. First, the subject matter portion of the objective needs to be elaborated and made explicit. This can be done by means of a list of key generalizations or a brief outline. It need not be more than the "bare bones ideas" you intend to consider in teaching one lesson.

LESSON PLAN FORMAT*

Teacher_____ Unit_____ Date_____

Specific measurable objective for this lesson

Initiation   (Your plan to build on a previous day's accomplishment and to commence today's activities; not what you plan to say but your plan for student activities)

Content	Estimated time	Materials	Plan of action	Special class arrangements
(Stated as generalizations or as short outline of the subject matter aspect of the objective)	(Based on your pre-lesson timing)	(Resources or teaching aids to be used)	(What the students will be doing as they practice the skill specified in the objective)	(Small groups singly, moving about?)

Culminating activities   How you will end the lesson so that students exhibit achievement of the
objective, i.e., their performance can be measured

Anticipated problems (what might go wrong?)	Possible solution (what could you do if something goes wrong)
For example, students are not prepared to participate in the activity planned for them.	Switch plans to an activity that can be carried out without preparation but is relevant to the stated objective.

_____

*Use this guide only as a structure for the presentation of your lesson plan. Do not attempt to fit your plan into the blank spaces.

A lesson plan, in essence, is like a well-organized story. It needs an interest-capturing *beginning* (the initiating activity that links today's plan to yesterday's achievement and whets the appetite for what is to come next). Next comes the *body* of the story (the description of what the students will be doing to practice the skill as they deal with the subject matter). Never assume that the students can carry out your plan without any effort on your part to provide them with the subject matter described. Indeed, the reverse is true. If the students can carry out your objective so competently that all you have to do is to arrange an opportunity that allows them to do so, there is no need for a lesson. In fact, what you have written in that event is an evaluation activity, not a learning opportunity.

Once you have decided on the subject matter you want them to learn, you must next decide the manner in which it will be provided them. Will you start the lesson by giving a short lecture, show them a film or a film strip that presents the information, ask them to report to you what they have learned by doing the reading you assigned for homework, or employ another technique? Research shows that everyone, youngster or adult, learns new material most quickly and easily if it is introduced at either the beginning or the end of a lesson. What does this suggest might sometimes be the focus of the culminating activity? Finally, a lesson plan has to have a good *ending* (the culminating activity that motivates the learner to summarize, draw conclusions, and makes him or her want to learn more about the subject. The quality of the culminating activity can make the difference between learning and confusion. Sometimes lessons never actually come to an end but just stop when the bell rings. The learner never finds out why the day's activities took place or what any of it had to do with what had been presented previously.

The plan that follows could be used either as a learning opportunity or a lesson, depending on the abilities and past learning experiences of the class. To achieve the objective, a primary student probably would first need to complete several en-abling activities. Intermediate-level students probably could bypass these and carry out the lesson in a single session. Study this plan. See if you can identify its unstated but implicit enabling objectives. What do the students need to be able to do before they can describe ways an individual can favorably affect and promote the health of others?

To develop one lesson absent the overarching logic of a stated framework of goals and a carefully designed scope and sequence plan is difficult to do effectively. However, an illustrative lesson on personal standards of behavior and their relationship to the welfare of others has been worked out, given these limitations. This topic is surely basic to desirable health behavior, although perhaps easy to overlook. This lesson illustrates the application of what the students have learned earlier about the ways in which personal actions can affect the well-being of others.

Outline of a Lesson

Objective: Describes ways an individual can favorably affect and promote the health of others.

Generalization: There are many ways by which an individual can contribute to the well-being of family, friends, and community. Choosing and carrying out a plan for some good action is an important step toward becoming the kind of person one admires.

Strategy: Using lecture-discussion and brainstorming to identify actions that can affect and promote the health of others.

Initiation activity: Introduce the concept of an individual's caring about the well-being of others by telling the story of Benjamin Franklin's plan for his day, as shown in his own diary. The question he posed to himself at the start of each day was, "What good shall I do this day?" Then he jotted down a proposed action. At the end of the day, in answer to the question, "What good have I done this day?" Franklin wrote a short description of the actions that he had taken that seemed to have been good ones.

Establish in brief discussion what Franklin probably meant by "good." Ask questions such as "What do *you* think 'good' means when used to describe an action?" or, "If no one ever did anything that was intended to help others, how could that affect your health and your family's health?"

Activity: Ask for volunteers to describe actions that young people or adults often take to help others and how these actions affect community health. If necessary, show pictures of helpful actions (e.g., a boy scout acting as school crossing guard or a volunteer reading to a young patient in a hospital) in order to get the ideas started. Begin by asking the students to comment on what is happening in the picture and to speculate about the motives and the rewards of such actions and lead them to think about actions they have noted themselves.

As each idea for a helping action is proposed, list the action on the chalkboard or on a transparency and ask the class to decide whether the action helped others at home, at school, or in the community. Then ask volunteers to tell about some action they have themselves taken that affected the well-being of another. Help each person to analyze how this made him or her feel as a result. Ask questions such as, "Did you do that because you wanted to or because it was required?" "Did you feel happy about what you had done?" "Would you do it again if you could?"

Culmination: When everybody who wanted to participate has been heard (and no one should be pressed to contribute unwillingly), ask the class to review the total list of actions that have been described and to speculate about what kind is most often chosen. Are they most often for people at home, at school, or in the community? Then ask each child to think for several minutes and decide on something good that she or he can do during the next day. Ask each of them to write or dictate to a teacher's aide or older student a brief description of the action they chose and how, on implementation, it affected the well-being of others, and have them hand it in at the next class meeting. Allow those who prefer to present their action in the form of a drawing or poster to do so. Devise some means of sharing the products of the assignment among the class members and help them to draw some conclusions about the whole experience.

Now that you have read the plan, decide whether students might be better equipped to participate effectively in the brainstorming that would be required if they had first completed lessons based on objectives like the following:

1. Define the meaning of "good actions."
2. Differentiate between actions that might enhance and those that might detract from the health of others.
3. Identify actions an individual could take that might promote community health.
4. Explain ways such actions contribute to the well-being of others.

Are there other objectives that might be necessary for younger children? How could you be sure if the students in your class were ready to deal with the principal objective of the lesson as it is? Chapter 7 considers some ways to measure readiness by means of pretests and other measurement techniques.

Every lesson needs to be planned. Whether a teaching plan is broad, as in the case of a learning opportunity, or specific, as for a lesson, it should be based on a measurable objective that is attainable by the students for whom it is intended; it should focus on process rather than information; it should be learner-oriented; and it should come to a meaningful ending.

SUMMARY

Application of the concepts, skills, and techniques discussed in this chapter depends on the depth of one's understanding of their interrelationships and their dependence on the ability to apply what was considered in the two preceding chapters. In order to develop effective teaching and learning plans you must first have studied the sources of a health curriculum (i.e., the learner, the community, and its body of knowledge); determined what the scope and sequence of the curriculum are to be; defined its goals; and based upon data obtained from the sources, inferred sets of feasible objectives by grade or level (i.e., primary, upper elementary, and middle school) to form a framework for the teaching-learning plans that might facilitate their achievement.

Chapter 5 has dealt with the final step in the curriculum planning process, which has to do with *how* the goals and objectives might be implemented effectively. Three fundamental problems must be solved. For any particular group of students, these are: first, deciding what is to be taught and learned; second, what the learner is to be doing in order to achieve the instructional objectives; and third, what the teacher will do in order to help the learner to do so.

A number of propositions have been discussed as considerations basic to lesson planning. Some of these are as follows:

Health behavior is the result of decisions, whether conscious or subconscious in nature.

Problem solving and decision making are skills with lifelong utility and total transfer to other situations.

Emphasis on process rather than information is essential in planning active teaching strategies.

Thinking skills can be taught and learned but cannot be fostered by telling and reciting activities.

The more senses involved in a learning experience, the greater its effectiveness as a teaching strategy.

Active participation in learning activities heightens the impact and increases the rate of learning.

Intellectual skills must be practiced if they are to be mastered.

The best teaching technique is the one that provides the greatest number of concurrent positive outcomes, matches the objective, is perceived as satisfying, and fits the abilities of the students for whom it is planned. Health education in schools tends to be evaluated on the basis of what is offered students in its name, rather than in terms of its philosophy and purposes as proposed by its specialists. We hope that you will perceive your health teaching assignment as an expression of trust. Any one course in health education can contribute only partially to the long-range goals set by the school. However, creative, thoughtfully conceived health lessons can make a difference in the lifestyle choices of students and can often change those of their parents as well.

QUESTIONS AND EXERCISES
Discussion questions

1. If you were asked what the content of health teaching should include during elementary school grades, what areas would you list? How would that list influence the lessons that you might plan?

2. In what situations would choice of a vicarious teaching technique have advantages over directly experienced activities?

3. Why is it essential that children comprehend the purpose of any values-clarifying activities? How could you determine whether or not they have in fact understood that purpose?

4. If you were limited to but one of the senses as your means of communicating with your students, which would it be and why?

5. What do you see as the advantages, if any, of buzz sessions over brainstorming as a means of quickly generating a number of good ideas relative to a health issue?

6. Suppose that your class wanted to visit a nearby health facility, but for several good reasons it could not be arranged. Suggest other ways that you could satisfy that interest but without the expense and other problems involved in making off-campus visits.

7. Health teaching in elementary schools is most often integrated with science courses and sometimes with mathematics or physical education. Suggest

some ways that, whatever scheduled instruction was provided, you could add to the curriculum by integrating certain objectives with other host subject areas, such as reading, writing, art, and history.

Problems and exercises

1. For each of Bloom's categories of cognitive objectives, write one instructional objective for an age group of your choice, employing as a behavior one of those defined on pp. 103-104. Next, for each of those objectives, suggest a teaching technique that would best implement that behavior.

2. Develop a health lesson for a specified elementary grade that includes each of the following components:
   a. An instructional objective
   b. A brief outline of the content to be taught
   c. An initiating activity
   d. A description of the principal activity required of the students.
   e. A culminating activity
   f. A list of possible problems that could interfere with the conduct of the lesson, along with ways that these could be quickly solved.

3. Exchange plans with a fellow student. Read the other's plan and judge its clarity (if you could not carry out the plan without asking for more information, it's not clear enough). Write your comments and questions directly on the plan and return it to the author for study and any necessary reworking.

4. For a given general objective, develop an outline of the related subject matter in the following two formats:
   a. Traditional outline form, main points and subpoints adequate to describe the content for a learning opportunity.
   b. A list of generalizations that express all of the key ideas implicit in the objective.

5. Select or develop an affective objective that interests you, and work out a lesson plan for its implementation, just as for the cognitive objective in exercise one. Be ready to explain your plan to the class.

REFERENCES

1. Association for Supervision and Curriculum Development: *Only the best*, Alexandria, VA, 1993.

2. Bandura A: *Social learning theory*, Englewood Cliffs, NJ, 1977, Prentice Hall.

3. Berges M: An apple for this teacher of teachers. Los Angeles Times, part 6, page 1, Jan. 26, 1986.

4. Blackwood PE: Science teaching in the elementary school. In: Hollson M: *Elementary education*, New York, 1967, Free Press.

5. Bloom BS et al: *Taxonomy of educational objectives: handbook I: cognitive domain* New York, 1956, David McKay.

6. Bloom BS, Hastings G, Madeus G: *Evaluation to improve learning*, New York, 1981, McGraw-Hill.

7. Bruner J: *The process of education*, Cambridge, 1960, Harvard University Press.

8. Combs A: What the future demands of education, *Phi Delta Kappan* 62:369, 1981.

9. Conrad D, Hedin D: National assessment of experiential education: summary and implications, *J Experiential Educ* Fall 1981, p 16.

10. Cotterall J: Viewpoint. *Educ.* 5:21, 1990.

11. Dorman SM: Evaluating computer software for the health education classroom, *J School Health* 62(1):36, 1992.

12. Feldman RD: What are thinking skills? *Instructor and Teacher* 8:95, 1986.

13. Gold, R. *Microcomputer Applications in Health Education*. Dubuque, 1990, WC Brown.

14. Goodlad JI: *A place called school*, New York, 1984, McGraw-Hill.

15. Hunter M: *Teach for transfer*, El Segundo, Calif, 1971, TIP Publications.

16. Hunter M: Great teaching is like conducting a symphony, *Education*, UCLA Graduate School of Education, Fall 1986.

17. James T: Learning as practice in theory, *Phi Delta Kappan* 62:185, 1981.

18. Kagan S: *Cooperative learning: resources for teachers, Inc*, 1992, San Juan Capistrano, Calif.

19. Kierstead J: Direct instruction and experiential approaches: are they really mutually exclusive? *Educ Leadership* 42:8, 1985.

20. Kolbe LJ et al: Propositions for an alternate and complementary health education paradigm, *Health Educ* 12:3, 1981.

21. Metropolitan Life Foundation, New York, 1991.

22. Mickler ML: Interviews with Ralph W Tyler, *Educ Forum* 50:1, 1985.

23. Moyer J: Child development as a base for decision making, *Childhood Educ* May/June 1986.

24. Oberteuffer D: *Concepts and convictions*, Reston, Va, 1977, AAHPER.

25. Parcel G, Barnowski T: Social learning theory and health education, *Health Educ* 12:3, 1981.

26. Parker PF, Rubin LJ: *Process as content: curriculum design and the application of knowledge*, Chicago, 1966, Rand McNally.

27. Resnik H: From social studies to social science, *Learning* 13:3, 1985.

28. Rowen H: Big blues for U.S. industry. *Washington Post Weekly*, Dec. 28, 1992, p. 5.

29. Wales CE, Nardi A, Stager R: Decision making: new paradigm for education, *Educ Leadership* 43:8, 1986.

30. White J: Decision making with an integrative curriculum, *Childhood Educ* 62:5, 1986.

SUGGESTED READINGS

Bensley R, Ellsworth T: Bulimic learning: A philosophical view of teaching and learning, *J School Health*, 62(8):386-387, Oct, 1992.

Cleary M: Restructured schools: challenges and opportunities for school health education, *J School Health*, pp. 172-175, April 1991.

Merch C et al: Effects of a take-home drug prevention program on drug-related communication and beliefs of parents and children, *J School Health*, pp. 346-350, October, 1991.

Moore B: The health information video project, *J School Health*, 61(6):265-266, August, 1991.

Pahnos M: The continuing challenge of multicultural health education, *J Health Educ*, 62(1):24-26, January, 1992.

Servela P et al: Applications software packages in the school health program, *Health Educ*, 20(2):43-49, April/May 1989.

Wallerstein N, Hammes M: Problem posing: a teaching strategy for improving the decision making process, *J Health Educ*, 22(4):250-253, July/August 1991.

6 Managing Categorical and Controversial Issues

When you finish this chapter, you should be able to:

- Explain why the potential for controversy persists in health teaching.
- Analyze opposing points of view as they affect curriculum decisions regarding content appropriate for health education.
- Synthesize a plan for deterring controversy when teaching health in schools.
- Describe methods for establishing policy guiding choices among materials and curricula that may be subject to criticism.
- Propose constructive ways of managing possible controversy.

As in every other discipline, curriculum, decisions in health education must be based on careful study of data gathered by analysis of its body of knowledge, as well as the needs of the students and the community. The task is complicated in health education, however, since health *is* based on learner needs. Human needs are personal, often intimate, and therefore emotionally charged. Probably no other area of the school curriculum is the center of greater community dissension or is pressured more insistently by special interest groups. The field of health education includes as many as thirty categorical health problems or behaviors, for example, addictive behaviors, or problem sexual behaviors, as well as teenage suicide, child abuse, abortion, sex education, and death and dying education. The inclusion of these topics is being urged on the schools by many pressure groups. Other pressure groups are working just as hard to get some or all of those aspects of health education *out* of the school curriculum.

Categorical health problems or behaviors are generally subsumed under one of the ten principal content areas but have particular relevance and implications for others. Sexual behavior has its roots in Family Life, but related concepts and problems are touched on significantly in other areas of the curriculum, such as Personal Health, Mental Health, Disease Prevention and Control, and Drug Abuse. Categorical health problems may or may not be controversial, but they do tend to be those about which there is greatest public and personal concern. For example, currently, there is little or no argument contesting the value of health education in schools as an important defensive weapon against HIV infection.

Any controversy stems from its unavoidable association with aspects of human behavior that some find objectionable or inappropriate for discussion with students.

Chapter 5 asserts that effective curriculum guides and lesson plans require attention to process-oriented rather than subject-oriented teaching. The goal is for the student to become engaged both cognitively and affectively in the subject matter being studied. In no other area of the curriculum will these planning skills be more critical than in implementing the content of lessons covering sensitive and private health-related personal behaviors. Although eating habits are personal and unique, nutrition is an accepted aspect of the health education curriculum. Yet eating habits are also public, acquired through imitative behavior (from parents and peers) and influenced by preferences of the family and its culture. The understandings and teachings about our sexuality, in contrast, are representative of the accumulation of nonpublic experiences and feelings that most often are not addressed by the family and almost never enacted (in the case of sexual intercourse) deliberately by parents for imitation by their children. In addition, nonverbal cues of family sex-related beliefs, either restrictive or approving, influence children's sexuality.

Other subjects besides sexuality and its related areas are just as intimate, personal, and private. Preventive approaches to such topics, intended to promote health, frequently are opposed by parents, community, and some school personnel. Why is this so in a nation so committed to staying healthy? It may be because most people don't think about their health until they lose it and because financial and governmental support is committed to treating rather than preventing disease. Another reason that the notions of prevention or health promotion have not been widely supported is that most people consider personal health to be solely a private matter, and they perceive education or information about health as an intrusion in their private lives. These individuals or groups often perceive health topics in general (from nutrition and safety to all or any references to reproduction or to sexuality) to be controversial.

It is impossible for any health education program to meet the needs and expectations of every parent and ethnic or cultural group. Therefore the existence of some areas of controversy, or the expression of opposing views, is highly possible if not inevitable. Yet controversy surrounding all or part of a health education program is not always bad for the program. Effectively managed, controversy can result in a stronger program that is more widely accepted and endorsed. It can also destroy part of a program or the entire program. The key ingredient for success in handling controversy is parental involvement and support.

SOURCES OF CONTROVERSY

Sources of controversy in health education are varied and complex. Several disputed areas included in the school's curriculum are considered in this chapter, many of which concern sexuality education, since this is the most difficult and significant controversial area. However, this emphasis does not obviate the importance of controversy in other areas. There is a long history of criticisms of topics that touch on personal health behaviors dating back to the early 1900s. Each generation of educators has had to recognize, respect, and attempt to overcome or negotiate such opposing views. It is an ongoing effort that must be continued over time if comprehensive health education programs are to continue as part of the school curriculum. Some community members may be just as concerned today about education in controversial areas, and teachers must be aware of possible conflicts involving personal values whenever such subjects are taught. Remember that the principles and practices to be discussed in this chapter are applicable to all areas of controversy in health teaching. Basic disagreements by parents and some community groups over each controversial area listed center around a number of common themes.

Fears That Sex Education Threatens Parental Rights

Many opposed to sexuality education in the schools are concerned that schools intend to take over the role of the parent as the primary sex educator. Proponents claim there is no basis for this fear and that the schools would only serve as a supplement to the education received at home. Gordon (7) and Brick (1) support this view; Gordon explains (7):

> The *primary* responsibility for educating children about sexuality from birth to adulthood always has been, and must remain, in the home. Parents provide love, warmth and caring that are the foundation of many future values and attitudes concerning sexuality; and family life is strengthened by parents who take an active role in communicating with their own children.

Researchers have found that peers often rank first as the source of information about sex, and, as can be imagined, the information from peers is often distorted. In the past this peer influence has been deplored. However, it is a fact that children, and many adults, turn to their friends and colleagues for health information before they seek traditional health care. Peer input is part of the fabric of a young person's life. It offers opportunities to debate values and express opinions about sexuality; drugs; STDs, including HIV; violence; home life; or whatever the group dynamic produces. Undue influence can only be balanced with what happens when parents, the schools, and community groups provide an alternate experience (5).

In a study of 1,152 teenagers, Thornburg found that the sources of sexual information after peers, in order of frequency, were literature, mothers, schools, experience, fathers, physicians, and religious leaders (19). Clearly, parents, schools, and religious leaders all should have a greater influence than that study indicates if they are to help children become responsible and sensitive adults in regard to sexuality.

MISCONCEPTIONS REGARDING VALUES-RELATED TEACHING STRATEGIES

Another frequently controversial issue revolves around how morals and values should be handled in the classroom. A value is a preference for an idea, thing, or behavior held by individuals and groups. There is the conviction that a certain idea or behavior is "right," at least for that individual or group. The problem is the lack of agreement regarding which or whose values are right for all of society. Although some values are generally accepted, diverse opinions exist in many areas of education. It is therefore difficult for a teacher to know how to address value-related ideas and behaviors in controversial areas of teaching.

There are two basic approaches to handling values regarding sexuality education in the classroom. One is to avoid dealing with values at all and teach only the biology of human reproduction, referring all other matters to parents. Many schools adopting this approach as a way to avoid controversy have been criticized and accused of teaching students the "what" of reproduction but giving them no direction and setting no limits (4). It is, however, an approach commonly employed in schools throughout the United States.

The other approach involves a methodology that helps children clarify for themselves what they value. This is different from trying to tell or persuade children what they value (16). Children are encouraged to investigate the values held by their family, religion, and culture and to use this information in deciding for themselves what they value. McNab explains (11): "The task of the sexuality educator is to present accurate information about sexuality so that individuals, based upon their cultural, religious, ethnical, and familial upbringing, can make responsible decisions regarding their own sexuality." Scales (17) also believes that the examination of values, in addition to factual information, is essential to sexuality education, and he adds the dimension of skill development. He says that increased communication and decision-making skills of young

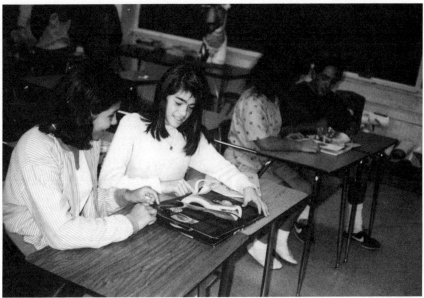

Matt Fischer

The biology of human reproduction is a commonly employed approach to human sexuality instruction.

people help them deal not only with sexual matters but also with all aspects of life. Young people practiced in these skills will have a heightened ability to make decisions concerning ethical behavior, to follow what they believe and support, to resist peer pressure, and to say no when that is what they believe is right.

A teacher should never try to impose a value system on children. Ideally, a school district policy should determine the fundamental or at least the publicly expressed values regarding sexuality education on which most community members agree. If such a list is formulated in a district, then a teacher is provided with written guidelines to the value system held by the district and community regarding sexuality education. Such a document provides the teacher direction and parameters for teaching in this controversial area. A modified list of such values or beliefs developed by Scales (17) is an example of fundamental values underlying contemporary sexuality education (see box on p. 152). This list exemplifies the kind of document that might be adopted by the

governing body of a school district as guidelines in determining its sexuality education program.

Scales listed the following other values that are appropriate for district staff and community members to consider when establishing a sexuality program:

1. Parents are the primary sexuality educators of their children, and schools and churches should supplement this role.
2. School districts should involve parents, students, and other community members in planning sexuality programs.
3. School districts should use trained health teachers who exhibit the highest standards of professional ethics and participate in regular continuing education programs.
4. In our society a wide range of values and beliefs about sexuality is to be expected.

The Fallacy of Sexuality Education Fostering Sexual Activity

There is a commonly accepted belief that if children are not told about sex, they will not become

> ## FUNDAMENTAL VALUES UNDERLYING CONTEMPORARY SEXUALITY EDUCATION
>
> 1. Sexuality is more than sex.
> 2. Knowledge and information about sexuality and family planning are essential.
> 3. It is important to examine one's own values in the area of sexuality and to respect the differing values of others.
> 4. Self-esteem is essential in making healthy and responsible decisions about sexual matters.
> 5. Each sexual decision has an effect or consequence.
> 6. Given the medical, psychological, and social ramifications of sexual intercourse, young teenagers are usually not ready for sexual intercourse.
> 7. It is wrong to exploit or to force someone into an unwanted sexual experience ("It's okay to say no").
> 8. It is beneficial when children can feel comfortable discussing sexual matters with parents and other valued adults.
> 9. Parenthood requires many responsibilities that adolescents are usually unable to assume and capabilities they usually do not have.

sexually active. It is also often expressed as: "If children are taught about sexuality, they are being taught how to have sex." Research demonstrates that neither case is true and that the more information children have about it, the less likely they are to experiment (7). Generally, it is agreed that children need a source of sexual information other than peers to be sure that they receive accurate information. Knowledge is always better than ignorance.

During the 1940s and 1950s there was some general public agreement that abusive and addictive behaviors were limited to the uneducated, underprivileged, unclean, and mostly nonwhite populations. Consequently there was no need for children in school to learn about these problems.

However, newly published data reveal that at that time drug use, teenage pregnancy, and child abuse crossed all demographic boundaries (meaning middle and upper class families) and had occurred for many decades. Protective parents found themselves overruled by public demands for special school and community programs to address these issues.

PARENTAL FEARS THAT THEIR OWN PROBLEM BEHAVIORS MIGHT BE EXPOSED

There are emotional overtones to all controversial topics, which for some parents cause deep anxiety and fear that they project onto their children. Parents who have had drug or alcohol addictions, unwanted pregnancies, eating disorders, or history of other abuse appear to be particularly threatened by classroom teaching about any such sensitive topics. Because they are secretive or feeling guilty, they fear that their children will want to discuss their school subjects or will suspect that their parents have or have had such problems.

UNREALISTIC EXPECTATIONS FOR SOLUTIONS

There are sometimes expectations that if a topic deals with a personal problem behavior, the problem will be "cured" or alleviated at the completion of the course. The school may be expected to show proof that this is the case. Teachers of civics cannot prove that their former students are now registered voters, which would at minimum demonstrate one expected outcome of such teaching that could be measured. The fact that voter registrations over the past 25 years has decreased has not brought demands that civics courses be removed from the curriculum. English courses being taught every year despite the falling literacy rate in the United States is another example. Few studies about drug use or sexual behavior can demonstrate that specific, related programs for elementary school children will prevent drug abuse or unwanted pregnancy in the future. However, at the late preteen and teenage level where a small number of programs were scientifically tracked, the pregnancy rate was shown to decrease (18).

AVOIDING PROBLEMS WHEN TEACHING CONTROVERSIAL TOPICS

First and foremost, school teachers must remember that they are employed by a school district and must follow the guidelines established by the district. Some teachers who have had problems in sensitive areas of the health curriculum have taken things into their own hands "for the good of the children." One example is a teacher suggesting to students that they "forget" to take home a letter notifying the parents of an upcoming lesson if they think their parents might object. Another is a teacher who decides that the approved text leaves out too much important information and brings in unapproved materials to help the children "really" understand the process of reproduction. In situations like these, the actions of one teacher can jeopardize an entire program or destroy a long-established one. In the long run, it is the children who are deprived of the education they need.

Problems teachers encounter while teaching sex education are described in Gilbert's thought-provoking list of "no-nos" (6). He says,

Without exception these teachers have been well meaning and have had the best interest of their students at heart. Poor judgment on their part, however, has often resulted in placing their sex education programs in jeopardy. Many supporters of sex education have become non-supporters because of incidents involving poor judgment.

The list offered in the box is by no means complete, but these points illustrate his argument.

THE HIV-AIDS EPIDEMIC

Teaching children how to avoid contact with a deadly virus should not be controversial. However, because the spread of HIV most often involves sexual contact or use of hypodermic needles to inject certain drugs, teaching about AIDS prevention is controversial by association. Currently, educators, public health officials, and policy makers are scrambling to address the AIDS crisis appropriately. However, there is still concern and controversy about the educational aspects of AIDS prevention, particularly regarding elementary school students. Even though the vast majority of elementary school students do not engage in high-risk behaviors for contracting HIV, programs specifically designed to be age-appropriate and to help keep them HIV-free are necessary. The US Centers for Disease Control (CDC) recommends that (3):

School systems should make programs available that will enable and encourage young people who *have not* engaged in sexual intercourse and who *have not* used illicit drugs to continue to—
- Abstain from sexual intercourse until they are ready to establish a mutually monogamous relationship within the context of marriage.
- Refrain from using or injecting illicit drugs.

Certainly all parents, educators, and public health officials agree that it is in the best interest of children and young people to abstain from sexual intercourse and from injecting drugs. Such responsible behavior prevents the spread of HIV, prevents teenage pregnancy, and promotes a healthier, drug-free lifestyle. Why then is there any controversy around AIDS education? The fact is that despite the rational reasons for saying no to sex and drugs, many young people engage in these risky behaviors.

The ultimate questions for educators and parents are: How should specific information be presented to students? At what age should it be provided and by whom? The answers to these questions need to be carefully considered by communities and schools. Some suggestions follow.

AIDS-Related Content

For children at the primary level, "AIDS education" consists of basic health education. It does

EASY WAYS OF GETTING INTO TROUBLE WHEN TEACHING SEX EDUCATION

1. *Teaching sex education with inadequate background.* Sex education is one of the few areas where teachers are held strictly accountable for what they teach. Let teachers of sex education make an error and you can bet they will hear of it. It isn't that they shouldn't be held accountable, because they certainly should, but such accountability is rare in education and a major challenge for sex educators. There are few nondedicated teachers teaching sex education for long, since it is a great deal of hard work. It requires a thorough background in the subject matter and continual reading to keep up to date. Making content errors will quickly result in lost credibility with students, parents, colleagues, administrators, and draw the fire of the anti-sex education group.

2. *Keeping your principal or administrator in the dark.* It is imperative that your principals and administrators be apprised of what is happening in your classroom. Keeping the appropriate administrator up to date for some will mean just a statement that your class is now studying sex education. For others it may mean detailed lesson plans from which you are not to deviate.

3. *Giving "secret" lessons.* A surefire way to get into trouble is to have secret lessons with students. Make a statement such as "Today's lesson is just between you and me—it is our little secret" and you can be certain many parents will hear of it. Never teach material you cannot defend as approved.

4. *Ignoring district or school policy.* This is clearly a violation of your responsibility as a teacher. Curriculum guides are set up to give you parameters to work within. In a general sense they reflect the wishes of the community. You must stay within those parameters no matter what you believe is "good" for your students. If you don't agree with the curriculum, you should certainly work to change it, and a great many curricula need improvement. Until you get it changed, however, you are bound by contract to reflect the existing curriculum.

5. *Using poorly constructed, home-made materials.* Parents especially do not find a poorly constructed penis model or free-hand drawings of genitalia appropriate or necessary especially for preteen students. Using anatomical drawings is certainly a legitimate exercise but use professional work duplicated for use with your students.

6. *Using questionable language.* Slang terminology is often all that children know of reproductive anatomy and physiology. They should not be reprimanded for using such terminology unless they use it deliberately to create a disturbance but should simply be taught the correct terms. Teachers who use slang terms generally to "get on their level" may soon be unemployed.

7. *Not previewing films or materials.* There should be a district committee to approve films, and you are courting disaster if you use any not on the approved list. It is always wise to preview films, but it is essential in sex education. One teacher who was not teaching health education by choice and consequently used a large number of films ordered the district approved-for-high-school film, "The Story of Eric" (an excellent film on Lamaze childbirth) for his class. As the film progressed he was not aware that an actual childbirth was included. Too late, he jumped in front of the projector, and his class witnessed a childbirth in vivid color on his white shirt! He had not previewed his film and was not qualified or willing to discuss childbirth.

8. *Not being prepared for opposition.* Most programs that are properly established suffer little opposition because the vast majority of Americans support sex education, but many programs have been attacked. All teachers should be able to verbalize the need for sex education when called on and should anticipate such encounters. Parents will have honest questions, and they deserve sincere, well-documented answers.

9. *Teaching by the joke.* Several instructors have gotten into trouble by telling or allowing students to tell "off-color" jokes in the classroom. Teachers telling inappropriate jokes can give the sex education classroom an improper atmosphere and denigrate sexuality at the same time.

Continued.

10. *Setting unrealistic goals.* Many programs have been set up with stated goals and objectives for the elimination of STDs divorce, and so on. Programs with unrealistic goals are often doomed to failure. A good example of this is when a program is expected to lower the STD rate. When a good sex education program is established, the STD rate often goes up! The reason for this increase is that people recognize signs and symptoms and go in for treatment. The rate may go down eventually, but it takes time and a more comprehensive curriculum than can be provided by so narrow a focus on any one human problem.

11. *Forcing teachers to teach sex education.* Mandating that all teachers must teach sex education is unwise. Assigning any teacher at all to teach health education leads to poor quality education and can lead to disaster. Many teachers will never be comfortable teaching sex education. Unwilling or embarrassed teachers can be turned to an anti-sex education position and should not be expected to serve as its advocate.

12. *Letting personal bias influence teaching.* Everyone knows what normal sexual behavior is—it is the way *they* behave. Open marriage, marriage at all costs, or any other lifestyle has no business being promoted in the classroom. We are all biased in some way. Recognize that bias and be careful not to try to convert your students.

13. *Using inappropriate guest speakers.* The selection of guest speakers must be done with great care. Inviting right-to-life groups to class with brutal pictures can be a traumatic experience for students. Certainly the antiabortion groups should have the right to express their point of view, but you as a teacher have the right and responsibility to screen how it is done. Inviting homosexuals to a junior high or high-school class is another example of an easy way to get into trouble. Certainly, they have the right to express their opinion, but the problem thus created might jeopardize a total program. Be sure you are clear on district policy before you allow guest speakers to visit your class. If the speaker's credentials and expertise matches the needs and interests of your students, inform the principal of the impending visit, as well as the subject matter that will be presented. Stay in control during the presentation to ensure that student questions don't lead to an inappropriate change in the subject matter.

14. *Citing personal sexual experience.* It may be difficult to believe that teachers need to be reminded that this is not okay, but it happens. Do not let students push you into discussing your personal life. It has no place in the classroom.

15. *Using nonapproved questionnaires of students' sexual experiences.* Finding out what is actually going on with your students may seem to be a good place to start your program. Your principal or administrator is likely to think differently. Remember that such questionnaires may be construed as a reflection of the performance of the school or district as a whole. Be certain to clear all questionnaires you use. They may provide useful information, but be careful they don't cost you your job or hurt the reputation of your school.

16. *Leaving nonapproved reading matter out for public view.* It is acceptable for you as a teacher to read anything you wish, but remember that the district has approved the materials for use with students. Do not leave nonapproved matter out where a student might it pick up or where an outsider might view it. Ask yourself if you are unnecessarily endangering your sex education program. Sex education is too important to be eliminated or watered down because of mistakes in judgment.

These situations offer sound and common sense advice to the classroom teacher of any subject, not just sexuality education. Unfortunately these experiences are not unusual. It is easy to see that some parents may have a legitimate concern. Teachers, administrators, and all health professionals need to ask themselves if they are part of the solution or the problem.

Modified from Gilbert G: *Health Educ.* 10(5):31, 1979.

not need to nor should it be explicit to AIDS. It should be age-appropriate and consistent with the developmental level of the child and woven into a planned comprehensive health education program. Although a detailed explanation of how HIV infection is acquired is not appropriate at the primary level, basic health concepts can serve as building blocks for later AIDS education. By laying a careful foundation of understanding of basic hygiene, we can give young children the tools they need for later, more sophisticated explanations of AIDS and other health issues. The CDC guidelines (3) do suggest some specific content for the primary level, saying: "Education about AIDS in early elementary grades should be designed to allay excessive fears of the epidemic and of becoming infected." For example,

- AIDS is a disease that is causing some adults to get very sick, but it does not commonly affect children.
- AIDS is very hard to get. You cannot get it just by being near or touching someone who has it.
- Scientists all over the world are working hard to find a way to stop people from getting AIDS and to cure those who have it.

Largely, the elementary teacher needs to be able to answer the questions about AIDS that will undoubtedly arise in the classroom. To respond to students appropriately, teachers must know and adhere to established district guidelines. Also, teachers must be comfortable enough with basic content about AIDS to answer questions calmly and knowledgeably.

For students in upper elementary and middle schools, the content addressed becomes more specific. However, "AIDS education" is still best taught within a planned comprehensive health education program. The CDC (3) recommends the following information be included in the curriculum:

- Viruses are living organisms too small to be seen by the unaided eye.
- Viruses can be transmitted from an infected person to an uninfected person through various means.

- Some viruses cause disease among people.
- Persons who are infected with some viruses that cause disease may not have any signs or symptoms of disease.
- AIDS (an abbreviation for *a*cquired *im*muno *d*eficiency *s*yndrome) is caused by a virus (HIV) that weakens the ability of infected individuals to fight off disease.
- People who have AIDS often develop a rare type of severe pneumonia, a cancer called Kaposi's sarcoma, and certain other diseases that healthy people normally do not get.
- About 1 to 1.5 million of the total population of approximately 240 million Americans currently are infected with HIV and consequently are capable of infecting others.
- People who are infected with HIV live in every state in the United States and in most other countries of the world. Infected people live in cities, as well as suburbs, small towns, and rural areas. Although most infected people are adults, teenagers can also become infected. Females, as well as males, are infected. People of every race are infected, including whites, blacks, Hispanics, Native Americans, and Asian/Pacific Islanders.
- HIV can be transmitted by sexual contact with an infected person, by using needles and other injection equipment that an infected person has used, and from an infected mother to her infant before or during birth.
- A small number of doctors, nurses, and other medical personnel have been infected when they were directly exposed to infected blood.
- It sometimes takes several years after becoming infected with HIV before symptoms of AIDS appear. Thus people who are infected with the virus can infect other people—even though the people who transmit the infection do not feel or look sick.
- Most infected people who develop symp-

toms of AIDS only live about 2 years after their symptoms are diagnosed.

- HIV cannot be caught by touching someone who is infected, by being in the same room with an infected person, or by donating blood.

The important theme for students in upper elementary and middle school involves understanding the nature of viruses in general and HIV specifically. This is fundamental to understanding the risk of HIV infection and the importance of preventive measures. For more detailed content concerning AIDS and HIV, see Chapter 14.

ADDICTIVE BEHAVIORS

Educating students to adopt responsible, nonabusive behavior related to drugs is an established aspect of the elementary health curriculum. Today the problem is even more critical because of the relationship between injecting illegal drugs and HIV transmission. Beyond the health-threatening aspects of intravenous drug use, there is also now the potential for acquiring HIV infection at the same time. Students need to learn that sharing needles between an infected person and a noninfected person amounts to a direct inoculation of the virus. Today, drug education programs, more often called prevention and intervention programs, are becoming important elements in elementary and middle school curricula across the nation. In 1986, the US Department of Education circulated *What Works: Schools Without Drugs* throughout the educational community and to every school in the country (20). This short book has been helpful to teachers in the effort to rid schools and communities of illicit drug use and alcohol abuse.

In the past, controversy affecting drug education in schools has often focused on the concern that education about drugs would encourage student experimentation. While this is still the concern of some educators and parents, the thrust of educational efforts has changed. Few programs consist of tedious studies of all the various drugs of abuse and their effects. Current approaches seek to help students build self-esteem and develop decision-making and refusal skills so that they can say "no" to drugs because they mean it and want to.

Following the guidelines outlined in *Schools Without Drugs*, many schools have implemented programs that involve the community and law enforcement (20). The document recommends that school districts set specific policies to clarify rules regarding drug use and include strong corrective actions. Teachers have the responsibility to understand and enforce the policies that are established by district officials. Care and sensitivity need to be given to students who come from homes where drugs of some sort are in use. The educational process should not promote guilt and fear among young people living in a home where parents use alcohol or other social drugs. Teachers should be aware of the possible difficulty that students in these situations face. These difficulties can range from uneasiness in hearing that their parents are involved in a behavior that is "wrong" to abuse situations related to drug use by parents or siblings. At all times it is the responsibility of the teacher to be sensitive to these situations and to be prepared to refer students for qualified counselling if necessary.

Legal Procedures for Combating Drug Use on School Grounds

Search and seizure of student lockers and desks is becoming more and more common in schools across the country. In the effort to rid our schools and communities of drugs, teachers and administrators have found themselves in the uneasy position of enforcer. Controversy over Fourth Amendment rights has taken search and seizure questions to the Supreme Court. A summary of the decisions regarding this issue follows (20):

- *What legal standard applies to school officials who search students and their possessions for drugs?*

  The Supreme Court has held that school officials may institute a search if there are "reasonable grounds" to believe that the search will reveal evidence that the student has violated or is violating either the law or the rules of the school.

- *Do school officials need a search warrant to conduct a search for drugs?*
  No, not if they are carrying out the search independent of the police and other law enforcement officials. A more stringent legal standard may apply if law enforcement officials are involved in the search.

- *How extensive can a search be?*
  The scope of the permissible search depends on whether the measures used during the search are reasonably related to the purpose of the search and are not excessively intrusive in light of the age and sex of the student being searched. The more intrusive the search, the greater the justification that will be required by the courts.

- *Do school officials have to stop a search when they find the object of the search?*
  Not necessarily. If a search reveals items suggesting the presence of other evidence of crime or misconduct, the school official may continue the search. For example, if a teacher is justifiably searching a student's purse for cigarettes and finds rolling papers, it will be reasonable (subject to any local policy to the contrary) for the teacher to search the rest of the purse for evidence of drugs.

- *Can school officials search student lockers?*
  Reasonable grounds to believe that a particular student locker contains evidence of a violation of the law or school rules generally justifies a search of that locker. In addition, some courts have upheld written school policies that authorize school officials to inspect student lockers at any time. Individual teachers should not take search and seizure tactics into their own hands. Any such action should be handled by administrators under the direction of the elected school officials. Policies and guidelines regarding these procedures must be established by local school boards of education (20).

EFFECTS OF CONTROVERSY ON SCHOOLS

Schools are run by school boards that are elected locally and are ultimately responsible for everything that happens in the district. In the United States the greatest amount of authority for education rests on the shoulders of local officials. Each school board must adhere to state mandates and laws, and "strings" usually are attached to state and federal money. But for the most part school districts are run by the community.

This local autonomy in the educational system of the United States can be positive in effect in that a school board can implement programs uniquely suited to the children in that specific district. Parents can have easy access to the board members because they are members of the community and often neighbors and friends, particularly in smaller school districts. However, this easy access to school board members sometimes results in drastic program changes as a result of controversy. Many times a program change is needed, but in other cases a vocal minority of the community can effect changes in school programs that do not represent the wishes of the majority. Most proponents of sexuality education have found that the great majority of people in the community favor such a program; however, often this positive preference is not communicated to the school board. A small but vocal and zealous group can pack a board room and make demands, which can be overwhelming for board members. If policies have not been established for making changes in the school curriculum, the school board may be persuaded to act on the concerns of a minority group without receiving input from other representatives of the community. For example, in one district a film was being considered for the sixth grade family life unit. Before recommending the film the health education committee (which consisted of teachers, administrators, and a school nurse) wanted to show it to the sixth grade parents. Eight hundred parents viewed the film and expressed their opinions on its possible inclusion in the program. Eighty-five percent of the parents surveyed approved of the film, so it was used in the unit. After a few apparently successful years of using the film, suddenly it was banned by the school board. On the night the board met, as usual, the relatively small room was packed with people, instead of the usual 10 to 20 persons. A vocal group of about 50 people demanded that the film be dropped from the sixth grade family life program because they objected to one frame of the film and one sentence of the sound track. The school board panicked and voted to drop the film from the program that night. There was no policy requiring that such changes be reviewed by a committee of advisors representing a cross section of community members, and there were no community representatives as voting members of the health education committee. Thus the result of controversy, in a district serving over 20,000 students, was that 50 people effected a change that did not represent the desire of the majority of parents surveyed.

CONSTRUCTIVE WAYS OF DEALING WITH CONTROVERSY

Fear of opposition to educational programs and materials is very real to district administrators, teachers, and board members. However, it is unlikely that opposition to some programs or materials, not only those for sexuality education, can be entirely avoided in a district. The way to deal with controversy is to know how to manage it, not to avoid it. Scales said, "It is apparent that moral conflict and political authority are at the heart of sex education controversies. Managing discontent, rather than trying to stifle it, is the key to success" (17). This can be applied to all curriculum issues. The following sections offer

suggestions to school district officials wishing to manage controversy.

Become Informed

Keeping apprised of the issues and concerns common to both national and local political efforts is essential for the school. It is naive to think that local communities are not affected by national issues. How other districts handle conflicts associated with these issues can be helpful in determining policies.

Review Current Policies

School policies are written procedures that have been adopted by the school board and must be followed by district employees. The district should have an explicit policy for the selection of materials, development and implementation of curriculums, how complaints are handled, and how teachers are selected to teach sensitive topics. If policies do not exist or are vague, a process for their development should be outlined. Examples of policies regarding selection and reconsideration of materials used in the classroom are presented in the box below and the box on p. 160.

THE SCHOOL SYSTEM'S POLICY ON MATERIALS SELECTION

The school system's policy on materials selection should include the following:
1. A statement on the school system's philosophy of resource and material selection.
2. A statement on the legal responsibility of the governing board and the delegation of authority to district personnel.
3. A description of resources and materials covered by the selection policy.
4. A listing of criteria for selection of all resources and materials.
5. A statement that all items will meet established criteria.
6. Procedures for selection.

THE SCHOOL SYSTEM'S POLICY ON RECONSIDERATION

The school system's policy on reconsideration should include the following:

1. A statement that the procedure applies to all requests for reconsideration (including those from school personnel and school board members).
2. The name of the person to whom the request for reconsideration should be directed.
3. An explanation of the use of the request for reconsideration.
4. An explanation of the reconsideration committee: names of members, how and when they are chosen or elected, length of terms, and so on.
5. An outline of the process used by the reconsideration committee with an indication of how long the process takes.
6. A statement about the status during the reconsideration process of the resource being questioned.

7. Criteria for the reevaluation of resources and materials.
8. A statement that the decision reached by the committee is to be based on the established criteria.
9. A statement indicating to whom the decision of the reconsideration committee is communicated (that is, the school board and the superintendent).
10. A statement of whether the decision relates to one grade level, one school, or the entire district.
11. A statement of whether the same resources or materials will be reconsidered more than once during a specified time period.
12. A provision for appeal of the decision.

Set Up a Curriculum Advisory Committee

The most productive vehicle for support of all educational programs, particularly those that may be controversial, is a curriculum advisory committee. Such a committee is usually comprised of representatives from the school district and community who recommend guidelines and execute subsequent board policies for the use of specific teaching methodology and materials. The committee should have the authority it needs to be effective. Hot issues should be discussed by the representative committee, rather than in a forum open to the entire community. There should also be a specific policy on the way issues are brought to the committee.

It is essential that all segments of the community are represented in the committee, including parents, students, and other interested citi-

zens. It is wise to involve parent-teacher groups in this effort, such as the National Congress of Parents and Teachers (NCPT), which has been participating in health education efforts throughout the United States since 1898 (2). Any vocal minority that may be opposed to certain educational programs or materials also should be represented. As Wagman and Bignell (21) have said:

> Most concerns about sex education stem not from opposition to sex education itself, but from a lack of understanding and/or mistrust of the particular program being presented by the school. If parents have been involved in program development, they will be more likely to trust the program.

Unfortunately there may also be a group of parents basically opposed to any sexuality education program. Their objectives do not arise entirely from personal, moral, or religious beliefs but are guided by political motives. This motive is to discredit the educational system in a particular community or district in order to later control it. These groups choose to demonstrate that the sexuality or other disputed health topics are *noneducational* subjects that the school system has irresponsibly included in the curriculum. Therefore the school system is being run incompetently and should have new Board members and new administration. This kind of attack situation is true for all health education programs, not only those for sexuality education.

Be Consistent and Calm

Once a policy has been agreed on, it should be followed consistently. If the process used to develop the policy included wide representation from the community, school personnel, and students, it should be sound. Policies should be flexible and changeable but not at whim nor without due process. Be calm and avoid shouting matches with concerned individuals. It is important to understand that they have a right to their point of view. Stay calm by standing firm on the policy established. Explain that any change in policy must follow certain procedures.

Hire Qualified Health Teachers or Health Supervisors

For potentially controversial subjects (such as sexuality education, AIDS education, drug education, and death education), qualified teachers should be hired or trained. Teachers should not be forced to teach these subjects if they do not desire to do so nor should they teach in these areas if they are not adequately prepared. At the elementary level, teachers with preservice experience in health teaching should be provided continuing inservice activities developed by a district health education supervisors. It is recommended that full-time school health teaching specialists be assigned this responsibility in middle schools.

Inform Rather Than Advertise

The community must be kept apprised of the programs and stands the district takes, but this is not the same as looking for attention. Informing parents of the sexuality education curriculum and urging them to review materials is one thing; issuing a press release announcing a new and wonderful comprehensive sexuality education program is quite another.

All state laws must be adhered to regarding notification to parents about sensitive topics taught in schools. This usually involves a letter to the parents explaining the program and inviting them to review the materials used. It is important to let parents know that other curriculum material besides health topics are also reviewed in this manner. As much as possible they should feel that the reviews are routine, rather than a special case. Most states allow students to be removed from classes if the parent wishes. No matter what the state law is regarding notification, every *effort* should be made to inform parents and to *remove* a child from a class if the parents request it. Appendix D is a sample letter to parents that announces future sessions dealing with sex education and STDs.

Few students will be denied parental permission to attend the class. However, in the event of even one such exclusion, the teacher must not forget the school's obligation to teach the same material to any youngster who must spend the class time in the library. Take time to prepare a contract that specifies materials the student is to read and the nature of a meaningful report or other product that is to be prepared and submitted at the end of the unit of study. Ask the student to read and sign his/her copy, as well as obtain the signature of the parents so that they are aware of the provisions that have been made in their child's behalf.

The Five Ps of Education

The categorical and controversial subject areas discussed in this chapter are but a few of those that may be included in a comprehensive health education curriculum. It is important for educators, parents, and the community to recognize that students of all ages receive many other "educations," both positive and negative, from other sources. Including the public school program, these major forces follow.

Parent Education. Whether or not parents ever say a word about sex; drugs; assault; STDs, including HIV; or any other health/risk behavior, they educate their children by their attitudes, affection, beliefs, and actions that provide verbal and nonverbal, positive or negative learning experiences. This is part of the parental contract that many parents are unaware that they agreed to when they became parents.

Peer Education. This is consistently the most authentic and authoritative education that individuals between 6 and 20 years of age receive. It is probably the most significant at any age. In over three decades that studies have been carried out, 80% of college-age students volunteer that as they grew up, their sex, drug, and alcohol information came from their friends, before or during their middle school years.

Public Media Education. There are almost no subjects of a controversial nature that have not been seen or discussed via radio, TV, magazines, books, and newspapers. These disclosures vary from the most thoughtful, research-backed presentations to the most blatant, sensational, manipulative, and commercial presentations permitted. Such words and images, both enlightening and distorting, permeate the learning atmosphere for most children throughout their early years. It is a powerful, if confusing, teaching/learning experience.

Public School Education. Like parents, the school system teaches categorical subjects whether or not the educators and staff desire to do so and whether or not these areas are ever presented in a classroom. Silence about these topics or their absence in the health curriculum conveys its own message to students. The message is that the system in which they are being taught is unaware of their needs, concerns, and interests; does not care about them; or deems the subjects too embarrassing or unfit for classroom discussion. It also demonstrates lack of trust in the learning abilities of its students.

Planned Public or Community Education. The fifth basic P may be still evolving in most communities. This concept allows all the previously listed education to continue (because it will) but strives to bring together all of the participants (parents, students, community leaders, professional educators, school administrators, and local media personnel) to develop comprehensive health education. Long-range goals would be to integrate the controversial topics into broader health education programs in the schools and to plan a similar community health education program in which parents, youth groups and church leaders, and the public would benefit.

SUMMARY

Effective health teaching is based on known human behavior and needs. That's the problem. Human needs are personal, often intimate, and therefore emotion charged. Categorical health problems such as addictive behaviors (use and abuse of alcohol, tobacco and other drugs), problem sexual behaviors, and other topics such as masturbation, teenage suicide, child abuse, sex education, death and dying education, and more are being urged on the schools by as many pressure groups. Other pressure groups are working just as hard to get some of those aspects *out* of the school curriculum. Inevitably there will be dissension in some areas because it is impossible for any health program to meet the demands of every parent or ethnic/cultural group represented in a school district.

The sources of controversy vary, but conflicts involving personal values are most often involved when such topics are taught in schools. Parents fear that their own authority over their children is being threatened. Some believe that discussion of personal values and morals does not belong in a classroom. There is concern that students will be motivated rather than deterred from experimentation with sex and drugs as a result of health education. Invasion of the privacy of the home and possible disclosure of certain parental past or present health-related behaviors is a common worry. Some parents demand that the school prove the efficacy of education planned to prevent illness or promote wellness.

The chapter provides many down-to-earth suggestions on ways to avoid problems in teaching about human sexuality. Guidelines and basic concepts direct development of a HIV/AIDs curriculum that meets recommendations for preventive learning activities while avoiding controversy. The dangerous link between intravenous drug use and HIV infection is explained. Legal procedures for the school personnel's use in combating drug use on campus are listed and described.

The role of local control of schools is discussed with attention to the effect of organized minority groups where there are no established policies in place to provide stability to board decisions.

Constructive ways of managing controversy if it occurs include:

- Being informed about controversial issues.
- Making certain that policies have been set governing textbook adoption, ways to handle complaints, development and implementation of a curriculum, and assignment of teachers for sensitive subjects.
- Setting up a curriculum committee representative of the entire community with authority to make recommendations that will be given serious consideration.
- Being consistent in following established policies.
- Being calm and considerate when dealing with individuals whose opinions differ from yours.
- Hiring qualified health educators whenever possible.
- Keeping parents and the community fully informed of new programs as they are developed and implemented.

Finally, be aware of the pervasive influence of the five Ps. (5). These are major educational forces that affect learning all the time, whether positively or negatively, and must be taken into account when planning a curriculum for health education. They include parents, peers, public media, public school education, and planned public, or community, education.

QUESTIONS AND EXERCISES
Discussion questions

1. Explain why the potential for controversy is so much greater in health teaching than for any other subject area considered in the public school curriculum.

2. Most schools ask parents to sign a note permitting their child to participate in planned sex education class sessions. For those youngsters what difficulties do you see as the class later covers problems such as STDs, including HIV infection; unwanted pregnancy; and abortion. How could you be sure that the subsequent learning activities were as effective for the entire class as for those excluded from the sex education unit of the curriculum?

3. In your own experience was the most effective sex education from your parents, your friends, your church, or other community-based group? Could the sex education you received at school be more effective, and if so how would you change and improve that instruction?

4. Why is the need for process-oriented lesson plans greater in connection with health behaviors that are personal and private?

5. Explain the difference between the condition termed *HIV positive* and a diagnosis of *AIDS*.

6. If you were asked to set up a health curriculum advisory group, whom would you select from among your colleagues in other disciplines? Whom would you want to represent the students in the health classes, and what community organizations you would want represented? Describe the special contribution you would expect of each member of the selected group.

7. Among the five Ps of education, studies show that probably the most significant is peer education. What could you do as a teacher with responsibility for health instruction to promote the quality of the information that your students gained from that source?

8. What do you see as the impact of practice in problem-solving and decision-making skills on the

every day behavior and related choices young people must make every day?

Problems and exercises

1. Interview a proponent and an opponent of sexuality or HIV/AIDS education in the schools. Then write a report presenting both views. Be as objective in your report as you can. Ask yourself, "Have I learned anything from this encounter? Was I able to accept an individual's right to have a point of view that is different from my own?"

2. Consult your state's education code to identify what laws, if any, control the range of subject areas that may be taught in local schools. Next visit your school district's office and talk with the health supervisor. Review district policy about the topics that must be taught and the requirements for the qualification of any one assigned to teach health. Are there established policies regarding selection of teaching materials or the inclusion or exclusion of specific health-related topics? What do you conclude about the need for additional policies if any?

3. Have policies been determined affecting the employment of HIV-positive personnel as teachers or staff in your district? If not, what would be a constructive way to prevent problems?

4. Assume that your school principal asks you to assemble a health education committee as a means of standardizing and upgrading the curriculum for all the students, K through 8. You have been selected because your experience and specifically your prior course work in health education make you the best qualified on the faculty. How many members of that committee would be ideal? Which grades and what other school personnel should be included? Prepare a short letter announcing the charge, the agenda for its first meeting, and the members of the committee.

5. Suggest ways to handle an irate parent who has demanded an explanation for a search of his/her child's locker. How could the problem have been avoided entirely by careful preplanning with the school health committee?

6. Attend a school board meeting. Familiarize yourself with the protocol of the board and the items that are handled in a meeting. At what point in this meeting can a community member voice a concern about teaching materials or curriculum issues? Does the school board have a curriculum committee to which these questions are referred? If so, who serves on that committee, and how does it handle various issues?

7. Obtain a sturdy loose-leaf notebook and begin accumulating clippings from news stories concerned with health topics, addresses of community support groups, or related health information from journals or professional organizations. Be sure to completely identify the sources of each of the entries so that they can be referred to when needed.

REFERENCES

1. Brick P: Sexuality in the elementary school, *SIECUS report* 12:3 January, 1985.
2. Carlyon P: The PTA's health education project and sex education in the schools, *J Sch Health* 51(4):271, 1981.
3. Centers for Disease Control: Guidelines for effective school health education to prevent the spread of AIDS, *MMWR* 37 (suppl no S-2), 1988.
4. Dickman IR: *Winning the battle against sex education*, New York, 1982, SIECUS.
5. Gendel E: *Human sexuality—the educator, the learner, and the society.* Paper delivered at the International Symposium on Sex education, 1972, Tel Aviv.
6. Gilbert G: Easy ways of getting into trouble when teaching sex education, *Health Educ* 10(5):31, 1979.
7. Gordon S: The case for moral sex education in the schools, *J Sch Health* 51(4):214, 1981.
8. Grady MI: Helping schools to cope with AIDS, *Med Aspects Human Sexuality*, January 1988.
9. Guttmacher A: *Risk and responsibility*, New York, 1989, The Institute.
10. Heller KS: Educational strategies to prevent AIDS: rationale. In Cohen PT, Sande MA, Volberding PA, eds: *AIDS knowledge base*, 1990.
11. McNab WL: Do's and don'ts in teaching sexuality education, *Health Educ* 13(6):31, 1982.
12. Neuten J: Comprehensive school health programs: surviving the moral smog, *J Sch Health* 62:2 February, 1992.
13. Parker B: Leadership: political battles offer you the challenge of a lifetime, *Exec Educator* 3(8):24, 1980.
14. Quackenbush M, Villarreal S: *Does AIDS hurt?*

Educating young children about AIDS, Santa Cruz, Calif, 1988, Network Publications.

15. Quackenbush M et al: *The AIDS challenge*, Santa Cruz, Calif, 1988, Network Publications.

16. Rath LE, Harmin M, Simon SB: *Values and teaching: working with values in the classroom*, Columbus, Ohio, 1966, Charles E. Merrill.

17. Scales PC: Sense and nonsense about sexuality education: a rejoinder to the Shornacks' critical view, *Family Relations* 32(4):287, 1983.

18. Thomas B et al: Small group sex education at school. In Miller B, et al: *Preventing adolescent pregnancy*, Newbury Park, Calif, 1992, Sage Publications.

19. Thornburg HD: Adolescent sources of information on sex, *J Sch Health* 51(4):274, 1981.

20. United States Department of Education: *What works: schools without drugs*, 1986, Washington, DC, The Department.

21. Wagman E and Bignell S: Starting family life and sex education programs: a health agency's perspective, *J Sch Health* 51(4):247, 1981.

22. Wilson P: *When sex is the subject*, Santa Cruz, Calif, 1991, Network Publications.

SUGGESTED READINGS

Ballard D, White D, Glascoff M: AIDS/HIV education for pre-service elementary teachers, *J Sch Health* 60(6):262-265, August, 1990.

Bramble DC, Bradshaw ME, Sklarew S: The sex education practicum: medical students in the elementary school classroom: *J Sch Health* 62(1):32-34, January, 1992.

Lively V, Lively E: Sexual development of young children, Albany, NY, 1991, Delmar Publishers.

Scales PC: Sexuality education in schools: Let's focus on what unites us, *J Health Educ* March/April 1993, ol 24:2 p. 121.

White D, Ballard D: The status of AIDS/HIV education in the professional preparation of pre-service elementary teachers, *J Health Educ* 24(2):68-72, March/April, 1993.

7 Health Education Evaluation

When you finish this chapter, you should be able to:

- Distinguish between the goals of evaluation and measurement.
- Compare the uses of formative evaluation with those of summative evaluation.
- Explain the interrelationships among objectives, learning opportunities, and evaluation procedures.
- Describe ways that changes in learner knowledge, attitudes, and practices can be assessed.
- Identify problems in evaluating health behaviors and attitudes.
- Apply evaluative criteria to the analysis of health teaching resources and materials.

What does the word *evaluation* mean to you? Does it arouse uncomfortable feelings of anxiety, stress, or expectation of criticism or failure? Perhaps you equate it with marking a score sheet and the effect that analysis of those marks can have on a course grade. Since you are a student at this time, your reactions may reflect both descriptions. Notice that the first interpretation is largely emotional and related to experience. The other confuses evaluation with measurement.

Generally, evaluation is a means of making an informed decision about a performance, person, or program. The fundamental activity involved is collecting and interpreting information. It is the ends that are sought that differentiate between evaluation and measurement. Measurement in education is determination of a quantitative index of individual performance with respect to a specified task. The goal of evaluation is always the same, whatever the object of scrutiny—to appraise the quality or worth of something or someone according to a specified standard.

Evaluation is not limited to whatever terminal procedure a teacher employs to assign a final grade to a student. That is termed **summative** evaluation. Neither is it solely concerned with a student's learning the subject matter and behaviors proposed for each unit of learning. Growth in social skills and emotional balance is no less essential among the goals of school health education. **Formative** evaluation may be the more worthwhile means of promoting desirable growth or change in ability and knowledge because it gives students feedback about their progress at a time when they can best use it. Formative evaluation is an ongoing process begun before instruction (pretesting) and carefully continued throughout the course. Short quizzes, accompanied by knowledge of results may serve as reinforcing experiences relative to growth in knowledge and cognitive skills (25). **Processing,** used as the closing activity in cooperative learning, is probably more effective in evaluating growth in interpersonal skills than analysis by the teacher. The fact that the students identify their growth or need for it is far more powerful an incentive to work for improvement than any other form of feedback could be.

Summative evaluation procedures are designed to elicit evidence of the end product of the course—the total change that has occurred from instruction. Final grades can not be appraised fairly by means of a single test or procedure but must represent a synthesis of significant data of several kinds. These data would include test scores, teacher observations of changes in attitudes and ability to work with others, and review of student portfolios containing course projects, notes, or products.

PURPOSES OF EVALUATION IN SCHOOL HEALTH EDUCATION

Ideally the purposes of evaluation in school health education include the following:

- To determine present health knowledge, attitudes, and practices as a basis for defining objectives for future instruction.
- To identify and diagnose sources of learning difficulties.
- To assess the effectiveness of teaching materials and strategies.
- To appraise the total health education curriculum.
- To provide continuing information about student achievement.
- To improve counseling effectiveness.
- To test the relevance of evaluation procedures to the stated course objectives.

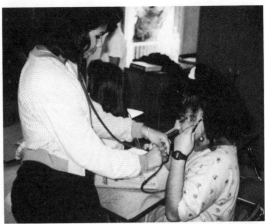

Matt Fischer

Evaluative data can include observations of students' abilities to work with others.

- To provide a basis for necessary modifications or improvements of all aspects of the school health program.

The focus of this chapter will be delimited to evaluation of the learners, the effectiveness of the teacher, and the quality, utility, and appropriateness of the health teaching materials and resources employed in the classroom. Evaluation of these elements of the teaching-learning task is essential at every level of implementation, whether it be the classroom, the program, or the curriculum, and whatever the age group for which a plan is designed and implemented. If health instruction is to keep pace with the rapidly escalating changes in society and in science, evaluation activity must be continuous and unending.

EVALUATION IS MORE THAN MEASUREMENT

A primary difference between evaluation and measurement is that the first is concerned with quality or value, while the second is concerned only with quantity. Evaluation is much broader in scope, and its outcome has far more weight in making decisions about the object of interest.

Cryan discusses the difference between the two in these words (5):

> Measurement is only part of the evaluative process, and testing is only one way of measuring certain characteristics. Because evaluation is continuous, comprehensive, and integral to the process of instruction, it must represent a variable set of procedures that are carried out daily as well as periodically. Those procedures accomplish purposes of: 1) preliminary diagnostic judgments to identify individual and group needs; 2) ongoing formative judgment of student and teacher progress toward instructional goals, and 3) concluding summative judgments of overall performance.

Popham describes measurement as *status* determination, while evaluation is *worth* determination. Evaluation is a comprehensive process, including both qualitative and quantitative descriptions of student behavior, as well as value judgments about that behavior (22). Evaluating health teaching and learning requires systematic assessment of the *total* performance of a student (quality of classroom participation, level of motivation evident, and ability to apply learned health concepts and information in solving real or hypothetical health-related problems). Although both formative and summative evaluation procedures are employed during the course of study, the formative is given the most attention, but always for feedback purposes rather than for ranking or grading.

RELATIONSHIP OF EVALUATION TO INSTRUCTIONAL OBJECTIVES

An evaluation activity or procedure, as an integral part of the instructional process, theoretically represents one side of an equilateral triangle, the other two sides being a given measurable objective and the learning opportunity designed to facilitate appropriate practice. (Figure 7-1). The dynamic interrelationships among them are not mutually exclusive. Each of these components affects and is affected by the other two. For example, just as objectives serve as guidelines to the development or selection of appro-

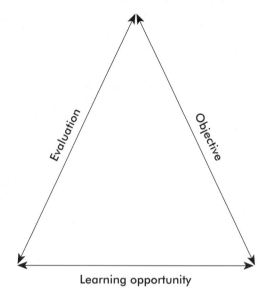

FIGURE 7-1
Relationship of evaluation to objectives and learning opportunity.

priate learning opportunities, so also do they suggest valid evaluation activities. There must be consistency between the two. On the other hand, evaluation yields information about the learner's performance and at the same time tells us which learning opportunities are working and even which objectives need to be revised or tossed out. Finally, learning opportunities often lead unexpectedly to new insights relative to student interests, community needs, and the like, which motivates the creation of new objectives.

Those three components of the total process of teaching and learning might also be expressed by means of three interrelated questions. (1) Where do we want to go?—the objective; (2) How can we get there?—the learning opportunity; and (3) How far have we come?—the evaluation activity. Specification of clearly stated objectives is an essential step in planning instruction in which evaluation is not only a means of measuring progress but also a contributing factor in the instructional process (2).

If the stated objectives are the *real* objectives,

it is impossible to separate them from planning for evaluation. Implicit in a measurable objective is the activity that is acceptable as evidence of its mastery. If the objective proposes that the student should be able to distinguish between illness and wellness, then the evaluation procedure must provide some means whereby the ability to do precisely that is elicited. Some instructors find it easier, in fact, to decide what they will accept as evidence that the student has learned what was taught and *then* choose the cognitive skill that fits the expectation. Teaching strategies or learning opportunities are the means by which the teacher helps the student to build a bridge of competence between "cannot do it" and "can do it."

An objective specifies a cognitive skill and some content to be learned. A lesson plan is designed to provide opportunities to practice that skill in connection with that content, until everyone in the class has mastered the objective. For example, if the objective stipulates that the learners will be able to explain *relationships* between certain environmental conditions and the health and safety of the community, it is neither fair nor logical to give them a test designed to measure the ability to name *sources* of pollution, to cite laws expected to prevent certain environmental problems, or to select from a list of federal and state agencies those charged with protection of the environment. Can you develop measurable objectives that would match the purposes implicit in the above three test problems?

WHAT CAN BE EVALUATED BY TEACHERS?

The problem of evaluation in health teaching is more perplexing than in most other school subjects because its desired outcomes are often not easily measured in the classroom. Tests of many kinds can provide data regarding growth in knowledge, but gains in information are not always transferred to the actions and attitudes that are important goals of health teaching. There is a wide difference between what a person knows

and does, as most of us will admit. Moreover, what can be taught in schools is severely limited in several ways—by the amount of time that is available, the interest of the teacher in teaching about health, and the amount and quality of professional preparation for the task the teacher has had, whether preservice or inservice.

Teachers are expected to appraise their students' performance subsequent to instruction, at least with regard to increases in knowledge. Positive shifts in health attitudes, correction of misconceptions, and evidence of new or reinforced desirable health practices are also hoped for. It is relatively easy to measure changes in knowledge, but it is possible to ascertain, to some degree, resulting changes in the other dimensions of health behavior as well. What children are thinking and feeling can't be measured as directly as knowledge, but a great deal can be inferred about these less quantifiable attributes from what children say and do. Among the ways these kinds of data can be gathered are: (1) direct observation, (2) interviews, (3) checklists, (4) questionnaires (these can be read to young children or administered to those with reading skills), and (5) portfolios of their work, drawings, and the like.

Hochbaum reminds us, however, of the many influences on health behavior other than those associated with education, most of which are outside the classroom and therefore outside a teacher's ability either to control or to counteract (12). In fact, some of those influences are not easily controlled by the individual who experiences them. Hochbaum says, "Social, economic, political, physical, environmental and a multitude of other conditions may render the chosen behavior possible and easy, or make it difficult or impossible."

The Learner

Evaluating Health Knowledge.   In planning instruction it must be decided what should be measured and how it will be assessed. The set of abilities or responses a teacher is willing to accept as evidence of a student's achievement becomes an operational definition of what she or he views as important, whatever the stated objectives may have been. Health knowledge is the aspect of health instruction that is easiest to measure, so knowledge tests are those most depended on by teachers. Although possession of information does not guarantee that its owner will use it, neither can it be denied that it is basic to making a reasoned choice.

Carlyon said that it is unrealistic and absurd to expect more from health education than from any other discipline offered in the schools; no one would try to teach children everything they need to know about mathematics or a language by means of a crash course once or twice during the public school years (4). He argues that:

> As I understand it, health instruction curriculum shares the overall goal of the entire school curriculum, which is to help students become knowledgeable, critical, independent learners. Health curriculum, more than the rest of the curriculum, focuses on knowledge, critical abilities, and learning skills related to normal growth and development and maintenance of well-being. It is assumed that people thus equipped are more likely to live healthful lives than those who are not.

Ways of constructing your own knowledge tests or identifying reliable standardized instruments are described in the next chapter. Remember that well-designed paper and pencil tests are not limited to the assessment of factual information but can be effective in measuring the ability to apply that information as well as in assessing attitudes and practices.

Evaluating Health Beliefs and Attitudes. The first step here is to try to distinguish between attitudes and beliefs. Attitudes usually are defined as being based on beliefs, and most people differentiate between the two. Green and Kreuter believe that an attitude reflects two concepts: (1) a rather constant feeling about a person, action, situation, or an idea; and (2) an inherent evaluation or good-bad dimension (11). They define a *belief* as a conviction that a phenomenon is true or real. Conviction about their truth is what is significant about beliefs. Those teaching about

health need to find out what students believe about it because often misconceptions, misperceptions, or outdated concepts are revealed that can be used as targets for lessons, for example, "fish is brain food," "a sip of brandy is an effective restorative for someone who has fainted," or "brown eggs are more nutritious than white eggs."

Unfortunately, evaluation of health attitudes and beliefs is difficult. There are several methods for doing so, all of which are subject to errors of perception and interpretation. The teacher can simply *ask* the student what his/her attitude is toward some health-related issue. However, although no one should know the answer better than the respondent, self-report is not dependably accurate. The individual may want to conceal a negative attitude and so says something that is not exactly true. The answer may reflect a belief rather than an attitude, or it may be influenced by what the student has learned is approved rather than reflect the real attitude.

Moreover, what many people *think* is their attitude toward something is often not their real attitude at all, although they may be quite sincere in their answer, for example, the individual who compliments a woman by saying that she thinks like a man.

A teacher can obtain information about students' attitudes from their peers, parents, or other adults who know the students well. Yet parents are understandably reluctant to report negative attitudes, and studies show that few parents can reliably report their child's actual attitude in any case.

A person's attitudes can be inferred from her/his reactions to issues and people. Observation can provide clues to attitudes, although the interpretation of observations, like beauty, depends a great deal on the eye of the beholder. In addition, a teacher must be cautious about making judgments about a child's attitudes based on his/her own attitudes.

Beliefs and attitudes also reflect values. Values reflect preferences or standards by which be-

HEALTH BELIEF CHECKLIST

	Very Important	Important	Fairly Important	Not Important
I believe I should				
Eat three meals a day				
Have my teeth checked by a dentist at least twice a year				
Have breakfast every day				
Eat eggs and bacon every day				
Be happy all the time				
Like myself				
Enjoy simple pleasures like food and nature				
Never snack between meals				
Accept disappointments calmly				
Show love of other people				
Trust my friends				
Feel responsible for other people				
Be able to laugh at myself when I am wrong				
Be glad if I am the largest person in the room				
Face problems and try to solve them				
Respect the differences I see in others				
Stand up for my ideas				
Not push others around				
Tell an adult when I don't feel well				
Take medicine when I don't feel well				
Do some strenuous exercise every day				

Modified from Nolte, AE and others: *Instructor* 81(1):47, 1971.

haviors, objects, qualities are judged by individuals or societies as being worthy or desirable. If it is known what children already believe and value relative to health and health practices, then not only can appropriate learning opportunities be arranged, but their effectiveness in changing misconceptions can also be appraised.

Typically, written health attitude tests ask the respondent to indicate feelings or opinions relative to specified health practices or issues. Most such instruments are designed in the form of answer-completion tests, checklists, or self-report devices such as Likert or semantic differential scales. Few, if any, standardized attitude tests that are appropriate for use with elementary school students are available. However, the previous example of a checklist regarding health beliefs could be used with young children as a pretest for health teaching and modified to serve as a summative test (18). Its authors do not claim that any of the items represent absolutes, nor do they specify which of them need to be interpreted or discussed further with the children.

The Semantic Differential Test of Meaning. Considerable use has been made of the semantic differential testing technique developed by Osgood, Suci, and Tannenbaum (20) in studies of children's attitudes toward health (26). A scale is used to measure the connotative meanings of concepts, as revealed by the respondent's rating of them on the basis of sets of bipolar adjectives. Connotative meanings reflect the attitude of the respondent toward a concept. Thus a student might be asked to rate health education or another such concept on a form like the one in the box below. The respondent is instructed to check the space that corresponds most closely to his/her feelings about the meaning of a word or concept.

Although some of the sets of adjectives appear to be totally irrelevant, a response is to be given for each, based on a quick reaction to the words themselves in association with the concept. If the student believes that health education is extremely useful, a check is made in the space closest to that adjective. A mark next to the opposing adjective records a negative attitude. The middle space allows a neutral feeling to be expressed, and the remaining spaces are used to indicate varying degrees of positive or negative feelings about the concept.

One way of scoring that is frequently used is to allot each position a certain number of points, the highest possible being seven points, neutral being four points, and the lowest rating being one point. Notice that the pairs are not always set up with the positive rating in the same direction so that the first score point for any pair of adjectives may be either seven or one. In this sample scale, the most positive attitude would yield 70

SEMANTIC DIFFERENTIAL MODEL

Health Education

Good	___ : ___ : ___ : ___ : ___ : ___ : ___	Bad
Fair	___ : ___ : ___ : ___ : ___ : ___ : ___	Unfair
Clean	___ : ___ : ___ : ___ : ___ : ___ : ___	Dirty
Fast	___ : ___ : ___ : ___ : ___ : ___ : ___	Slow
Hard	___ : ___ : ___ : ___ : ___ : ___ : ___	Soft
Sharp	___ : ___ : ___ : ___ : ___ : ___ : ___	Dull
Strong	___ : ___ : ___ : ___ : ___ : ___ : ___	Weak
Sad	___ : ___ : ___ : ___ : ___ : ___ : ___	Happy
Nice	___ : ___ : ___ : ___ : ___ : ___ : ___	Awful
Useless	___ : ___ : ___ : ___ : ___ : ___ : ___	Useful

points, the most negative attitude 10 points, and a neutral attitude 40 points.

There is no right answer in this situation, but there is a positive direction. All the interpretations of the sets of adjectives are based on extensive analyses conducted by Osgood and his colleagues (20). The scales permit comparisons between individuals and groups relative to their attitudes toward specified persons, concepts, or issues. This test can be used to see how similarly one individual perceives a number of related concepts, and to measure changes in attitudes after a course in health education. Even young children can be asked to respond to a scale like this, either verbally or by checking spaces. For elementary school children it may be wise to limit the possible intervals to five, however.

A major advantage of the semantic differential assessment of affect or meaning is that the sets of adjectives are not based on obvious or seemingly relevant comparisons, so the responses are less vulnerable to faking.

Likert Scales.   The Likert scale is probably the most widely used among available affective scales. Typically, the Likert scale offers the respondent a five-point rating scale ranging from strongly agree *(SA)*, agree *(A)*, uncertain *(U)*, disagree *(D)*, and strongly disagree *(SD)*, relative to a series of positive or negative statements. With young examinees, only three (e.g., yes, maybe, and no), or two (yes or no), ratings may be elicited. The scoring scheme depends on the number of ratings in the scale and awards the most points to the most positive response to positive statements and the most negative response to negative statements. The major advantages of the Likert scale are its relative ease of construction and scoring and the reliability of its results. Following is a scale constructed for use with elementary students that is focused on their attitude toward smoking.

Evaluating Health Behavior.   Health behavior has to do with the actions customarily taken by an individual that have an impact on personal and community well-being. A goal of health education is to promote desirable behaviors and

---

The questions below ask about different people you don't know. Circle the word that shows what you think about a person.

YES = The person probably smokes
MAYBE = Not sure if the person smokes
NO = The person probably does not smoke

YES MAYBE NO Greg has many friends. Do you think he smokes?
YES MAYBE NO Cheryl almost never looks good. Do you think she smokes?
YES MAYBE NO Raymond is a very good runner. Do you think he smokes?
YES MAYBE NO Linda is not healthy. Do you think she smokes?
YES MAYBE NO Keith usually feels healthy. Do you think he smokes?
YES MAYBE NO Tony has a hard time when he runs. Do you think he smokes?
YES MAYBE NO The other kids don't like Valerie. Do you think she smokes?
YES MAYBE NO Jimmy is the best-looking boy in the class. Do you think he smokes?

Adapted from An Evaluation Handbook for Health Education Programs in Smoking, Centers for Disease Control, Atlanta, 1983.

---

practices (personal health care actions that may not always be consistent but that are at least the result of decisions one way or another), either through change or by reinforcement of existing desirable patterns. This is not easy, since (1) behaviors can only be assessed at a given point of time and (2) only certain health practices can be observed at school. Nobody knows if what was observed was typical or if it will be different if noted under other circumstances. As in the case of attitude assessment, if the only feasible ways of determining a person's health-related behavior are self-reports and questionnaires, the results may be biased due to conscious or unconscious "bending" of the truth. The respondent may report a behavior that reflects what is the best behavior rather than the usual behavior. The response may be slanted for a number of reasons, for example, knowledge of best behavior, desire to appear to good advantage in the instructor's eyes, prior experience, or even for fun or to shock the teacher (27).

Certain informal procedures can be used to supplement information gathered through structured means. Casual but direct observation of student behavior in the classroom, cafeteria, or school grounds can yield information to be incorporated in health records in anecdotal form. Making such notations is easier and more efficient when a checklist or other such form has been prepared for this purpose.

A weakness inherent in some techniques for appraising behavior is their dependence on verbal descriptions of actions. Words do not mean the same thing to all people or even to the same people at all times. For example, self-report instruments typically ask the respondent to judge the frequency of specific health behaviors. The individual may be asked to indicate whether between-meal snacks are eaten (1) often, (2) frequently, (3) sometimes, (4) seldom, or (5) never. Only the last of these frequencies is dependably interpreted the same way by everybody. One person's "often" may be another's "frequently" or vice versa. "Sometimes" may mean once a month to Tom and once a week to Joanne. Unless the directions for each alternative are carefully written to ensure uniformity of interpretation, it is impossible to draw any valid conclusions from the answers; yet it is difficult to construct such an unambiguous instrument that is comprehensive enough to be useful and at the same time feasible in terms of the time needed to administer it. Another common problem is the irrelevance of what is measured to the actual concern, that is, health behavior. *Knowing* what to do is not evidence of application, yet overemphasis on content is reflected in the measurement techniques used in many classrooms. An analysis of typical teacher-made tests revealed that 8 out of 10 measured knowledge of specific facts only (3). Even though questions may offer choices among several possible health actions, the correct answers are designed to reflect knowledge primarily. It cannot be otherwise if the intention is to evaluate retention of factual material covered in the course.

Finally, because health behavior does not begin or end in the classroom, and because certain kinds of behaviors cannot be evaluated during the school year ages, the outcome of some instruction may not be demonstrated for many years. Ironically, it is even possible that the most significant impact on health behavior may never be recorded. For example, how do you measure the amount of undesirable behavior that never happened because health instruction reinforced health practices learned at home or prevented the later emergence of some that were potentially harmful?

It is probable that what can be learned about children's health behavior is more useful and meaningful as the basis of decisions relative to the health content and teaching techniques employed, than as evidence supportive of the effectiveness of health instruction. Veenker says that it is not knowledge but the many factors and forces in school, home, and community life that determine the kind of health practices an individual follows (27). To claim that any change is directly and solely attributable to a course in health education is foolish. Teachers can accomplish wonders in the little time allotted for their efforts, yet they cannot and should not be expected to counter the many forces that promote negative health behaviors in our society.

Hochbaum agrees, saying (13):

> In school health education, for example, the appropriate criteria [of effectiveness] are certain cognitive and affective changes in children and in some cases in their parents and other significant persons. While these are already well accepted objectives, there is always the lingering notion that the "real criteria" are to be found in actual behavioral change. This poses unrealistic demands on available evaluation methods . . . It may, moreover, infuse in the health educator a sense of failure and futility, when the expected behaviors do not occur, while in reality he or she may have succeeded su-

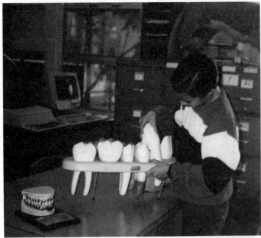

Matt Fischer

Health instruction reinforces health practices learned at home.

premely well in accomplishing all that education can accomplish: create conditions favorable to the desired behaviors though without assuring the emergence of such behaviors.

EFFECTS OF EVALUATION ON THE LEARNER

Evaluation can have both positive and negative effects on the learner. A good evaluation activity can be as much a learning opportunity as it is a procedure for the appraisal of results. Look at any textbook or curriculum guide that lists ideas for learning opportunities and notice how many of them are in fact evaluation activities (27). The principal difference between the two is in the assumptions on which each depends. The assumption underlying a learning opportunity is that the students *do not* know the subject matter and part of the plan has to provide for its provision in some manner. The assumption of the evaluation activity is that the learner *does know* the information needed to carry it out, and that it has been learned as an outcome of earlier experiences in the classroom. Moreover, it is expected that the student has also had practice in dealing with the content as specified in the objective.

An evaluation activity (where *activity* refers to the use of a realistic problem as a means of assessing ability) requires the learner to apply this new information in a new but hypothetical situation. As a result, skill in problem solving is reinforced, information about the problem is reinforced or even added to, and the learner does not have to be told where her/his strengths or weaknesses lie. Motivation to learn is increased when evaluation is used either to estimate progress or to gauge total achievement following a series of lessons.

If evaluation is seen as a threat, it can have negative effects, not only on present learning, but also on the students themselves, because it influences their attitudes toward health education as a course and the promotion of health as a valued pattern of behaviors. For example, the pressure of test taking, particularly when the results are used to determine positions on a grading scale, may be motivating for a few. For others, the result may instead be frustration, dependence on test-taking tricks, cheating, and what is the worst, perhaps, feelings of defeat and apathy.

Testing procedures must be planned carefully so that the effect will be positive in as many ways as possible. After administering a test, it helps to go over it, item by item, and allow the students to give their reasons for having answered any item differently from what you have intended to be the correct response. Often you will discover that another answer was just as good or that the item was so ambiguous in meaning that other answers are just as acceptable as the "right" one. This can be painful for you if you wrote the test, but it is worth it. All of your students will have learned the correct answers, which ones they missed and why, and where to focus further study. If there was any difference in opinion regarding certain items, the issue has been faced and resolved on the spot. You will feel satisfaction in knowing that learning has been the outcome, even more than assessment. You will have earned your students' respect by your willingness to accept criticism and deal with it fairly. And it is a quick way to evaluate the test itself and improve it for the next application.

EVALUATING THE CURRICULUM PLAN AND THE TEACHER
Evaluating the Curriculum Plan

The curriculum plan in a school or district is the result of a great many decisions made by administrators and teachers that specify how health education will be organized, how much time it is allotted, what subject matter it will be included or omitted, at which grades it will be taught, whether specialists or special resources will be provided, a statement of the system of beliefs about health education as a basic course of study, and more. Some of these elements are written, others are specified as part of school administration. All of these should be reviewed continually and revised as needed as means of assurance that the plan reflects the state of the art and not some outdated, no longer adequate curriculum.

A handbook prepared for state policy makers detailing recommendations for school health education suggests standards by which programs may be examined. Many of the above problems are addressed directly in this document (8). Another publication, *How Healthy Is Your School?* contains a wealth of material for the evaluation of the school health program, including ways of assessing student achievement and the curriculum (17).

Most often, health teaching in grades K through 6 is integrated in organization. As such it works quite well in effecting cognitive and affective changes that influence children's health behavior. Direct teaching is even more successful and is usually the pattern in middle schools, but whichever plan is specified, evaluation must be an ongoing process. The procedures of evaluation are much the same whether they appraise the learner's progress or the success of a lesson, unit, or entire curriculum. The only real difference is *what* is being evaluated and whose values determine the criteria to be applied. Any appraisal technique can yield data that are useful in making a formative evaluation of organized

programs of instruction. Indeed, formative evaluation provides the best perspective from which to view instructional programs. Most subject areas have goals and objectives that are not fixed but change over time. Valid summative program evaluation is therefore difficult and maybe too late. Nor is it possible to evaluate a program without considering the skill and interest of the instructor and the characteristics of the student who is being taught.

Parts of the plans made for the curriculum are often specified in formal documents termed "frameworks" or "guides." Goodlad's large scale study of schooling in the United States found that those prepared at state or district levels were of minimal effectiveness (10). However, those curriculum guides developed for the guidance of teachers in specific subjects were quite good. He reports:

> Three of our seven states produced subject-oriented guides intended to be helpful not just to local districts, but to individual teachers. Indeed, some of these could be used with very little modification or extra effort, as frameworks for entire courses. However, there were no trends in our data to suggest that teachers in the 18 schools we studied in these three states, more than teachers in the other 20 schools, perceived their curriculum guides as useful. Overall, teachers in our sample viewed state and local curriculum guides as of little or moderate usefulness in guiding their teaching.

Written curriculum plans differ considerably in what is provided to guide the process of instruction. There is wide variation in the specificity of the plans. Some focus on content, others on choices among student activities; some are suggestive ("the teacher might"), while others are prescriptive ("the teacher must"). Guideline questions for describing the kinds of decisions suggested as appropriate for more specific plans such as curriculum guides follow.* These guidelines, published first twenty years ago are as valid today because they focus on plans designed specifically for the classroom teacher. Notice the

---

*From Payne A: *The study of curriculum plans*, Washington, DC, 1969, National Educational Association.

word "specific" throughout these questions.

1. Does the plan provide the outline for organization and sequence of the course or curriculum area?
2. How specific is the treatment of subject matter (unit topics, daily topics, specific examples, etc.)?
3. Does the plan include specific activities for students? If so, are the activities described in sufficient detail to suggest what the student is actually to do and the related cognitive process? What is the general emphasis in types of activities described?
4. Does the plan give specific activities or methods for teachers? What is the general emphasis in types of activities?
5. Does the plan specify the materials to be used in instruction? Are there descriptions of what is to be done with the materials?
6. Are there any explicit statements about the nature of learning and the conditions under which it occurs (e.g., statements about motivation, learning environment, maturation and capacity, cognitive processes)?
7. Are there any explicit views on the structure of the subject matter? Are the criteria for selecting and organizing subject matter and materials given?
8. Is there a statement of objectives or desired results of instruction? To what degree of specificity have these been developed (course, unit, or activity)?
9. What are the suggested purposes for evaluating students? What evaluation methods are recommended? Are the specific procedures given? Is there a proposed schedule for evaluation? What suggestions are provided for the analysis and use of the evaluation?

Payne adds that two evaluative criteria are essential in appraising curriculum plans: clarity of meaning and internal consistency. An important check on internal consistency is to compare the stated objectives with the learning opportunities and evaluation procedures provided for their implementation. Clarity depends on the care with which these facilitating activities (both for learn-

ing and evaluating) have been described. She asserts that where this important quality is neglected, it is not possible to judge the validity of any curriculum decisions.

It is the clarity with which learning opportunities and evaluation procedures are described that often fall short of excellence. Learning opportunities tend to be less than carefully developed, and sometimes there are no stated objectives whatever. What you get are a lot of very good ideas that lack any stated purpose other than supposed relevance to the subject matter. Example: "Have the students bring in products made especially for children and discuss their uses in class." That's not enough, particularly when there is nothing to tell the teacher what the purpose of that activity is to be. There are similar problems when objectives exist but the evaluation is fuzzy or weak. For example, here's an objective: "The student identifies positive and negative effects of stress." That sounds worthwhile if the learning opportunity arranges for its implementation. But what is the suggested evaluation activity to match? "Have the students identify positive and negative effects of stress." Obviously that matches the objective. The only thing wrong with it is that it is no help at all. If you are interested in learning how that might be done, you are on your own. The questions that are unanswered are how do you test for achievement of the objective and what do you accept as evidence of success.

If you find it difficult to explain an evaluation activity, but you have an objective to work with, it becomes easy to explain. Simply describe a learning opportunity that matches the objective but assumes that the students learned how to do that somewhere or some time earlier. Then all you have to do is decide upon the criteria to be applied to the product of that activity.

Evaluating Teacher Effectiveness

Today we are asking teachers to start teaching students how to apply skills, how to understand concepts, and solve problems, how to work collaboratively, and how to take responsibility for learning (6).

Evaluating teacher effectiveness has been the purpose of a vast amount of research (1). No one has yet been able to devise an evaluation scheme that is not plagued with faulty assumptions, as well as uncontrolled or uncontrollable sources of error that threaten the reliability of any conclusions that might be drawn from the obtained data. In general, three approaches have been employed. These include (1) psychometric analysis of the relationship between measures of teacher behavior based on comparisons between pretest and posttest scores on standardized achievement tests, (2) systematic observations of teacher behavior, testing its consistency with specified criteria of acceptable performance; and (3) self-reports obtained by means of structured interviews or questionnaires.

Most state-wide studies of teacher effectiveness are based on the first of these approaches. Typically, mean scores on standardized achievement tests obtained in individual school districts are compared with their previous scores and also with other districts. Any difference, however slight statistically, is by inference used as irrefutable evidence of the quality of teaching for that year, in that school district. Some monumental assumptions are never admitted, the least of which is the assumption of common curriculums.

Individual teacher performance has tended to be based almost entirely on the observations noted by a busy administrator during a routine, quick visit to a randomly selected class. Any growth in teaching effectiveness has largely depended on a teacher's self-motivated efforts to discover better ways of achieving course objectives.

Currently, however, parental dissatisfaction with the quality of public education has resulted in "back to basics" and accountability demands. And this in turn has sparked increased attention to the quality of education in individual schools and districts, as well as to the specification of criteria defining teacher competencies on which appropriate inservice development programs can be based. For example, educators in Orange County, Virginia, have replaced annual teacher evaluations with professional growth assessments tied to comprehensive master teaching training programs. Instead of focusing on identifying the 2% of the teaching staff deemed incompetent, full attention is given to the other 98% to improve their instructional effectiveness (9).

The first step in this process was the identification of 15 performance indicators, described as "Procedures for Effective Teaching" (PET), applicable to all teaching situations and content areas (see box on p. 179). These were stated in terms specific enough to serve as guides but flexible enough to allow for individual teacher style and creativity. These teacher behaviors include:

Ample time and opportunity for success are provided, in that teachers are given 5 years and 30 observations in which to demonstrate and assess their proficiency with all the performance indicators. The observations are made by individuals who are themselves classroom teachers. Selection of the teaching skill to be demonstrated, the day, and the class to be visited is up to the teacher to be evaluated. The observers are directed to document only the teaching strengths present during the visit. Subsequent reports of the visit are reviewed by the teacher and observer for completeness and accuracy before they are submitted to the school administrator. Use of other classroom teachers as observer/raters would appear to avoid teacher complaints that principals' ratings tend to be biased according to their own values, and personal teaching experiences, hence less than valid as measures of teachers' effectiveness (23).

Zahorik has said that there is no one view of good teaching that everyone accepts (28). He believes that supervisors need a definition that describes how a teacher behaves while displaying good teaching. The following definition is proposed therefore, "Good teaching is teaching that is purposeful, consistent, and skillful."

A broader study of teacher effectiveness evaluation standards was reported by Johnson and Orso (15). A survey of evaluation instruments used in large school systems in each of the 50 states was undertaken, and 48 systems in 48

KEY TEACHER BEHAVIORS—PET

1. A model of courtesy is exhibited.
2. Positive associations are used with enthusiastic or humorous statements.
3. The teacher circulates among students inviting participation.
4. The teacher mediates or redirects incorrect responses.
5. Students are asked to describe the learning objectives.
6. Concrete examples are used to link learning objectives to prior learnings.
7. Guided practice with teacher-shaped responses is used.
8. The teacher monitors student readiness to proceed to independent practice.
9. Student independent practice without grades is used to determine the success of instruction.
10. Questioning techniques are used to assess fluency and stimulate divergent thinking.
11. Transition strategies for group and class changes are established.
12. Expectations of behavior and routines are explained.
13. The teacher anticipates student behaviors instead of reacting to them.
14. Nonverbal communication techniques are used to encourage appropriate behavior.
15. The teacher makes a statement to the whole group and then directs it to an individual.

From Edwards CH Jr: An effective teaching approach to teacher evaluation and staff development, *ERS Spectrum* 4:2, 1986.

states responded. Analysis of these instruments yielded a group of categories of teacher behaviors and criteria for their evaluation that were common to all of them.

Five categories of behavior were identified as follows: (1) instruction, (2) classroom management, (3) professional responsibilities, (4) personal characteristics, and (5) interpersonal relations. Ten criteria are listed relative to the first four of these categories and five for the last. For the category of instruction the following were criteria commonly specified in all of the instruments studied, along with the percentages of systems that specified them (15):

1. Employs a variety of instructional media and instructional techniques (100%).
2. Implements the district's instructional goals and objectives (100%).
3. Provides for attention to individual differences (100%).
4. Evaluates students effectively and fairly on a regular basis (93%).
5. Shows written evidence of preparation for classes (78%).
6. Is knowledgeable of subject matter being taught (76%).
7. Reviews test results with students (53%).
8. Motivates students (53%).
9. Actively involves students in learning (44%).
10. Provides positive reinforcement whenever possible (44%).

Examples of the criteria for other categories include for classroom management, "establishes an environment conducive to learning" (100%); for professional responsibilities, "participates in professional development activities such as workshops, courses, other school visits, etc." (80%); for personal characteristics, "uses clear speech" (53%); and for interpersonal relations, "establishes positive relationships with students, parents, and community" (78%). It was concluded that, important as instruction skills are, teachers have difficulty in instructing effectively unless these other categories of teacher behavior are mastered as well.

Probably the most reliable gauge of a teacher's effectiveness is whether or not the instruction has enabled most, if not all, of the students to demonstrate successful achievement of the course objectives. Theoretically, most students can master every educational objective identified by the teacher and students as worthy of achievement. Bloom, Madaus, and Hastings believe that, for most students, aptitudes are predictive of the *rate* of learning rather than of achievement potential and that, with enough time and appropriate help, the grade of A could be earned by 95% of students (2). They also suggest that a teacher's effectiveness needs to be evaluated on the basis of the ability to present, explain, and order the elements of the learning task so that mastery is the outcome for all students. Such an outcome may not be acceptable in most schools because many people are conditioned to the system in which the full range of grades, A to F, is expected, and a teacher who rewarded 95% of the students with an A would be regarded with suspicion and disapproval. Nonetheless, it certainly is an ideal toward which teachers should aspire. We will discuss this suggestion further in the section on grading in the following chapter.

The self-evaluation checklist on p. 181 has been suggested for the elementary teacher's use as criteria for evaluating effective teaching of any subject. Obviously, the desired answer in every instance is "Yes."

Evaluating Teaching Materials and Resources

Textbooks. A textbook can be a valuable resource for teaching and learning if it is accurate, up to date, and written at the vocabulary and reading level of the students for whom it is intended. Education in the United States traditionally is so textbook-oriented that everybody—teachers, students, and parents—seems to feel more secure about the quality of instruction if there is a book from which information can be drawn and assignments made. Goodlad (1984) found that, in the classrooms observed across the country, textbooks continue to be the most common medium for teaching and learning. However,

since health education is so dynamic a field, even the newest text will be out of date in some respect the very year it is published.

The first step in evaluating a textbook is to check its publication date. If more than 5 years have elapsed since it was copyrighted, it has been at least seven years since it was written. Unless it is entirely concerned with relatively timeless facts, there is likely to be newer information now. For example, physiological facts such as the names of bones or body parts are not likely to change, whereas theories or current information about nutrition or health promotional techniques or practices may have changed considerably. Even when it is new, a textbook can never be regarded as the best or only source of information, but only one among many to be investigated.

The next step is to examine the table of contents to see if the book is over-concerned with human physiology and anatomy or focuses on causes and prevention of diseases and disorders rather than the promotion of a healthful life style. Does the list of chapter topics approximate the scope of the curriculum framework adopted by the school or district? If the book is to be useful, the content should be compatible both in content and philosophy of health education with accepted best practice.

A continuing problem in every discipline is that some children cannot read at the level expected for their age and grade. In such situations it is possible to secure texts prepared for younger students or specially written for slower readers. One health educator, when transferred to an inner-city school, found that his accustomed use of the textbook as a data source for his students was hindered by the number of non-readers (many of them recent immigrants) in his classes. To solve the problem he first identified sections of the book that seemed to be the most clearly and simply written, as well as the best suited to his objectives. He tape recorded those sections, speaking as clearly and carefully as he could. Then, as each section of the book was needed to help meet the objectives, he helped his students follow each word in the text by eye, as the ear

CHECKLIST FOR TEACHERS

Yes	No	
____	____	I encourage students to express different ideas and values.
____	____	I encourage students to explore their ideas and values.
____	____	I prepare for the wide range of ideas and values students may express.
____	____	I select learning opportunities to stimulate student curiosity.
____	____	I select a wide variety of resources and materials for student use.
____	____	I support the right of a student to express an idea or value which may not be universally accepted or agreed upon and with which I may not agree.
____	____	I provide opportunities for students to use and apply the facts and information they gather.
____	____	In health education, I emphasize the idea of a variety of practices followed by different groups of people.
____	____	I encourage students to explore and examine a range of ideas and practices.
____	____	I encourage students to examine the results of taking certain actions regarding health.
____	____	I am a continuous learner along with the children.
____	____	I involve children in the process of learning.
____	____	I am more interested in how children react and behave than I am in how many facts they know as the result of health instruction.
____	____	I use varied cultural backgrounds and experiences in positive ways as I teach.
____	____	My instruction is organized around specific objectives.
____	____	I use some kind of planning system to help me use time more effectively.
____	____	My methods of teaching focus on the students and not on myself as the teacher.
____	____	My health teaching focuses upon the total child, his or her actions, his or her feelings, and the context in which he or she lives, as well as his or her physical well-being.
____	____	I use characteristics of the children in the teaching-learning process.
____	____	One of the criteria I use in choosing teaching methods is based on what I hope to accomplish.
____	____	When children are immersed in the learning process, I observe their reactions.
____	____	I provide opportunities for students to bring their own experiences into the learning process.
____	____	I help children clarify their responses to questions rather than declaring them right or wrong.
____	____	I provide opportunities for children to assume responsibility in accomplishing specific learning opportunities.
____	____	Children in my class are aware of the actions they are taking in trying to accomplish health objectives.
____	____	I am aware of the strengths and weaknesses of the children in my class.
____	____	I know the varied cultural and ethnic backgrounds of the children in my class.
____	____	I have identified the varied occupations of the childrens' parents.
____	____	I am aware of health problems the children may have or encounter in others.
____	____	I know the variety of religions represented by the children in my class.
____	____	I vary class organizational patterns for instructional purposes by using individual, small-group, large-group, or other patterns.
____	____	I involve children in teaching others who may be younger than themselves.
____	____	I help children feel that they are worthwhile as individuals.
____	____	I keep up with recent professional literature that will assist me in teaching.
____	____	The children in my class are aware that I do not know all the answers.

Modified from Nolte AE et al: *Instructor* 81(1):47, 1971.

CHECKLIST FOR EVALUATION OF PRINTED MATERIALS

Sample Criteria

A. Suitable teaching material meets all of these criteria

	Yes	No
1. Is appropriate to the course of study	____	____
2. Is a reinforcement of other materials	____	____
3. Is significantly different	____	____
4. Is impartial, factual, and accurate	____	____
5. Is up-to-date	____	____
6. Is non-sectarian, non-partisan, and unbiased	____	____
7. Is free from undesirable propaganda	____	____
8. Is free from excessive or objectionable advertising	____	____
9. Is free or inexpensive and readily available	____	____

B. Pamphlets

	Excellent	Good	Fair	Poor
1. Readability of type	____	____	____	____
2. Appropriateness of illustrations	____	____	____	____
3. Organization of content	____	____	____	____
4. Logical sequence of concepts	____	____	____	____
5. Important aspects of topic stand out	____	____	____	____
6. Material directed to one specific group such as teachers, pupils, or parents	____	____	____	____
7. Reading level appropriate for intended group	____	____	____	____
8. Based on interests and needs of intended group	____	____	____	____
9. Positively directed in words, descriptions, and actions	____	____	____	____
10. Directed toward desirable health practices	____	____	____	____
11. Minimal resort to fear techniques and morbid concepts	____	____	____	____
12. In good taste; avoids vulgarity, stereotypes and ridicule				
Total rating	____	____	____	____

Adapted from Osborn BM, Sutton WF: *J Sch Health* 34(2):72, 1964. Copies of the sample criteria rating scale to evaluate health education materials were distributed throughout Los Angeles County. Additional copies are not available for mailing. Anyone who desires to use this scale is most welcome to reproduce it singly or in quantity through the courtesy of the Tuberculosis and Health Association of Los Angeles County.

CHECKLIST FOR EVALUATION OF PRINTED MATERIALS—CONT'D

Sample Criteria

C. Posters

	Excellent	Good	Fair	Poor
1. Realistic and within experience level of students	——	——	——	——
2. Appeals to interest	——	——	——	——
3. Emphasizes positive behavior and attitudes	——	——	——	——
4. Message clear at a glance	——	——	——	——
5. Little or no conflicting detail	——	——	——	——
6. In good taste	——	——	——	——
7. Attractive and in pleasing colors	——	——	——	——
Total rating	——	——	——	——

D. Recommended for use
  1. For use by:
     a. pupils____ b. teachers____ c. parents____ d. adults____
  2. Appropriate grade level:
     a. primary____ b. elementary____ c. junior high school
     d. secondary____ e. college____ f. adult____

E. Not recommended for use
   Why not?_____

Date_____Evaluated by_____

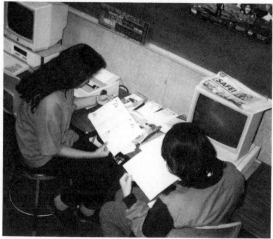

Matt Fischer

The use of computer-assisted health instruction is increasing.

heard it. The students were elated by their success in understanding the new material and the language. They were learning to read, learning to listen with comprehension, and learning about health practices at the same time.

Supplementary Teaching Materials. A wealth of written materials, produced by voluntary health agencies, industrial organizations, public health agencies, and other health-concerned groups, is freely available for classroom use. For example, the American Cancer Society via every one of its offices offers a wide array of program packages, including film strips, cassettes, records, films, video tapes, pamphlets, resource lists, and posters. All are available to schools and cover many health topics. An interagency School Health Alliance of eleven national voluntary health agencies in Los Angeles county have prepared a guide with sections on speakers, printed materials, in-service education programs, and special health programs. It is likely that alliances of this nature can be found in many metropolitan areas. Appendix E is an example of an analysis checklist for educational audiovisuals.

The problem is not how to find enough current pamphlets, booklets, and other supplemen-

QUICK HEALTH-PROMOTION SOFTWARE REVIEW

1. Have you conducted an appropriate needs assessment and determined that this program meets your needs?
2. Is there evidence of a good health-education basis for the software? (Author's credentials in health, appropriate advisory help, etc.)
3. Is the manual easy to follow, and have you been able to find answers for two or three questions without difficulty?
4. Have you personally tried the software, or do you have recommendations from more than two people whom you trust and who have similar needs?
5. Is the cost reasonable for what you will receive?
6. If the program costs one hundred dollars or more, is there a helpline, and have you called it to see what kind of help is available?
7. Does the program use the capabilities of the computer, or would it be just as effective as a book or other medium?
8. Has the program been pilot tested with an audience comparable to your intended audience, with good results?
9. Will the program run on your system, or does it warrant purchase of special hardware?
10. Are you reasonably certain that this is the best program you can find to accomplish this task? (It is very upsetting to find another, better, program at lower cost a few weeks after making an important purchase.)

If you cannot answer yes to all questions, it is time to reevaluate your selection. Do not purchase until you can answer yes to all questions.

tary printed matter for health teaching but how to select the most relevant and appropriate from among them. Often a school or district has an established policy that teachers must follow in choosing materials for use in their classrooms. Where no clear-cut guidelines exist, the criteria in the box for the evaluation of such printed materials can be applied.

Microcomputer Software. Recognizing the fast growing popularity and use of computer-assisted instruction in the health classroom, Dorman offers the following recommendations to help teachers in choosing among the available health-related software packages (7).

- Consider the characteristics of your students and their particular educational needs.
- Examine the courseware for content accuracy and instructional methodology. Does the content meet the curricular needs you will address? Are methods used in the courseware appropriate from a learning theory perspective?
- If possible, before purchase, ask the distributor for a demonstration copy of the courseware and try it with a group of students to assess their response.
- Examine the courseware for additional software or hardware that might be required.
- Assess the technical merits of the courseware. Does the program make effective use of sound, color, graphics, and music? Is the courseware free from programming errors or "bugs"?
- Consider ease of use for the courseware and any documentation or help available to you as the teacher.
- If another teaching technique could present the material in a more motivational and educationally sound fashion, use it rather than the courseware.

Dorman's suggested software evaluation form with adaptations for health educators is based on a synthesis of other software evaluation forms. This evaluation form can be found in Appendix F. In addition to Dorman, Gilbert has formulated a quick check list to help teachers assess their software needs (see box on p. 184).

SUMMARY

Evaluation is the term used in education to describe what is happening during the process of appraising the worth of the products, procedures, people, and materials involved in schooling. Measurement is the part of that process concerned with gathering specific information quantifying specified aspects of the object of interest. Measurement is often mistaken for evaluation because scores on tests or rating scales are cited as an index of student performance. But a score, however high or low it may be, does not tell us anything about the worth of a performance. It simply reports a measurement. It is status determination. This does not mean that values are not operating in any way when measurements are designed and applied. Very few measurements are absolute, and even if so, only at a given point in time (e.g., age, weight, height). Although the measurement possibilities may be of the either-or kind, somebody's values influenced the decisions involved in designing the instrument, as did those of the people up and down the line who approved its application.

Surveys show that at the elementary level, less emphasis is placed on measurement per se than on evaluation activities. Teachers of children in the primary grades report that observation and interaction are their favored evaluation techniques. Among experienced teachers at the primary level, about two thirds say that they have gained a general feel for their students' abilities within the first week or two, or within the first month to nine weeks (24).

What should be remembered is that neither evaluation nor measurement is adequate in describing the quality of a performance or product. Evaluation is not as comprehensive as it must be without measurement, and measurement cannot be substituted for the insightful observations and interpretations of behaviors that cannot be measured but must be inferred.

For the teacher who must make decisions about lesson planning during the course and who must assign a letter grade symbolizing the learner's success, it is essential that measurements and observations be frequent and that the student receive immediate feedback from the results. The younger the child, the more dependence on evaluative observation of behavior and products of learning and the less dependence on paper and pencil testing. Cryan has some very nice suggestions. He says that one should evaluate children's behavior first by describing how it fits with what is reasonable to expect (5). He recommends that you observe, interview, interact, take notes, and write down your goals for their learning. He also recommends that you use your own collected information as the true picture of the child's performance, and measure specific behaviors only when it is necessary to diagnose entering ability or when transitions to more complex material are required. To reduce both your own and the child's anxiety level, he advises keeping the extent of "testing" to an absolute minimum. Finally, Cryan warns against what Goodlad calls "CMD" (Chronic Measurement Disease), preoccupation with pulling up plants to look at them before the roots take hold. He reminds us that learning will develop its roots if the conditions provided for learning and the kinds of learning supported are as important as what is being taught.

QUESTIONS AND EXERCISES
Discussion questions

1. Why is it more difficult to evaluate the effectiveness of health education than of most other school subjects?

2. Differentiate between the purposes of formative and summative evaluation procedures. If you were required to limit your evaluations to one of the two kinds, which would you choose, and what would be your reasons for that choice?

3. Some educators are willing to stipulate in advance of instruction that a certain amount of achievement of an objective will be adequate evidence of its success, for example, "By the end of the course, the student will be able to state at least three reasons why cigarette smoking is dangerous to one's health." In this event, is the focus on measurement or evaluation?

4. Can absolute mastery of the objectives defined for health instruction be a reasonable goal if the objectives themselves are in all ways feasible for the students involved? Explain.

5. Knowles, a physician whose pronouncements derogating the value of school health education are often quoted by those wishing to do the same, said that "School health programs are abysmal at best . . ." and "There are no examinations to determine if anything's been learned" (16). If you were asked to respond to such an accusation by describing what an appropriate evaluation plan should cover, what would you propose? List the procedures you would recommend be adopted, and briefly describe the kinds of things that should be evaluated.

6. What might be some difficulties you would encounter if you were forced to develop an evaluation plan based on objectives stated too ambiguously to provide any guidance, such as, "knows", "understands," "appreciates," etc.? How might you resolve this problem?

7. If you were asked to describe an effective way to appraise the health beliefs of primary school children, what would you recommend, and why? Would your answer be different if the problem involved middle school children? In what way?

8. Should a summative evaluation activity address primarily cognitive outcomes, or should equal emphasis be given to assessment of changes in attitudes or behaviors? What is your rationale for your answer?

9. If a teacher employs a wide range of measurement techniques during a semester course and determines the course grade on the basis of all of the resulting scores, summarized and weighted carefully, is the final outcome an evaluation or is it measurement? Why?

Exercises

1. For each of the following situations decide whether the action involves measurement or evaluation and explain why it is so.
   a. A principal wishes to select an elementary health textbook series that will provide a comprehen-

sive view of the subject matter, that is up to date, and that fits the increasing level of reading skills and vocabulary expected at successive grades. A teacher committee is asked to analyze three available series and submit their recommendations relative to the best choice among them.

b. A teacher gives a standardized knowledge test as a means of determining the relative background in health information of each individual in the class before instruction, so that plans can be tailored to class needs.

c. As the school year comes to an end, a teacher reviews the complete record of each student, looking at knowledge test scores, quality of participation, growth in problem-solving skills, change in attitudes as revealed by both observation and measurement techniques, and a host of other significant data accumulated during the past year's activities.

d. To demonstrate individual differences in physical growth rates, a teacher determines the height and weight of each sixth grade student during the first week of school and again during the final week. The change in the two sets of figures is announced and a chart constructed to show comparisons.

2. Select a health-concerned pamphlet, booklet, textbook, or any other material prepared for use in elementary health education teaching. Adapt any of the guidelines proposed in this chapter appropriate for the purpose of evaluating its utility and acceptability. Prepare a brief report of the results of your analysis, and include the set of criteria you applied.

3. Obtain a copy of a recent district curriculum guide prepared for the elementary health instructional program, K to grade 7. Apply Payne's questions to the analysis of the plan as proposed. How well does it adhere to the criteria implicit in those questions? On a scale of one to ten, how would you rank the document for its adequacy of description? What are its strengths, and what are its weaknesses in your view?

4. In association with a classmate, choose an instructional objective listed among those in the guide as the focus of this exercise. Decide, between you, who will develop a learning opportunity that would provide appropriate practice for the objective and who will design an evaluation strategy that would allow the students to demonstrate mastery of the objective. Each of you must work independently so that neither knows what the other is planning. When the proposals are finished, study the results together. Would completion of the learning opportunity have prepared the learners to fulfill the requirements of the evaluation activity? Does each plan match the intentions of the objective? What are your conclusions? Would you have been measuring or evaluating the outcome of the learning opportunity?

REFERENCES

1. American Educational Research Association. In Wittrock MC, ed: *Handbook of research on teaching*, ed 3, New York, 1986, Macmillan.
2. Bloom BS, Madeus GF, Hastings JT: *Evaluation to improve learning*, New York, 1981, McGraw-Hill.
3. Burns R: Objectives and content validity and tests, *Educ Technology* 8(23):18, 1968.
4. Carlyon WH: The seven deadly sins of health education, *Health Values* 13:1, spring/summer, 1981.
5. Cryan JR: Evaluation: plague or promise? *Childhood Educ* 62(5):344-350, 1986.
6. David JL: Restructuring and technology: Partners in change, *Phi Delta Kappan* 73(1):40, 1991.
7. Dorman, S: Evaluating computer software for the health education classroom, *J Sch Health* 62(1):35-37, January 1992.
8. Education Commission of the States: *Recommendations for school health education*, report no 130, Denver, 1981, The Commission.
9. Edwards CH Jr: An effective teaching approach to teacher evaluation and staff development, *ERS Spectrum* 4:2, 1986.
10. Goodlad JI: *A place called school*, New York, 1984, McGraw-Hill.
11. Green LW, Kreuter M: *Health promotion: An educational and environmental approach*, Mountain View, Calif, 1991, Mayfield.
12. Hochbaum GM: Behavior change as a goal of health education, *Eta Sigma Gamman* 13(2):3, 1981.
13. Hochbaum GM: Certain problems in evaluating health education, *Health Values* 6(1):14, 1982.
14. IOX Associates: *Evaluation handbooks for health education programs*, Culver City, Calif, 1983, The Associates.
15. Johnson NC, Orso JK: Teacher evaluation criteria, *ERS Spectrum* 4(3):33-36, 1986.

16. Knowles J: The responsibility of the individual, *Daedalus* 106:57-80, Winter 1977.

17. Nelson S: *How healthy is your school*, New York, 1986, NCHE Press.

18. Nolte AE et al: Values for your children, *Instructor* 81(1):47, 1971.

19. Osborn BM, Sutton WF: Evaluation of health education materials, (adapted) *J Sch Health* 34(2):72, 1964.

20. Osgood CE, Suci GJ, Tannebaum PH: *The measurement of meaning*, Urbana, Ill, 1957, University of Illinois Press.

21. Payne A: *The study of curriculum plans*, Washington, DC, 1969, National Education Association.

22. Popham WJ: *Educational evaluation*, ed 2, Englewood Cliffs, NJ, 1988, Prentice Hall.

23. Riner PS: A comparison of the criterion validity of principals' judgments and teacher self-ratings on a high inference scale, *J Curr Superv* 7(2):149-169.

24. Salmon-Cox L: Teacher and standardized achievement tests: what's really happening? *Phi Delta Kappan* 52:9, 1981.

25. Scriven M: The methodology of evaluation. In *Perspectives of curriculum evaluation*, Chicago, 1967, Rand McNally.

26. Thygerson AL: Task analysis: determining what should be taught, *Health Educ* 8(2):8, 1977.

27. Veenker HC: Evaluating health practice and understanding, *Health Educ* 16(2):80-82, April/May, 1985.

28. Zahorik, J: Good teaching and supervision, *J Curr Superv* 7(4):393-404, Summer 1992.

SUGGESTED READINGS

Contento I, Kell D, Keiley M, Corcoran R: A formative evaluation of the American Cancer Society: Changing the course of nutrition education curriculum, *J Sch Health* 62(9):411-416, November 1992.

English J, Sancho A: *Criteria for comprehensive health education curricula*, Los Alamitos, Calif, 1990, Southwest Regional Laboratory.

Gold R, Parcel G, Walberg H, et al: Summary and conclusions of the teenage health teaching modules evaluation, *J Sch Health* 61(1):39-42, January 1991.

Maeroff G: Assessing alternative assessment, *Phi Delta Kappan* 73(4):273, 281, December 1991.

Robinson J III: Criteria for the selection and use of health education reading materials, *Health Education* 31-34, August/September 1988.

Taggart V, Bush P, Zuckerman A, Theiss P: A process evaluation of the District of Columbia: Know your body project, *J Sch Health* 60(2):60-66, February 1990.

Worthen B: Is your school ready for alternative assessment? *Phi Delta Kappan* Feb 1993. 74(6):455-456, February 1993.

8 Designing Classroom Tests and Evaluation Activities

When you finish this chapter, you should be able to

- Define the meaning of key measurement terms.
- Design a test blue print.
- Develop a functional set of test specifications.
- Identify ambiguities or other common errors in proposed test items.
- Construct an achievement test appropriate for use with a specified age group of children.
- Describe activities designed to assess specified competencies
- Explain ways differing referencing frameworks affect the meaning of course grades.

Just as evaluation is not limited to measurement, measurement is not limited to testing; yet very probably most people think of *test* as a word that is synonymous with both of those terms. Tests have been used to assess achievement and competence as long as there have been teaching and learning. The most frequent use of educational tests has been to assess the learning status of individual students in order to make instructional and other decisions concerning those students. Predominantly, the tests used as means of determining course grades and endorsing promotion to the next grade are teacher-made. This means that every teacher needs to know how to plan a test, prepare valid test items, and correctly interpret scores resulting from administration of tests. It isn't easy. And sometimes it is an anguishing responsibility. Whether a test is a good and

fair assessment of learning or one that is ambiguous, poorly planned, or otherwise inadequate, can result in the difference between a satisfied, motivated learner and one who is frustrated and apathetic about the whole business of schooling.

Elementary and middle-school teachers need to be just as knowledgeable about test construction as those at any other level of instruction. The Goodlad study of schools found that test taking in early elementary grades accounted for 2.2% of total class time and that upper elementary grades spent 3.3% of their time in test taking (5). That may not sound like very much testing activity until you learn that even middle-school students spent merely 5.5% of class time and senior high school students only a bit more than that (5.8% of class time) in testing.

It is not possible within the purview of a text

concerned with teaching about health to provide much more than a brief overview of the concepts and skills involved in educational measurement. We hope that if you are not lucky enough to have been provided at least a semester's course work in this important aspect of your teacher preparation program, you will do some independent reading in one of the very good texts available to you, for example, Ebel and Frisbie (4): *Essentials of Educational Measurement;* Wiersma and Jurs (17): *Educational Measurement and Testing;* Mehrens and Lehmann (10): *Measurement and Evaluation in Education and Psychology;* or one of the most enjoyable textbooks you will ever experience, Popham (13): *Educational Evaluation*, second edition.

Because measurement people employ a great many terms not common to other fields of education, it seems worthwhile to introduce and explain some of them before we begin. We will limit the definitions to those for reliability, validity, content validity, objectives-referenced, norm-referenced, achievement tests, and standardized tests.

Reliability refers to the extent to which a test is consistent in measuring what it measures, its stability over time. The longer the test and the more representative the items, the greater its reliability.

Validity refers to the extent to which a test actually measures what it purports to measure, or more precisely, the extent to which interpretation of its measures fits its purported purpose. A test that is not reliable can never be valid, although a test can be reliable without content validity.

Objectives-referenced tests are those used to ascertain the extent to which an individual's score compares with the maximum possible as a measure of the performances proposed by a set of objectives.

Norm-referenced tests are those used to measure a student's performance relative to that of other students taking the same test.

Criterion-referenced tests are those used to measure a student's status in relation to a set of clearly defined behaviors. In contrast to norm-referenced tests that emphasize relative comparisons among those examined, criterion-referenced tests are *absolute* measures, designed to determine, as precisely as possible, what an examinee can or cannot do, without reference to the performance of others (6).

Achievement tests are sets of items or questions representative of the knowledge or skills associated with a given content area or discipline and are designed to measure a student's comprehension of that knowledge or competence in those abilities.

Standardized tests are instruments commercially prepared and scrupulously validated by experts in measurement and the subject matter of concern. Such tests are supported by manuals detailing uniform procedures to be followed in administering, scoring, and interpreting the results. Scoring is typically objective, and established norms are provided (10).

FUNCTIONS OF CLASSROOM TESTS

Ebel and Frisbie believe that the primary function of teacher-made tests is to provide precise measures of achievement that can be used to report learning progress to students and to their parents (4). Scores on a good test do provide a teacher with quantitative evidence on which grades can be defensibly based, and students do want to know what grades they have received. For several years, Middleton was charged with responsibility for teaching health to all of the seventh grade students in a junior high school. This meant that every day she met five or six separate groups—some thirty classes each week. Grades were not a requirement of this staggering work load; merely a "pass" or "fail" notation was called for. But after a few years, the plan was changed. Students were not happy with just "pass" as recognition of their work, nor were their parents. A passing letter grade communicates much more about the learner's effort and ability than the word pass, especially when all that "pass" tells you is that the student did not fail. A good grade is a source of pride and pleasure. More than that, as a matter of record, it can be an asset long after school days are over.

A movement toward the development and use of assessment tools other than pencil and paper tests is currently widespread. Altogether some 40 states, notably Rhode Island, Kentucky, California, and Vermont, are planning at least some form of **alternate assessment** at the state level. Several labels have been proposed to describe alternatives to standardized tests. Those used most commonly are performance assessment, authentic assessment, and alternative assessment. All of them are viewed as *alternatives* to traditional multiple-choice, standardized achievement tests; all refer to *direct* examination of student *performance* on significant tasks that are relevant to tasks outside of a school (16). For the purposes of this discussion, we will use the term *alternative assessment* to describe activities that can be exhibited or viewed in the classroom for purposes of evaluating growth in abilities and knowledge as the outcome of health teaching and learning. These are not intended to supply data intended for use in compiling school, district, or state level achievement reports. The assessment task is specific to each student and evaluated and reported individually.

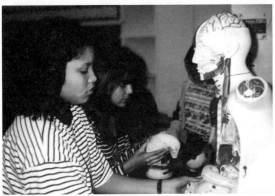

Matt Fischer

Alternative assessment activities can be used to evaluate health teaching.

Performance assessment refers to testing methods that require students to create an answer or product that demonstrates their knowledge or skills. Performance can take many forms, such as writing short answers, an essay, carrying out an experiment, presenting an oral argument, or assembling a portfolio of representative work.

Portfolios are made up of records of each student's work, tests, worksheets, notes from a journal, descriptions of demonstrations, field trip observations, or any written work that records the student's learning experiences during the course. A collection of work seen as a whole provides the teacher with an opportunity to view the range of health information and abilities possessed by a student. Assessment of achievement based on such an accumulation provides far better evidence of growth than individual pieces of work seen separately. This does not suggest that no evaluation be made of the components as originally submitted, however.

Obviously there is no quick and easy way to rate large numbers of performance-based tasks, portfolios, or interviews. Even the number of such assessments required for one class would be a workload far beyond reasonable. Another problem is the fact that since the content of a portfolio depends on the assignments made by the teacher; in essence the assessment tasks are part of the instruction. That means that in a very real sense the portfolio is an evaluation of the teacher as well. Still, the major problem is cost versus benefit. That cost is not just in money, which is considerable, especially if the intent is to arrange mass applications of the assessment tools. It is also measured by the tremendous amount of time needed to determine the criteria and assess the outcomes.

Given that assessment of achievement and awarding of grades should not be limited to analysis of scores on tests, alternatives to testing must be used with care and with full realization of their shortcomings. Observations, however specific and objective, have value in assessing achievement, but they are not adequate as total replacements for *good* classroom achievement tests. Imperfect as tests may be, they are typically more reliable, objective, and valid than the alternatives tend to be. The answer seems to be to use the best of each to counteract the weaknesses of the others.

Expectation of testing, particularly among upper elementary and middle school students, prompts review and sharpened attention to important aspects of what has been studied and what is to be covered in the test. Just the experience of *being* tested—working through the questions, and receiving feedback on its results—adds significantly to every student's store of knowledge, whatever the prior level of achievement may have been.

Finally, and not least among the functions of testing, is its influence on and contribution to the quality of planning the teaching it requires. To construct an acceptably valid test you have to think carefully about your goals and objectives *before* you plan either your lessons or your tests. When you know what you want your students to be able to do after your instruction, lesson planning is much easier and test questions simply have to match your objectives.

KINDS OF ACHIEVEMENT TESTS

Ebel and Frisbie categorize achievement tests broadly by the type of test-score interpretation they yield, as content-referenced, group-referenced (norm-referenced), or criterion-referenced (4). Because teachers are typically concerned with their students mastering specific content and skills, content-referenced tests would appear to be appropriate for both student and teacher needs. A content-referenced interpretation is made when the performance level of individuals is assessed in terms of a test focused on an explicit content area, without regard to how other examinees have scored. A special kind of content-referenced interpretation is termed *objectives-referenced*. When the test items adequately correspond to the instructional objectives of interest to the test user, scores can be interpreted in terms of mastery of these objectives.

The use of instructional objectives as guides to valid evaluation has already been discussed in Chapters 4 and 7. Scores on teacher-made tests, whether interpreted in relation to mastery or not, are usually also ranked in determining grades.

PLANNING TESTS

Ideally, test construction is based on a set of specifications established as the first step in the total process. Decisions must be made and explicitly set down as guides to the development of the instrument regarding the kinds of items to be used, the number of items of each kind; the kinds of tasks the items will require, the level and range of item difficulty, the time the test will take for completion, and the amount of direction that will be necessary. Few of these are mutually exclusive. The decision shaping one aspect of the test is influenced by decisions made about the others. For example, the number of items in a test depends somewhat on the amount of time available for its administration. The kinds of items used depends on the maturity and cognitive skills of the examinees. The areas of content chosen for emphasis depend on what has been studied during the period for which the test is being constructed. The level of difficulty (whether the items can be answered correctly by only the better students or by most of the students) depends on whether the purpose of the test is to rank-order the examinees according to their scores or to determine the number of students whose achievement approaches mastery, and so on.

CONSTRUCTING TEST BLUE PRINTS

Often two-way grids, sometimes called test blue prints, are employed as preliminary plans for test construction. The purpose of the grid is to guide the format of a completed instrument, not to summarize. In a typical grid, the content to be covered is listed at the left in a column, and cognitive behaviors or objectives are listed across the top in a row. For example, the left hand column for a test in health education might list the content areas, with cognitive behaviors such as Bloom's (1) knowledge, comprehension, application, and perhaps analysis as well, set across the horizontal axis. A content outline has been adapted from a health textbook designed for upper elementary school students. Items are assigned to each of the columns and rows as illustrated in Table 8-1.

Notice that the content dimension covers the total scope of health; hence such a test would be summative in purpose. Formative tests would be limited to one or two of the listed content areas, more items would be allocated to each, the test would be shorter, and less time would be needed for its administration and scoring.

A test instrument based on such a grid would result in nearly even consideration of the subject matter involved. Instructional objectives would specify behaviors according to their planned distribution among the four levels of cognition indicated. Another technique used in developing test specifications for norm-referenced measures is to list only the content categories along with the number of items intended to be provided for each. The list could similarly be limited to the set

of objectives employed in the instruction and items allocated to measurement of their achievement (12). If instructional objectives are used in this case, they should specify behaviors drawn from the proposed four levels of cognition.

In the simplest situation, where instruction has been based on a single textbook designed for a specified grade, the book's section headings may well provide a usable list of topics as outlines of the content. Given that the sections are about equal in the importance given them, items could be constructed on the basis of topics systematically selected from that list.

PREPARING TEST ITEMS

Once the specifications are determined, appropriate items have to be constructed. "Appropriate" is a word often used in this context but less often explained. It stands for the degree to which the tasks implicit in each test item match the content or objective they are supposed to elicit. The decisions made so far only serve as guidelines to the listed aspects of test construction. Still to be decided is which kind of test will be developed, for there are generally only two kinds of cogni-

TABLE 8-1

Content Outline for Test Items

	Number of Test Items for Each Cognitive Level				
	Knowledge	Comprehension	Application	Analysis	Total
Content Areas					
Growth and development	2	2	1	0	5
Consumer and personal health	3	2	0	1	6
Physical fitness	2	2	2	0	6
Nutrition	3	2	1	0	6
Safety and first aid	2	2	1	0	5
Mental and social health	2	2	2	1	7
Environmental and community health	2	1	1	0	4
Diseases	2	2	1	0	5
Drugs	2	3	1	0	6
TOTAL	20	18	10	2	50

tive test formats, free response and structured response. When that decision has been made, the items particular to the kind of test chosen must be written. And this is a task fraught with difficulty and pitfalls.

First, what are the kinds of tests between which you can choose? Written tests are usually categorized as either **free-response** or **structured-response,** sometimes instead as **essay** or **objective,** or as Popham (12) prefers, as **constructed** versus **selected.** A free-response or constructed item is one that requires examinees to use their own words to respond in writing to a relatively small number of questions. The results are judged more or less subjectively, depending on the form. The test requiring the most subjective analysis is the least structured of all, the essay test.

Tests referred to as having structured or selected responses are those in which the students can only *select* an answer from a limited number of alternatives. They are asked to read all the proposed answers and then to check the one that either is the one correct answer or is the *best* among those offered. The score is obtained by comparing the responses to these kinds of items with a standard key.

Free-response tests require recall of information in order to prepare an answer, whereas structured responses appear to depend more on a student's ability to recognize the correct answer among those provided, all of which seem plausible to anyone who does not have the needed information. When skillfully constructed, both kinds of tests demand recall and reasoning. Whether a given response represents rote recall or reasoning depends on how the student has been taught, not solely on how the question is written. When facts have been the focus of instruction, possession of facts will be the end product, and this limitation is perpetuated by fact-specific questions.

In general, the use of free-response tests is limited in the elementary grades to older children who have learned to read and write well enough to comprehend the questions and construct an answer in their own words. Structured-answer tests can be devised or are available in standardized form for use with nonreaders. Teachers or aides read the questions, and the students point to pictured alternatives or tell the teacher which answer is correct. The television series "Sesame Street" uses this sort of pictured format with great success.

Next, what are the mistakes to be avoided? Choosing between these two categories is relatively easy. As long as the test items are carefully designed, are relevant to the instruction and subject matter, and fit the format, you should be successful in developing a good test unless, in writing the items, you make what Popham terms a "A lot of dumb mistakes" (12). Fortunately these are mistakes that can be avoided if you keep them in mind as you write your questions.

1. **Unclear or inadequate directions.** Don't assume that your students know exactly what you want them to do with each item or even that they know how to do it. Write the directions for answering each kind of item first, not last, and if possible try them out on a few students of the same grade level before you prepare the final copy of your test.

2. **Ambiguity.** Probably everyone has experienced the frustration that an ambiguous test item causes an examinee. For example, consider this true-false item: "When both parents are working, they often have difficulty with disciplining their children because they are seldom home at the same time." There are two "theys"; does either of them refer to the children, or do both of them refer back to "parents?" How can the respondent tell which meaning is correct? The item writer knows, but the respondent has to be a mind reader.

3. **Specific determiners, or unintended clues to the right answer.** There are several ways that an item can unintentionally point to the right answer or at least delimit those that can be right. Sometimes only some of the distractors in a multiple-choice test fit the stem grammatically; sometimes distractors are irrelevant, illogical, or otherwise impossible, for example: "Sleep is

soundest during the: (a) first 2 hours; (b) before midnight; (c) after midnight; (d) last 2 hours; (e) after the first 2 hours." Only two of these alternatives fit with the last word of the premise, "the." Some words, such as "always," "never," or "all," typically seen in true-false items, are giveaways to experienced test takers who know that very few things are always or never anything. Another clue to the right answer is furnished when one statement is very much longer than the others, in the attempt to make certain that what has been said is absolutely correct.

4. **Complicated sentences and unfamiliar vocabulary.** Overlong statements may be perceived as clues that they are true, but the situation may simply be that the writer didn't know how to say what he or she wanted to say more succinctly. Overuse of unfamiliar or difficult words also tends to discourage the reader, thereby motivating the choice of an answer that is simply a quick guess in order to get past the item and get on with the test. Try this one for example: True or False? "Qualified physicians such as those specializing in healiocosmopathology have accomplished unusual cures with their methods of treatment."

Some of these common mistakes are probably more easily avoided than others, but keep all of them in mind as you write each of your test items. The items you develop will vary according to the age and past experience of your students, of course, but because you have been their teacher and know what they have studied and can do, you will be better qualified than anyone else to write items that will be right for them.

Teacher-made tests and the kinds of items of which they are composed are nothing new to anyone who has attended school in this country. But this time you must approach testing from the other side of the desk. Therefore review of the most often used kinds of teacher-made tests follows.

Free-Response Tests

Free-response tests are composed of essay and short-answer or completion kinds of items. *Es-*

say tests take much less time to prepare than do objective tests, but they require a great deal of time to score. Moreover, good essay questions are not all that easily written. They must ask the student to exhibit the cognitive skill or process that was stipulated in the objectives. If the behavior was "explain," the question has to require explaining, not listing, comparing, describing, or any other behavior. The question has to be written in such a way that it cannot be answered by filling in memorized sections of the material provided in the textbook. Instead it must require application of what has been studied in a different context than as considered during the learning opportunities.

A poorly or carelessly constructed essay item is more likely to measure a student's ability to figure out what it means than her/his knowledge about the subject matter. An item such as, "Discuss the importance of various locations of accidents," is not only impossibly global but baffling as well. Does it mean that the respondent should itemize locations and describe their importance as factors in the incidence of accidents? What does "importance" mean? Should locations be ranked according to the probability of an accident occurring there? What is meant by "discuss?" How many is "various?" Is there a location where an accident could *not* occur? That item, taken from a teacher's manual for a health textbook, is so ambiguous that suggestions for its improvement are limited to tossing it out. A good way to ensure that every student will perceive the task similarly is to pose a problem situation and then ask a series of questions based on that situation. For example:

> Accidents claim more lives of school children than all other causes of death combined. Explain how each of the following serves to prevent an accident: (1) traffic signals, (2) pedestrian walk markings, (3) bicycle lights and reflectors, (4) safety rules, (5) fire drills, and (6) crossing guards.

An essay item structured in this way is more easily scored because the possibility of misunderstanding the question is minimized and the range of possible answers is delimited. Still, the student is given freedom in composing answers, and the requirement that knowledge about these factors be applied to the explanation of accident prevention among peers makes it meaningful and relevant to their own needs and interests.

Examples of other simply but clearly posed essay items are the following:

> How a person grows and develops is influenced by two important factors: heredity (determined by the genes we receive from our parents) and the environment (physical, social, mental, and emotional) in which we live. Write a short paragraph that describes some important traits that make you different from other people but that can only be the result of your environment.

> For each of the following foods, (1) name an acceptable substitute food that could supply the same nutrient, and (2) give at least two reasons why this kind of food is essential to a balanced diet: (a) whole milk, (b) meat, (c) oranges, (d) bread, and (e) spinach.

Essay tests are difficult to score and require a lot of time to do it. Moreover, the obtained scores are notoriously unreliable. Many biasing factors, some of them entirely unrelated to the quality of the answers, influence the judgment process. Some of these include whether a paper is read before or after a poor or excellent one; whether the handwriting is legible, the spelling correct, and the paper neat; how tired the teacher is when reading the papers; how the student perceived the meaning of the questions compared with the teacher's intention; how well designed and comprehensive the directions are; and what the teacher already knows about the student's past performances and personality. Some students are so good with words, and even with redirecting the discussion toward a related topic about which they know more, that the reader is lulled into believing that the assigned topic has been addressed.

Teachers often vary in their evaluation of the same paper at different times. Astonishingly, research shows that the same paper can be awarded every grade from A to F depending on

who reads it. And, in addition to its being laborious and time consuming to read a great number of essay papers, so few questions can be asked that the resulting sample of a student's achievement may not adequately represent his/her grasp of the material or the course. Given other essay questions, a student who has done poorly might have done very well, and vice versa.

The advantages of essay questions are that they give students an opportunity to show ability to analyze a problem and prepare a solution in their own words and at their own pace. Some students do not perform well when under pressure to read and answer a long list of questions, nor do they like to be restricted to a few prepared responses in choosing an answer.

Scoring is more likely to be consistent when a set of criteria for evaluating the answers can be predetermined. Papers should be read without knowing who has written them so that any subjective set toward their authors can be avoided. The answers to each item should all be read at the same time and evaluated and scored relative to the performance of every examinee on that question. In this way a student gets credit for the quality of the answer to each question rather than one score arrived at on the basis of some generalized accomplishment index based on a quick reading of all of the items at once.

Another technique is to skim all the papers quickly, sorting them roughly into piles labelled *excellent*, *good*, *fair*, and *weak*, or something similar. Next, each paper is carefully reread, with shifts made between the preliminary assignments to higher or lower ratings as seems more appropriate. Each paper is thus judged along with others that are similar in quality to see if it belongs in that category or if it should be rated higher or lower.

The evaluation of essay papers is even more complex when students are allowed to select from a list of alternative questions. In effect, each student has taken a different test. In addition, since it cannot be demonstrated that essay items are equally representative of the same amount and kind of learning, what happens is that not only different tests but different *kinds* of tests may have been assembled as a consequence of the choices. Certainly, there being fewer answers to any one of the items, there is less possibility of making valid comparisons among the few.

Short answer and *completion tests* are a more restricted form of the free-response test and may be better suited and easier for children whose writing skills are limited or not yet developed. Such an instrument can be duplicated and distributed to each child or read aloud by the teacher for the entire class. In the same way, answers can be written by the individual students or agreed to in discussions by the total group. Short answer tests are composed of specific questions that can be answered with one word or a very short statement, for example:

Meat and nuts are foods representing which class of nutrients?_____
What most often causes tooth decay?_____
How many chromosomes are contained in the nucleus of a human cell?_____

A direct question is better for short answer items than an incomplete statement, especially when used with young children, because they are used to that format. In addition, it forces the teacher to prepare items that have one and only one right answer. Incomplete sentences invite ambiguity because the author, knowing the word wanted, assumes that everyone else will think of that word and no other. In actuality, there may be several alternative words that would finish the statement just as logically, even if differently.

Completion items are similar to short answer questions but usually are written as incomplete sentences rather than as questions, for example:

Pathogens (germs) that cause diseases such as colds, measles, and flu are called_____.
Blood vessels that carry the blood away from the heart are termed_____.
Twins who develop from the same single cell are termed_____?

The blank should be placed at the end of the statement, otherwise the student may have for- gotten what was wanted by the time the entire statement has been read. Limit the blanks to one or at most two in any one item. Make the blank long enough to permit the word to be written legibly and as nearly as possible equal in length to the others in the list of items. When one blank space is noticeably different, it provides a clue to the expected answer.

The advantages of the short-answer and completion tests are that they can be more easily and quickly scored, and a great many more questions can be asked than is the case with essay questions, thus providing a better sample of a student's knowledge and comprehension. The learners still have to produce their own answers and must recall the information needed to do so. Because these kinds of items must be so specific, they are best used in testing factual material, such as dates, definitions, and terminology, and are not useful in appraising problem-solving skills.

How accurate the answers to these kinds of free-response items can be depends on the way they are written. Teachers sometimes unwittingly reward rote recall and penalize creative thinking when only one answer is accepted—the one that uses the exact words from the text. An example of this is, "There are more than _____ bones in the human skeleton." The answer wanted is "200", but actually *any* number less than 200 would be correct. Some other weaknesses to guard against in constructing items include over-emphasis on trivial information, for example, "Your hair grows about _____ inches a month," or "The current population of the world is in excess of _____," or calling for inconsequential words such as, "The first teeth to _____ are called baby, or primary, teeth." Another pitfall is that the desired answer may be factually incorrect, as in "Good dental health is ensured when we visit our dentist _____ times a year." Good dental health cannot be ensured by *any* means, and, although biannual visits generally are recommended, people vary in their needs, and unexpected problems often occur.

No item should omit so much that it is incomprehensible as a statement, for example, "Most microbes can be killed by _____, by _____, and by _____." Without the missing words "sunlight, dryness, and very high temperatures," the item is a guessing game, not a test of knowledge.

Short answer tests should not be scored solely by comparison with a prepared key. Keys need to be supplemented with a qualified scorer's ability to judge whether a different answer is equally appropriate and correct.

Structured Response Tests

Tests that require the student to choose among already prepared alternative answers to questions are usually termed **objective,** although actually only the scoring procedures are objective. Subjective judgment is always involved in devising the questions, and it influences the selection of the material that is considered important to test, as well as the choice of the right answer. The most commonly used objectively scored tests are the binary-choice (so called because they offer only two choices) such as true-false, right-wrong, yes-no, agree-disagree, etc., multiple choice, and matching-item tests.

True-False Tests.   The true-false test item is simply a statement that the student reads and judges to be one or the other. It might be described as a two-response, multiple-choice item, although the opposing statement (that the statement is or is not true) is unstated. Such an item can be written in a slightly different form so that the correct answer is yes or no, right or wrong, agree or disagree.

Another variation is to require the student to explain *why* an item is false, or to correct any item that has been judged false in part or entirely. This is supposed to minimize the effect of guessing, but it costs a great deal of teacher time in order to evaluate the correctness of the explanation and in effect changes the test from structured to a combination structured and free-response style.

True-false items are those most often chosen by teachers for their tests and quizzes. They ap-pear to be easy to write but actually the creation of concise, unambiguous items that are unmistakably and unarguably either true or false is not easy at all. Critics of the true-false format hold that, with only two alternative answers, anybody can get 50 percent of the items right without knowing anything at all about the subject matter. This is true only if you have but one item to answer. The longer the test, the less the possibility that guessing has much effect. For example, it has been demonstrated that chances are only 2 in 100 that a person who has guessed blindly on a 15-item test will get 80% or more of them correct. On a 25-item test, there are only 2 chances in 1000 of getting 80% or more correct by blind guessing, and the odds drop to 3 in 100,000,000 of getting all 25 right (11). Don't forget that if there is a 50% chance of getting an item right by chance, there is also a 50% chance of getting it wrong.

Ebel has long championed the use of true-false tests as means of measuring a wide variety of meaningful propositions far beyond trivial or single fact-related information. The rationale for this belief is summarized in the four statements that follow:

1. The essence of educational achievement is the command of useful verbal knowledge.
2. All verbal knowledge can be expressed in propositions.
3. A proposition is any sentence that can be said to be true or false.
4. The extent of students' command of a particular area of knowledge is indicated by their success in judging the truth or falsity of propositions related to it (3, 4).

It was Ebel's belief that if true-false items are held in low esteem, it is not because the binary-choice format is inherently limited to assessment of trivial information, rather it is because the form is so often used ineptly by unskilled item writers.

There are the usual pitfalls into which the careless or inexperienced writer can fall. Often statements from the textbook are copied as is or doctored with a negative word to make them

---

ITEM-WRITING TIPS OR GUIDELINES

1. Keep the word length of all items as even and short as possible.
2. Select statements that are representative of important ideas or generalizations.
3. Make certain that each item is true or false beyond question.
4. Construct about the same number of binary response items of either kind.
5. Write statements as clearly, concisely, and simply as possible.
6. Paraphrase rather than copy statements verbatim from the book.
7. Do not use a negative as means of altering statements. If the negative is essential to a true statement, underline or capitalize the word, and *never* use double negatives.
8. Don't try to trick the examinee into giving a wrong answer.

---

false; yet it cannot be assumed that every statement in the book is true. And even if true, such statements, taken out of context, may not be able to stand alone, as they must be good true-false items. Also, this places too much emphasis on memorization, and the items picked in this way tend to focus on trivia. Words such as *never, all,* and *always* are often employed to make an item false, and students quickly learn to mark any statements with one of those words as false when they are guessing. They may also be tricked into marking a statement false when it is true, for the same reason, because sometimes "never," "always," or "all" may be correct. Another tip-off for the test-wise is the wordiness that sometimes accompanies true statements as the writer attempts to make them definitively so. If these kinds of items are frequent, test scores are more likely to reveal which students are practiced test takers than which of them are better prepared and more knowledgeable.

Another dubious practice is to use phrases like "the best way to," "the chief reason for," or "the best method of," which forces the student to make a judgment when the alternatives are unknown. The student has to ask, "the best way compared to what?" The most aggravating fault, from the students' point of view, is the attempt to trick them into missing the item, as in, "Walter Reed is the physician credited with the discovery that malaria is transmitted by mosquitos." The disease with which his name is associated is

not malaria, but yellow fever. Even the student who knows that, may miss it in the pressure to read and react to a long list of true-false statements.

The purpose of a test is to find out how much the student knows; it is not a contest to find out whether a clever use of words can trick students into making a mistake. Ambiguity is a frequent fault in item writing. For example, look at this statement: "The best way to help a drowning man is to jump into the water and save him." Certainly saving a drowning person is the best way to help him, but the student must weigh that part against the part about jumping into the water, which may or may not be helpful to either the victim or the would-be rescuer. Another foolish ploy is to make the correct answer depend on knowledge about some unessential word, as in the statement, "The cochlea is a part of the inner ear." This item does not test anything other than knowledge about the anatomy of the ear; to answer, the student has to possess knowledge about the cochlea, which has little to do with health behavior or knowledge except in a trivial way.

These are some of the weaknesses in test construction to keep in mind when writing true-false items or any structured test problems. Actually the distractors in a multiple-choice or matching-item test are simply a cluster of true-false items related to the same premise or stem. It follows that each distractor in a multiple-

A

Mark an X on the picture that shows the health worker who takes your temperature and helps you get ready to see the doctor.

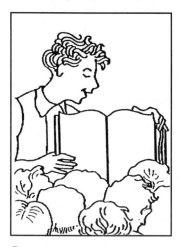 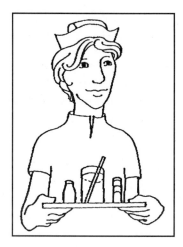 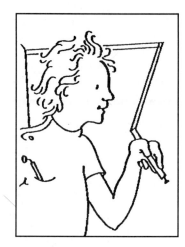

B

Mark an X on the picture that shows the health worker who you go to see when you are ill (sick).

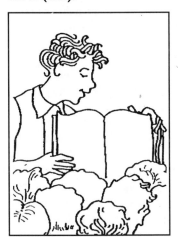 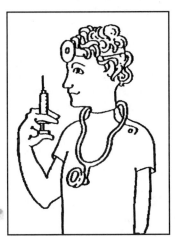 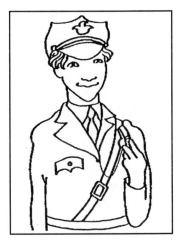

FIGURE 8-1

Health knowledge test for preschoolers. This pictorial, multiple choice instrument has 45 items developed for use with 4-, 5-, and 6-year-old children. The test is group administered and read to children by a teacher or aides. Each child has a booklet with the items as follows and a crayon with which to mark the picture selected as the best or correct answer. The teacher reads the words that are provided above each set of pictures in the examiner's booklet.

C
Mark an X on the picture that shows where garbage should be kept.

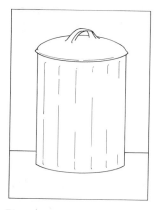
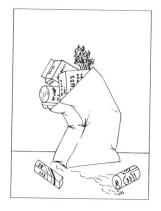
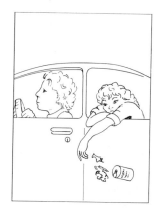

D
Mark an X on the picture that shows what you should drink to help your teeth grow healthy and strong.

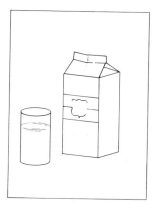
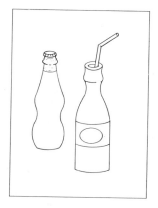
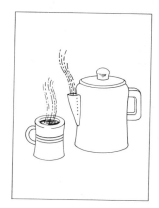

FIGURE 8-1   cont'd
For legend see opposite page.

choice test must be written with attention to the same guidelines as in the case of the true-false item.

As in the case of any test, true-false tests can be read to young children, whose responses are verbal or recorded by simple marks, such as plus or minus signs. The distinguishing characteristic of true-false statements designed for young children is the simplicity of the language and concepts with which they are asked to deal. A 3-picture format to which a child could point was used by Jubb (8) and Hendricks, et al. (7) to as-

sess the health knowledge of 4-, 5-, and 6-year-old children enrolled in early childhood programs. Face validity of the test was established through consensus of a 10-member panel of experts. Items are based upon objectives inferred from wide review of health curricula and instructional materials appropriate for this age group. Figure 8-1 is an example of Jubb's 3-picture format test.

Multiple-Choice Tests.   A multiple-choice item consists of an incomplete statement or question called the **stem** and, at the elementary level, usually no more than three or four alternatives from which the student is directed to choose either the correct or best answer that fits the stem. When incomplete statements are used, the responses (called **distractors**) are written so that they fit into and complete the sentence, for example, "If you are nearsighted, you can see objects near you (1) better than those far away; (2) less clearly than those far away; (3) as well as those far away." Or, an item can ask the student to indicate the best of several proposed answers, for example, "What is the best time to brush your teeth in the morning? (1) as soon as you get up, (2) while you are bathing and dressing, (3) after you have eaten your breakfast."

An advantage of the multiple-choice item is that the desired choice does not have to be the one answer deemed true, although it does have to be defensibly best among the alternatives provided. It can be constructed to call for problem-solving skills such as interpretation, analysis, application, and other cognitive processes, as well as simple recall of information. Construction of this type of test is perhaps the most time consuming. In a very real sense, each item represents three or four questions, depending on the number of distractors. A 50-item multiple-choice test is the equivalent of a 200-item true-false test when there are four distractors. As a result, since there are more questions, the potential reliability of the test is increased. Of course, reading time is also increased, which can lead the student to make errors even though she/he may have known the answer, because when the *best* answer is the correct answer, the student often chooses the first *good* answer without reading all of them. This problem can be dealt with most effectively by carefully constructing the instructions that precede multiple-choice items.

Another challenging task is to write three or four distractors that are so plausible that only an individual who really knows the answer can choose among them with confidence. A distractor so unreasonable as an answer that no one chooses it is termed **non-functioning.** In the following example, which distractor would you predict would seldom if ever be chosen? "Between 1975 and 1985, air pollution in major cities in the United States (1) was largely caused by automobile exhaust; (2) was the cause of 1 million deaths per year; (3) decreased; (4) increased in some places and decreased in others."

You must be careful to prepare distractors that sound logical, are similar in nature, and either complete a partial statement or answer a stated question. The stem must include enough of an incomplete statement (and all of a question) so that the alternatives that are to complete it or answer it are readably short and about the same length. An example of a typically inadequate stem is, "Aspirin is (1) harmless, (2) addictive, (3) harmful, (4) rarely overused." The stem is inadequate because it does not tell the examinee anything about the problem. As a consequence it is nothing other than a cluster of four true-false questions, each of which begins with the words "aspirin is." A better question might be, "The most likely effect of heavy overuse of aspirin would be (1) stomach ulcer and bleeding; (2) physical addiction; (3) tolerance, or the need to take more of the drug each time; (4) severe skin rash or loss of hair."

Frequently, you will see options consisting only of "all of the above," "none of the above," or "A and B only." These may be alternatives worth the student's consideration, or they may simply be evidence of the difficulty involved in writing four good distractors. When "none of the above" is the desired answer to such an item, and the student picks it, what has been revealed is that the individual knew that the others were wrong but not whether he or she knew the correct answer, which leaves the teacher nowhere as far as knowing the status of student learning is concerned.

Depending on your decision regarding the number of distractors, take care to construct every item with that same number of alternatives. Otherwise the student may mark the last one on the answer sheet, while the correct answer was the third of a four-alternative question.

Another way to design the response pattern

for a multiple-choice test is to develop distractors, all of which are correct but one. The examinee is to pick out the one that is wrong. This system potentially provides the teacher with a lot more feedback on the student's fund of knowledge. Can you see why?

A variation of the multiple-choice test is a combination of its usual form with a matching test. The same three or four alternatives are used in connection with a longer list of related items, for example:

Matching-Item Tests. In another variation of a multiple-choice test, for each item in a list of terms, topics, or other elements, a word is chosen from another list that describes, defines, or somehow relates to it. Usually a list of terms is placed to the left and the list of alternatives to the right. The list of alternatives should be longer than the terms so there is no automatic answer to the last item. For young children the second list should not be longer than five or six items, so the search for the matching answer each time is not complicated or long. For the student to quickly grasp the relationship of the items to the alternatives, all the elements in the first column should have some clear connection, rather than being an assortment of unrelated terms or ob-

jects. Finally, the directions should clearly explain the task. The following is an example of this type of test item.

Directions can be varied to say, "Draw a line connecting each item in column I with its function listed in column II." For the primary grades, matching tests can be developed in the form of pictures, real objects, or models (Figure 8-2). In the simplest form, one item represents column I, and three pictures or real objects are used in place of column II.

"Sesame Street" uses this technique in reverse with its singing game, "One of these things is not like the others," in which four or five pictures are shown, and the children try to discover which one is unrelated to the others. What they are doing is classifying, which is basic to conceptualizing. Matching tests are best used to measure growth in knowledge of facts and of important terminology.

STANDARDIZED TESTS

Standardized tests are those whose validity and reliability have been determined by means of rigorous statistical and other procedures and for which norms have been established (9). Norm-

---

MATCHING ITEM TEST FORMATS

Directions: Beside each of the substances in the following list, place the letter from the key that matches the nutrient it represents. You may use any item more than once.

Key: A—Vitamin, B—Protein,
C—Carbohydrate, D—Mineral

Substances

1. Calcium   _____
2. Meat   _____
3. Niacin   _____
4. Sugar   _____
5. Milk   _____
6. Iron   _____
7. Thiamine   _____
8. Gelatin   _____

Directions: Beside each item in column I place the number that is given for its function in column II. Any of the functions may be selected more than once, or not at all.

I Organ	II Function
____ Heart	1. Excretion
____ Brain	2. Movement
____ Lungs	3. Structure
____ Skeleton	4. Digestion
____ Muscles	5. Circulation
____ Kidneys	6. Reproduction
____ Skin	7. Coordination
____ Stomach	8. Respiration
	9. Perspiration

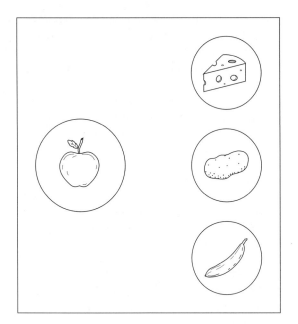

FIGURE 8-2
Pictorial matching test. Verbal instructions, "Which one is like the one on the plate?"

referenced tests are, by definition, a means of comparing one student's performance with that of others of the same age group or grade. The advantage of using standardized tests is that, used correctly, they are presumed to be valid and can tell you how your students compare with others who have taken the test. A disadvantage is that the test may not be appropriate for your needs. It may not match the objectives that structured your teaching. Another problem is that any one test can only be a sample of the entire domain of achievement items that might have been asked of your students. Consequently, any conclusions based on the resulting scores are likely to depend on too little information. For example, administration of one standardized test of health knowledge showed that nutrition was the content area in which students appeared to be weakest. This judgment was based on the fact that more people missed nutrition questions than those in any other of the areas tested. Still, since there were only five questions concerning nutrition, the pos-

sibility exists that five different questions might have yielded quite different results. The longer the test of any particular subject or sub-topic thereof, the more reliable and valid it will be.

How useful standardized test scores are to elementary teachers is debatable. Perhaps the question should be, what use do elementary teachers make of the information they receive as an outcome of standardized testing?

Salmon-Cox studied a group of 68 school teachers in urban and suburban school districts who administered and received test results from a standardized test of student achievement (14). She found that about half of them used the information only as a supplement to or in confirmation of what they already knew about their students through interaction with them, observation of classroom performance, and application of teacher-made tests. Generally, the teachers had more confidence in their own measurements and judgments than in standardized test scores when the results of the two appeared to be divergent. All of them believed that no single source of information about student achievement could be dependably employed as a summative assessment, especially not a standardized test.

EVALUATING TESTS

Textbooks on measurement provide many more suggestions for constructing tests than can be discussed here. Remember that no test is so good that it does not need continual evaluation and revision to keep it up to date and as valid as possible. A practical way to do this is to study the results of every administration. If time is taken to tabulate the scores and responses to a multiple-choice test, analysis quickly reveals which distractors are not functioning. Let the children take part in this activity. Hand back the papers and have them, with a show of hands, tell you how many got each item right, and even how many picked each of the distractors. Any alternative not chosen by at least 3% of the class is not functioning and needs to be replaced. Another valuable source of information is a survey of the missed items. Which ones were missed by most of the respondents? Were those who missed a question the students whose test scores were highest or those whose scores were low? Which wrong distractors were selected most frequently as the correct answer? The answers to these questions tell the teacher a great deal about the item itself and about the students' knowledge or lack of it regarding that item.

An instrument that has evolved and been improved as an outcome of this kind of scrutiny can be used with some confidence as a pretest. It can provide guidance to the development of lessons appropriate to the special needs of the students in a given class. And it can be used as a summative test to demonstrate the amount of change that has taken place as a consequence of the instruction. Don't forget, however, that a student who has done well on a pretest cannot show as much improvement as one who has missed most of the questions earlier. As a matter of fact, if a great many people do very well on a pretest administration of an instrument, it is too easy and should tell you that you are planning to teach what your students already know. This is a good thing to find out *before* you plan your semester's work. But, it means that a new test will have to be devised to match the changes you wish to make in your teaching plans.

EVALUATION ACTIVITIES

Measurement of the achievement of students should not be restricted to pencil and paper instruments, however valid and well designed they may be. Written tests have their special uses, but hypothetical situations requiring practical application of what has been learned are uniquely suited to health education, especially when comprehension, problem solving, and decision making have been the goals of instruction. In a sense, such evaluative means as these are criterion-referenced, in that students are required to show that they can or cannot demonstrate competence.

For example, in testing for comprehension,

assume that the objective is that the student will be able to "Identify factors that contribute to the abuse of drugs." One way to evaluate that competence would be to divide the class into small groups of two or three. Then distribute cards, each of which lists one of the factors that have been identified in preceding lessons. Ask each group to plan a dramatization of their factor in operation. When the resulting skits are presented to the total class, they should be able to easily identify which factor is being shown. If the presenting group cannot do that, or the class cannot recognize what they are illustrating, you will know which factors need further study and how many students need more instruction. Another way to evaluate achievement of this objective is to develop a series of short stories about drug abuse or misuse and ask the children to suggest what the causative factor could have been in each case. The answers may vary because the factors involved in drug use problems are rarely one-dimensional. What is important is that the suggested causes are possible and relevant.

Comprehension of the key idea related to an objective such as, "Describes ways children resemble their parents," could be measured by asking each child to draw a picture that illustrates some ways in which a child resembles his or her parents. The special features illustrated can be labeled or highlighted by some means, and the pictures need not be restricted to humans. You will be able to see at once whether the concept of heredity has been understood.

Success in motivating understanding of the often trivial reasons why people begin to smoke and the forces that keep them smoking despite the publicity given the very real ill effects of the habit could be appraised by asking students to write a letter to a friend who has not yet thought of smoking. In the letter, they would be asked to tell that person why the decision not to begin smoking should be one that every young person ought to make.

Problem-solving ability can be appraised in many ways. Present the children with a health-related problem that elicits demonstration of

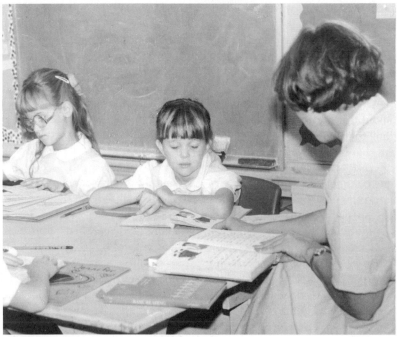

Armi Lizardi

Testing reading and comprehension skills.

competence in dealing with it. The examinee must either have the knowledge needed or know how to find it and know how to apply it in thinking about and working out a good solution. For example, if the objective specified that a student should be able to infer relationships between malnutrition and the growth and development of children, a description of a diet poor in protein and other nutrients can be presented. The task is to analyze that diet and predict what its effect would be on the development and well-being of children with no other foods to eat. Another approach to the same objective would be to describe a child with an existing nutrition-related health problem, and ask the students to suggest or infer which of the essential nutrients are probably lacking in the individual's diet and propose solutions to the problem that could be effected by the addition of specified nutrients to the daily diet.

Decision-making ability can be measured in many other ways, for example, if your objective is to have the students develop practical criteria to be applied to the selection of any health-affecting products, set up an exhibit of eight to ten kinds of toothpaste, soap, painkillers, shampoos, etc. (actual samples or empty packages of such products may be used), and ask the students to indicate which ones, if any, they would choose from each category and to name the criteria they applied in making that decision.

Role playing can be used as effectively in an evaluation activity as in a learning opportunity. Health problems can be presented to small groups who are to work out the solutions and then dramatize both the problem and the solution. The criterion of their success could be the ease with which their fellow students are able to recognize the problem being presented and to agree that the solution is a good one.

Any learning opportunity with which you are comfortable or that you might see described in a guide or text can be adapted for use as an evaluation activity. All you have to do is be sure that the students have already learned what the learning opportunity was intended to teach. This usually means that the information and skills needed to carry it out have been learned elsewhere or at another time. In fact, the majority of "learning opportunities" as written are based on the unstated assumption that the students already know what they need to know in order to carry them out.

EVALUATION OF AFFECTIVE OBJECTIVES

Health education objectives that specifically address the affective domain and are concerned with the development of positive health attitudes and values need to have matching evaluation activities, just as do cognitive objectives. Tyler (15) suggests ways that this can be done. He says:

The definition of a value as an object, activity, or idea that is cherished by the individual which derives its educational significance from its role in directing his interests, attitudes, and satisfactions implies that an assessment should furnish opportunity for the students to make choices that can be perceived as connected to particular values . . . . Hence, the testing situation appears to require opportunities for choices, and for the student to state why he made those choices . . .

Perhaps the most direct evidence is obtained in group discussions, or informal interviews in which the choices are examined in various ways, and different alternatives are proposed. The feeling of the individual can be inferred from his voice, the content of his comments, and the persistence of the same choice in spite of questions regarding other alternatives. With good rapport, the student's report of how he feels about the choice is likely to be sincere.

Attitudes and cognitive changes often can be assessed simultaneously by means of evaluation activities. For example, student-created posters, pictures, and other artifacts reveal far more than

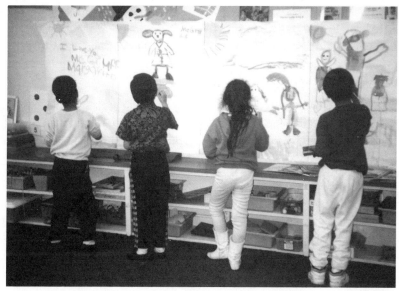

Angela Loya

Student-created posters can reveal attitudes and feelings, as well as knowledge.

knowledge, since they reflect attitudes and feelings about the worth and meaning of what is depicted. Behavioral choices reflect changes in attitudes, too. Once students have completed related learning opportunities, do they volunteer to participate in health-concerned community programs? Do they use seat belts without being reminded? Do they urge their parents and friends to do so? Do they often bring newspaper clippings to class that illustrate some of the health problems or issues that have been discussed? All these actions are indicative of success in the affective, as well as the cognitive domains, yet these changes are more powerfully revealed unintentionally by means of evaluation activities than by scores on objectively scored tests.

Evaluation activities chosen for their relevance to actual health problems that students of any particular age group face every day or are concerned about bring health education and health behavior to life. Reading about health in a book and hearing about it from a teacher or visiting speaker is one thing, but using what one has learned as a consequence can be exciting and deeply satisfying even to young children. They discover that what they have learned works! On top of that, demonstrating competence in coping with a real health problem is a lot more fun than checking the right answer on a piece of paper.

GRADE, GRADING, AND GRADES

In the United States, the word *grade* is used in various ways in speaking about schools and school work. One sort of grade is a division or segment of schooling, representing a year's work. Most college students have completed thirteen of them—kindergarten and twelve more. *Grades* usually refers to test scores or the marks given to completed assignments, such as written reports or projects. Grades of this kind are of a formative nature and cumulatively serve as an important source of judgments about a student's overall performance and ability. Final grades are summative and become a part of a student's record and form the primary basis of the decision to promote a student to the next grade. *Grading* has to do with ranking, is done by the classroom teacher, and reflects that person's judgment of a youngster's achievement as it relates to his or her capabilities.

The meaning of any grade given a student depends on the referencing framework within which it has been assigned. Commonly there are three of these: first, task-referenced or criterion-referenced, which is based on absolute standards of achievement; second, group or norm-referenced, which is based on relative standards in that the student's grade reflects her or his ranking compared with every one else in the group or class; and third, self-referenced, which reflects a comparison between a pupil's performance and the teacher's perception of that individual's capability (11).

Elementary and middle school grading is more comprehensive in scope than grading at the secondary school level. Judgments are not limited to a single letter grade or percentage figure as a summation of a semester's work. Instead, teachers are required to indicate a wide range of judgments based on observations of the child's social and personal development, study habits, and attitudes, as well as her or his cognitive progress and achievements.

The responsibility of a teacher at every level of education is to take care that course grades indicate a student's competence relative to the instructional objectives that have structured the work. Only behaviors that reflect academic achievement should be used to determine grades. Grades must never serve as tools of discipline, or as rewards for pleasant personalities, good attitudes, or skillful apple-polishing.

To exclude such things as obvious effort and level of motivation, writing and speaking skills, and personality in making judgments about a student's academic progress is not an easy thing to do, yet accurate and meaningful grades depend on it.

The following was published more than 20

TEACHER EVALUATION OF STUDENT BEHAVIORS AND SKILLS

Pupil Name _____

DESCRIPTORS MARKED (+) BEST DESCRIBE YOUR CHILD'S PERSONAL STRENGTHS AS OBSERVED AT SCHOOL.

Your child is:

	Trimester		
	1st	2nd	3rd
Flexible..............			
Helpful..............			
Honest..............			
Imaginative..............			
Inquisitive..............			
Respectful..............			
Self-directed..............			
Tolerant of differences in others..............			

Your child demonstrates:

Ability to communicate feelings..............			
Desire to improve..............			
Leadership..............			
Positive self-image..............			
Sense of humor..............			

EXPLANATION OF SYMBOLS USED:

+	shows strength		✓	needs to improve
	satisfactory performance			not graded at this time

PERSONAL AND SOCIAL DEVELOPMENT

Follow school routines and procedures..............			
Respects personal and public property..............			
Shows courtesy..............			
Cooperates with adults and peers..............			
Follow through on responsibility..............			
Demonstrates self-control..............			

STUDY HABITS AND STUDY SKILLS

Listens attentively..............			
Follows directions..............			
Manages time effectively..............			
Works independently..............			
Checks work carefully..............			
Completes daily assignments on time)..............			

LANGUAGE ARTS

Reading

	Trimester		
	1st	2nd	3rd

Instructional level
[Grade   1st   2nd   3rd]
[Text level 2-9   8-11 10-12]

Effort..............			
Uses word attack skills..............			
Understands word meaning..............			
Comprehends what is read..............			
Does competent follow-up..............			
Reads orally with fluency..............			
Enjoys independent reading..............			
Applies reading skills to other subject areas..............			

Listening

Effort..............			
Listens with understanding..............			

Communication (Oral and Written)

Effort..............			
Expresses complete thoughts..............			
Uses correct grammar/mechanics..............			
Exhibits creativity..............			
Uses appropriate vocabulary..............			

Spelling

Effort..............			
Learns assigned words..............			
Applies spelling skills to written work.			

Penmanship

Effort..............			
Forms letters and numerals correctly..............			
Writes neatly..............			
Applies skills consistently..............			

MATHEMATICS

Instructional level
[Grade 1st, 2nd, 3rd]

Effort..............			
Masters arithmetic facts..............			
Understands math concepts..............			
Works accurately..............			
Applies problem solving skills..............			

SOCIAL STUDIES

	Trimester		
	1st	2nd	3rd
Effort..............			
Contributes to discussions/class activities..............			
Understands concepts taught..............			

SCIENCE/HEALTH

Effort..............			
Contributes to discussions/class activities..............			
Understands concepts taught..............			

FINE ARTS

Participates in activities..............			
Exhibits creativity..............			
Appreciates works of others..............			
Uses appropriate arts skills..............			

PHYSICAL EDUCATION

Demonstrates sportsmanship..............			
Participates in activities..............			
Develops physical skills..............			

*SPECIAL PROGRAMS_____

COMMENTS

ATTENDANCE

Days absent..............			
Days tardy..............			

PLACEMENT FOR NEXT YEAR: _____ Grade

_____
Teacher Signature   Principal Signature

_____
Parent Signature   Date

years ago, but it is as meaningful today as then and ought to be required reading for every teacher every time grades are due.

> Teachers should not be in a position merely to declare that students are improving or not improving. They ought to contrive situations in which they will be trying to find out whether improvement occurs and how much. In other words, they should approach the task of evaluation not with the arrogance of a judge, but with the humility of an enquirer. The proper frame of mind for evaluation is fear and trembling. Then, if everything turns out all right, the relief of the teachers should be even more stupendous than that of the students! (2)

SUMMARY

Elementary and middle-school teachers need to be as knowledgeable about test construction as those at any other level of education. Admittedly, the more advanced the grade, the more paper and pencil tests are employed in assessing classroom achievement. But objective tests can be and commonly are constructed and administered effectively at every grade, even preschool (7). The complexity of the items and the difficulty of the concepts being explored vary according to the age group concerned, but the principles of test construction stay the same.

It is probably safe to say that teacher-made tests constitute a primary source of information regarding a child's growing competence as a learner throughout his or her elementary school experience. Whether the tests constructed and administered by successive teachers are good, poor, or indifferent can have a lot to do with the quality and rate of a child's achievement along the way. And wherever paper and pencil tests are scored and reported, they tend to have more influence on course grades and promotion recommendations than all other sources of performance data put together.

Test construction is a skill that must be learned like any other. Competence in teaching and command of the subject matter to be tested are essential elements of, but do not themselves assure competence in, test construction. What are the skills that teachers need if they are to be able to construct a good achievement test for their students?

At a minimum you need to be able to demonstrate basic test construction techniques. You have to know how to write test instructions clearly and concisely enough that students will be able to follow them easily and without error. You must be able to differentiate between what is worth knowing and what is trivial or irrelevant and strive to focus on the former at all times. You need to know how to design a blueprint and specifications for a test that will be balanced in content emphasis as well as be appropriate to the abilities and experience of your class. You must be able to write clear and unambiguous items. You will need to have a working knowledge of the form in which each of the principal kinds of items is expressed, whether free-form or structured. And you must know which sort of item is best suited to measure achievement of the skills and information with which your class has been dealing, which means that not only do you need to know which kinds of items are best for a given purpose but their limitations as well. You must be willing to revise, refine, and evaluate the success of every item before it is administered as well as again and again after use.

No less essential to the development of a good teacher-made achievement test is the desire to give the time and energy it takes to accomplish the many tasks associated with its evolution. It might be argued that all of this effort could be avoided if standardized tests were employed rather than teacher-made tests. Be sure that you are familiar with the strengths and limitations of standardized tests and that you know how to interpret scores obtained from their administration properly.

Other measurement techniques, such as evaluation activities, require students to demonstrate, in contrived situations, competence in applying what has been learned. In this sense, the activities are criterion-related, for they are typically derived from the objectives of the preceding instruction, and the student either can or cannot carry out the proposed tasks. The rigors of design and writing that typify paper and pencil tests are not such a problem in devising evaluation activities. If you can clearly communicate a learning opportunity in writing, you should have no difficulty in writing an evaluation activity. Ideally, both paper and pencil and situational evaluation activities will be employed in assessing student achievement.

Grades are the ultimate evaluation symbol, and it is the teacher who must analyze all of the obtained evaluation data and make the assignment. It is often difficult to make decisions about grades, but the more valid the tests and evaluation activities you have applied and recorded, the easier it will be to justify what you decide is the fairest representation of each student's achievement.

QUESTIONS AND EXERCISES
Discussion questions

1. A test can yield only a sample of what has been learned by a student, so at best it provides only an estimate of his/her achievement. Can a final grade be reliably based on tests alone, and if not, what supplementary evidence would be acceptable and how could it be recorded?

2. In your view, what is the best kind of instrument to be used in assessing achievement in health education? Would you favor one that requires the student to construct answers or one that allows selection of answers from provided alternatives? What aspects of a particular grade level would have to be considered in making a choice?

3. What are the principal advantages and disadvantages of evaluation activities as indicators of learning as compared to paper and pencil tests?

4. How might the validity of an otherwise well written and designed test be lessened by unconscious biases of the teacher who has written it? How could the risk of such an unwanted influence be diminished?

5. If you were able to obtain a standardized test that matched the objectives of the health instruction planned for the children in your class, when would you administer it and how could you best use its results?

6. What is the relationship between clearly stated and measurable objectives and the development of valid tests?

7. Many instructors use multiple-choice tests almost exclusively for several reasons, one of which is the fact that they can be machine-scored. What advantages do you see in giving students a chance to react to both free and structured response items?

8. Explain why reliability is a necessary condition of a valid test, whereas a test can be completely reliable without being valid.

Exercises

1. For a health content area and grade level of your choice, develop two or three examples of each of the following test items: essay, short answer, completion, true-false, multiple-choice, and matching items of at least five pairs. Which are the least time consuming in development? What difficulties did you encounter? How could you test the items for clarity and representativeness of the subject matter?

2. Construct a two-way grid and plan a 60-item instrument designed to assess a health science unit provided for a grade and level of your choice (primary, upper elementary or middle school). Make sure that there is a balance among the items specified for each of the columns, according to the scheme that you choose (e.g., as the horizontal axis is divided, whether by objectives, cognitive skills or whatever).

3. Choose a measurable cognitive objective from any published list proposed for elementary students, develop a problem-solving situation for its administration, and develop criteria for determining the quality or product of that activity. A criterion does not just describe *what* is to be measured but also *how* it is to be done. For example, you will often see suggestions that creativity, or thoroughness, or worthiness be measured, but no explanation to help you know how to do that or how the quality is to be defined.

4. Describe an evaluation activity that would be capable of eliciting both the cognitive and the expected affective outcome of a specified plan for health instruction.

REFERENCES

1. Bloom BS, et al: *Taxonomy of educational objectives.* Handbook 1: The cognitive domain, New York, 1956, McKay.
2. Diederich PB: The classroom teacher and the teacher-made test, *Educ Horizons* 43(1):20, 1964.
3. Ebel R: *Essentials of educational measurement,* ed 3, Englewood Cliffs, NJ, 1979, Prentice Hall.
4. Ebel R, Frisbie D: *Essentials of educational measurement,* ed 4, Englewood Cliffs, NJ, 1986, Prentice Hall.
5. Goodlad JI: *A place called school,* New York, 1984, McGraw-Hill.
6. IOX Assessment Associates: An evaluation handbook for health education programs in smoking, Culver City, Calif, 1983, The Associates.
7. Hendricks M, et al: Reliability of health knowledge measurement in very young children, *J Sch Health* 58(1):21-128, January, 1988.
8. Jubb W: The development of an instrument to assess health knowledge of children prior to first grade, *Evaluation Instruments in Health Educ,* 1986, AAHE.
9. Mehrens W, Lehmann I: *Measurement and evaluation in education and psychology,* ed 3, New York, 1984, Holt, Rinehart, & Winston.
10. Mehrens W, Lehmann I: *Using standardized tests in education,* ed 4, New York, 1987, Longman.
11. Nitko A: *Educational tests and measurements: an introduction,* New York, 1983, HBJ.
12. Popham J: *Modern educational measurement,* Englewood Cliffs, NJ, 1981, Prentice Hall.
13. Popham J: *Educational evaluation,* ed 2, Englewood Cliffs, NJ, 1988, Prentice-Hall.
14. Salmon-Cox L: Teachers and standardized tests: what's really happening, *Phi Delta Kappan* 62:631-34, 1981.
15. Tyler R: Assessing educational achievement in the affective domain, *Measurement in Education,* National Council on Measurement in Education, Spring 1973.
16. Worthen BR: Critical issues that will determine the future of alternative assessment, *Phi Delta Kappan* 74(6):444-454, February 1993.
17. Wiersma W, Jurs S: *Educational measurement and testing,* Boston, 1985, Allyn and Bacon.

SUGGESTED READINGS

Badger E: More than testing, *Arithmetic Teacher* 39:9 May 1992.

Bracey G: Sense, non-sense, and statistics, *Phi Delta Kappan* 73(4):335, December 1991.

Hill JR: Apathy concerning grading and testing, *Phi Delta Kappan* 72(7):540-545, March 1991.

Maeroff G: Assessing alternative assessment, *Phi Delat Kappan* 73(4):273-281, December 1991.

Schick J: Those tantalizing textbook tests. I. *Health Educ* 18(6):42-45, Dec/Jan 1988.

Schick J: Those tantalizing textbook tests. II. *Health Educ* 20(2):18-22, April/May 1989.

Young M, Chudley W, Bakema D: Area-specific self-esteem scales and substance use among elementary and middle school children, *J Sch Health* 59(6):251-254, August 1989.

PART TWO

Content and Practice

9 Personal Health and Fitness

When you finish this chapter, you should be able to:

- Define the complexity of health.
- Describe the basic structure and function of the major body systems.
- Explain important behaviors that promote personal health and fitness.
- Develop learning opportunities for elementary and middle school students in the area of personal health and fitness.

Recognizing, valuing and adopting good health practices establishes the foundation for a healthful lifestyle. These practices are best learned early in life. Personal health goes beyond cleanliness and hygiene to the affective dimensions of feeling good about practices that promote health and fitness. Good health is a personal responsibility. It is the individual who makes the daily decisions that promote or adversely affect health.

It is important to keep in mind that health status constantly changes, the desired goal being to adopt habits that promote general health as a basic value in life. It is not possible to be in a state of "excellent" health at all times in one's life, but it is possible to be working consistently toward the highest possible level of wellness as deter-

mined by hereditary and environmental factors.

In exploring personal health and fitness topics, there will be two levels of information. Most of the information is aimed at adults. However, since there are many developmental issues and topics that relate to health, specific information that is for children and youth is found in boxes labeled "What About My Students?"

WAYS TO THINK ABOUT HEALTH

When people think about health they think of different things. Often, health is associated with the physical, more tangible factors that relate to body functioning. Health is actually viewed in a very dynamic way. As mentioned in Chapter 1, the most recognized definition of health was re-

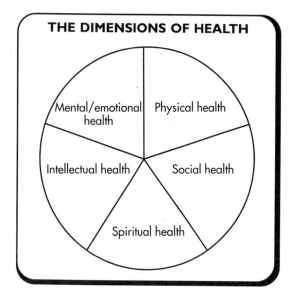

THE DIMENSIONS OF HEALTH

Mental/emotional health · Physical health · Intellectual health · Social health · Spiritual health

leased in 1947 by the World Health Organization (WHO). It states that "Health is a state of complete physical, mental, and social well-being and not merely the absence of disease and infirmity," (3).

This definition clearly indicated that health was more than not being sick. It opened up the mental and social dimensions of health. Since that time, other aspects of health have been identified. Payne and Hahn (1) offer the following:

> Health is the blending of your physical, emotional, social, intellectual, and spiritual resources as they assist you in mastering the developmental tasks necessary for you to enjoy a satisfying and productive life.

HEALTH CHOICES

Accurate information about health is critical to establishing patterns and choices that affect health in a positive way. However, the information about health is constantly changing. What we know and believe as "fact" today may change as technology and science progress. Think about things that you know today about health. Did you know that at one time there was no connection

between cleanliness and disease? And, when cigarettes became popular during World Wars I and II, it was not known that this habit could be harmful to health. As science and technology move even faster, it becomes a major task to stay current about the latest health information. Therefore as a teacher it is important to remember that the subject of "health" is not static.

In the United States today, the major health problems involve conditions that are related to personal choices about lifestyle. These include conditions and diseases, such as cardiovascular disease, cancer, unintended and intended injuries (including suicide and violence related injuries), and sexually transmitted disease (including HIV).

To make positive changes in our health behavior, we need to *personalize* the information. It is important to recognize that *you* are (or could be) at risk for a certain condition or disease. For example, if you don't think that you could get a sexually transmitted disease even though you are sexually active—you have not personalized the risk. And, because you do not *believe* that it can happen to you, it will affect your behavior. You could choose not to use a form of protection "just once" during sexual intercourse because you have not personalized the risk.

Another important factor influencing health behaviors is that of *information*. Using the same example, if you *do* believe you are at risk for a sexually transmitted disease, you need information to protect yourself from infection. Certainly, the knowledge that you cannot become infected if you avoid sexual intercourse is widely available. However, if you choose to become sexually active there is a great deal of information that you need. This would include knowing the various methods of protection, the effectiveness rates of each method, and the cost and the availability of each method. This information is not widely known to everyone who needs it.

Finally, you need skills to make positive health behavior changes. In our example about sexually transmitted disease, let's assume that you have personalized the risk and have obtained the information that you need about methods for protection. There is a level of skill that will be needed to be comfortable with this health behavior. If the method to use condoms in conjunction with a lubricant containing the sperm killing chemical, nonoxynol-9, has been chosen, the skill is learning how to use the condom and the lubricant. Similarly there is skill involved in brushing and flossing teeth.

Positive health behaviors result from a dynamic process that involves personalization of risk, accurate health information, and the skill to apply information. We will be specifically addressing most of these topics in separate chapters in this section.

PHYSICAL HEALTH
Growth—More Than Physical Changes

There are predictable growth periods in a person's life. One critical factor to keep in mind for yourself and as a teacher is that growth is unique. We all grow in different ways, and growth involves not only the obvious physical changes but the mental/emotional and social aspects of our lives.

Achieving positive social and emotional growth of children are important goals in the elementary curriculum. It is important for children to mature emotionally and learn how to get along in the classroom in addition to society. Additionally, students in elementary and middle schools are growing physically as well. The most pronounced kind of growth for students is physical growth during puberty. This is a period of very rapid physical changes that can start as early as age 10 for some students and as late as 16 or 17 for others. They are growing physically, emotionally, and socially. Often students worry that they are too short, too tall, too heavy, too thin, or are abnormal in some way. Not all parts of the body grow at the same time, so for a while hands and feet may seem out of proportion. It also takes time to get used to the changes in body size and shape. Everyone grows and develops on his or her own timetable. Girls generally start their growth spurts at an earlier age than boys.

Many of the concerns we have as adolescents going through puberty carry over into adult lives. Body image is a common concern of children, adolescents, as well as adults.

Growth involves three basic things: heredity, environment, and behavior. *Heredity* is the passing of traits from parent to child. A person's looks, growth patterns, and special talents are traits that are influenced by heredity. *Environment* refers to everything in a person's surroundings. The types of food that are eaten, where a person lives, and daily experiences influence physical, emotional, and social growth.

Behavior involves actions or responses to the environment. Each person can control their behavior to a greater extent than their heredity or environment. Maintaining a healthy diet, performing regular exercise, and making friends are examples of behaviors that can influence growth and health.

BODY SYSTEMS

To teach health concepts, some general background information about the human body is essential. Following are brief descriptions of major body systems, including organs and their functions. There is not space in this text to provide a great deal of information about each system, but an overview of the major structures and functions is provided.

Respiratory System

The respiratory system (Figure 9-1) includes the lungs and tubes that convey air into the body and help eliminate gaseous wastes. The body must have oxygen from the air to stay alive. Oxygen enters the body in a process called *inhalation*. During inhalation the diaphragm (a large tentlike muscle) under the lungs contracts with certain rib muscles to make the chest expand. When the chest expands, air is sucked into the body through the nose.

The nose prepares the air for the lungs by filtering out some of the microorganisms and large dust particles by means of the nose hairs. Mu-

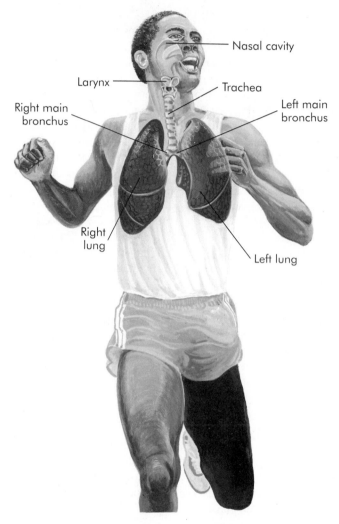

FIGURE 9-1
The respiratory system.

cous in the lining of the nose also helps to collect germs and dust, as well as moistening the air that is breathed in.

The pharynx is a funnellike structure at the back of the mouth that allows the air to pass from the nose into the trachea or windpipe. The trachea extends down the neck and then divides into two large branches called bronchial tubes.

One of these branches goes to the left lung, the other goes to the right lung.

The lungs are where the exchange of oxygen and waste products takes place. The bronchial tubes inside each lung branch into smaller and smaller tubes resembling an upside-down tiny tree, finally ending in balloonlike air sacs. The oxygen from the air goes through the thin walls

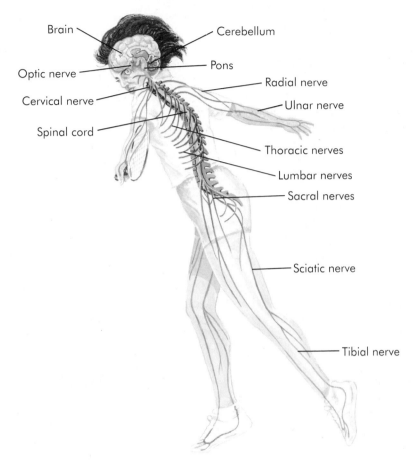

FIGURE 9-2
The nervous system.

of the air sacs and into the capillaries that surround them. At the same time, wastes, such as carbon dioxide, pass from the capillaries into the air sacs where they are exhaled from the body.

In the process called *exhalation*, the diaphragm and the rib muscles relax to make the chest become smaller. Air is forced out of the chest as the ribs and diaphragm push on the lungs. A person does not have to think about breathing most of the time because the nervous system controls the breathing movements.

Nervous System

The nervous system allows us to receive, interpret, and react to the messages we receive from our senses. The brain, spinal cord, and nerves make up the nervous system (Figure 9-2).

The nerves are special "transmitter" cells that send messages to and from the spinal cord. The "sensory nerves" transmit the signals that come into the body from the sense organs (eyes, ears, nose, skin, and tongue). The "motor nerves" take messages to the muscles if action is needed.

The spinal cord extends from the base of the brain down the back. It is protected by a chain of bones called the vertebrae or backbone. The spinal cord carries messages to and from the brain.

The brain is a soft, spongy organ that is protected by the skull bones, three coverings or membranes, and a special fluid. The brain interprets the messages that come into the body and decides what to do about them.

The nervous system is sometimes called the "master system" of the body because it controls many of the processes that are necessary for life. Besides making sure that our muscles move, the nervous system controls breathing, heart beat, and other vital organ functions.

Circulatory System

The circulatory system moves blood around the body so the cells can receive nutrients and oxygen and get rid of waste products. The heart, blood vessels, and blood are the parts of the circulatory system (Figure 9-3).

Your heart is about the size of your closed fist and is located behind the ribs in your chest. The heart is made of a special kind of muscle that constantly beats and rests. The human heart has four chambers. The upper chambers, the atria, receive blood from the body (right atrium) or lungs (left atrium). The lower chambers, ventricles, pump blood to lungs for oxygen (right ventricle) or to the rest of the body (left ventricle). When the heart beats, the ventricles contract. Blood that is low in oxygen is pumped to the lungs. At the same time, blood that has returned from the lungs rich in oxygen is pumped throughout the body. When the ventricles contract, the atria relax and fill with blood. When the atria contract, the ventricles relax and receive blood. Thus when the heart pumps blood, it does not contract completely. Valves keep blood from flowing in the wrong direction.

A network of vessels carries blood throughout the body. Blood vessels called "arteries" carry blood away from the heart. Blood in most arteries is rich in oxygen. Blood vessels called "veins" carry blood back to the heart. The blood found in most veins carries carbon dioxide and other waste products. (The only exceptions are the pulmonary artery and vein.) The smallest blood vessels are capillaries. Body cells receive materials, such as nutrients, from the blood as it passes through the capillaries. These cells give up wastes that are picked up by the blood and carried to lungs or kidneys for elimination.

Digestive System

The job of the digestive system is to convert the food you eat into substances that can enter the blood and be used by all body cells. The process of digestion begins with the mechanical grinding action of teeth. When food is swallowed, it travels from the esophagus into the stomach, where major chemical digestion begins. Digestive juices, such as hydrochloric acid and enzymes, break down large food molecules. Mucous protects the stomach from digesting itself. Food is channeled from the stomach into the upper part of the small intestine where it is further broken down by chemicals from the pancreas and the lining of the small intestine. Bile, a chemical produced by the liver and stored in the gall bladder, is necessary for proper fat digestion. As food moves into the lower part of the small intestine, the nutrients are absorbed through the walls into the blood. This nutrient-rich blood travels first to the liver, which stores and often repackages nutrients before releasing them into the general circulation. Food substances, such as plant fiber, that cannot be digested and absorbed by the digestive tract pass into the large intestine (colon) from which they are eliminated from the body. Figure 9-4 shows the digestive system.

Muscular and Skeletal Systems

Bones in the skeleton provide a framework for supporting the body and protecting the internal organs (Figure 9-5). Over 200 bones make up the human skeleton. The skeleton has joints that allow the "framework" to move. Bones are made of an inner layer of spongy tissue surrounded by material hardened by deposits of the minerals

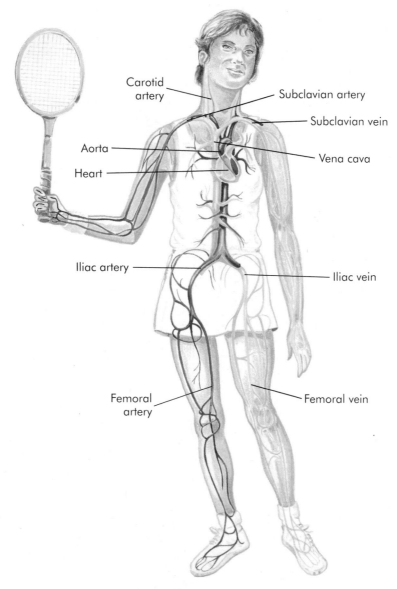

Carotid artery

Subclavian artery

Subclavian vein

Aorta

Vena cava

Heart

Iliac artery

Iliac vein

Femoral artery

Femoral vein

FIGURE 9-3
The circulatory system.

calcium and phosphorus. Exercise, heredity, and what we eat influences the quality of a person's bones.

There are approximately 650 muscles in the human body (Figure 9-6). Without muscles, movement would be impossible. Some muscles attach to bones by tendons, and as they contract, muscles move bones in different ways. These muscles are called "voluntary" because they work as a result of conscious commands sent by

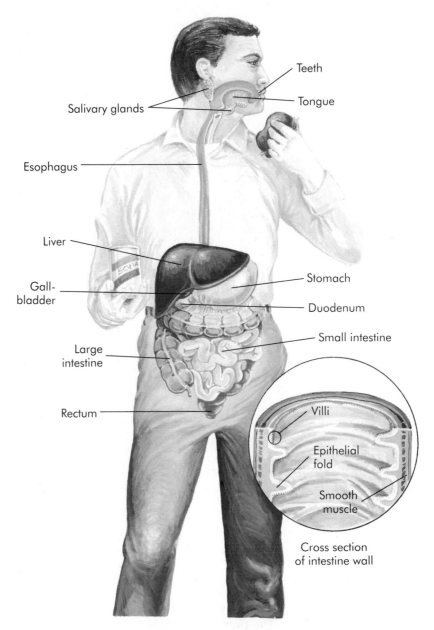

FIGURE 9-4
The digestive system.

the brain. Other muscles like those of the intestines are called "involuntary" because they work without our having to think about them. The heart muscle is referred to as "cardiac muscle." It is made up of several powerful muscles that contract in a particular sequence. The only way to build muscles is to exercise them. Furthermore, nonuse causes them to shrink (atrophy). This is one reason that regular exercise is healthful.

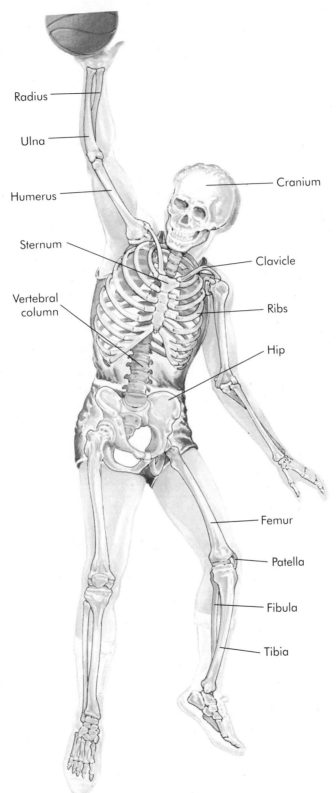

Radius

Ulna

Humerus

Sternum

Vertebral
column

Cranium

Clavicle

Ribs

Hip

Femur

Patella

Fibula

Tibia

FIGURE 9-5
The skeletal system.

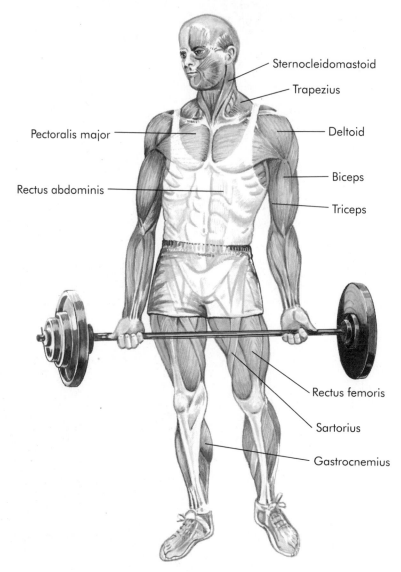

FIGURE 9-6
The muscular system.

Skin (Integumentary System)

The skin is called "one of the body's most complicated structures" and is an obvious feature of any individual. Skin, hair, and nails make up this system. A closer look at the skin reveals three layers of skin cells (Figure 9-7). The outermost layer is the *epidermis*. The epidermis forms an important body defense against infection by keeping microorganisms out of the body. Folds and creases in the epidermis make it possible for the skin to stretch easily when the body moves. Tiny oil glands open onto the epidermis and sup-

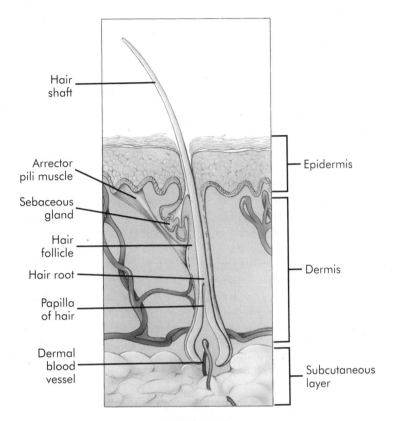

FIGURE 9-7
Layers of skin.

ply oil that keeps the skin soft, smooth, and waterproof. The lower part of the epidermis makes millions of new cells each day, replacing the old cells that die as they are pushed to the surface. These dead cells compose the upper layer of skin that is seen and felt. Dead cells are shed daily; in fact, much of the dust in our homes contains our old skin cells! The next layer of skin is the *dermis*. Nerve endings, blood vessels, and glands are located in this layer. The nerve endings are important for sense of touch. Blood vessels, arteries, veins, and capillaries supply oxygen and nutrients to keep the skin cells of the dermis alive. Two types of glands are located in the dermis, sweat glands, and oil glands. The sweat glands take in liquid from the spaces around the

skin cells and send the liquid up to the skin surface through the pores. Sweating cools the body and carries off small amounts of waste materials. The fatty layer below the dermis cushions the body and helps hold in body heat.

One of the most interesting features of the skin is the ridges that form fingerprints. No two people have the same pattern, so fingerprints are a good method of identification. Fingerprints never change even if fingers get burned. When the skin heals the same fingerprint will appear. Each of the ten fingers show a different fingerprint. Hair and nails are a form of protein called keratin. The body is covered by hair; most hair is fine, nearly invisible. The only place where hair does not grow is on the lips, the palms of the hands, and soles of the feet. These structures are not "alive"; ads that claim a particular shampoo "feeds" hair are misleading. The hair grows from a follicle in the skin that has a blood supply. Plucking or shaving hair does not make it grow thicker or coarser.

A major function of skin is to serve as a sense organ. Imbedded in the skin are various types of special nerves, referred to as sensory receptors. There are receptors for cold, hot, pain, and pressure. Information from these receptors is relayed to the spinal cord and brain. Much of the information from the environment is ignored. But as most of us know, a brush with a hot iron causes an immediate response away from the danger.

Related to skin are the membranes that line body cavities. One type, mucous membranes, line exposed places such as body openings where skin does not cover. These membranes produce a slippery material, mucous, that keeps the structures moist and soft. For example, the insides of the mouth, eyelids, and vagina are lined with mucous membranes.

Endocrine System

The endocrine system is made up of glands that secrete hormones. Hormones are chemical messengers produced in one part of the body, usually by a gland. When signalled by the nervous system, glands release hormones which travel to another organ and convey some message. For example, insulin is a hormone produced in the pancreas. It is released after meals and signals cells to take in the simple sugar, glucose. Hormones signal many vital body activities including growth, reproductive cycles, and energy use. Figure 9-8 identifies hormone-producing glands.

Urinary System

The kidneys, urinary bladder, and urethra are parts of the urinary system (Figure 9-9). This system is needed to excrete waste products that result from the work that cells perform. The kidneys filter waste products and extra water from the blood forming urine. Urine is stored in the bladder until one feels the urge to urinate.

Immune System

The immune system includes the white blood cells, lymphatic system (a kind of second circulatory system), and the fluid the surrounds cells. The role of the immune system is to protect the body from disease-causing microorganisms and foreign materials, collectively called antigens. Two major groups of special cells, T cells and B cells work together in this effort. When a foreign material or microorganism enters the body, a series of cellular reactions known as the immune response occurs. This response often allows the body to fight the infection and control it. In many cases, a specific response occurs, preventing future infections by that particular invader. This is referred to as immunity. Immunity to many diseases can be created when one is exposed to parts of antigens in the form of a vaccine. The body responds to the vaccine as though it is the natural antigen. For example, polio vaccine causes an immune response that protects the individual from developing polio when exposed to the naturally occuring virus.

Reproductive System

Both males and females have biological structures that contribute in unique ways to the process of renewing life. These structures enable males to impregnate; females have the ability to become pregnant, give birth, and nourish infants through breastfeeding. Chapter 11 includes a detailed description of the male and female reproductive systems.

HEALTHFUL PRACTICES

There are many practices children need to be taught to be healthy and socially acceptable. The following information provides basic information concerning hygienic behaviors.

Cleanliness

Cleanliness is often associated with "health." Rightly so! The single most important hygiene habit is frequent handwashing. As simple as it seems, this one behavior is often not given the

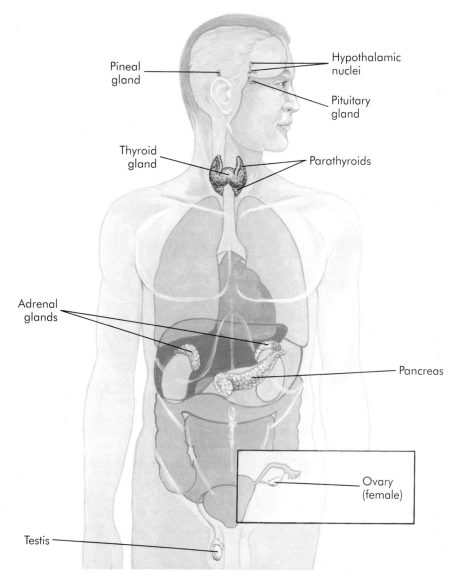

FIGURE 9-8
The endocrine system.

important "credit" it needs in the fight against the spread of disease. Washing with soap and water removes many of the microorganisms that cause disease. Simple rinsing with water is not adequate. Thorough washing will remove or kill most disease-causing microbes that may have been picked up by the hands. It is particularly important to wash hands after going to the bathroom and before eating or preparing foods. It is also important to avoid sharing items that can carry disease causing microorganisms. Combs, brushes, toothbrushes, towels, tissues, cups,

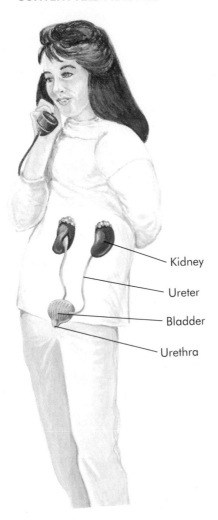

Kidney

Ureter

Bladder

Urethra

FIGURE 9-9
The urinary system.

to perform all of its functions. Keeping the skin clean is an important healthful behavior. The face needs a thorough washing with soap and water at least once a day. The rest of the body can be cleaned by bathing or showering several times a week. Many people bathe once a day. Just how often a person bathes or showers depends on how dirty a person gets, whether the skin is dry or oily, the temperature outdoors, and personal preference. Young children and the elderly may experience excessive drying of the skin if they bathe too often.

Avoiding sunburn is another way of caring for the skin. Wearing protective clothing like hats and long-sleeved shirts provides protection when one is exposed to sunshine for long periods of time. Sun screen preparations are also effective in preventing sunburn.

Acne

During puberty, the oil glands in the skin become more active and often manufacture more oil than is needed. When too much oil is produced, the ducts that transport the oil become clogged often forming a blackhead. The dark color is due to a chemical reaction that occurs when the oil is exposed to the air. If the excess oil remains in the oil gland and is not exposed to air, a "whitehead" is formed. In acne, the oil glands and ducts become swollen and infected, forming "pimples." The face, neck, shoulders, and back are common

glasses, and other eating utensils can be the means of transmitting disease from one person to another. Additionally, being clean is a pleasant feeling for many people. Good grooming, including maintaining clean, neat hair, clean teeth, and trimmed fingernails, wearing clean clothes, and bathing regularly not only promotes health but is socially desirable.

Skin Care

Taking care of the skin is an important part of making sure that the skin stays healthy and able sites for acne because many oil glands exist there. Most experts believe that the extent of acne is due to hereditary and hormonal factors, not diet.

Teeth and Gums

Teeth are necessary for eating the wide variety of foods we enjoy (Figure 9-10). Dental health is an important aspect of general health. It is also a major health topic of study in elementary schools. Establishing correct and consistent toothbrushing and flossing habits can help prevent dental caries and gum disease. Flossing and toothbrushing help to prevent the build up of plaque on the teeth. Plaque is a film of certain bacteria that grows rapidly from the presence of sugar in the mouth. These bacteria use sugar for food and produce acid by-products. If allowed to build up on the teeth, the acid destroys the tough enamel layer and attacks the softer tissue underneath, forming a dental cavity.

Malocclusion

Malocclusion is a condition in which the teeth are poorly aligned so that chewing ability or appearance is affected. Malocclusion results from hereditary factors or premature loss of deciduous or permanent teeth. Poorly aligned teeth can contribute to faulty nutrition, tooth decay and gum disease. Orthodontists are specially trained

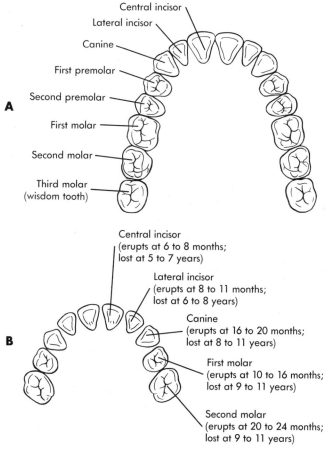

FIGURE 9-10
Teeth. A, Adult teeth. **B,** deciduous (baby) teeth.

FLOSSING AND BRUSHING TECHNIQUES

Flossing Teeth

- Floss your teeth before you brush them.
- To floss the teeth, break off about a foot and a half of dental floss and wind most of it around one of your middle fingers.
- Wind the remaining floss around the middle finger of the other hand.
- Steady the floss between your hands with your thumbs and forefingers.
- Leave about 1 to 4 inches of floss between your thumbs to get between your teeth.
- Move the floss between your teeth, and gently guide it into the space between your tooth and gum.
- Bend the floss toward each tooth as you scrape the floss up and down against the sides.
- Do the same thing for *each pair* of teeth, *using a new piece of floss as needed.*

Brushing Teeth

While there are several different methods suggested for brushing teeth, one good way is described below. Always use a flat, soft-bristled toothbrush.

Starting with the brush near the gum line, use the top surface of the brush in a back and forth motion.

1. Brush the outside surfaces of the upper teeth.
2. Brush the outside surfaces of the lower teeth.
3. Brush the tops of the upper and lower teeth.
4. Brush the inside surfaces of the upper and lower teeth.

Using the tip of the brush and brushing gently with an up and down motion, brush the inside surface of the top front teeth and the bottom front teeth.

Then rinse the mouth with water. Flossing and brushing are desired after every meal, but it is not always possible. At least once a day is recommended. Special care should be taken to brush after eating foods containing sugar. While it is obvious that cakes, candies, and cookies are high in sugar, other foods, such as apples, raisins, and oranges, also contain sugar.

dentists who can correct occlusion problems by using braces made of wires, bands, tiny springs, and elastic devices. During orthodontic treatment, gentle pressure is exerted on the teeth to move them through the bone tissue until they are correctly aligned. This process takes from 1 to 3 years. While under orthodontic treatment, practicing good dental hygiene is important to keep the teeth and braces free of food debris that can contribute to tooth decay and bad breath.

Sleep and Rest

Adequate sleep is necessary to keep mentally alert, to maintain a good disposition, to stay physically well, and to maintain proper growth. Sleep needs vary from one individual to the next; however, most adults need from 7 to 10 hours of sleep at a time. A simple way to determine if you have had enough sleep is to see if you feel rested and energetic during the day.

Children need anywhere from 8 to 11 hours of sleep per night. The actual amount of sleep needed is different for each individual and usually decreases with age. Lack of adequate sleep will interfere with a child's ability to learn and achieve. Fatigue can be physical or mental. Knowing how to relax after play or stressful events is an important skill and should be related

WHAT ABOUT MY PRIMARY LEVEL STUDENTS?

Young children need practice in the techniques for effective brushing and flossing. Using oversized models of teeth and toothbrushes to demonstrate the techniques is both fun and informative for children. If invited, dentists and dental hygienists will often be willing to come to primary level classrooms to provide such instruction.

Children in the primary grades will be losing primary teeth and cutting permanent teeth. This is a normal body process that proceeds on a child's individual timetable. Comparisons between and among children should be discouraged with the explanation that each child will lose primary teeth whenever the body is ready for this to occur.

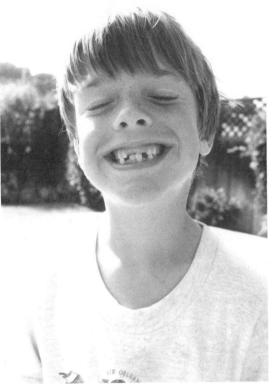

John Sabo

What a smile!

to personal interests. Engaging in "quiet time" activities, such as reading, playing with puzzles, creative writing, and listening to music are enjoyable and restful for children.

Another important practice is relaxation. People engage in a variety of activities just for relaxation. Many activities can relieve stress and contribute to fitness. These include exercise and sports, hobbies, listening to or playing music, talking to friends, and meditating. Children can also engage in these activities for relaxation purposes.

Posture

Posture is the alignment of body parts while maintaining an upright position. Posture reflects an individual's health status and is particularly important during adolescence because it is during this time postural faults often develop. Poor posture is often seen in students who are self-conscious about height. However, some postural defects are physical in origin. *Scoliosis* (curvature of the spine) can cause defects in posture. Additionally, poor muscle tone resulting from a recent injury or illness

may contribute to slouching or slumping. These types of posture defects can often be corrected under the advice of a physician through surgery, exercises, or a combination of surgery and exercise.

There is no one perfect standing, walking, or sitting posture for everyone, since individuals differ in skeletal and muscular structure. Proper posture involves sitting, standing, and walking without appearing out of alignment by being slumped over, rigidly erect, or uncomfortable. Diet, fitness levels, and emotions affect posture so the best way to ensure good posture is to enhance health in general. Also, being conscious of one's posture and lifting heavy objects properly to avoid injury will aid in the development of good posture.

Exercise and Fitness

Physical fitness is an important component for the maintenance and enhancement of personal health. Physical exercise can become an integral part of everyone's life. For exercise to be incorporated into an individual's lifestyle, it should be fun and interesting. Anyone, regardless of physical ability, can establish a regular exercise regime that will be beneficial. Exercises for children should be age-appropriate, building on coordination skills and including a variety of activities that involve all parts of the body. While individual definitions of fitness may vary, fitness has three basic components.

Flexibility is the range of motion that joints allow. As children develop, they become more flexible until adolescence, when gradual loss of joint mobility begins. Individual flexibility depends upon many factors; age, sex, posture, and fat/muscle distribution in the body. Flexibility can be increased through regular stretching exercises that are done properly. The safest way to stretch is "static" stretching, which is a relaxed, gradual stretch that is held for a short time. When stretching, reach to the point of discomfort, then back off slightly, allowing the muscle to adjust for 20 to 30 seconds. Hold the stretch until the feeling of tension diminishes. Concentrate on the feeling of the stretch rather than the flexibility you want to attain. Some good exercises to increase flexibility include:

- *Knee-chest pull*—Lie on your back, clasp one knee and pull it to your chest. Hold for 15 to 30 seconds, then repeat with the other knee. Perform at least five repetitions with each knee.
- *Wall stretch*—Stand three feet from a wall with your feet slightly apart. Put your hands on the wall and lean forward for 10 seconds then repeat five times.
- *Side stretches*—Stand in a comfortable stance. Stretch arms up and bend the upper body to each side slowly. Count to ten as you stretch. DO NOT BOUNCE. Straighten up and bend to the other side. Do several sets of the side stretches up to ten.

- *Seated toe touch*—Sit on the floor with your legs extended to the front. Point your toes and slide your hands down your legs until you feel the stretch. Holding this position, slowly lean forward and try to touch your toes. Hold for ten seconds, then repeat five times.
- *Foot-buttocks roll*—Lie on your stomach, reach back and grasp one foot. Bend your knee and pull your foot toward your buttocks. Hold the stretch for 15 to 30 seconds. Repeat with the other foot.

Cardiovascular stamina is the second component of fitness. It is maintained and increased through "aerobic" exercise that conditions the heart and lungs. Aerobic exercises are activities that use the large muscle groups of the body and that keep your pulse at the " target heart rate" for at least 20 minutes. Aerobic activities include walking, jogging, swimming, cycling, skipping rope, cross-country skiing, aerobic dancing, and skating. Children enjoy running, jumping, hopping, rope-jumping, rollerblading, skating, swimming, biking, and climbing.

The best way to make sure that you are working hard enough but not overdoing is to use your heart rate as a guide. Calculate your target heart rate (THR) by using this formula:

220 − your age = maximum heart rate (MHR)
MHR × 75% = THR

Find your pulse at the carotid artery by tilting your head slightly back and to one side. Slide your forefinger and middle finger into the groove to the side of your "Adam's apple" and feel for your pulse. Don't use your thumb because it has a pulse of its own. Learn to find your pulse quickly and easily.

About 3 minutes into your exercise, take your pulse for 6 seconds and multiply by ten. If your pulse rate is higher than your target heart rate, slow down. Speed up your exercise if your pulse rate is lower than your target heart rate zone. Monitor your pulse at several intervals during your workout to make sure that you are exercising at the proper intensity.

No matter which aerobic exercise you choose, your workout should follow the same steps:

1. *Warm-up* gradually to prepare your body for more vigorous exercise. Jogging in place is a good example (5 minutes). Stretching is also used to loosen muscles and prevent injuries (5 minutes).
2. *Exercise* at your target heart rate (20 minutes).
3. *Cool down* by gradually decreasing your activity (5 minutes). Similar to warm-up activities, these are "slow-down" ones. Instead of stopping vigorous aerobic activity abruptly, stretching and balance activities are recommended. Stretching prevents soreness (5 minutes).

One-foot balance—While standing, stretch your arms out straight to the sides. Slowly lift one leg and balance for a count of ten. Repeat with alternate legs up to five times.

Muscular strength and endurance are the components of fitness that enable an individual to handle everyday tasks, like raking leaves. Exercising to increase muscular strength and endurance enables muscles to work efficiently and reliably and to give shape and tone to our bodies. Muscle tissue never stays the same. If it is used, it grows stronger. If it is unused, it breaks down. The only way to develop muscle tissue is to demand more work of it than it is used to performing.

Muscular exercises are classified as either "isometric" or "isotonic." Isometric exercises are those in which you pull or push against a stationary object, for example, pushing your ankles against the legs of a chair. Isotonic exercises involve moving a moderate load several times. Weightlifting and calisthenics are examples of isotonic exercises. Few repetitions of heavy weights are best for producing muscular strength. Low resistance and frequent repetitions are best for developing flexibility, coordination, and muscular endurance.

Regular exercise, including aerobic, endurance, strength, and flexibility exercises, contribute to a sound body. In particular, the respiratory, circulatory, musculoskeletal, and nervous systems benefit from exercise. And, since all systems must work together, the body as a whole benefits. It is also proven that regular exercise relieves tension and that physical fitness is usually accompanied by feelings of well-being.

BODY WEIGHT

Many people feel that they either need to gain or lose weight. This is a serious undertaking. We are influenced heavily by media to adhere to rigid criteria for an attractive body. There is a common perception among girls and women that thinness equals physical attractiveness and for boys and young men in particular, that a muscular body equates to physical attractiveness. Weight loss and weight gain diets can be very hard on the body. Particularly "quick" loss or gain diets. Any kind of weight loss diet or weight gain diet should be gradual and should include both healthful eating guidelines in addition to exercise. Before embarking on any program to alter body weight, it is important to have a physical examination by a physician to determine if a gain in body weight or a loss of body fat is warranted. Weight-loss diets are usually not recommended at all for children and adolescents. Exercise in combination with healthy eating is recommended.

If the individual is truly underweight, the physician will try to determine physical causes that contribute to the condition. Lack of proper diet, emotional problems, or failure to get enough sleep and rest can be contributing factors. It is possible that some underlying disease is the cause. If weight loss or inability to gain weight results from a faulty diet, the doctor will suggest ways to increase the amount of calories consumed.

A health examination is also important before anyone attempts to lose weight; it is particularly important for a young person is attempting to lose weight. Experts realize that body weight alone is not an accurate indicator of overweight. The amount of body fat is an important determinant of obesity. Altering diet at this age can be dangerous because, without a nutritious daily diet, the child's body may be deprived of essential nutrients needed for growth and development.

REFERENCES

1. Payne W, Hahn DB: *Understanding your health*, St Louis, 1992, Mosby.
2. Seeley R, Stephens T, Tate P: *Essentials of anatomy and physiology*, St. Louis, 1991, Mosby.
3. World Health Organization: *Chronicle of the world health organization*, 1:29-43, 1947.

LEARNING OPPORTUNITIES FOR PERSONAL HEALTH AND FITNESS

GENERAL STUDENT OBJECTIVES

Primary Level K-3

The student:
1. Names habits that promote health and wellness.*
2. Identifies physical, mental, and social benefits of good health.
3. Explains why daily dental care is essential for the healthy growth and development of teeth and gums.
4. Describes how decision making affects personal health practices.

Intermediate Level 4-5/6

The student:
1. Explains how personal health behavior is influenced by friends and family members.*
2. Describes the relationship of personal health behavior to the optimum structure and functioning of the body.
3. Explains the relationship of physical fitness to sound body function.

Middle School Level 6/7-8

The student:
1. Analyzes the relationship between diet choices and fitness.
2. Designs personal health care and fitness programs to meet individual needs and interests.*
3. Describes both immediate and long-range effects of personal health care choices.

---

*These objectives are illustrated by sample learning opportunities.

This section presents several fully developed health education learning opportunities. To provide examples for a variety of developmental levels, learning opportunities appropriate for primary, upper elementary, and middle school have been presented. They are designed to meet objectives selected from the example scope and sequence plan in Chapter 5. Each learning opportunity described here is an example of *one way* to meet a specific objective.

Although the teaching plans in this chapter do not represent a comprehensive health education program, they do provide examples for the creation of plans when developing one. The teaching plans for the primary level have been designated as either for those for children in kindergarten and grade 1 or grades 2 and 3. This is due to the fact that the capabilities of the kindergarten child are so different from those of the third grade child. Learning opportunities are based on the assumption that the second and third grade students have some reading and writing abilities.

The teaching techniques have been chosen carefully for their appropriateness for the developmental level of the student. The components of the teaching plan, as well as the teaching technique used, are consistent with those described in Part I. Plans include an objective, content generalizations ("big ideas"), initiation activity, sample learning activities, and an evaluation activity relating to the objective. The last activity in each lesson serves as the culminating activity. Other helpful components included are vocabulary words, suggested integration possibilities, lists of specific materials and resources needed, and actual worksheets, patterns, and bulletin board examples for the activities described.

In developing these learning opportunities, teachability was of primary concern. Each has a beginning, a logical sequence, and an ending that evaluates the stated objectives. Teachers must add, delete, and modify activities to meet specific student needs. The actual time needed to teach the activities will vary for every classroom situation, and teachers will need to plan accordingly. It can be assumed, however, that several days will be required to complete all the activities included in each plan.

It is important to note the health lessons do not fit neatly in a content area. While we have choosen to provide examples that fit within the content area of personal health and fitness, the activities described here show the interrelationships among health content areas. For instance, activities for disease prevention and control are also appropriate for personal health and fitness. Community health workers could be discussed in relation to community health, consumer health, accident prevention and safety, disease prevention and control, and so forth. This overlapping demonstrates the dynamic nature of effective health education. A skilled teacher will recognize these interrelationships and use them to promote the concept wellness.

PRIMARY LEVEL

OBJECTIVE: The student names habits that promote health and wellness.

LEVEL: Kindergarten and grade 1

INTEGRATION: Art, writing, coming to conclusions

VOCABULARY: Habits, health, protect

CONTENT GENERALIZATIONS: Habits, such as washing hands before eating, covering sneezes, using clean eating utensils, limiting or avoiding contact with sick people, and staying home from school when sick help to keep diseases from spreading. These habits promote health and wellness for children and others.

INITIATION: "Mystery Health Bag"
Fill a bag with items that often are used when practicing good health habits. Identify the bag as the "Mystery Health Bag." Use a bag that will allow the students to feel the items when they handle the bag (such as a pillowcase, opaque plastic bag, or cloth bag). Place the bag in a prominent spot in the classroom, or set up a table display using the bag in the center and placing items around the bag as they are discussed. Printed name signs for the items can be made for the table display.

Allow a student to feel the outside of the bag and guess what might be in it. Then pull out one item. Ask the students to identify the item and tell about its use. Supplement their answers as necessary. Repeat this for two or three items a day. Ask the students to bring items that might go into the "Mystery Health Bag."

MATERIALS
Pillowcase, plastic bag, or cloth bag.
Items for bag: Brush, soap, toothbrush, shampoo, tissue, etc., raincoat.
Optional: Name signs for each item for table display.

ACTIVITIES

1. Stay Well

Put up a bulletin board display, *Stay Well!*, with Miguel Mouse in the center. Tell students that there are many things we can do to help stop the spread of disease, and these habits all help us and others stay well.

MATERIALS

Bulletin board display: *Stay Well!* (Figure 9-11)

2. "Dirty and Clean" Demonstrations

Rotate small groups of students into a demonstration on washing hands, preferably near a sink. Explain to them that proper handwashing is an important health habit to learn.

- Have students rub a few drops of salad oil on their hands.
- Then they should sprinkle some cinnamon on their hands.
- Have them wash their hands with water *only* and observe. Ask, "Are your hands clean?" (No.) "How can you tell?" (The cinnamon is still sticking.) "Does washing hands with just water get hands clean?" (No.)
- Now have the children wash their hands with *soap* and *water* and observe. Ask, "Are your hands clean now?" (Yes.) "How can you tell?" (The cinnamon is gone; they smell clean.) Ask the students to draw some conclusions on proper hand washing. Ask, "What is needed to get hands clean?" (Soap and water.)
- Ask the students if they know when to wash their hands. Explain that sometimes we cannot see the dirt, so it is important to wash hands even if they do not look dirty, particularly before we handle or eat food and after we go to the bathroom.
- Ask the students if they can think of other items that should be washed before use. (Dishes, utensils, combs, brushes, clothes.) Ask, "What is the best way to get these objects clean?" (Wash them with soap and water.)

MATERIALS

Sink or bucket of water, salad oil (not in glass container), cinnamon, paper towels.

3. Covering Sneezes Experiment

In another small group conduct an experiment about covering sneezes. Fill a spray bottle with water with several drops of red food coloring added, and set it on the table. Hand students the worksheet, *Look What Happens When I Don't Cover My Sneeze!*, and have them draw pictures of their family members or friends on the worksheet. Then have the students take turns using the spray bottle to squirt their picture. Suggest that they say "ah choo" when they squirt. Then the students should try it again using a tissue to "catch" the spray. (More than one tissue may be needed if the spray is strong.) This activity could be done outside.

MATERIALS

Spray bottle with colored water (use several drops of *red* food coloring), tissues, worksheet: *Look What Happens When I Don't Cover My Sneeze!* (Figure 9-12).

4. Well Child, Sick Child

a. Use a flannel board and figures to create a story or a discussion about the difference between wellness and illness.

b. Ask children how staying home when you are sick helps their health as well as the health of others. (It protects others from catching the sickness you have and protects you from getting sicker.) Ask what they can do to stay well if they have a friend who is sick. (Stay away until their friend is well; do not play with a sick friend.)

MATERIALS

Flannel board figures: *Stay Well!* (Figure 9-11); *Well child* (Figure 9-13); *Sick child* (Figure 9-14)
Flannel board

EVALUATION: "Miguel Mouse Says"

Have the students form a circle. Start out saying, "Miguel says . . ." and then all the students say "Stay well!" Then spin a bottle in the middle of the circle, and the student to whom the bottle is pointing must name a health habit studied. Then that student spins the bottle, and the next student replies. They may name a habit mentioned before but not the one named the turn before. Continue until all students have participated.

NOTE: You may wish to use a name other than Miguel if there is a student with that name in the class.

MATERIALS

Bottle

FIGURE 9-11

Bulletin board display   Name _____

Protect Yourself, Protect Others

Directions: Make a large Miguel Mouse for the center of the board. Fill the board with good health habits and pictures that represent each habit. Leave enough room to mount student work.

Miguel says,

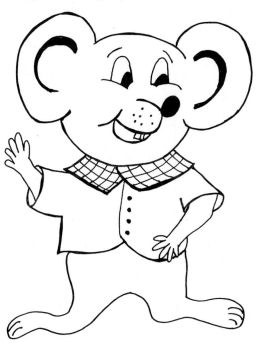

STAY WELL !

FIGURE 9-12

Worksheet

Name _____

Look What Happens When I Don't Cover My Sneeze!

Directions:
1. Draw a member of your family.
2. Draw a friend.
3. Write their names above their pictures.

_____ _____

_ _ _ _ _ _ _ _ _ _ _ _ _   _ _ _ _ _ _ _ _ _ _ _ _ _

_____ _____

FIGURE 9-13

Flannel board figures   Name _____

Well Child

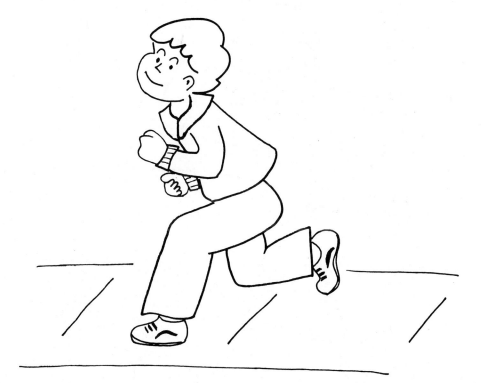

FIGURE 9-14

Flannel board figures   Name _____

Sick Child

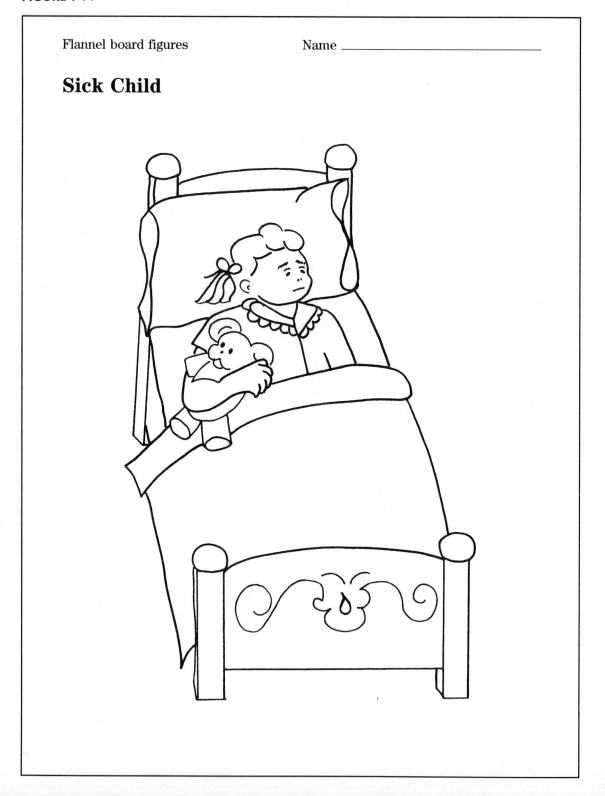

INTERMEDIATE LEVEL

OBJECTIVE: The student explains how personal health behavior is influenced by friends and family members.

LEVEL: Grades 4 to 6

INTEGRATION: Language arts

VOCABULARY: Lifestyle, peer pressure, influence

CONTENT GENERALIZATIONS: The personal health behaviors chosen greatly influence the quality of life. The adoption of a healthful lifestyle or an unhealthful lifestyle is a personal choice that is influenced by a number of outside variables. Initially personal health behaviors are learned from parents and family members. When children enter school, they learn about other habits perhaps not practiced in their family. Particularly in the adolescent years, peer pressure has a strong influence on health behaviors. It is not unusual to see great changes in personal health behaviors of adolescents because of peer pressure. These changes can be positive, such as the adoption of better grooming habits or a personal fitness and sports program. The changes also can be negative, such as the adoption of drug habits or risk-taking behaviors. Whatever the final lifestyle chosen, the health behaviors determining the choice have been greatly influenced by friends and family members.

INITIATION: Habits—Word Puzzle
Hand out the worksheet for the students to solve. When they are finished, go over the solution to the puzzle. Then ask how many students got everything correct. (Most students will do *very* well on the puzzle.) Ask, "Why did you do so well filling in the missing words when we have not studied anything about health habits in class yet?" Students probably will have answers, such as, "I learned it last year in Mr. Garcia's class," or "My mom always tells me to brush my teeth."

Explain to the students that we learn what good health behavior is from many places. This starts when we are very young. Ask the students if they can think of a health habit that a parent has been telling them about for as long as they can remember. Also ask them "Just because you know you should do something (such as wash your hands after using the restroom), do you always do it?"

Have the students consider the following questions for discussion.

1. Can personal nutritional choices be influenced by friends and family members?
2. How can personal nutritional choices be influenced by friends and family members?
3. Can the influence of others be positive, as well as negative?
4. How can you reinforce positive health behaviors in your family or friends?
5. How can you resist friends or family influencing you to develop a negative health habit?

ACTIVITIES
1. A Story About Maverick
a. Tell the students they are going to hear a story about a 10-year-old boy celebrating his straight-A report card. Ask them to think about what the boy, Maverick, does to celebrate his success.

MATERIALS
Worksheet: *Habits—Word Puzzle* (Figure 9-15)

MAVERICK CELEBRATES

Maverick flew into his house calling out, "Mom, Dad, Grandpa, come look. I got all A's on my report card, not even one A-. And the teacher's comments were great. Ms. Chin said that I was exceptional in completing my assignments and a model student in class. Listen to what she said about my health lessons: 'Maverick learned his health lessons and actually applied them in class. He bought fruit and milk every day during the nutrition break. Maverick successfully led our *I don't smoke cigarettes* campaign in school and received the highest grade in the class on all his nutrition, science, and health examinations.'"

"Great!" exclaimed Maverick's dad. "You weren't kidding when you said you could get straight A's by studying after dinner every night."

"What a difference from last year when you didn't study and got all C's," said Maverick's mom. "You did better than get straight A's. It sounds as though you're the star in school, particularly in health."

Maverick could scarcely hold in his joy. He was jumping up and down and shouting, "I did it!"

Grandpa said, "I'm proud of you too, Grandson. I'm going to give you $5 to save or spend. A smart boy like you will know the right thing to do with $5."

Maverick thanked Grandpa, Mom, and Dad and ran upstairs to get ready for a party at his friend's house. Maverick brushed and flossed his teeth, put on a clean shirt, and stuffed the new $5 bill into his jeans pocket. He dashed out of the house, whistling as he walked to the party.

On the way Maverick ran into Albert, who was headed to the party also. Albert said, "Didn't you hear? The parents won't be home during the party. I'm bringing beer so that we can really celebrate. You especially have to celebrate your straight-A report card."

"No thanks, I don't drink beer," said Maverick.

When they arrived at the party, Maverick noticed that the music was turned up loud, some people were drinking beer, and others were chewing or smoking tobacco. Maverick turned down several offers to chew or smoke tobacco or drink beer. But he did not turn down Albert's last offer.

Albert said, "Maverick, are you too good to celebrate with us just because you got all A's? You're not really one of us any more unless you have a couple of beers and a few cigarettes."

Maverick could not resist. He wanted to be one of the gang—their friend. They were all drinking and smoking, so why shouldn't he?

On the way home from the party Maverick had an upset stomach. He felt sick partly because he had had two beers and three cigarettes, but mostly because he had let himself down. As Maverick walked home alone, he was thinking, "Why did I have those beers and cigarettes? I really didn't want them, so why did I have them?"

b. Discussion questions
- Why did Maverick drink two beers and smoke three cigarettes?
- Why was Maverick able to turn down Albert the first time but not the second time?
- Did Maverick's friends have anything to do with his decision to drink and smoke?
- How could Maverick have avoided drinking beer or smoking cigarettes without jeopardizing his friendship with the others?

2. **Let's Do It Together**
   Identify a group health behavior that the class would like to collectively practice. It might be related to safety (not running in halls or putting away classroom materials that could cause someone to trip), environment (a litter cleanup campaign or a "be quieter in the lunchroom" campaign), nutrition (no junk food at school), or another area of health. Students should develop an approach to positively support and influence one another in practicing this positive health habit.

EVALUATION: "The Apple and the Candy Bar"

WHICH SNACK?
Read the following story aloud to students:

Latoya has to make a snack choice. Her friend Sandra is going to have a SuperCocoCarmel Bar and thinks Latoya should have one, too. Sandra says to Latoya, "It's new and so good. Everyone has to try the SuperCocoCarmel at least once."

Latoya has just returned from the dentist and has more cavities than she would like to admit. Her dad told her to eat apples instead of candy because they are naturally sweet and good for her. Besides, Latoya likes apples.

Ask the students to explain the influences Latoya is feeling before she makes her choice. The explanation can be done as a paragraph or a drawing.

MATERIALS
Worksheet: *The Apple and the Candy Bar* (Figure 9-16)

FIGURE 9-15

Worksheet   Name _____

Habits—Word Puzzle

Directions: Fill in the missing word in each sentence on the blanks to the
              right. Use all the letters that are in a circle to complete the secret
              message at the bottom of the worksheet.

1. Always _____ your hands after
   using the restroom.

2. Cover your nose when you _____.

3. B _____ and F _____ your teeth
   regularly.

4. Eat nutritious _____ for a strong
   body.

5. Fitness and strong muscles come
   only if you _____.

6. Wear clean C _____ every day.

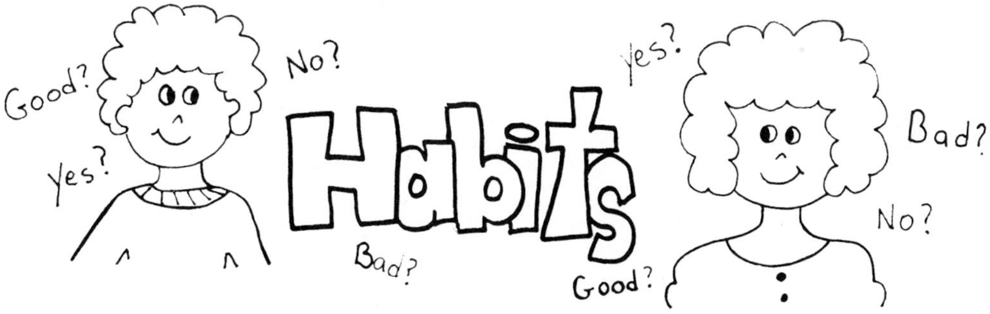

Secret   First put all the circled letters below. Then use those letters to
message: finish the message at the bottom.

THESE ARE HABITS _ _ _ _   _ _ _ _ _ _ _ !

FIGURE 9-16

Worksheet   Name _____

The Apple and the Candy Bar

Directions: Listen to the story as your teacher reads about Latoya and Sandra.
Then write about or draw the influences Latoya feels.

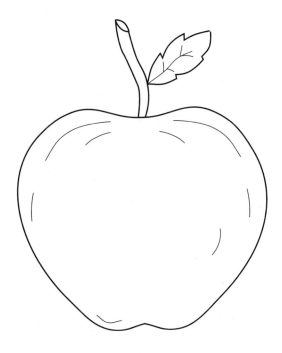

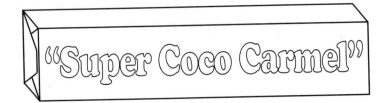

MIDDLE SCHOOL LEVEL

OBJECTIVE: The student describes personal health and fitness programs to meet individual needs and interests.

LEVEL: Grades 6 to 8

VOCABULARY: Lifestyle, heredity fitness, aerobic

CONTENT GENERALIZATIONS: Often people take better care of their automobiles than they do of their body. Personal health care habits contribute to overall well-being, physically, mentally and socially. Developmentally, students in these grades are very conscious about the way that they look. Their interest is high in the area of physical appearance. Linking personal health and fitness to appearance is often a key for health-related decisions made by these students. Care of teeth, eyes, ears, and skin will enhance attractiveness and contribute to physical and mental well-being. Adequate amounts of sleep and exercise are needed as well for mental and physical fitness. An important aspect in the success of a program of personal health care and fitness is that it must be valued by the individual. Exercises that the individual enjoys and health practices that he or she views as important are more likely to be incorporated into a lifestyle.

INITIATION: My Ideal

Ask the class to identify an adult who most students in the class consider "ideal." Ask "Who in sports, on television, or in the movies is particularly attractive? Who is the 'picture of health?' " Write the names of persons who students identify on the board. Tell the students to look in magazines and cut out pictures of these people or of any person they think looks attractive and healthy.

MATERIALS

Magazines (brought in by students)
Scissors

ACTIVITIES

1. Picture of Health

a. Tell the students to use the picture they recently cut out to observe healthy characteristics. Explain that people are attractive for many reasons, and different people think different traits make a person attractive. Most people think that being and looking healthy makes a person look attractive. Tell students to look at the pictures and try to determine why these particular people look attractive and healthy.

b. Write the words *heredity* and *lifestyle* on the board. Explain that certain factors influencing our health are inherited from our parents, and others, *environmental* factors, are the result of the way we live.

c. Hand out the worksheet, *Picture of Health.* For each question on the worksheet, have students check the box that they think most contributed to the attractiveness and health of the person in their picture. Explain that they may not know exactly in each case, but they should suggest possible reasons. In many cases, both heredity and lifestyle will apply.

d. After students have attempted to judge which characteristics were caused mostly by heredity or lifestyle, review each question. Have students make corrections on their worksheets, as necessary. Emphasize that these worksheets are for awareness and reference; they were not expected to know the correct answers to all questions. The answers are as follows.

- Color of eyes is hereditary.
- Sheen of hair is both, but largely lifestyle. Clean hair shines.
- Color of skin is largely hereditary, but a tan is a result of lifestyle.
- Complexion is both. However, lifestyle habits of cleanliness and proper nutrition usually can help even the most difficult complexion problems.
- Clean teeth are due to lifestyle. Brushing and flossing teeth regularly not only help

teeth look clean but also remove plaque that causes tooth decay.

- Build of body is both. You inherit a basic body type, but exercise and eating habits will determine the muscle development and contours of the body.
- Cavity-free teeth are both. You may inherit a tendency toward developing dental cavities or not, but eating habits, brushing, flossing, and regular visits to the dentist also are important behaviors.
- Clean body is lifestyle. Washing removes dirt, oil and germs that cause odor and disease. Being clean is both attractive and healthful.
- Have students look at all the items that have *lifestyle* or *both* checked. Explain that all these characteristics are ones we *can* control in our lives. We can choose a lifestyle that contributes to health and appearance. Ask if there is one important health habit that was not mentioned. (Sleep.) Ask them if they think getting enough sleep also can contribute to attractiveness and why or why not.

MATERIALS
Worksheet: *Picture of Health* (Figure 9-17)

2. What A Workout!
Explain to students that a good exercise program is planned and tailor made for the individual. A complete program includes exercises for flexibility (i.e., stretching), endurance (i.e., aerobic), and strength (i.e., lifting and repetitious). Aerobic activity increases heart and lung capacity and functioning. For exercise to be aerobic, it is necessary for the heart to beat hard continuously for at least 20 minutes. Tell them they are going to check their pulse rate before, immediately after, and 3 minutes after exercise.

a. Have students place two fingers (not the thumb) on the side of their neck and feel for a pulse. When they have all found their pulse, have students determine their pulse rates. Tell them to count the beats of their pulse to themselves while the teacher times exactly 30 seconds on a stopwatch or watch with a second hand. Say "stop" when the 30 seconds have passed. Ask the students to multiply the number of beats counted by 2 to determine their resting pulse rate.

MATERIALS
Stopwatch or watch with a second hand

b. Pass out the worksheet, *What A Workout!* Have students record their resting pulse rate on the worksheet. Then ask them to run in place for 1 minute. Have them check their pulse rate the same way by counting the beats for 30 seconds and multiplying by 2. Have them record that number on the worksheet as well. Then have students rest for 3 minutes and take the pulse rate again. Tell the students that the faster your pulse rate returns to normal after exercising, the better. Hand out the worksheet, *Step Test*, and suggest they try it with their parents at home. This test is an adaptation of the Harvard step test.

MATERIALS
Worksheets: *What a Workout!* (Figure 9-18); *Step Test* (Figure 9-19)

c. Find out from students what the highest and lowest pulse rates were for the three measurements. Record the highest and lowest rates on the board. Point out that this range shows the individual differences that exist in one class. It reinforces the point that all programs should be tailored to individual needs.

d. Brainstorm and establish the kinds of exercises that students enjoy. Record them on the board. Ask if there are any on the board that get the heart working hard. (Jogging, dancing, basketball, swimming, skating, bicycle riding, jumping rope.) Explain that these are called *aerobic* exercises and should be done at least three times a week. Stretching and strength exercises should be added to round out the workout. Have the students fill in the worksheet *What a Workout!* as you explain that during a workout one should do the following.

- Warm-up exercises (stretching) such as touching toes and stretching arms to the sky for 5 to 10 minutes
- Some endurance and strength exercises such as pushups, sit-ups, and possibly weight lifting for 5 to 10 minutes
- Some aerobic exercises such as swimming, running, dancing, jumping rope, bicycle riding, and quick walking for 15 to 20 minutes
- Some cool-down exercises like the warm-up exercises for 5 to 10 minutes

MATERIALS
Worksheet: *What a Workout!* (see Figure 9-18)

EVALUATION: Checking Myself
Hand out the worksheet, *Checking Myself.* Explain that this is very personal. They have learned a great deal on health care habits and exercise. This worksheet is a way to see how well they personally do with various health habits. These papers should be checked only to see if the assignment was completed, not for correct responses. Encourage students to be honest in this activity. Tell them that this is a 2-week project. Give them about 2 minutes each day in class to work on these worksheets. Allow students to choose one person in the class as a partner. It should be someone with whom they feel comfortable. Allow the pairs to talk to each other about their findings. Tell the students that they only need to share information they feel comfortable sharing.

Have the students talk with their partner regarding health care habits that may need improving and develop a written plan about how to do so. Students should write a sentence on why this program works for them. Students should review their success in the exercise program as specified on their plan with their partners. Assess plans for student's ability to propose a plan that meets their personal needs and interests.

MATERIALS
Worksheet: *Checking Myself* (Figure 9-20)

FIGURE 9-17

Worksheet

Name _____

Picture of Health

Directions: To which can you attribute the following characteristics for the person in your picture? Check either HEREDITY or LIFESTYLE or BOTH.

	HEREDITY	LIFESTYLE	BOTH
1. Color of eyes	☐	☐	☐
2. Sheen in hair	☐	☐	☐
3. Color of skin	☐	☐	☐
4. Complexion of skin	☐	☐	☐
5. Clean teeth	☐	☐	☐
6. Build of body	☐	☐	☐

Answer the following even though you cannot see these characteristics in the picture.

7. Cavity-free teeth	☐	☐	☐
8. Clean body	☐	☐	☐

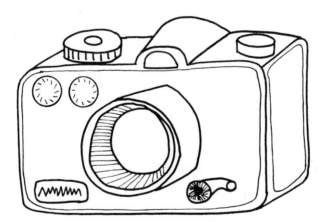

FIGURE 9-18

Worksheet   Name _____

What a Workout!

Pulse rate: Resting _____ After exercise _____
                 3 Minutes after exercise _____

Pulse rate
1. My resting pulse rate was _____ beats per minute.
2. My pulse rate immediately after exercise was _____ beats per minute.
3. My pulse rate 3 minutes after exercise was _____ beats per minute.
4. Did your pulse rate drop 10 to 15 beats per minute after 3 minutes? _____

- -

The parts of a workout

1. _____ exercises such as _____

   _____

   for _____ minutes

2. _____ exercises such as _____

   _____

   for _____ minutes

3. _____ exercises such as _____

   _____

   for _____ minutes

4. _____ exercises such as _____

   _____

   for _____ minutes

- -

Working out for 2 weeks
On the back of this worksheet draw a calendar for 2 weeks, and fill in your progress as in the example below. (Record the aerobic exercise only, but do warm up and cool down.)

Monday	Tuesday	Wednesday	Thursday	Friday	Saturday	Sunday
After-school jog, 20 minutes						

FIGURE 9-19

Worksheet   Name _____

Step Test   Modified from the Harvard step test.

Test your heart's capacity to adapt to and recover from strenuous exercise.

1. Use a platform 14 to 17 inches high. Step up and down 30 times per minute for 4 minutes.

2. Start by placing the left foot on the platform at the command up. Then step up with the other foot, so both feet are on the platform. Then step down, using the same rhythm. Use a marching count: up, 2, 3, 4. The signal *up* comes every 2 seconds.

3. Exercise for 4 minutes. Then sit down and remain quiet.

4. One minute later the pulse rate is taken for 30 seconds.

5. Two minutes after exercising the pulse rate is taken for 30 seconds.

6. Three minutes after exercising the pulse rate is taken for 30 seconds.

7. Add the total of all three 30-second counts.

RECOVERY INDEX

Total count	Index	Your response
199 or more	60 or less	Poor
171 to 198	61 to 70	Fair
150 to 170	71 to 80	Good
133 to 149	81 to 90	Very good
132 or less	91 or more	Excellent

This test taxes the cardiorespiratory resources of the individual and is approved by the American Medical Association.

FIGURE 9-20

Worksheet   Name _____

Checking Myself

Directions: This worksheet is a personal record to help you see how well you do
                with your health care habits. Put a check mark in the box for the days
                that you did those activities. It is not necessary to do all activities every
                day to have good personal health habits. Some are daily habits; others
                are not. This will help you see how often you perform each habit. Then
                you can determine whether it is often enough.

	DATE									
1. Brushed teeth										
2. Flossed teeth										
3. Slept 8 to 9 hours										
4. Washed hair										
5. Washed clothes										
6. Changed sheets										
7. Changed towels										
8. Scrubbed fingernails										
9. Clipped toenails										
10. Washed face										
11. Showered or bathed										

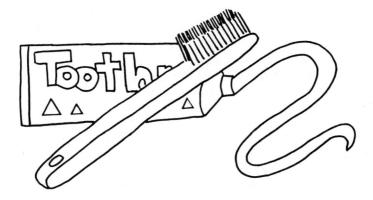

10 Mental and Emotional Health

When you finish this chapter, you should be able to:

- Define mental and emotional health.
- Analyze the importance of self-esteem for individuals and educators.
- Describe appropriate content in the area of emotional health for elementary and middle school students.
- Develop learning opportunities for elementary and middle school students in the area of mental and emotional health.

As we saw in Chapter 9, health is a dynamic state reflecting the interactions between a person's physical, social, spiritual, intellectual, and emotional resources. This chapter looks at one of the more abstract parts of a healthy lifestyle: the development of emotional or mental health. For the purposes of this text, the terms mental and emotional will be used interchangeably.

Unlike good physical health habits, good emotional health habits are difficult to define. The emotional, intellectual, physical, spiritual, and social aspects of the individual are interrelated. What affects the individual physically most likely will affect him or her emotionally and socially as well. For example, a broken leg certainly has physical effects, but, in addition, during the physical mending process the individual cannot participate in normal social activities because it is more difficult to get around. Therefore emotional strain is expected. Although the health

problem is physical, the ramifications to the whole person are emotional and social as well. This interrelationship can be seen in all health-related circumstances and choices.

Central to the development of good mental health are high self-esteem; the capacity for emotional growth; the ability to maintain healthy social relationships; the mastery of effective ways of coping with stress; and the capability to make good decisions. These are the topics we will explore in this chapter.

DEFINITIONS

What are the characteristics of an emotionally healthy person? Emotionally healthy people are resilient. While they may experience stress, frustration, and feelings of self-doubt or failure, they are able to recapture a sense of mental wellness within a reasonable period of time.

More specifically, the National Mental Health

Association describes mentally healthy individuals as follows:

- *They feel comfortable with themselves.* Mentally healthy people experience the full range of emotions—fear, anger, love, jealousy, guilt, joy—but are not incapacitated by them. They can take disappointments in stride.
- *They feel good about other people.* They feel comfortable with others and can give and receive love.
- *They can meet the demands of life.* Mentally healthy people can deal with their problems, accept responsibility, plan ahead, and establish realistic goals.

Mental health is built on all experiences since birth. Future experiences will also contribute to mental health status. This means that it is possible to improve mental health through increased understanding of self and others. Some keys to establishing or improving mental health include the following:

- Maintaining good relationships with family and friends
- Communicating with the people you care about
- Feeling good about yourself
- Becoming involved in activities that are interesting to you
- Appreciating individual differences
- Determining the personal values by which you want to live

It is normal and healthy to experience a range of emotions. Some of these feelings are pleasant, while others are uncomfortable. You may feel angry, happy, sad, uncertain, confident, excited and afraid—all in the same week or even the same day. Feelings are usually reactions to circumstances that occur in life and should not be viewed as "good" or "bad." Emotionally healthy people experience uncomfortable or sad feelings as temporary and are able to regain their emotional equilibrium.

It is normal for feelings to cause physical changes as well. Being aware of these changes can help you to recognize your emotions. For instance, when anger is experienced, an upset stomach or a headache may be the body's response. Being called on in class may make your heart race and your palms perspire in response to the felt anxiety. This is the body's way of preparing you for a stressful situation that requires a reaction. You can control the physical response by learning to recognize feelings of stress and to deal effectively with such situations. Stress is discussed later in this chapter.

A particularly common mental health concern among college students and others is depression. While everyone feels "down" at times, depression is characterized by being persistently depressed. Since depression can be helped with a variety of therapies, it is important to be able to recognize the symptoms in yourself as well as in others. Some of the common symptoms are shown in the box below. Keep in mind when emotional extremes such as depression persist, it may be important to seek professional help. Universities often have mental health counselling and treatment services offered by the campus health center. Other mental health resources available in communities include hospitals, health departments, and private psychologists and psychiatrists who can be identified by personal physicians or through the yellow pages of the telephone directory.

**COMMON SYMPTOMS
OF DEPRESSION (4)**

Persistent sad moods

Feelings of hopelessness or pessimism

Loss of interest or pleasure in ordinary activities, including sex

Sleep and eating disorders

Restlessness, irritability, or fatigue

Difficulty concentrating, remembering or making decisions

Thoughts of death or suicide

Persistent physical symptoms or pains that do not respond to treatment

Suicide Prevention

If severe and untreated, depression can result in suicide. Teenagers, young adults, and the elderly are more likely than any other age groups to commit suicide. The American Psychiatric Association estimates that there has been more than a threefold increase in the rate of suicide among adolescents in the past 25 years. Suicide is now one of the leading causes of death for teens and young adults.

Usually, a person considering suicide gives clues that can serve as warning signals. Among young persons, common signals or precursors of suicide are the following:

- Increased moodiness
- Seeming depressed or uncommunicative
- Feelings of worthlessness
- Withdrawal from normal activities
- Writing and/or talking about death
- Specific suicide threats
- Breaking off friendships
- Failure or poor school performance
- Increased drug and alcohol use
- Failed love relationship
- Giving away prized possessions

There are steps you can take to help an individual who is considering suicide. Perhaps most importantly, talk to them and show that you care. Don't ignore or dismiss their feelings that life isn't worth living. Suggest some possible solutions to their problems. Often, desperate people do not see any alternatives. Help them make future plans. If they remain convinced that suicide is the only solution to their problems, have them promise they won't do anything to harm themselves without calling you first. Refer them to a professional who can help. Most major cities have crisis centers that a suicidal person can call 24 hours a day for help. For help with depression or suicide the National Runaway Switchboard (1-800-621-4000) is a valuable resource.

Self-Esteem

Simply put, self-esteem is the way we feel about ourselves. When we have high self-esteem, we are able to feel a sense of satisfaction that comes from our own inner resources. For both children and adults, having high self-esteem means that we feel good about ourselves. We feel a sense of security and are willing to explore the world. High self-esteem helps us to take risks, communicate with friends, even deal with stress, set goals, and make decisions. Low self-esteem may mean that we do not feel comfortable raising our hands in class, having friends, trying out for a role in a play, or even choosing what we want for lunch.

Clearly, raising self-esteem is important not only for the sense of mental and emotional well-being that it creates but also is necessary for developing the ability to make decisions—such as choosing healthy behaviors—and setting goals—such as the goal of living a healthy lifestyle. Low self-esteem has been found to be a common thread for many of the problems of children and youth, particularly substance use and abuse, (see Chapter 17.)

Conditions of Self-Esteem.   According to Bean, there are four important conditions or feelings we need to experience in order to have high self-esteem (1). People with high self-esteem experience all of these feelings frequently, in different circumstances and with a high level of intensity. People with low self-esteem have difficulty feeling one or more of the four feelings. When one or more of these feelings is missing, feeling "bad" is the result. Persistently feeling bad is a sign of low self-esteem.

A *sense of connectiveness* is the ability to gain satisfaction from the people, places, or things we feel connected to. When we have a high sense of connectiveness, we feel that we are a part of something, that we are important to others, and we feel comfortable with our bodies (feel connected to ourselves).

A *sense of uniqueness* is the feeling that we have qualities that are special and different. When we have a high sense of uniqueness, we feel that we are valued for who we are, and we are able to respect ourselves.

A *sense of power* enables us to believe in ourselves, feel competent, and feel comfortable with responsibility. When we have a high sense of power, we are able to feel in control of ourselves despite pressures that we might experience and able to feel that others can't make us do things we really don't want to do.

A *sense of models* is the ability to refer to human, philosophical, and operational models to help make sense of the world. People with a high sense of models feel confident that they can tell right from wrong and good from bad. They have consistent values and beliefs guiding their actions in different situations, have a sense of their own standards, and are able to organize their environment to accomplish a task.

Clemes and Bean identify some strategies for improving self-esteem (2):

- *Maintain satisfying group relationships.* A good way to do this is to become affiliated with existing groups, such as voluntary or professional organizations, church groups, or any other group that will provide a sense of "belonging."
- *Set and reach realistic goals.* Achieving goals can allow you to feel a sense of personal power and control over yourself. Goals can be related to your health, your academic progress, your social relationships, or any other dimension of your life.
- *Appreciate your uniqueness.* Enjoy compliments you receive. Each day, consider your special strengths and abilities and remind yourself of your uniqueness.
- *Maintain contact with a mentor.* Mentors are role models who can give you advice, as well as support and encouragement.

It is important to remember that there is no "perfect" self-esteem profile. Everyone has areas that are strong and areas that are more challenging for them. The goal should be to learn to work well with what you've got and to make changes where you can. If you take some time to examine your own self-esteem, you'll be able to better understand how your self-esteem and children's interact to affect the learning process, as well as your own feelings of comfort and satisfaction in the classroom.

The Teacher's Role in Developing Self-Esteem. Teachers can influence their students' self-esteem, not only by acting as models but also by encouraging students to develop in all of the above areas. As one expert in this field has noted, it is simplistic to say that you can't raise another person's self-esteem unless you have high self-esteem yourself. Instead, there is a more complex relationship between teacher and student self-esteem.

Teachers are more likely to nurture in their students the particular self-esteem conditions that are strongest in themselves. For instance, a teacher with a high sense of connectiveness feels good about close relationships with children and highly values them in the classroom. The climate for connectiveness is good in this teacher's classroom. This teacher is sensitive and compassionate; children who come into this class with a low sense of connectiveness will benefit from being with this teacher.

If this teacher also has a low sense of power, however, children who also have a low sense of power won't experience the conditions necessary for growth in that area. As a result, some children's self-esteem will improve in this classroom, while others' may not.

Appreciating Similarities and Differences. All people are alike in certain basic ways. As part of the "human community," we share similarities in our physiological makeup, as well as our emotional experiences and needs. Yet we are also unique individuals with our own body type, personality, abilities, and interests.

Beyond our individuality, we may share with our family a specific cultural or ethnic heritage—or combination of these—that differs from that of our neighbors or friends. In an educational environment, young children must learn to appreciate these differences to prevent the development of stereotypes and prejudices that in turn can lead to unjust treatment of people who are "different." Self-acceptance and acceptance of others are cyclical; the more children's self-esteem and confidence in themselves increases, the easier it is for them to become accepting of others.

CLASSROOM ACTIVITIES FOR ENHANCING SELF-ESTEEM (3)

Connectiveness

Ask children to share things about their families and their ethnic backgrounds. Point out similar interests and common values as you go along.

Have children work together in cooperative projects.

Allow children to plan special events and incorporate cultural diversity into these projects (for instance, play games or music from different cultural traditions).

Uniqueness

Encourage children to do ungraded assignments that allow personal expression (for instance, fantasy books or scrapbooks about themselves or their families).

Provide opportunities to share positive ways in which children are different from one another.

Help children see their affiliation with an ethnic group as a source of values and pride in who they are. Be aware that in some cultures, individual uniqueness is not a positive attribute; in these cases, reinforce the uniqueness that comes from being a part of a family, a community, and an ethnic group.

Power

Help children identify their skills and abilities, viewed broadly (for instance, include friendliness as a skill and a sense of humor as an ability).

Involve all children in setting rules for the classroom.

Introduce group decision-making processes such as voting, consensus, or using representatives.

Models

Emphasize visible, everyday role models available to children.

Introduce children to leaders from diverse cultural and ethnic groups.

Provide children with age-appropriate models for making decisions, setting goals, and resolving conflict.

Personality

Personality is the combination of a person's physical, mental, and social traits that makes a person unique. Since everyone's personality is different, there is a wide range of personality traits. Personality is shown in how a person reacts to the people, things, and events in his or her environment. An individual's personality will change throughout life, but most experts believe that the early years of a person's life are the most important. Heredity, personal experiences, self-concept, and the environment are factors that contribute to the formation of personality.

Friendship and Social Support

Friendship and social support are important for maintaining both physical and mental health. Friendships can help people manage the effects of stress. Recent studies of elderly people and people with heart disease suggest that friendship may strongly influence health. Heart patients without a spouse or close friends were three times more likely to die within five years of their diagnosis than those who were married or had a close friend. In a study of healthy older people, those with close friends were better able to fight disease.

Friendship is an important concept especially for primary level children to understand. Many different kinds of friendships can be studied, including close relationships with classmates, family members, neighbors, and pets. Students can identify some of the characteristics of good friends, such as shares toys, treats you with courtesy, can be trusted with secrets, and will help each other out when necessary.

Stress

In the simplest terms, stress is the feeling of being under pressure. Stress is the body's response to any physical or mental demand. Whatever triggers this response is called a stressor.

Stressors: Life Events and Daily Hassles. Stressors affect people in many different ways.

In fact, many researchers believe that the effects of stress are related more to each individual's reactions than to the specific stressors themselves. For one person, missing a train can cause extreme agitation, while another might use the time to read the paper—and enjoys it.

For adults, stress may be triggered by major "life events" such as a job change, a new baby, or a divorce. But it is not just major life events that trigger the body to react. Research now shows that even daily hassles—the repetitive, routine problems of daily life—can be significant stressors for some people. These hassles may be *emotional,* such as unresolved arguments or conflicts between people; *physical,* such as chronic lack of sleep; *occupational,* including a demanding or repetitive job; or *spiritual,* such as moral dilemmas.

Responding to Stress. People who are experiencing stress notice certain predictable body signals. Their heart rate increases, their throat becomes dry, their palms sweat, and they feel dizzy or light-headed. They may also feel sick to their stomachs. This typical physiological response to a stressor has been described as a three-stage reaction called the *general adaptation syndrome* by Selye (5):

- *Alarm stage:* involuntary hormonal changes cause blood sugar levels, blood pressure, heart and breathing rates to increase. The body releases the hormone, adrenaline, to prepare for the "fight-or-flight" response.
- *Resistance stage:* the body tries to combat the stressor by reducing the initial response.
- *Exhaustion stage:* following long-term exposure to a stressor, physiological function can deteriorate. However, when a stressor lasts a short time and a person can relax afterward, blood pressure and hormone levels can quickly return to normal.

Long-term stress seems to reduce the body's ability to fight disease. During the alarm and resistance phases of the general adaptation syndrome, the immune system can become suppressed, resulting in increased vulnerability to infections. There is also evidence that high levels of stress are linked to hypertension and heart disease. Stress may also contribute to other disorders, such as diabetes, cancer, and depression.

Types of Stressors. Stressors can be both positive and negative. While stressors produce the same generalized physical response whether they are perceived as positive or negative, the behavioral response experienced will be different. Selye coined the word *eustress* for the reaction to positive stressors. This kind of stress is associated with enhanced longevity, productivity, and life satisfactions—for example, the stress you feel while exercising. Negative response to stressors Selye calls *distress*. Some examples are chronic pain, depression, and anxiety.

It is important to remember that stress is inevitable. We cannot "avoid stress," but we can learn to identify the stress levels at which we function best and to take actions that improve our ability to cope with the stressors in our lives.

Coping with Stress. How one chooses to cope with the "alarm" response is significant. Coping mechanisms can be healthy or destructive. One common destructive reaction to stress is the use of alcohol or other drugs to calm and mask the alarm response. Some other responses we sometimes use to protect ourselves from uncomfortable thoughts or feelings are "defense mechanisms." Some of the ways we defend ourselves include the following:

- *Repression*—keeping threatening memories, feelings, or wishes from becoming conscious. For example, "forgetting" to feed the dog after once being bitten.
- *Denial*—refusing to accept a painful fact. For example, refusing to believe that someone you love is dying of cancer.
- *Rationalization*—substituting "good" reasons for the real motivations of behavior. For example, saying you can't come to a friend's house because you have to study, when the real reason you won't go to her

house is because you are angry at something she said.

- *Projection*—attributing your own unacceptable feelings to someone else. For example, saying that your girlfriend or boyfriend broke up with you because he or she wanted to date someone else, when you were really the one who wanted to date other people.
- *Displacement*—redirecting feelings from their true object to a substitute. For example, snapping at your closest friend when you are really angry with your parents.

Rather than relying on defense mechanisms, healthy and more productive coping skills can be used. Some healthy ways to cope include the following:

1. *Physical activity.* Since the hormone adrenaline is released during stressful times and therefore muscles are tense, physical activity is useful in burning up the pent-up energy. Regular physical exercise programs—particularly aerobic exercise programs—have been shown to be useful in reducing stress levels.

2. *Talk things out.* Using a friend's ear just to get things off your chest can be very helpful. It is not even necessary for the friend to offer useful suggestions; just the chance to talk to someone about what is worrying you is helpful.

3. *Take things one at a time.* When a problem seems overwhelming, break it into small pieces and consider one step at a time.

4. *Don't try to win every time.* Life has ups and downs. We cannot always have things our way. Accepting the fact that sometimes things do not work out the way you want them to is one way of coping with stress.

5. *Balance work with play.* Be sure to take the time to do things that you enjoy doing. Find a balance.

6. *Take a break for yourself.* Plan a certain

amount of time each day for yourself. It may be only 15 to 20 minutes, but do something you like to do such as read a magazine, listen to music, or even daydream. The important thing is to have some planned time just for you.

Payne and Hahn suggest approaching life with a "tough-minded optimism," since life will never be stress-free(4). Since most people's lifestyle is necessarily fast-paced and demanding, the following are some perspectives that can help us to stay realistic yet positive in our outlook:

- Anticipate problems and look for solutions: see yourself as a "problem solver."
- Take control of your own future; don't see yourself as a victim.
- Identify and steer clear of negative thought patterns. Don't generalize difficulties from one area into another.
- Rehearse success without disregarding the possibility of failure. Focus on what's necessary and possible to ensure success.
- Accept that some things can't be changed, coping as effectively as possible with events you can't control.
- Live each day well. Balance responsibility with play; celebrate special occasions.
- Act on your capacity for growth; undertake new experiences and use them to gain new information about yourself.

Stress for children often is not caused by the day-to-day activities of home and school but by being in situations where their options have been taken away or reduced. The same skills for managing stress that can be learned and practiced by adults can be used by children. For example, children can learn how to communicate their emotions without hurting others, decision-making and problem-solving skills, realistic goal setting, and valuable social skills.

In general, a constructive way to cope with stress is to develop a healthy lifestyle, focusing on both mental and physical health. When a person is generally healthy, the body is more resistant to the effects of prolonged stress. A healthy lifestyle includes eating well, exercising for fitness, getting enough sleep, and learning ways to relax. Living with a positive and flexible mental outlook is also helpful in coping with stress.

Decision Making

Learning to make decisions and take actions that reflect one's beliefs and values helps to maintain and enhance self-esteem. If decisions are contradictory to strongly held values, stress and emotional conflicts arise. Decision-making patterns and resulting actions give valuable clues about an individual's value system. Good mental health can be promoted by learning to make decisions through consideration of one's own beliefs and values.

DECISION MAKING AND CULTURAL DIVERSITY (4)

Students who learn the elements of decision-making from a very young age have an advantage when it comes to achieving life goals.

When helping young children to develop decision-making skills, remember that:

- Different options in decision making depend on one's cultural background and perspectives.
- The best decision for the same situation may be different for each student based on experience and cultural background.
- Consequences of an action or decision may be seen differently by children based on their experience and cultural background.
- Exploring consequences with children should include discussing how the decision might affect their families and their relationship with family members.
- Ability to implement decisions is influenced by ethnic background as well as economic or educational levels, language, and resources.
- Students should be encouraged to consider family values as well as individual strengths and desires when making decisions.

Good decision making involves several specific steps:

1. Identify the exact decision to be made.
2. Consider all the possible outcomes.
3. Evaluate each outcome. Ask yourself what will happen if you choose that outcome. Consider how that decision will affect you and other people.
4. Make the decision that seems the best. Remember that you are responsible for your decisions.

SUMMARY

In this chapter we explored some of the conditions that are essential for the development of good mental and emotional health: high self-esteem, the capacity for emotional growth, the ability to maintain healthy social relationships and cope with stress, and the capability of making good decisions.

Being emotionally healthy means being resilient—able to recapture a sense of wellness within a reasonable period of time after experiencing stress, frustration or feelings of self-doubt or failure. People with good mental health feel comfortable with themselves, feel good about other people, and feel that they can meet the demands of life.

Four conditions of high self-esteem were identified, including the senses of connectiveness, uniqueness, power, and models.

Responses to stress are highly individualized; what is stressful for one person may be merely challenging or even enjoyable for another. While we cannot avoid stress in our lives, we can learn to identify the stress levels at which we function best and take actions that improve our ability to cope. Good mental health can also be promoted by learning to make decisions that are consistent with one's beliefs and values.

In the section that follows are examples of learning opportunities that are appropriate for primary level, intermediate level, and middle school students, as well as objectives indicating scope and sequence of content for this area.

REFERENCES

1. Bean R: *The four conditions of self-esteem*, Santa Cruz, Calif, 1992, ETR Associates.
2. Clemes H, Bean R: *Self-esteem: The key to your child's well-being*, New York, 1981, GP Putnam.
3. Matiella A: *Positively different. Creating a bias-free environment for young children*, Santa Cruz, Calif, 1991, ETR Associates.
4. Payne W, Hahn D: *Understanding your health*, ed 3, St. Louis, 1992, Mosby.
5. Selye H: *Stress without distress*, New York, 1974, JB Lippincott.

SUGGESTED READINGS

Berryman J, Breighner K: *Modeling healthy behavior*, Santa Cruz, Calif, 1993, ETR Associates.

Branden N: *The psychology of self-esteem*, New York, 1983, Bantam Books.

Emotional and mental health, *MacMillan Health Encyclopedia*, vol 5, New York, 1993, MacMillan.

Maslow A: *Motivation and personality*, ed 3, New York, 1987, Harper & Row.

Stung L, Miner K: *Mental health: health facts for teachers*, Santa Cruz, Calif, 1994, ETR Associates.

LEARNING OPPORTUNITIES FOR EMOTIONAL/MENTAL HEALTH

GENERAL STUDENT OBJECTIVES

Primary Level K-3

The student:
1. Classifies social behaviors as acceptable and unacceptable.
2. Differentiates between pleasant and unpleasant emotions.
3. Illustrates ways to show friendship.*

Intermediate Level 4-5/6

The student:
1. Explains the difference between physical well-being and mental and emotional health.
2. Identifies positive and negative effects of stress.
3. Proposes acceptable ways to deal with strong negative emotions.*

Middle School Level 6/7-8

The student:
1. Identifies constructive ways to manage stress.*
2. Analyzes the influence of peer pressure health related choices.
3. Describes the importance of setting realistic goals.
4. Explains the interrelationships among physical, mental, emotional, and social well-being.

*These objectives are illustrated by sample learning opportunities.

PRIMARY LEVEL

OBJECTIVE: The student illustrates ways to show friendship.

LEVEL: Grades 2 and 3

INTEGRATION: Reading, problem solving, drawing conclusions

VOCABULARY: Friendship, feelings, sharing, enjoyment

CONTENT GENERALIZATIONS: Friendship is an important aspect of life, but it has a different meaning for different people. A friend is usually someone you like to be with. Often friends enjoy the same activities, like playing baseball, roller skating, going shopping, or dancing. A friend is also someone who cares and helps out when needed. A friend is someone who shares possessions (such as toys, books, and cookies) and feelings (such as happiness, sadness, frustration, and anger).

INITIATION: Reporting on "Friendship"
Ask for a volunteer to play the part of a television reporter. This student is to go around the room surveying other students in the class about friendship. The question should be something like, "What are some ways that you show you are a friend?"

MATERIALS
Optional: Prop microphone

ACTIVITIES
Ask the students if anyone in their survey said that sharing was a part of friendship. If no one did, explain that many people believe it is a very

important part of being a friend. Tell them that the next activity will give them an opportunity to practice sharing.

1. A Crayon for my Friend

    a. Allow the students to form groups of five or six. A working space is needed for each group, ideally a table with six chairs or a table the children can stand around. Each working space should have six crayons of different colors: red, green, blue, yellow, orange, and purple.

    b. Explain the task to the students before handing them the worksheets. The task is to color each crayon pictured on the worksheet the correct color. Since there are six children in a group and only six crayons, the members of the group will have to share the crayons for all to finish the worksheet.

    c. Hand out the worksheet, *A Crayon for My Friend*, and circulate around the room, observing the sharing in each group. Stop at each group and ask how they are doing.

    d. When everyone has finished, ask a person from each group to tell about his or her experiences with the activity. Ask the students, "What are some other ways that you share and show friendship?"

MATERIALS

Crayons: red, green, blue, yellow, orange, and purple (1 set per group)

    Worksheet: *A Crayon for My Friend*, Figure 10-1

2. Showing Friendship

Tell the students they are going to practice some more ways to show friendship. Use the worksheet, *Showing Friendship*, which portrays a situation where friendship can be demonstrated. Students are to read about the picture and draw or write a way that the character in the picture could be a friend. Post the finished worksheets on the bulletin board.

MATERIALS

Worksheet: *Showing Friendship*, Figure 10-2
Crayons

EVALUATION: "Friendship Mural"

Have the students cooperatively make a large mural on friendship. Each student in the class must participate by painting one way to show friendship on the mural. Mount the mural in the classroom or hallway of the school.

MATERIALS

Large piece of butcher paper
Poster paints

FIGURE 10-1

Worksheet   Name _____

A Crayon for My Friend

Directions: Color the crayons the correct color. Share crayons.

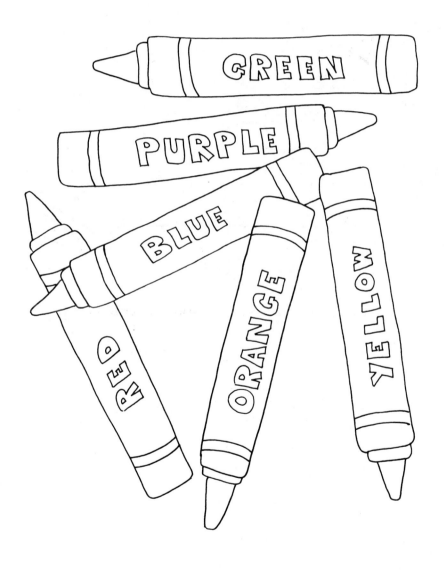

FIGURE 10-2

Worksheet   Name _____

Showing Friendship

Sam has two fish. Coco has none.
Both cats are hungry.

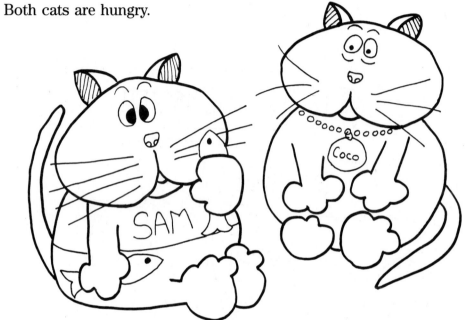

How can Sam be a friend? Draw or write below.

INTERMEDIATE LEVEL

OBJECTIVE: The student proposes acceptable ways to deal with strong negative emotions.

LEVEL: Grades 4 to 6

INTEGRATION: Art, language arts

VOCABULARY: Conflict, emotions, resolve, anger, appropriate, inappropriate

CONTENT GENERALIZATIONS: Conflict in our lives often due to a difference in opinions, ideas or values can result in strong negative emotions. Anger and frustration, arise, causing a stressful situation. Unacceptable ways that people deal with conflict and anger anger include fighting, swearing, breaking objects, and pouting. It is also unacceptable to "hold it in" and do nothing. Acceptable ways to deal with anger include exercise, "getting it off your chest" by talking it out, long walks, shouting into a pillow, and taking deep breaths. Some sort of physical exercise is probably the most effective. It is important to understand that anger is a normal emotion which everyone experiences. All these ways to deal with anger also can be used to deal with any stressful situation.

INITIATION: "It Really Makes Me Angry . . ."
Ask the students to think about various things that make them angry using the worksheet, *It Really Makes Me Angry . . . .* Explain that they are to write down situations which make them angry. An example is, "I get angry when my little brother breaks the airplane model I spent 3 hours working on." Ask the students what they might do in this anger-causing situation. Ask for volunteers to tell what they really do when they get angry. Make no value judgment at this time regarding the appropriateness of their actions. Explain that anger is normal. We need to learn how to deal with anger and other negative emotions because life is filled with both good and bad emo-

tions. The good ones are easy to deal with; the negative ones are more difficult. Tell the students to hold on to their papers for use in later activities.

MATERIALS
Worksheet: *It Really Makes Me Angry . . .* (Figure 10-3)

ACTIVITIES

MATERIALS
Worksheet: *Ways to Deal With Anger* (Figure 10-4)

1. **Ways to Deal With Anger—Part I**
   Write the words *acceptable* and *unacceptable* on the board. Explain to the students that anger can be dealt with in an acceptable or unacceptable way. Ask them to help you determine what is acceptable and what is unacceptable. Generally, unacceptable can be defined as any action that damages people, property, or feelings. Anything violent is unacceptable.

   Hand out the worksheet, *Ways to Deal With Anger.* Individually allow the students to read each situation in part I and determine if the action was acceptable or unacceptable. Tell them to leave part II blank for now.

MATERIALS
Worksheet: *Ways to Deal With Anger* (with part I completed) (see Figure 10-3)
Transparency (1 sheet per group)
Transparency pens (at least one per group, but preferably several colors)

2. **Ways to Deal With Anger—Part II**
   When students are done with the individual work on part I, put them in groups of four or five to discuss their choices. Part II is to be completed as a group. First, students should discuss and defend their choices in part I. Then, as a group, they should decide on an acceptable behavior for the situation described

in part II. Everyone in the group must agree that the behavior chosen is acceptable. As a group, they should design a way to present their ideas to the class on a transparency. They can draw a cartoon, write a paragraph, or act it out as a skit.

The groups should elect a representative to present their ideas orally to the class.

MATERIALS

Overhead projector
Transparencies (completed by groups)

3. "Angry Feelings" Boxes

a. A few days before this activity tell the students to bring to class an empty half-gallon milk carton. (Small milk cartons from the school cafeteria could be used if necessary.)

b. Tell the students they will be making "Angry Feelings" boxes. First they are to decorate a milk carton as follows.

- On one side print the word *acceptable*.
- On another side print the word *unacceptable*.
- On the two remaining sides draw two pictures of acceptable ways of dealing with anger.

MATERIALS

Half-gallon milk cartons (1 per student)
Construction paper (light colored)
Stapler
Felt pens, colored pencils, or crayons

c. Then every day for a week or so, at the beginning of class they are to write down the various situations that made them angry the day before. Each instance is written on a separate piece of paper, including the way that they handled their anger in that situation. Each piece of paper should be placed into the milk carton.

MATERIALS

"Angry Feelings" boxes (previously made by students)
Scratch paper

d. After about a week of collecting information about situations that make them angry, the students should draw out a slip of paper from the milk carton. The students should read each situation to themselves and consider whether the action taken was an acceptable or unacceptable way of dealing with anger. Students should paste a star on the "Angry Feelings" boxes either under *acceptable* or *unacceptable*, whichever applies for that particular situation. They continue the same process for each slip of paper in the box.

MATERIALS

"Angry Feelings" boxes filled with descriptions of anger-causing situations
Stars (all one color; at least 5 to 10 per student)

4. Dealing With My Angry Feelings

a. Ask the students to count the stars on their boxes. Ask, "Which side has the most stars? How well do you do at handling anger in an acceptable way?" Hand out the worksheet, *Dealing With My Angry Feelings*. Ask the students to use one of the situations where they behaved in an unacceptable way and to write a suggestion of a different way to behave in the same situation that would be acceptable. Allow them to work on this assignment in pairs if they desire. Review the written suggestions, and give them back to the students with comments.

MATERIALS

Worksheet: *Dealing With My Angry Feelings* (Figure 10-5)

b. Have the students collect another week's worth of anger-causing situations and behaviors in their "Angry Feelings" boxes. At the end of the week they should analyze their behaviors again and give themselves a star on either the *acceptable* or *unacceptable* side. Ask if they improved during the second week. Explain that this is a very difficult behavior to learn and they should try not to be frustrated if they are having problems. Tell them it might be helpful to talk to someone they trust about further suggestions of appropriate ways to handle anger.

MATERIALS

"Angry Feelings" boxes (filled with anger-causing situations)

Stars (all one color but a *different* color than used previously; at least 5 to 10 per student)

5. Take a Breather

Practice deep-breathing exercises with the students. Tell them this is often a very effective method of dealing with strong emotions, especially when it is difficult to do any physical exercise. Have the students sit up straight and inhale deeply from the abdomen. They should try to inhale slowly through their nose and bring their shoulders back slightly during inhalation.

A slow inhalation should take at least 5 seconds. Then have them exhale for 5 seconds *slowly* through the mouth. Have the students try this two or three times in class. Tell them to teach it to their parents if they like. **NOTE:** For this activity you may want to consider playing soft music, darkening the room, and having the children close their eyes and get comfortable. This will help the students relax. You could suggest that they try this type of relaxation at home if it is not possible at school.

EVALUATION: "What I Can Do When I'm Angry?"

Ask the students to look at the worksheet, *It Really Makes Me Angry . . .* , completed at the beginning of these activities. For each statement about what makes them mad, the students should write at least one acceptable way to deal with their negative emotions. Encourage them to use those behaviors when the anger-producing situations arise again.

MATERIALS

Worksheet: *It Really Makes Me Angry . . .* (completed earlier) (see Figure 10-3)

FIGURE 10-3

Worksheet   Name _____

It Really Makes Me Angry

1. When _____

_____

_____

_____

_____

2. When_____

_____

_____

_____

_____

3. When_____

_____

_____

_____

_____

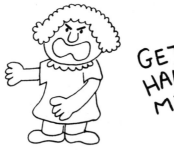

GET YOUR HANDS OFF MY STUFF!!

FIGURE 10-4

Worksheet   Name _____

Ways to Deal with Anger

Part I

1. Susan has a new dress. She wore it to school for the first time on Monday.
   When she went to the cafeteria, one of the boys accidently squirted catsup
   on the dress. She grabbed the catsup bottle and squirted catsup all over his
   shirt.

   ACCEPTABLE   UNACCEPTABLE

2. Mary was working hard in her garden. She had just planted new seedlings.
   She had several neat rows of vegetables. Suddenly, Joe's large dog saw a cat
   and ran through the new garden. The seedlings were mashed but not too
   damaged. She shouted, "Oh, no!" and took a long walk around the block.
   When she came back from her walk, she asked Joe to help her replant the
   seedlings.

   ACCEPTABLE   UNACCEPTABLE

3. Rena was skating down the sidewalk. She hit a little pebble on the sidewalk
   and fell down. She got up and started to swear at the pebble. She picked up
   the pebble and threw it as hard as she could. She was so mad that she did
   not even look to see where the pebble landed.

   ACCEPTABLE   UNACCEPTABLE

4. Ken came home from school to find that his little brother Patrick had been
   looking through his closet again. He went downstairs and told Pat in a firm
   voice, "Please stay out of my closet." Then he went outside to play a hard
   game of touch football.

   ACCEPTABLE   UNACCEPTABLE

Part II

Myrna studied hard for the mathematics test. She took her book home every
day for 2 weeks. She had her brother quiz her on fractions. On the day of the
test, Sam looked over her shoulder and copied her answers. The teacher graded
the tests as the students finished them. Myrna did well, but Sam did the best in
the class. Myrna was very angry. When she got out of class, she went over to
Sam and gave him a good punch.
*Was Myrna's behavior acceptable? What other ways could Myrna have handled
this situation and dealt with her anger?*

FIGURE 10-5

Worksheet

Name _____

Dealing With My Angry Feelings

Unacceptable
★ ★ ★ ★

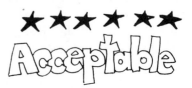

★ ★ ★ ★ ★ ★ ★

Acceptable

OBJECTIVE: The student identifies constructive ways to manage stress.

LEVEL: Grades 6 to 8

VOCABULARY: Stress, coping, adrenaline, conflict

CONTENT GENERALIZATIONS: Stress is a normal part of life. It is an outcome of both physical and mental tension. Stress occurs during the more serious parts of life such as death of a loved one or the divorce of parents, but it is not necessarily all bad. Sometimes stress can help us perform better in the face of a challenge. It is important that we learn what situations in our own lives produce stress and how we react in those situations. Successfully coping with stressful situations contributes to both mental and physical health.

MATERIALS
Dictionaries

INITIATION: Stress—What Does It Feel Like?
Write the word *stress* on the board. Tell the students that we will be spending some time talking about stress. Ask them to look up the word in a dictionary and write a definition of it in their own words. Inform them that this is to be a quiet activity.

While the students are concentrating on their work, set up one of the following situations to produce "stress" in their lives at that moment. Two options are suggested:

1. Walk to the back of the classroom. Make certain that no one is looking, then make a sudden loud noise by slamming a door or dropping tin cans or books on the floor. Practice ahead of time with several items to see what makes a good loud noise.
2. Announce to the class that a very important test will be given the next day. It will

be several pages long and involve at least two essay questions that will have to be a full written page in length.

Tell the students of your hoax. Then ask what physical feelings they experienced. Write them on the board. Such reactions will include fear, pumping heart, butterflies in stomach, and anger at teacher. Tell the students that they have just experienced a stressful situation and that the reactions they are describing are normal responses to stress.

ACTIVITIES

1. Cope With Stress
Using a transparency and worksheet, explain various ways to deal with stress. Hand out the worksheet, *Stress—Don't Let It Get You Down*. Tell the students to write the various ways to deal with stress on their worksheets as they are explained in class. Use the transparency, *Cope With Stress*, as an aid in the brief lecture.

MATERIALS
Worksheet: *Stress—Don't Let It Get You Down* (Figure 10-6)
Transparency: *Cope with Stress* (Figure 10-7)
Overhead projector

After explaining each of these coping strategies, ask students if they can think of any others. Tell them to go home and ask parents and other adults how they cope with stressful situations. They should record ideas on their worksheets as they are discovered.

2. Stress—Don't Let It Get You Down
Allow students to work in pairs to complete this activity. Explain that you will be telling them about two stressful situations. Each pair of students should discuss ways to deal with stress in that particular situation and either draw or write a suggested course of action. It may be helpful to the students to write the situations on a transparency and project them on the screen while they are working.

MATERIALS

Worksheet: *Stress—Don't Let It Get You Down* (partially completed by students) (see Figure 10-6)

Blank transparency

Transparency pen

Overhead projector

SITUATION A

Andrea had a large report due in her social studies class. She was so nervous about the report that she did not play after school or watch television. She forced herself to work instead, but she just sat in her room staring at her books. She had butterflies in her stomach and was having a hard time sleeping. What could she do?

SITUATION B

Stevie's friend Dave was having a party. Everyone important would be there, but Stevie did not get an invitation. When he thought about it, his heart started pounding. He knew that he should never have loaned his favorite record to Dave. What can he do?

When the students are finished, ask each pair what suggestions they have for Andrea and Stevie.

3. Stress Test

Hand out the worksheet, *Stress Test*, and allow the students to chart their personal reaction to various potentially stressful situations. Emphasize that stress is a normal part of life. (There is no correct answer for this test. It is designed to help them see how stressful their life is and to see what situations cause the most stress.) Then ask the students to brainstorm other potentially stressful situations. Choose a few to discuss in class.

MATERIALS

Worksheet: *Stress Test* (Figure 10-8)

EVALUATION: Dealing With Stress

Hand out plain paper to the students. Have them divide the paper into four equal sections. Use the eight situations in the *Stress Test*, or make up eight new ones for this evaluation. Ask students to identify a way to deal with each stressful situation. They can either draw or write about a coping strategy for each situation. Tell them that they may choose to use a strategy more than once. It is important, however, that they identify an acceptable coping strategy they would personally use.

An option is to have the students use two pieces of paper, putting four drawings on each piece. Then they can cut out the drawings and staple them together in a booklet. They should put a title page on the booklet, such as "Dealing With Stress," and take it home to their parents.

MATERIALS

Plain paper

Felt pens, crayons or colored pencils

FIGURE 10-6

Worksheet   Name _____

Stress—Don't Let It Get You Down

Part I   Fill in ways to deal with stress below as they are discussed in class:

1. _____   6. _____
2. _____   7. _____
3. _____   8. _____
4. _____   9. _____
5. _____   10. _____

Part II   Draw or write a way to deal with the stressful situations explained in class.

SITUATION A	SITUATION B

FIGURE 10-7

Transparency master Name ______________________

Cope with Stress

Cope With Stress

1. Get some physical activity.
2. Talk things out.
3. Take things one at a time.
4. Don't try to win every time.
5. Balance play with work.
6. Take a break for yourself.

FIGURE 10-8

Worksheet   Name _____

Stress Test

Directions: Read each situation. Give yourself a stress score for each situation
based on the way you think you would react to that particular situation.

1. You just found out that there is a "pop" quiz   A   B   C   D   E
   in mathematics class.

2. Your favorite record got scratched.   A   B   C   D   E

3. You see the girl or boy you like talking to   A   B   C   D   E
   someone else.

4. You have to give an oral report in social   A   B   C   D   E
   studies tomorrow.

5. Your team in physical education is tied for   A   B   C   D   E
   first place, and the play-offs are today after
   school.

6. Your English teacher says he or she would   A   B   C   D   E
   like to speak with you after class.

7. Just as you hear your mother's car drive up,   A   B   C   D   E
   you remember that you are supposed to
   sweep the porch.

8. You walk into the house after going to the   A   B   C   D   E
   movies and hear arguing.

To find out your stress score, complete the following:

How many As did you circle? _____ Multiply by 1 = _____

How many Bs did you circle? _____ Multiply by 2 = _____

How many Cs did you circle? _____ Multiply by 3 = _____

How many Ds did you circle? _____ Multiply by 4 = _____

How many Es did you circle? _____ Multiply by 5 = _____

TOTAL SCORE

40 to 33   Your life is extremely stressful.

25 to 32   Your life is very stressful.

17 to 24   Your life is moderately stressful.

 9 to 16   Your life is not very stressful.

Under 9   Your life must be pretty boring.

IF YOU WISH: On the back of this paper list items that are stressful to
               you personally.

11 Family Life

When you finish this chapter, you should be able to:

- Define the diversity of family and family living.
- Describe sexuality, reproduction and birth.
- Explain the complexity of sexual victimization.
- Analyze the effects of behavior on prenatal health.
- Develop learning opportunities for elementary and middle school students in the area of family life.

Family living in some form is a necessity in all societies to ensure physical, economic, and emotional well-being. Shelter, food, safety, protection, love, a sense of self-worth, and socialization and education are some of the specific life needs that families help provide.

Many different family structures occur throughout the world. Family structures, from nuclear to extended and childless to single-parent, fulfill the individual needs of a specific population. As our society becomes increasingly complex and varied, it is all the more important to recognize and accept a wide range of types of family structures.

WHAT IS A FAMILY?

Family is a term used to describe a group of two or more persons who are related by blood, marriage, or adoption who reside together. A *nuclear* *family* is composed of members who usually live together; they are dependent on one another economically; and they are usually self-sufficient.

An *extended family* includes the members of a nuclear family along with other family members—most commonly grandparents, aunts, uncles, or cousins. Extended families traditionally live under the same roof, in a family compound, or in geographical proximity to one another. A small number of people form extended families by having more than one wife or husband. Within their societies this is normal and acceptable practice.

Single-parent families headed by a mother or a father are common in the United States today. A couple may have chosen to live separately or divorce, or an unmarried woman may choose to have children and live separately from the father of the child. *Blended families* are becoming more common in our society; these join two single parents (or a single person and a single parent) and create a family with stepparents, stepchildren, and stepbrothers or sisters.

Many people are choosing to live together or marry without having children (establishing a *childless family*). Reasons for this choice include concern with overpopulation, financial interests, inability to reproduce, and joint pursuit of careers.

More and more people are choosing to live alone or remain *single* rather than marry or live with someone. While this category does not fit a strict definition of a family, it is an important category to consider when looking at the overall structure of families in our society.

SEXUALITY AND REPRODUCTIVE SYSTEMS

Our sexuality is an important part of our being, affecting the way in which we interact with the world and plan for our life goals, relationships, reproductivity, and role in society. Sexuality has biological, emotional, psychosocial, and cultural dimensions. Biological changes related to sexuality include the onset of puberty and development of sexual maturity, changes associated with pregnancy and birth, and changes related to the aging process.

All of these changes require emotional and social adjustments. For example, it is common for adolescents to experience depression, confusion, and sometimes loneliness and isolation. The high rate of teenage suicide can be related to this difficult emotional time.

Sexual intimacy can be one of the most stressful areas of life for many young adults. Being comfortable with your sexuality involves acting on the basis of your core values. Because sexuality includes interacting with other people, developing social skills is critical.

Reproductive Systems

The reproductive system enables humans to reproduce. Not only are the male and female external reproductive organs (genitals) different,

but internally the organs are different, too. Figure 11-1 identifies the structures that make up the male's reproductive organs. The two testes, or testicles, are the main sex organs (gonads) in the male. In the mature male, testes produce millions of sex cells called sperm. Sperm production requires temperatures that are cooler than normal body temperature; the testes are located in a pouch called the scrotum that hangs outside the body. There are many other male organs associated with reproduction. The penis, prostate, and seminal vesicles are unique to males. The prostate and seminal vesicles produce nourishing and protective fluids that are added to sperm when the male achieves the highest level of sexual arousal, ejaculation. At that time, muscular contractions forcibly move sperm from the storage area in the testicles and out of the penis. Along the way, the fluids from prostate and other glands are added. The mixture is called semen. In the fertile male, over 200 to 500 million sperm are ejaculated at a time.

The urinary system and reproductive system of the male are related. The penis is composed of columns of spongy tissue. It contains the urethra, which serves as a passageway for sperm to leave the body. Urine is also eliminated through the urethra. During sexual arousal, the spongy tissue fills with blood, stiffening the penis and lengthening it (erection). The organ can then be inserted into a female for reproductive purposes. No urine can be eliminated while the penis is erect. Before ejaculation, a few drops of fluid are secreted into the urethra from the Cowper's glands. This fluid neutralizes any acid from urine that may be present in the urethra. Acid kills sperm so this neutralization process is an important step in preparing the urethra for ejaculation.

The female's reproductive organs are primarily on the inside of her body (Figure 11-2). The two ovaries contain the female sex cells called eggs. The uterus is a muscular and hollow organ that used to be called "the womb." The uterus looks like an upside down pear. On either side attached to the top part of the uterus are thin structures called fallopian or uterine tubes. The

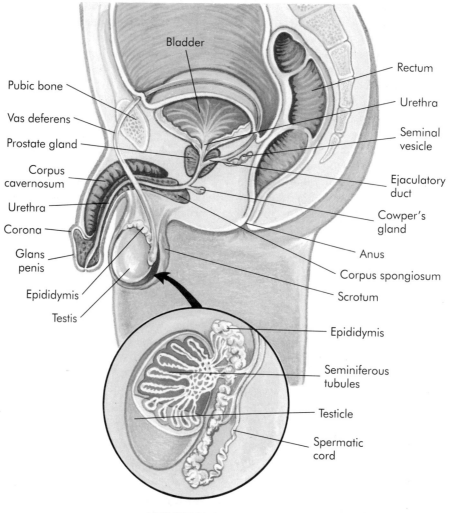

FIGURE 11-1
Male Reproductive System.

smaller part of the uterus is called the cervix. The cervix is attached to a sleevelike structure called the vagina ("birth canal"). The vagina holds the erect penis during the sex act. During the natural birth process, the baby passes through the vagina on its way to the outside world. Later in this chapter, you will read more about pregnancy and parenting.

Each month, the inside wall of the uterus thickens with a rich blood supply in preparation for pregnancy. If pregnancy does not occur, the uterine lining breaks down and is shed through the vagina, a process called menstruation. This occurs due to hormonal cycling that eventually stops (menopause) by the time the woman is in her fifties. In males, sperm production occurs daily from about the age of 15 into old age.

The ovaries and testicles are also considered members of the endocrine, as well as reproductive system. Ovaries produce the hormones, es-

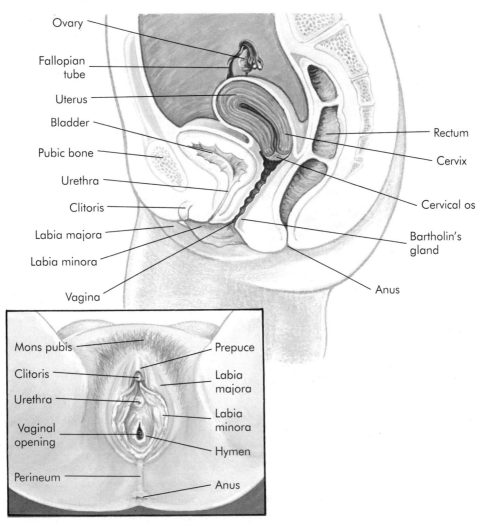

FIGURE 11-2
Female Reproductive System.

trogen and progesterone; testicles produce testosterone. These hormones play important roles in sexual development and behavior.

Puberty

Puberty involves an important series of events in the growth and development of an individual. It is the period when girls and boys sexually mature into young women and men who are able to have children of their own. Stimulated by hormones—estrogen in girls and testosterone in boys—the secondary sexual characteristics for males and females emerge. Both sexes experience a growth spurt, thickening of the skin, a new interest in the opposite sex, and growth of pubic and other body hair. The amount of body hair that develops is largely inherited.

Breast development, widening of the hips, and menarche (the onset of menstruation) are significant physical changes that occur for girls.

Boys grow more muscular, their voices get deeper, and they begin to experience nocturnal emissions, or "wet dreams," which are releases of semen during sleep. It is important that adolescents realize that they will develop and mature at their own rate; there is no right time for puberty to begin, since everyone is different.

For instance, while the average age at menarche is 13, a particular girl's development may vary from this average by two years in either direction. During the past 160 years the average age at menarche has dropped considerably; in the 1830s the average age was 17 years. It is thought that improvements in nutrition and health care may be responsible for this change.

Around the time of menarche the ovaries begin to produce mature eggs, and a girl is then capable of becoming pregnant. During adolescence, both boys and girls develop oilier skin, often resulting in the development of acne, and their body odors become stronger. They are also likely to experience rapid but uneven growth in different parts of their bodies. Because of these rapid physical changes, many young people feel awkward, self-conscious, or confused.

Confusion in the social realm may also result, since a person going through puberty is no longer a child but is not yet an adult. In many societies this transition from childhood to adulthood is marked by "puberty rites," or rites of passage. Through these rites, boys and girls gain adult status by participating in symbolic initiation ceremonies. In our society, high school graduation ceremonies and some religious rituals such as the Jewish Bar Mitzvah (for boys) or Bat Mitzvah (for girls) and the confirmation ceremonies of some Christian denominations serve a similar function.

Gender Identity

Gender identity is a person's sense of being male or female. Developing one's gender identity as a child and young adult is considered to be a crucial step in the development of an adult self-image and adult identity. Research indicates that gender identity is largely learned through the adoption of socially approved sex roles. As people get older, their views of what constitutes appropriate behavior for men and women may change.

Gender Stereotypes and Changing Sex Roles. In recent years, there has been an increased awareness of some gender stereotypes and their negative effects. For example, activities formerly limited to boys, such as Little League baseball, are now open to girls, and more girls and women are participating in competitive sports. Many women now choose careers previously considered closed to them, such as law, medicine, and business. Similarly, men have some traditionally feminine careers, such as nursing, open to them, and it is generally more acceptable for men to take a primary role in child rearing and homemaking activities—although such roles are far from the norm. Research suggests that people who assume a lifestyle with less rigidly defined sex roles are more flexible, have higher self-esteem, and demonstrate more social skills and motivation to achieve.

Despite social and cultural changes that break down some gender stereotypes in American society, discrepancies still exist. For instance, in general, women's salaries are not yet equal to men's, and many jobs still have a "glass ceiling" preventing women from adequate representation at the upper levels of authority. As another example, the enduring popularity of Barbie dolls among young girls for the past 30 years attests to the continued strength of many gender-based stereotypes formed early in life.

Transsexuality. A psychological gender identity in opposition to a person's biological sex is called transsexuality. Most transsexuals are men who feel that they are "trapped" in a man's body and believe that they should be women. While the cause of transsexualism is unknown, it is thought to be related to a hormone imbalance during prenatal and early childhood development, as well as a strong identification with the opposite sex during childhood. Some transsexuals undergo reconstructive surgery, or sex change operations, to refashion their sex organs to match their gender identity.

Sexual Orientation. Sexual orientation refers to the way in which people express their sexuality. Heterosexuality is sexual attraction to and activity with members of the opposite sex. This is the most common sexual orientation. Bisexuality, which is attraction to and activity with persons of both sexes, and homosexuality, which is attraction to and activity with persons of one's own sex, are less common. The term *gay* is used to describe both male and female homosexuals; homosexual women are also called *lesbians.*

Why some people are attracted to the opposite and some to the same sex is not known. Both biological and environmental factors are thought to influence sexual orientation, which is developed early in life and is probably impossible to change. Studies have also demonstrated that there is a wide range of normal human sexual behavior, and no one orientation should be considered to be more "normal" than the others.

Many teenagers experiment with both homosexual and heterosexual experiences, and these experiences do not necessarily predict adult sexual orientation. Because of myths about homosexuality and the lingering attitude that it is "wrong," homosexuals still experience many forms of discrimination and are becoming increasingly politicized as a result. While the extent of homosexuality in our society is unclear, recent estimates are that about 3% to 10% of Americans are homosexual and up to 50% have experimented with homosexual activity.

DATING AND MATE SELECTION

Dating allows persons to interact and become better acquainted with one another. It also provides an opportunity to learn how to make conversation and to share feelings and opinions. Your definition of an ideal date may change from one month to the next as you experience dating with people who have a variety of different traits.

What factors bring people to be attracted to one another? Several factors seem to be at work in this process. First is *homogamy:* similarities in age, ethnic and familial background, educational goals, and possibly religious preference. *Physical proximity*, or closeness in terms of places of residence, employment, and recreation, is another important factor. Long-distance relationships are difficult to maintain.

Sometimes people are drawn to those with *complementary* characteristics—for instance, a quiet man may be attracted to an outgoing woman who makes him more sociable; a woman may seek him as a partner for the balance he provides to her gregariousness. These are people whose needs are different from one another's.

Others are attracted by *compatible* needs—needs that are the same as one another's. Although we like to say that "opposites attract," it is those with compatible needs whose attraction tends to be the strongest.

Dating provides an opportunity to explore sexual identity. This is why it is not unusual for adolescents to choose a date by appearance alone. Sexual attraction may bring couples together where they may discover commonalities or may break up after the initial attraction cools. It is often difficult to sort out emotional feelings from sexual desires, but eventually each person must make decisions about sexual behavior in relationships. The first step in making a responsible decision is respecting your own sexual values and those of your partner.

Payne and Hahn propose a three-stage, dating-mate selection model to describe the process of selecting a partner:

- *Stage 1: Marketing:* Both you and the new person you've met construct an "ideal" image of yourselves to transmit to each other. Infatuation, an intense and often shallow attraction, may be strong during this stage. For most, this stage is relatively short.
- *Stage 2: Sharing:* Partners have discovered a compatibility and wish to explore underlying beliefs and feelings beyond what is

"marketed" in Stage 1. This stage can be observed as "steady dating" with movement toward permanence.

- *Stage 3: Behavior:* In this stage you determine whether your behaviors are consistent with the values and beliefs you shared in Stage 2. This involves a maturing process that results in mutual commitment.

CHOICES FOR FAMILY LIVING

Marriage

Marriage is a basic social institution that functions as the basis of the traditional family unit. In marriage, two people make a formal and public commitment to share their lives as intimate partners. For most people (though not for all), marriage provides the most acceptable framework for parenthood. It also helps people fulfill other emotional and material needs. Alternatives to traditional married life are also becoming more common and more socially acceptable.

During the past 20 to 30 years there have been significant changes in our attitudes toward marriage. Recent trends show that most adults in American society are or have been married; approximately 80 percent of adults age 18 and older are married, widowed or divorced. A relatively recent change is the age at first marriage. Now the average age at first marriage for men is almost 26 years. Women are also waiting longer to get married and tend to be more educated and career oriented. The average age at first marriage for women is nearly 24 years.

Alternatives to Marriage

Many people are choosing other alternatives to marriage. Increasing numbers of people are now remaining unmarried or are choosing not to remarry after a divorce. Living together, or *cohabitation*, has become more common, particularly for people ages 25 to 44 years; according to the U.S. Census, in 1989 almost 1.7 million unmarried couples in this age group were living together.

Some gay and lesbian couples who live together decide to formalize their commitment through marriage ceremonies, even though these marriages are not legally recognized. (This denial of legal status is now being challenged in some states—notably Hawaii.)

Divorce

Almost half of all marriages end in divorce. The rate of divorce has steadily increased over the past two decades, although since the late 1980s there appears to be a decline. Marriage experts do not have a clear answer to the question of why divorce is so common in our society. They suggest that, in part, it is a reflection of unfulfilled expectations of marriage on the part of one or both partners. Some experts propose that it is unrealistic to expect a marriage to remain the same over time and that to be successful a marriage should be viewed as a continually evolving process. Suggested guidelines for "reinventing" a marriage so that it can stay current follow:

- Remember that people can unlearn behaviors that no longer work or are self-defeating.
- Eliminate judgmental labeling of one another.
- Make a conscious attempt to be kinder to one another.
- Don't try to read a partner's mind or make assumptions about what he or she is thinking.
- Learn to identify the underlying meanings of expressed emotions.
- Cultivate the art of receptive noticing.
- Practice forgiveness; allow for fresh starts.
- Cultivate a you-never-know attitude; you may be pleasantly surprised!
- If needed, seek out a good marriage counselor.

SEXUAL VICTIMIZATION—STRATEGIES FOR PREVENTION

While sexual intimacy ideally is a mutual form of communication between two people, it is sometimes approached as an aggressive, hostile behavior directed toward a victim. This is the case with rape and sexual assault, sexual harassment, and the sexual abuse of children.

Rape and Sexual Assault

Rape is forced sexual contact, including sexual intercourse, oral sex, or anal sex. Women are the most common victims of rape, although men and children also are sometimes raped. While it is popularly believed that rapists are strangers who attack women, the reality is that more than half of all rapists know the people they attack, and about one third of all rapes occur on dates *(date rape)*. Most rapes occur in the victim's home. It is now recognized that rapists are not motivated by sexual desire but by the need to exert power and control using violent means.

People at greatest risk of being raped include women between the ages of 18 and 25, poor people, and blacks. The risks can be reduced by learning to recognize potentially dangerous situations and by being especially cautious.

Many people believe that date or *acquaintance rape* is a result of miscommunication about sex between men and women. Sometimes men believe that women say no to sex when they really mean maybe or yes; and sometimes women believe that they are expected to say no at first, even when they intend to have sex with a partner. There are some things that you can do to avoid getting into a sexual situation that could lead to acquaintance rape. For men, some guidelines are:

- Know your sexual desires and limits.
- Communicate those desires and limits clearly.
- Don't assume that a woman wants to have sex because of the way she is dressed, because she is friendly, or because she has been drinking.
- Listen to what a woman says. Assume that she means what she says and accept her sexual limits.
- Don't think that rejection of sex means rejection of you as a person.

- Avoid excessive alcohol and drug use. In most acquaintance rape cases, both the rapist and the victim had been drinking and/or using drugs.

Some guidelines for women follow:
- Know your sexual desires and limits.
- Communicate these clearly. Say what you mean and mean what you say.
- If you feel uncomfortable in a situation, pay attention to this feeling.
- Be alert for any warning signs of aggression or lack of respect for women.
- Avoid excessive alcohol and drug use.

If you are in a situation where you are at immediate risk of being raped, the following are strategies to use that may help:
- Try to stay calm; it will be easier to think clearly.
- Be assertive; pleading and crying are not likely to help.
- Use active resistance if possible—fighting, screaming, or running away.
- Use passive resistance—say that you have a sexually transmitted disease, such as herpes or AIDS.
- Trust your intuition about the situation you are in. Sometimes submission is necessary to avoid more serious injury.

It is estimated that fewer than 10% of all rapes are reported. Nearly all rape victims experience anger as well as some embarrassment, fear, depression, humiliation and guilt. The important thing is not to blame oneself for being the victim of a crime. It is essential to seek help from someone who can provide support.

If you have been raped, it is also important to seek medical help. You may be at risk for sexually transmitted diseases and pregnancy. In addition, medical evidence will be needed if you decide to press charges against the rapist. Help from people trained to assist rape victims is available from counselors at women's centers or sexual assault centers, from rape hotlines, from emergency room staff, and from the police (who now often use specially trained officers, many of whom are women).

Sexual Harassment

Sexual harassment includes any unwelcome sexual advances, requests for sexual favors, or other verbal or physical conduct of a sexual nature, especially when the behavior comes from someone with obvious power over you. The person might be an employer, a supervisor, or a teacher. Others, such as coworkers or fellow students, can also be guilty of sexual harassment.

Most victims of sexual harassment are women. Many women do not report sexual harassment, for a variety of reasons. A woman may not be aware that she has the right to report it, or she may be afraid of losing her job or getting a bad grade. She may also worry that no one will believe her if she does report it. Some employers and schools have a policy against sexual harassment, although many still do not.

Some steps to take if you believe that you are a victim of sexual harassment are:

1. Seek support from someone you trust.
2. Say no to the harassment.
3. Find out if others also have been harassed and might be willing to come forward to confront the person, as well.
4. Keep written records, including dates and exact events.
5. Find out if sexual harassment policies and procedures are in place. Sexual harassment is a form of illegal sex discrimination, violating Title VII of the Civil Rights Law of 1964.

At places of employment, you can report sexual harassment to the personnel office. In school or college settings, seek help from the counseling center, guidance office or affirmative action office. Realistically, there may be some risks to reporting. Whether or not to do so is up to the person who is harassed. But this problem will only begin to be solved when more women become aware of it and report it when it happens.

Child Sexual Abuse

Sadly, children are especially vulnerable to sexual abuse because of their dependent relationships with adults, including parents, relatives and caregivers. Child sexual abuse is sexual contact or activity between a child and an adult.

Child sexual abuse may often go unreported, making accurate statistics impossible to gather. Of the cases that are reported, over 90% of abusers are not strangers but rather persons known to children. Almost half are members of the child's family. One out of 5 girls and 1 out of 11 boys experience some form of sexual abuse before the age of 18. The peak age for abuse is between 8 to 12 years, although children under age 5 are also at high risk for being abused.

While abusers may use physical force, they are more likely to be a trusted friend or relative who bribes, tricks, or threatens the child to participate and remain silent about the incidents. Children can learn to protect themselves by learning the following:

- To identify good, bad, and confusing touch according to how they feel about it
- To trust their intuition
- To say no to adults
- That they "own" their own bodies
- That secrets between adults and children aren't always appropriate, especially if they are confusing
- To tell someone if they feel bothered, bad, or confused

BECOMING A PARENT
Conception and Pregnancy

Pregnancy begins with two cells: a sperm cell from the male and an egg cell, or ovum, from the female. These two cells come together inside the uterus after millions of sperm cells are deposited inside the vagina during sexual intercourse. While each ejaculation contains only about a teaspoon of semen, this small quantity holds between 200 and 500 million sperm cells.

In the fertilization process, a sperm penetrates an ovum and the two cells merge into one, creating a fertilized egg called a zygote. Since a woman ovulates about once every 28 days, ovum and sperm are not always present at the same time. If either are not present, fertilization or conception cannot occur. However, fertilization can result from intercourse that occurs almost any time during a woman's menstrual cycle. This is because of unpredictable month-to-month variation in the timing of ovulation and because sperm can remain alive in a woman's body for 5 days or longer.

Individually the ovum and sperm each hold 23 chromosomes containing thousands of genes. These genes transmit hereditary characteristics from the parent to the child. When the ovum and sperm merge, the two sets of chromosomes combine to form the full set of 46 chromosomes required by human beings. As a result, children inherit characteristics from both parents. This genetic material determines such traits as sex; eye, hair and skin color; body type; facial features; and, in part, mental ability and personality.

Multiple births, such as twins, occur if two or more eggs are released into the fallopian tube and fertilized by different sperm or if one fertilized egg splits to form two or more zygotes. If the latter process occurs, the children will be identical because they are inheriting the same genetic material.

As the zygote travels to the uterus and implants in the uterine wall, it becomes a blastocyst and then an embryo as the cells divide and multiply. The embryo begins to look somewhat like a tiny human. After the twelfth week it is called a fetus (although some call it a fetus at all stages of development). Early in pregnancy the outer layer of cells develops into the placenta, which provides the embryo and fetus with nourishment from the mother's blood supply.

The placenta is a large organ containing many blood vessels that is attached to the wall of the uterus. Through the placenta, nutrients and oxygen are provided to the embryo and fetus, and waste products are taken away. Drugs, including nicotine, alcohol, and caffeine, also can pass through the placenta to the developing embryo and fetus.

Pregnancy lasts approximately 40 weeks and is usually described according to 3-month intervals, or trimesters. During each trimester, the fetus reaches specific growth and development milestones. Some of these key developments include the following:

First trimester: weeks 1 to 13
- Arms, legs, hands, fingers, feet and face are completely formed.
- Brain and muscles coordinate.
- All internal organs are formed and functioning.
- Fetus is about 2½ inches long and weighs about ⅝ ounce.

Second trimester: weeks 14 to 27
- Facial features are fully developed.
- Fetus can swallow and pass urine.
- Fetus can hear voices, music, and other external sounds.
- Fetus is about 13 inches long and weighs about 1¼ pounds.

Third trimester: weeks 28 to 40
- Lungs mature during this trimester.
- Body begins to plump out.
- Eyes are open and the fetus is aware of light.
- Fetus descends into the pelvis and head engages in preparation for birth.
- Fetus is about 19 to 21 inches long and weighs about 6 to 9 pounds.

Birth

There are three basic stages of birth, when the baby moves out of the mother's uterus through the vagina into the world. In the first stage, contractions begin, and the cervix opens wide enough to allow the baby's head to pass. In the second stage the baby is pushed completely out of the uterus. In the third stage the placenta is expelled from the uterus; this is called the afterbirth.

There can be complications during birth. Sometimes caesarean deliveries (caesarean sections, or C-sections) are necessary; surgery is used to remove the baby from the uterus. Rea-

sons for needing a caesarean section include the
following:

- The fetus is improperly aligned for a vaginal delivery, for example, the head is not positioned to come out first.
- The mother's pelvis is too small.
- The fetus is especially large.
- The fetus shows signs of respiratory or cardiac problems (distress).
- The umbilical cord is compressed.
- The placenta is being delivered before the fetus.
- The mother's health is at risk.

While in 1980 caesarean sections accounted
for 17% of all deliveries, in 1990 they accounted
for 25%. While some experts have questioned the
need for so many C-sections, others believe that
they are justified based on the need criteria listed
above.

Prenatal Health

Because the outcome of a pregnancy is strongly
influenced by the health status of the parents,
particularly the mother, it is important to be
aware of the effect a woman's health habits may
have upon childbearing.

Nutrition. Eating a well-balanced diet is
critical for the development of the unborn baby
and the health of the mother. No vitamin/mineral
supplement can replace the nutrients that a varied diet can provide. It is usually recommended
that the mother gain from 20 to 30 pounds during the course of the pregnancy.

Exercise. Exercise is recommended for the
pregnant woman throughout the pregnancy. As a
general rule, women should engage in the same
activities they enjoyed before becoming pregnant
(swimming, jogging, and playing tennis are examples). As the uterus enlarges, some women
may find vigorous activities to be uncomfortable
and may substitute brisk walking.

Rest. Adequate rest is essential for the pregnant woman. If frequent urination during the
night or other discomforts keep the woman from
getting enough sleep, she may need to nap or
schedule rest periods during the day.

Smoking. Women who smoke during pregnancy increase their risk of having a miscarriage
or delivering a baby who is premature and has
low birth weight. The more cigarettes smoked,
the greater the risks.

Alcohol. When consumed by a pregnant
woman, alcohol passes through the placenta and
into the baby's bloodstream. Children who are
born to mothers who have drunk heavily during
pregnancy are at risk for *fetal alcohol syndrome.*
These babies suffer low birthweight, mental retardation, cardiovascular disorders, and specific
facial characteristics. There is no safe level of alcohol consumption for pregnant women; therefore, health professionals recommend that
women who are pregnant, or are trying to become pregnant, avoid alcohol.

Drugs. Any drug that is taken into the body
of a pregnant woman can affect the baby in some
way. To avoid the risks of birth defects and complications surrounding delivery, drugs should be
avoided unless prescribed by a physician who is
aware of the pregnancy.

Age. The "best" time to have a healthy baby
is between the ages of 25 and 29. Teenage mothers and their babies are at increased risk of physical and psychological problems. Pregnant teens
are more likely to have premature babies and to
have difficult labors. Newborn babies of teenage
mothers are less likely to survive.

Environmental Risks. High levels of radiation and pollutants have been associated with
birth defects. As research continues in this area,
women are advised to be cautious about environmental conditions that constitute hazards to unborn children.

Adoption

Adoption is the legal process allowing a person
who is not a child's biological parent to raise
the child as his or her own. Most adoptive
parents are couples who have not been able to
conceive children of their own. Children may
be adopted when their biological, or birth, parents die or abandon them, or when the parents
decide that they cannot care properly for a child

and decide to give the child up for adoption.

There are several different types of adoption. Adoptions usually occur through adoption agencies which may be public or private. Adoption agencies screen potential adoptive parents and often offer counseling and other help to the birthmother. *Independent or private adoptions* are usually arranged by physicians or lawyers. Sometimes relatives choose to adopt children in *family adoptions.*

Traditionally in American society birth and adoptive parents have chosen *closed adoption,* in which the birth parents and adoptive parents do not meet or learn each other's names. The records are sealed by an adoption agency, and the birth parents have no further contact with the child. In *open adoption,* a more recent development, the birth parents help select the adoptive parents and are able to remain in contact with the adoptive parents and the child, although they still give up their legal rights to the child.

Adoption raises emotional issues for all those involved. Adoptive parents must decide when and what to tell the child about their adoption and their birth parents. Adopted children may have feelings of rejection by their birth parents and may begin to search for them when they grow older. Birthmothers also may experience emotional difficulties with their decision and decide to seek out their children later in life. In some states, adoption registries have been established allowing children, adoptive parents and birth parents to agree to be contacted by one another.

FERTILITY CONTROL

An important issue for many individuals and families is controlling fertility, or *birth control.* Birth control is a broad term referring to all of the procedures you can use to prevent the birth of a child. Birth control includes available contraceptive measures, as well as sterilization, use of the intrauterine device (IUD) to prevent conception, and abortion procedures.

Contraception is a specific term used to describe any procedure used to prevent the fertilization of an ovum. Some examples of contraceptive methods are the use of condoms, oral contraceptives (birth control pills), spermicides, and diaphragms. Other birth control methods are periodic abstinence, withdrawal or coitus interruptus, and subdermal implants (such as Norplant).

Abortion refers to the induced premature termination of a pregnancy. The decision to abort a fetus is a highly controversial and personal issue. On the basis of a landmark U.S. Supreme Court case, *Roe v. Wade,* in 1973 the United States joined many of the world's most populated countries in legalizing abortions within certain guidelines. For the first 3 months of pregnancy, or first trimester, the decision lies with the woman and her doctor. In the second trimester, the state may regulate abortion as it relates to maternal health. In the third trimester, a viable fetus would be considered a live birth and would not be allowed to die.

The political atmosphere in the United States with regard to abortion has been changing, and a woman's right to abortion has been challenged by some. Each year, approximately 1.5 million women decide to terminate a pregnancy through abortion. Almost all (90 percent) are done in the first trimester. The decision to terminate a pregnancy is a highly personal and often emotionally difficult one.

THE LIFE CYCLE

The life cycle extends from birth to death, and the stages are universal and predictable. It can be said that aging begins at conception and continues until death. The stages of the life cycle are as follows:

- Infancy—a time of total dependency.
- Toddler stage—a time of rapid physical and mental changes and growth in independence.
- Early childhood—a time to explore the world and test abilities.
- Middle childhood—a time when greater responsibility and independence are assumed

and typically children develop a sense of accomplishment from being successful in tasks at home and at school.

- Adolescence—the transition from childhood to adulthood, when peers are highly significant and physical sexual maturity is reached.
- Early adulthood—a time to take total responsibility for oneself, to build intimate relationships with friends and perhaps a member of the opposite sex.
- Middle adulthood—typically a time to have a family, to develop a sense of accomplishment with work, and to become a contributing member of a community.
- Later adulthood—a time to relax, often to retire and pursue creative interests that time did not allow previously, such as returning to school, reflecting on one's life, and enjoying grandchildren

Dying and death are a part of the life cycle as well. It is common and normal to fear death and to avoid talking of such a depressing subject. However, most experts believe that the study of death and dying will enhance life and living.

Kubler-Ross (6) observed five stages that terminally ill patients go through—although all persons do not go through all stages, and the stages may not be sequential: *denial* of imminent death, *anger* about dying (often called the "why me?" stage), *bargaining* to buy a little more time, *depression* at the realization of losing all loved ones and mourning one's own loss of life, and *acceptance* of the inevitable.

Death is when all life signs disappear. It has been increasingly difficult to define the exact time of death as medical science improves its abilities to forestall death. The most often agreed on determination of death is a flat electroencephalogram (EEG), which means that no brain waves can be measured.

When death occurs or is imminent, it is essential for family members and friends to grieve. Grief is a human reaction to loss. We grieve not only for the sake of the person who has died, but also for the loss of that person in our life. Just as dying and death are a normal part of life, so are grief, mourning, and coping with the death of friends and family members.

SUMMARY

The focus of this chapter was on a variety of biological, psychosocial and emotional experiences that are a part of family life. Families are shown to come in a wide range of sizes and types—and new types of families, such as those formed by gay and lesbian couples—are also emerging.

Biological, psychosocial, and cultural aspects of sexuality were covered, including the onset of puberty, male and female reproductive systems, gender identity, and sexual orientation. Dating and mate selection were discussed, leading to choices for family living and the variety of choices that people make. The unfortunate reality of sexual victimization of both adults and children was described, along with prevention and coping skills.

Conception, pregnancy, and prenatal health were covered in the section on becoming a parent. Becoming a parent through adoption is another alternative open to those who are unable to conceive children of their own. An important issue for many individuals and families is controlling fertility through a variety of birth control methods.

We briefly discussed stages of the life cycle from birth to death. Learning to cope with death and loss is a necessary part of life, and it is important to grieve when we are faced with these events.

Some classroom activity ideas covering some of these issues follow. They address the specific developmental needs of your primary, intermediate, and middle school level students.

REFERENCES

1. Ashley R: *Human anatomy*, New York, 1976, John Wiley.
2. Clark K: *Adult's guide to Touch Talk!* Santa Cruz, Calif, 1985, ETR Associates.

3. Eshleman JR: *Family, an introduction*, Boston, 1988, Allyn & Bacon.

4. Hiatt J: *Pregnancy facts*, Santa Cruz, Calif, 1989, ETR Associates.

5. Krantzler M, Krantzler P: *The 7 marriages of your marriage*, San Francisco, 1992, Harper San Francisco.

6. Kubler-Ross E: *On death and dying*, New York, 1967, Macmillan.

7. Ogletree R: *Acquaintance rape*, Santa Cruz, Calif, 1993, ETR Associates.

8. Payne W, Hahn D: *Understanding your health*, ed 3, St. Louis, 1992, Mosby.

9. Post J: *Living in a family*, Santa Cruz, Calif, 1989, ETR Associates.

10. *Pregnancy basics*, Bethesda, Md, National Institute of Child Health and Human Development.

11. *Sexuality and reproduction*, Macmillan Health Encyclopedia, vol 6, New York, 1993, Macmillan.

LEARNING OPPORTUNITIES FOR FAMILY LIFE

GENERAL STUDENT OBJECTIVES

Primary level K-3

The student:
1. Defines the meaning of family.
2. Identifies responsibilities and privileges of various family members.
3. Describes ways family membership changes.*
4. Explains that all living things come from other living things.

Intermediate Level 4-5/6

The student:
1. Proposes constructive ways to solve conflicts with friends and family.
2. Interprets changes in social activities as family members mature.
3. Describes the progression of the individual through the life cycle from birth to death.
4. Identifies growth and developmental characteristics common in puberty*

Middle School Level 6/7-8

The student:
1. Predicts physical, emotional, and social changes that occur during adolescence.
2. Explains why growth and development is individual, although predictable.
3. Describes the reproductive processes.*
4. Identifies social and cultural factors in the development of responsible health behavior.

*These objectives are illustrated by sample learning opportunities.

PRIMARY LEVEL

OBJECTIVE: The student explains ways family membership changes.

LEVEL: Grades 2 and 3

INTEGRATION: Mathematics, social studies, creative writing, art

VOCABULARY: Family, increase, decrease

CONTENT GENERALIZATIONS: The membership of different families is varied, and the composition of an individual family is dynamic. Family membership can involve many combinations of people, such as mother, father, siblings, uncles, aunts, grandparents, and cousins. Many people consider pets to be family members too. The membership in any one family can grow from one to many members. The changes in the family are usually a result of marriage, birth, death, and divorce. Moving from one location to another also can affect family membership.

INITIATION: "Family Portrait"

Ask the students, "What is a family?" After they have given their responses, explain that we are all part of a family and everyone's family is different. Hand out the worksheet, *Family Portrait*, and ask the students to draw their family. (Some children will include pets.) Tell them to count the number of persons (and pets) in their family.

Ask the students if this number was always the same for their family, and if not, why it was different. (My little sister was born. My grandfather died. My parents got divorced. My mother remarried, and now I have a father and a stepfather.)

MATERIALS
Worksheet: *Family Portrait* (Figure 11-3)
Crayons

ACTIVITIES

1. Our Families

a. Construct a bulletin board display, *Our Families*.

- Mount a class picture, individual school pictures, or both on a bulletin board.
- Have the students mount their completed worksheets, *Family Portrait*, randomly around the class picture.
- Instruct them to draw, color, and cut out the same number as there are family members i 'eir picture. When finished, they shoula 'nt their number next to the family por. .s.
- Help the students connect a string from their picture in the class picture to their family portrait.

b. When finished with the bulletin board, ask the students to count and record on a piece of paper the number of families with two members, three members, four members, and so forth. Then ask which number was the most common and which was the least common. Finally, explain to the students that all families are unique and that there is no "right" number of members in a family.

MATERIALS
Class picture or individual school pictures
Worksheet: *Family Portrait* (completed) (see Figure 11-3) or actual family photographs brought from home
Scissors
Crayons
String

2. The Story of Two Families

a. Tell the students they are going to meet two families: the Red Family and the Blue Family. Prepare a flannel board with the two families side by side as follows:

Red Family   **Blue Family**
(mount pictures here)

b. Read or present a story such as the following to the students. Have a student put pictures of the characters and their names on the flannel board as they are introduced and remove them as they leave.

TWO FAMILIES

I'd like you to meet two families: the Red Family and the Blue Family. The Red Family is composed of Grandma Red and Rick, who lives with his Grandma. The Blue Family is composed of Father Blue, Mother Blue, and their daughter Beverly. How many people are in each family? [Place each number on the board.] Which family has more members? Which has less members? One day Grandma Red received a telephone call from her daughter Dorothy and son-in-law Samuel. Dorothy and Samuel were moving to Grandma's town, where they have jobs. Grandma says, "Come live with Rick and me in our house. Join our family. We have plenty of room." So Samuel and Dorothy moved in with Grandma and Rick. The Blue Family changed too. Mother Blue was pregnant—she was going to have a baby. One day Mother and Father Blue went to the hospital. When they returned home, they introduced Beverly to her new baby brother. Now how many are in each family? Which family has more members? Which has fewer members? [Change the numbers on the board.] Grandma Red got another telephone call. One of her oldest friends, Mrs. Lettie Yellow, said that her husband Mr. Yellow had died. Lettie Yellow said she did not like living by herself. Grandma Red said, "Come over and live with us. We have plenty of room." So her friend, Lettie Yellow, moved in too. How many are now in the Red Family? Which family has more members? Which has fewer? [Change the numbers on the board.]

c. Discussion questions
  ▪ Did the membership of the two families remain the same, increase, or decrease? (Both increased.)
  ▪ In what ways did family membership increase? (Birth, friends moved in, and relatives moved in.)
  ▪ How could family membership decrease? (Someone moves out when grown, to get a job, to go to school, or after getting married; or death.)

MATERIALS
Flannel board
Pictures of family members (cut from magazines or group pictures)
Name signs for family members to mount on flannel board:
  Grandma Red
  Rick Red
  Daughter Dorothy
  Son-in-law Samuel
  Mrs. Yellow
  Mother Blue
  Father Blue
  Beverly Blue
  Baby Blue
  Various numbers to mount on flannel board

3. How the Green Family Changes
Then have the students write their own illustrated story about the Green Family. The Green Family changes from *three* members, to *two* members, and then to *four* members. Have the students draw a picture and write about the members of the Green Family in each stage—3, 2, and 4 members—and how the membership changed. (**NOTE:** Students may do each third of this assignment on three separate days.) Allow them time to tell the class or each other in small groups about their stories.

MATERIALS
Paper
Pencils or crayons

EVALUATION: "Families Change"
Each student should complete the worksheet, *Families Change*, and explain two ways family membership can increase and two ways it can decrease.

MATERIALS
Worksheet: *Families Change* (Figure 11-4)
Pencils

FIGURE 11-3

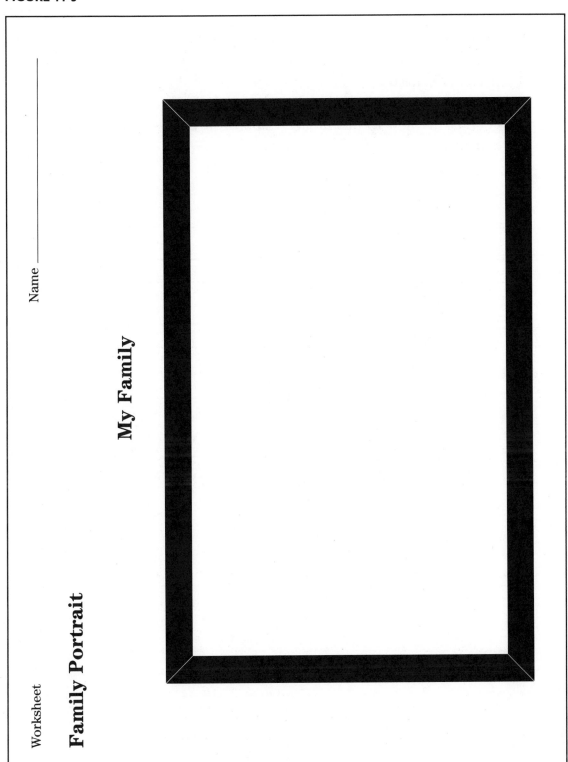

Worksheet

Family Portrait

My Family

Name _____

FIGURE 11-4

Worksheet   Name _____

Families Change

Two people are new to this family. List two ways this *increase* might have happened.

1. _____

- -

_____

2. _____

- -

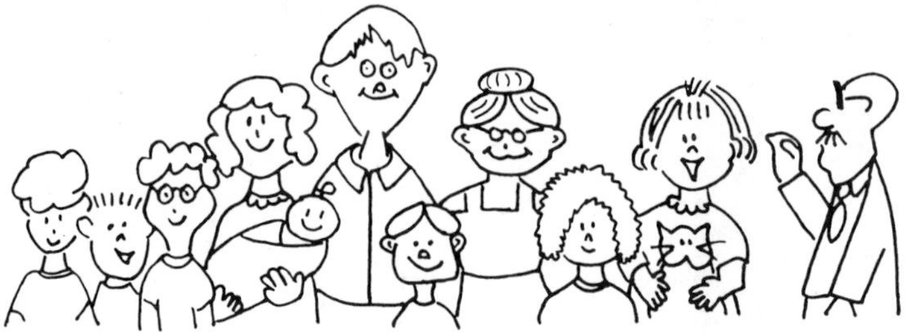

_____

List two ways this family might *decrease*.

1. _____

- -

_____

2. _____

- -

_____

INTERMEDIATE LEVEL

OBJECTIVE: The student identifies growth and developmental characteristics common in puberty.

LEVEL: Grades 4 to 6 (more appropriate for grade 5 or 6)

INTEGRATION: Science

VOCABULARY: Puberty, hormones, menstruation

CONTENT GENERALIZATIONS: As boys and girls mature into men and women, many physical and psychological changes occur. Puberty is when these changes occur, and the result is the capability of sexual reproduction. Although puberty does not commence or end at the same time for each individual, the pattern of change is predictable. Puberty is a slow and gradual process that begins with a signal from the pituitary gland that stimulates the production of sexual hormones. These hormones in turn signal various parts of the male or female body to start growing and changing. Puberty is also a time when boys and girls begin to become more interested in each other. Generally, girls are about 2 years ahead of boys in both the physical and psychological changes of puberty.

NOTE: Before teaching any lessons regarding sexuality, state and local school district guidelines should be studied. It is highly recommended that parental consent forms be sent out with the help and advice of the school principal.

The teaching plan presented here deals primarily with puberty. Depending on the previous exposure of the students to information on reproductive processes, more or fewer activities may be required.

These activities are probably more appropriate for grade 5 or 6 (if grade 6 is housed in the elementary school). These lessons should be taught by a teacher who feels comfortable dealing with this material. It is also important to be sensitive to possible student anxiety and embarrassment.

INITIATION: "My, Have You Changed"
A few days before starting these activities, ask the students to bring in a baby picture of themselves. It should be one that they don't mind others seeing. (The best pictures are of students when they were toddlers rather than infants.)

Put up the bulletin board display, *My, Have You Changed!* Students should give you the picture *without* showing it to anyone else in the class. Allow the students to study the pictures on the bulletin board. Then have them number on their paper from 1 to whatever number of students there are in class. Ask the students to try to match each picture with a student's name. When they are finished listing names corresponding to the numbers next to the baby pictures, have all the students in the class go to the bulletin board and mount a slip of paper printed with their name under their baby picture. Have the students check their lists to see how many baby pictures they were able to identify correctly.

MATERIALS
Bulletin board display: *My, Have You Changed!*
    Slips of paper with each student's name
    Student pictures as babies
    Ask students the following discussion questions:
    1. Were you able to identify all the pictures correctly? Why or why not?
    2. What are some of the ways that most students have changed since the picture was taken? (Taller, heavier, possibly more hair.)
    3. Can you think of any changes that will occur in the next few years?

ACTIVITIES
1. What Is Puberty?
    Conduct a short lecture on puberty. Bring out the following points in the lecture. As each of the words in italics is explained, write it on the board, and have the students write it on a piece of paper for use later.

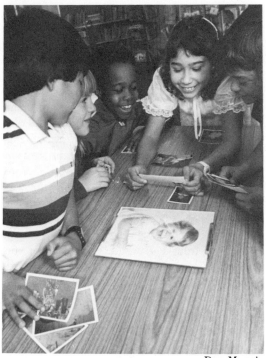

Don Merwin

a. *Puberty* is triggered and regulated by the *endocrine system.*

b. Chemical "messengers" called *hormones* regulate growth and development. They determine when and how you grow and change during puberty.

c. The *pituitary gland* is a part of the endocrine system and is located at the base of the brain. This gland signals the body when puberty is to begin.

d. The pituitary gland signals the female *ovaries* and the male *testes* to start producing hormones.

e. One of the first signs of puberty is the *secondary sexual characteristics.*

1. For the boy:
   ▪ Body hair (face, underarms, legs, pubic area, and possibly chest)
   ▪ Deeper voice
   ▪ Enlargement of penis and testes
   ▪ Production of sperm
   ▪ Broadening of shoulders

2. For the girl:
   ▪ Development of breasts
   ▪ Body hair (underarms, legs, pubic area)
   ▪ Widening of hips

f. Both boys and girls start producing mature sex cells: *sperm* in boys and *ova* in girls. (In girls all the eggs are present and begin to mature and be released at puberty.)

g. An important part of puberty for girls is the onset of *menstruation.* This is a cyclical discharge of blood and *endometrial cells.*

h. The changes that happen during puberty are natural and normal. Everyone will experience these changes at their own rate.

   At the end of the lecture ask if there are any questions. It may be helpful to set up a question box so students can write questions anonymously on slips of paper.

MATERIALS
Paper
Pencils

2. **Steps to Growing Up**
   Hand out the worksheet, and explain that these are the usual steps (sequence of events) in puberty. Have the students complete the questions at the bottom of the page. Orally review the answers to the questions on the worksheet, *Steps to Growing Up.* Tell the students to take the worksheet home and keep track of the changes as they occur in their own body.

MATERIALS
Worksheet: *Steps to Growing Up* (Figure 11-5)

EVALUATION: "Changes, Changes"
Students identify on *Changes, Changes* the growth and developmental characteristics that occur during puberty.

MATERIALS
Worksheet: *Changes, Changes* (Figure 11-6)
Teacher resource: *Changes, Changes* (Figure 11-7)

FIGURE 11-5

Worksheet   Name _____

Steps to Growing Up

Directions: The steps below happen during puberty. Girls and boys go through
different changes during this time. When each change happens will
depend on your own individual body. Look at the steps. Answer
the questions on the bottom of the worksheet. Then find a picture
of a young boy and young girl (preferably about your age). Paste
the pictures above the words boy and girl. Find a picture of an
adult man and woman. Paste those pictures above the words
woman and man. Use magazines to find the pictures.

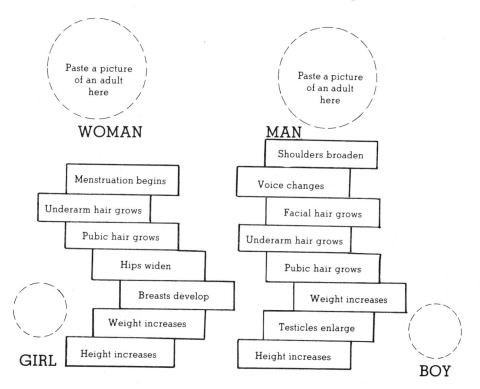

1. Which of the changes are the same for both boys and girls?_____
   _____

2. Which of the changes are different? Put a check mark next to the steps
   above that are different for girls and boys._____
   _____

FIGURE 11-6

Worksheet   Name _____

Changes, Changes

Directions: The two people below have both grown up. What changes did
                their bodies experience during puberty? Circle the characteristics
                of puberty for boys and girls.-

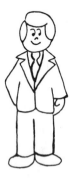

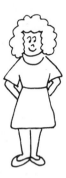

Boys	**Girls**
Weight increases	Weight increases
Pubic hair grows	Pubic hair grows
Underarm hair grows	Underarm hair grows
Hips widen	Hips widen
Menstruation begins	Menstruation begins
Voice changes	Voice changes
Testicles enlarge	Testicles enlarge
Breasts develop	Breasts develop
Facial hair grows	Facial hair grows
Shoulders broaden	Shoulders broaden
Height increases	Height increases

FIGURE 11-7

Teacher resource   Name _____

Changes, Changes

Directions: The two people below have both grown up. What changes did
their bodies experience during puberty? Circle the characteristics
of puberty for boys and girls.

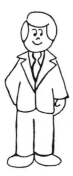   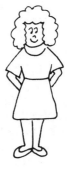

Boys	**Girls**
Weight increases	Weight increases
Pubic hair grows	Pubic hair grows
Underarm hair grows	Underarm hair grows
Hips widen	Hips widen
Menstruation begins	Menstruation begins
Voice changes	Voice changes
Testicles enlarge	Testicles enlarge
Breasts develop	Breasts develop
Facial hair grows	Facial hair grows
Shoulders broaden	Shoulders broaden
Height increases	Height increases

MIDDLE SCHOOL LEVEL

OBJECTIVE: The student describes the reproductive processes.

LEVEL: Grades 6 to 8

VOCABULARY: Reproduction, ovum (ova), sperm, fertilization, conception, embryo, fetus

CONTENT GENERALIZATIONS: Reproduction is a complicated process involving the production of egg cells in women and sperm cells in men. The fertilization of the ovum by a sperm cell is called "conception." The fertilized egg implants in the uterus and grows as a fetus in the body of a pregnant woman. In approximately nine months childbirth occurs, and a baby is born.

NOTE: When teaching about reproduction, it is important to be fully aware of the recommendations and guidelines for your school or district. The activities presented here are conservative and simply designed. Traditional teaching methods involving lectures, discussions, books, and audiovisual materials are the most effective and appropriate approach. However, it cannot be emphasized enough that any books, films, videos, charts, or transparencies used in teaching about reproduction should be submitted to review by parents.

INITIATION: "Parent Letter"
Explain to the students that the class will be studying about human reproduction and birth. Tell them that you would like them to invite their parents to a meeting where they can meet the teacher and talk about the program. Explain that it is often hard for parents and children to talk about this subject. Possibly, if reproduction is discussed with the parents at school, it will be easier for parents and children to talk about it at home.

Hand out a letter from the teacher for students to take home to their parents. Use the *Sample Parent Letter* for a reference. It is sug-

gested that parents be asked to respond to the letter in one of two ways. (The way that parents should respond already may be a specified guideline for your state or district.)

1. Ask the parents to sign and return the letter if they *do* give their permission for their child to be in class during the discussions on reproduction. In other words, only allow a student to stay in the class if you have written permission from the parents.
2. Ask the parents to sign and return the letter if they *do not* give their permission for their child to be in class during discussions of reproduction.

Suggest to the students that they ask their parents a few questions about their own birth, such as the following:

Was my birth normal, breech, or caesarean?
Was my father present at the birth?
How long was mother in labor?

NOTE: Teachers should be sensitive to the differences in families and the presence of adopted children in class. Therefore the questions to ask parents should be voluntary.

MATERIALS
Teacher resource: *Sample Parent Letter* (Figure 11-8)

ACTIVITIES
1. The Question Box
Explain that a *question box* will be a part of the activities for the next several days. Display a question box you have prepared. (A decorated shoe box with a slot at the top or any other decorated box of similar size will work well.) Explain that the box will be used every day to collect questions they may have. These questions will be answered the following day in class. All students will get an index card (or a slip of paper) each day. If the students have a question, they are to write it on the card and put it in the box. If they do not have a question, they are to put a blank card into the box. This method ensures that the

questions are anonymous. Each day read the questions and prepare answers for the next day in class. Some questions may not be suitable for answering in a full group situation. In those cases tell the class, "There were a few questions that we did not have time to address in class. If you are concerned that your question was not answered, please see me after class or after school, and I will attempt to provide an answer." This process helps the teacher sort out the questions that are "planted" to embarrass him or her (which does happen). Also, you may get questions like, "Hi!" "How are you?" and "This class is boring!" Deal with these in a light and friendly manner. After a few days of using the question box students may become comfortable asking questions aloud in class. You need to decide then whether to field these questions openly in class or ask students to continue to put their questions in the question box. This will depend entirely on the skill, experience, and confidence of the teacher.

MATERIALS
Question box (decorated shoe box, teacher-made)
Index cards or slips of paper

MATERIALS
Film/video: district approved titles
  Film projector or video monitor

2. **Film or Video**
Show a film or video on reproduction. The school or district may have titles that are recommended. Tell students to note questions after the film for the question box.

  If the students have not yet been exposed to activities regarding growth and puberty, it may be wise to address these topics now.

3. **Male and Female Reproductive Organs**
Review the anatomy of the male and female reproductive organs, using the transparencies indicated in the margin. Hand out worksheets, and have the students record the anatomical locations on their worksheets as each organ is reviewed.

MATERIALS
Worksheets and transparencies: *The Female Reproductive Organs* (Figure 11-9); *The Male Reproductive Organs* (Figure 11-10)
Overhead projector
Transparency pen

4. **Mini-lecture on Pregnancy and Birth**
Address the following points in a lecture on pregnancy and birth. Use whatever visual aids possible to dramatize these points. **NOTE:** Students are often interested in the topics of pregnancy and birth. They certainly will ask questions about abnormal births. Try to avoid long discussions on abnormalities, and emphasize that most births are normal.

Fertilization, or conception, occurs when a male sperm cell enters a female ovum. This happens after a man and woman have had *sexual intercourse:* an erect male penis is placed into the woman's vagina. Sperm is ejaculated out of the man's body into the woman's body.

One of the first signs that a woman may be pregnant is the skipping of a menstrual period.

The fertilized egg is first called a *zygote,* then, as it multiplies, a *blastocyst,* and then an *embryo.* It grows very rapidly. The embryo implants onto the wall of the uterus and continues to grow. The growing organism is called an embryo for the first 3 months of pregnancy.

The life-support system that connects the baby and mother is called the *placenta.* It is a large organ housing many blood vessels that is attached to the wall of the uterus. Through the placenta, nutrients and oxygen are provided to the embryo, and waste products are taken away. Drugs, including nicotine, alcohol, and caffeine, also can pass through the placenta to the developing embryo.

About the fourth month the developing baby is approximately 3 inches long. It now is called a *fetus.*

Movement of the fetus can be felt around the

fifth month. The heartbeat usually can be heard by a physician earlier than the fifth month. By the end of the sixth month the fetus is about 12 to 14 inches long.

During the last 3 months of pregnancy the fetus grows rapidly. A *premature* baby (one born too soon, whose weight is less than normal) may survive if born during the last 3 months of pregnancy.

Birth is the process when the baby moves out of the mother's uterus through the birth canal (vagina) into the world.

There are three basic stages of birth. In the first stage contractions begin, and the cervix opens wide enough to allow the baby's head to pass. In the second stage the baby is pushed completely out of the uterus, and in the third stage the placenta is expelled from the uterus. This is called the *afterbirth*.

There can be complications during birth. Sometimes caesarean births are necessary, where surgery is used to remove the baby from the uterus.

EVALUATION: "Where Did I Come From?"

Ask the students to write a report answering the question, "Where did I come from?" Tell students to pretend they have to explain reproduction to a young child. It must be done simply but factually. Suggest that they visit their local library and read a few books about this subject written for young children. In evaluating the reports, look for descriptions of fertilization of an egg cell, implantation in the wall of the uterus, growth of an embryo and fetus, and birth.

FIGURE 11-8

Name _____

Sample Parent Letter

Dear Parent:

In a few weeks we will begin our family life unit in health class. This unit was carefully designed to fit the needs of the students in our school district. A curriculum committee consisting of teachers, parents, administrators, and community members was involved in the development of the program.

We would like to invite you to a meeting at the school on the evening of _____ at _____ P.M. At this time you will have the opportunity to view the films and filmstrips used in the program and review all other materials. It will also give you a chance to meet and talk with your child's teacher.

We encourage students to participate in the family life program. Nevertheless, it is voluntary. If you do not wish your child to be involved in the classroom activities, complete the bottom portion of this letter, and send it back to school. We will remove your son or daughter from health class during the unit and involve him or her in an independent study activity dealing with some other aspect of health.

Sincerely,

_____
(Principal)

_____
(Teacher)

- -

To the Principal of _____ School:

I do not wish my son or daughter _____ to
(Name)
participate in the family life unit in health class. Please remove him or her from class during those activities and assign an independent study assignment on some other aspect of health. Thank you.

Signed_____
(Parent)

Date_____

FIGURE 11-9

Worksheet and transparency master   Name _____

The Female Reproductive System

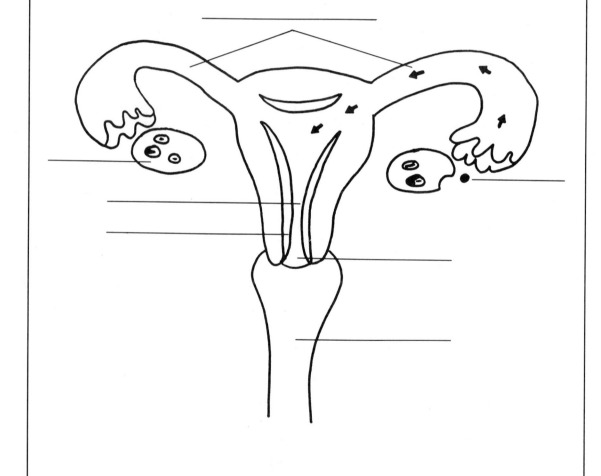

FIGURE 11-10

Worksheet and transparency master   Name _____

The Male Reproductive System

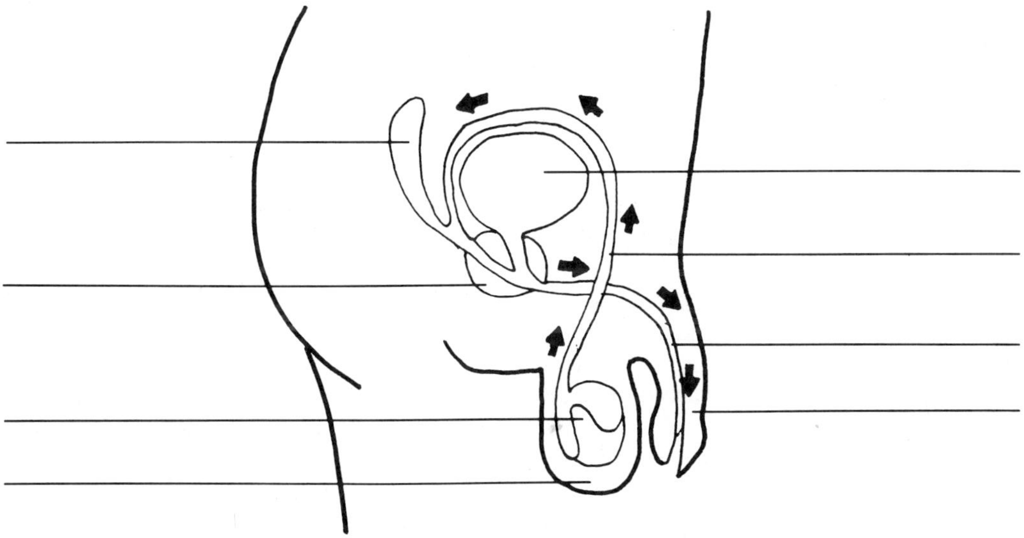

12 Nutrition

When you finish this chapter, you should be able to:

- Describe the importance of the six classes of nutrients.
- Evaluate diet according to recommended servings in six food groups.
- Analyze issues related to weight, body image, and eating disorders.
- Compare the effectiveness and healthfulness of various weight loss diets.
- Develop learning opportunities for students in the area of nutrition.

People eat for many reasons—because they are hungry, for enjoyment, and for social interaction. Food provides the body with the materials it needs to work, grow, and repair itself.

Because of the linkages between nutrition and health, over the years various professional and governmental organizations have developed dietary guidelines for the American public. As our understanding of these linkages has changed over time, so have the recommendations. In the 1940s, nutritionists and health care professionals were concerned about inadequate nutrition in the population. Today, the concerns are more with the *excess* consumption of certain foods and the long-term effects of these food habits.

The most current and widely used recommendations are the Dietary Guidelines for Americans, updated in 1990 by the U.S. Department of Agriculture (USDA) and the U.S. Department of Health and Human Services. Based on the connections between diet and chronic illnesses, such as heart disease and cancer, the report made the following recommendations:

- Eat a variety of foods.
- Maintain healthy weight.
- Choose a diet low in fat, saturated fat, and cholesterol.
- Choose a diet with plenty of vegetables, fruits, and grain products.
- Reduce sugar and salt intake.
- If you drink alcoholic beverages, do so in moderation.

Actually putting these guidelines into practice may not be so simple. We need to have a few basic building blocks in place to learn healthy food habits. First, we must learn to eat in response to body hunger cues and to stop eating in response to feelings of satiety. As we get older, external cues may confuse our natural ability to regulate our food intake. For example, we may have learned to become "hungry" in response to turning on the television. Next, we must accept the fact that although our society places a premium on being thin, in reality there is wide variation in body size, shape, and weight—a result in part to genetic differences, eating habits, and activity levels. And finally, to learn healthy eating habits we must understand basic nutrition. This chapter covers basic information on nutrition, including discussion of the nutrients that are required for health, the food choices we make and how to improve them, the importance of meal and snacking patterns, and dieting and weight control.

NUTRIENTS

Foods contain substances called *nutrients* that are essential for good health. Nutrients build, maintain, and repair body tissues; regulate body processes; and provide fuel for energy. Over fifty essential nutrients are grouped into six main classes. Three of these—carbohydrates, fats, and proteins—are called *macronutrients*, since they are nutrients that the body needs in large amounts. They provide calories, which are sources of energy. A calorie is a unit of heat energy and is used to measure both stored energy (as in food) and energy expended (as in exercise). Technically, a calorie is really a *kilocalorie*—the amount of heat needed to raise the temperature of 1 kilogram of water 1 degree Centigrade. (Kilocalories are sometimes expressed as *C*alories.) Your body needs enough calories from food to provide adequate fuel for all of its energy needs.

All foods have calories, and different foods have different caloric values. The body needs a certain amount of calories a day to function, since every activity of life from jogging to breathing requires energy. *Basal metabolism* refers to the minimum amount of energy required to maintain vital body functions and muscle tone. If an individual is balancing the calories eaten daily with the calories used daily, body weight will stay the same. If more calories are consumed than are used daily, weight will increase.

Carbohydrates are the most important source of energy for all body functions. Depend-ing on their chemical structures, they are either *simple* (sugars naturally produced in plants such as fruits, as well as refined sugars) or *complex* (starches in foods like breads, pasta, and rice). Each gram of carbohydrate provides 4 Calories. It is recommended that 60% of our daily calories—about 1200 Calories—come from carbohydrates, especially complex carbohydrates. In particular, athletes find it helpful to eat a diet rich in complex carbohydrates for several days before an athletic event. This "carbohydrate loading" creates energy reserves in muscles and extends the time that the body is able to maintain strenuous activity. Most forms of fiber are carbohydrates, but the body cannot digest fiber. Fiber provides bulk, which helps the digestive tract function.

Fats provide energy and carry vitamins A, D, E, and K throughout the body. Fats also cushion kidneys and other internal organs against sudden shock and insulate the body against loss of body heat. Each gram of fat contains 9 Calories, compared with the 4 Calories per gram in carbohydrates and proteins. This is what makes fats the most "fattening" foods to eat. In the right amounts, fats are just as necessary as carbohydrates and proteins, as they provide the body's long-term energy reserve, while reserves of carbohydrate energy are limited and are easily exhausted.

Different types of fats have different effects on health. *Saturated* fats are fats that are solid at room temperature and come from both animal and plant sources; meats, dairy products, and coconut oil are examples of foods high in this type of fat. This type of fat contributes to high blood cholesterol levels that increase the risk of heart disease and stroke. *Unsaturated* fats are usually liquid at room temperature. Some of these fats can help lower blood cholesterol levels; olive, canola, corn, sesame, and safflower oils are examples. It is recommended that no more than 30% of daily calories come from fats, and no more than 10% of daily calories should come from saturated fats. Cholesterol is a fatlike substance that is found only in animal foods.

Proteins are essential for the growth and repair of tissue. Protein is a part of every cell in the body and is an important part of the structure of body tissues, such as hair, skin, and muscles. Proteins contain *amino acids*, which are chemicals called the "building blocks" of the body. While about 22 amino acids build human proteins, 9 of them are called *essential* amino acids because we must get them from the food we eat. The body manufactures the other amino acids from substances in food.

A food that contains all 9 essential amino acids is called a *complete protein*. Examples of foods with complete proteins are milk, cheese, and eggs. *Incomplete protein* foods (generally from plant foods) do not contain all 9 essential amino acids. They can be combined to make complete proteins—for example, combining peanut butter and bread or milk and cereal. Nutritionists recommend that 15% of our daily caloric intake be from protein. Protein deficiency can cause fatigue and irritability and make a person prone to infection. Prolonged protein deficiency may cause anemia and liver disorders. In less developed countries, malnutrition caused by protein deficiencies is often seen in a disease called *kwashiorkor*.

Minerals regulate body functions, such as blood clotting and muscle contraction, and they are needed to build strong bones and teeth. There are more than 60 minerals found in the body; about 21 of these have been identified as essential for human health. There are two categories of minerals in the body: *macrominerals*, which are found in large quantities and include calcium, potassium, and sodium; and *microminerals*, or *trace minerals*, found in smaller amounts. Trace minerals include iodine, zinc, and fluoride.

Most **vitamins** regulate chemical reactions in the body. The 13 known vitamins are A, C, D, E, K, and the 8 "B-complex" vitamins. All vitamins have scientific names, for example, vitamin B 1 is called thiamin. They are required in small amounts generally found in a balanced diet. However, in certain circumstances, such as during pregnancy or while breastfeeding, the body's need for vitamins increases and vitamin supplements may be required.

Water may be the most essential nutrient, since it makes up more than half our body weight and without it, humans can survive for only a few days. Water has no caloric value; it is present in and vital to the functioning of every living cell and tissue. It helps eliminate wastes, regulates body temperature, and carries dissolved nutrients to the cells. Most people require from six to eight glasses of water a day.

FOOD CHOICES

The foods we eat often have too little to do with the nutritional needs of the body. The food choices of parents and siblings usually become the food choices of younger children. These eating patterns, once established, are not easy to change. For example, having potato chips and soft drinks as an after-school snack is not easily changed to eating a banana and drinking a glass of milk. Food customs are also influenced by ethnic beliefs and traditions. Jews may refrain from eating pork or may eat only kosher foods. Mexican Americans may prefer tortillas to sliced bread. Young children enjoy learning about different cultures and trying new foods. Primary level students can learn to identify the various characteristics of foods by tasting them.

Food Groups: Guides for Nutritious Eating

Food groups are ways of grouping foods of similar nutrient content to help people plan for good nutrition. Ensuring a well-balanced diet with adequate amounts of essential nutrients can seem very complex. Grouping foods according to what they have in common makes this task easier.

Nutritionists have developed several food grouping systems. Each system suggests eating certain amounts or servings from the food groups it includes. The goal of all of the systems is to ensure that an individual's diet includes all the essential nutrients in appropriate quantities. Since no one food group provides all of these nutrients, variety is the key to good nutrition.

In the mid-1950s the USDA food group system contained four groups: milk, meat, fruits and vegetables, and breads and cereals. Twenty-five years later, food group classification was revised and a fifth group containing fats, sweets, and alcoholic beverages was added. In 1991, the USDA again revised the food guide as "A Pattern for Daily Food Choices." In this plan there are six food groupings, which are graphically depicted as a pyramid (Figure 12-1). The groups are roughly the same as those in the five food groups system, except that fruits and vegetables become two separate groups, and the recommended amounts of these and of breads and cereals is increased. The goal of the changes is to provide most dietary energy intake from carbohydrates while limiting fat intake.

The pyramid shape depicts the relative quantities of the foods in the different food groups that should be consumed in a balanced diet. Foods that are at the broad base of the pyramid should form the largest part of the diet; those in the middle of the pyramid should be eaten in moderate amounts; and those at the top are foods that should be eaten sparingly. While initially there was some controversy over this way of showing food groupings (e.g., some argued that people might misconstrue the meaning of the various groups' placements within the pyramid), its advantage is that it reminds people at a glance which foods to focus on and which to eat sparingly and how to create a balanced diet.

The six food groupings are as follows:

- *Milk, yogurt, and cheese* group contains all milk products (except butter). This group contributes high-quality protein and calcium, required for bone and tooth development. Whole milk, low-fat milk, yogurt, cheese, and ice cream are included. Low-fat milk products are recommended over high-fat milk products. While they provide similar nutritional benefits, high-fat milk products contribute excess fat, cholesterol, and calories.
- *Meat, poultry, fish, dried beans and peas, eggs, and nuts* group is essential for its protein, iron, and B vitamins.
- *Fruits* food group includes all fruits and fruit juices. They provide vitamin A, vitamin C, carbohydrates, and fiber in our diets. According to the American Cancer Society, this food group may play an important role in the prevention of certain forms of cancer.
- *Vegetables* also provide vitamin A, vitamin C, complex carbohydrates, and fiber. Foods included in this group are dark green, yellow, and orange vegetables; canned or cooked vegetables; and salads. Cruciferous vegetables, such as broccoli, cabbage, brussels sprouts, and cauliflower, may be helpful in preventing certain types of cancer.
- *Breads, cereals, pasta, and rice* group is important for its B-complex vitamins, iron, and carbohydrates. According to some nutritionists, use of these foods promotes protein intake, since many of the foods in this group are prepared with other foods to make a complete protein (for example, macaroni and cheese or cereal and milk).
- *Fats, oils, and sweets* are foods that contain many calories from fat and sugar but few other nutrients—such as candies, cakes, pies, cookies, chips, and soft drinks. For this reason, they are often referred to as "junk foods." They should not be eaten in place of a food in one of the other important food groups and should be eaten only occasionally.

The box on p. 312 describes serving sizes and lists the recommended minimum number of servings for three different groups of people.

Fast foods are mass-produced foods usually served in drive-through or walk-in restaurants. Typical fast foods are hamburgers, french fries, pizza, fried chicken, hot dogs, and tacos. Most fast foods are high in calories, fats, salt, and sugar but low in other nutrients. However, the

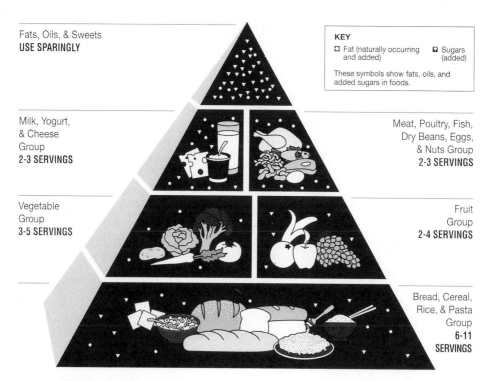

Fats, Oils, & Sweets
USE SPARINGLY

Milk, Yogurt,
& Cheese
Group
2-3 SERVINGS

Vegetable
Group
3-5 SERVINGS

Meat, Poultry, Fish,
Dry Beans, Eggs,
& Nuts Group
2-3 SERVINGS

Fruit
Group
2-4 SERVINGS

Bread, Cereal,
Rice, & Pasta
Group
**6-11
SERVINGS**

KEY
▫ Fat (naturally occurring   ☑ Sugars
  and added)   (added)
These symbols show fats, oils, and
added sugars in foods.

FIGURE 12-1
Food guide pyramid.
How many servings are right for me?   The Pyramid shows a range of servings for
each food group. The number of servings that are right for you depends on how many calories you need, which in turn depends on your age, sex, size, and how active you are. Almost
everyone should have at least the lowest number of servings in the ranges. The following
calorie level suggestions are based on recommendations of the National Academy of Sciences and on calorie intakes reported by people in national food consumption surveys.
For adults and teens   1,600 calories is about right for many sedentary women and some
older adults. 2,200 calories is about right for most children, teenage girls, active women, and
many sedentary men. Women who are pregnant or breastfeeding may need somewhat more.
2,800 calories is about right for teenage boys, many active men, and some very active women.

HOW TO USE THE DAILY FOOD GUIDE*

What Counts as One Serving?

Breads, Cereals, Rice, and Pasta

1 slice of bread
½ cup of cooked rice or pasta
½ cup of cooked cereal
1 ounce of ready-to-eat cereal

Vegetables

½ cup of chopped raw or
  cooked vegetables
1 cup of leafy raw vegetables

Fruits

1 piece of fruit or melon wedge
¾ cup of juice
½ cup of canned fruit
¼ cup of dried fruit

Milk, Yogurt, and Cheese

1 cup of milk or yogurt
1½ to 2 ounces of cheese

Meat, Poultry, Fish, Dry Beans, Eggs, and Nuts

2½ to 3 ounces of cooked lean
  meat, poultry, or fish
Count ½ cup of cooked beans,
  or 1 egg, or 2 tablespoons of
  peanut butter as 1 ounce of
  lean meat (about ⅓ serving)

Fats, Oils, and Sweets

LIMIT CALORIES FROM THESE
  (especially if you need to lose
  weight)

How Many Servings Do You Need Each Day?

	Women and some older adults	Children, teen girls, active women, most men	Teen boys and active men
Calorie level†	About 1,600	About 2,200	About 2,800
Bread group	6	9	11
Vegetable group	3	4	5
Fruit group	2	3	4
Milk group	‡2-3	‡2-3	‡2-3
Meat group	2 for a total of 5 ounces	2 for a total of 6 ounces	3 for a total of 7 ounces

*The amount you eat may be more than one serving. For example, a dinner portion of spaghetti would count as two or three servings of pasta.
†These are the calorie levels if you choose lowfat, lean foods from the 5 major food groups and use foods from the fats, oils, and sweets group sparingly.
‡Women who are pregnant or breastfeeding, teenagers, and young adults to age 24 need 3 servings.

nutritional value of fast foods can vary greatly. Many fast food restaurants have altered their menus to include salads, lower-fat meats, and low-fat milk products. Every day, about one third of the foods Americans eat are fast foods.

Nutrient Density

Good nutrition involves eating a wide variety of "nutrient-dense" foods. These are foods with good nutritional value (vitamins, minerals, protein, and complex carbohydrates) in relationship to their caloric value. Foods with low nutrient density, the so-called "junk foods" have little nutritional value in relationship to their caloric value.

Within each of the food groups, foods can be categorized as having high nutrient density, good nutrient density, or low nutrient density. Most of the foods we eat should fall into the category of high nutrient density. Some examples of high nutrient density foods in each of the food groups are low-fat cheeses, skim milk, skinless chicken or turkey, tuna canned in water, all fresh fruits and vegetables, and whole grain breads and cereals.

Meals and Snacks

Another key to developing healthy eating habits is establishing regular meal patterns. In particular, it is important to eat a nutritious and balanced breakfast because of the time that has elapsed since the evening meal, and breakfast (meaning "break the fast") is the first meal of every day. It helps get the body going and provides energy for the day's work and play. Sometimes the foods thought of as "breakfast foods" are not appealing in the morning. But there are no "right" or "wrong" foods for breakfast. The important thing to remember is to eat foods from at least three of the food groups. For example, if a menu of toast, scrambled egg, and orange juice is not appealing, a peanut butter and jelly sandwich with a glass of milk may be more tempting while fulfilling the same nutritional needs.

Snack foods can be part of a balanced diet, as long as nutritious foods with high nutrient density are chosen most of the time. Snack food is any food that people eat between meals. They provide people with energy and may be particularly important for primary level children who are not able to eat the large quantities of the foods they need at one mealtime. For this age group, snacking may actually provide a significant part of the day's nutrition. Quick, ready-to-eat snacks that are healthful include fresh fruits, raw vegetables, nuts, seeds, yogurt, cheese slices, and unbuttered popcorn. Fruits, vegetables, and grains contain fiber, as well as needed vitamins, minerals, carbohydrates, and proteins; the fiber is filling and helps to satisfy the appetite until the next meal.

ASSESSING THE QUALITY OF YOUR DIET

Comparing personal food choices with recommended servings in each of the four food groups is one way to analyze eating habits. Often teenagers and young adults find that they eat too few servings in one or two of the groups. Or they may be eating foods with a lower nutritional quality within a food group. For example, ice cream is classified in the milk group, but it is lower in nutrient density than milk. Teenagers may also find they are eating several foods in the fats, oils, and sweets category and are taking in "empty" calories.

A more specific way to assess the quality of your diet is to keep track of what you are eating each day by writing it down in a "diet record." You can assess the quality of your diet by checking your daily intake of servings from the major food groups. If your intake meets the recommended number of servings, you are probably obtaining adequate amounts of nutrients from food.

MODELING HEALTHY FOOD HABITS

Teachers can have a significant influence on children's food choices and on children's perceptions of appropriate foods by what they model for children on a daily basis. Not only do children observe what adults do and compare it with what they say, they also depend on adults to set standards and, when they are very young, provide the foods from which to choose. This is especially true when the adults are authority figures. For example, a teacher who eats carrot sticks as a snack teaches students about healthy choices. The teacher who snacks on candy throughout the day, as children watch, is sending a message that such snacking is an acceptable way to eat.

Schools can model healthy food choices in a number of ways. They can develop a clear, written policy regarding the nutritional value of food served at school. Many schools have already put such policies into place. Ideally, this policy would be a part of a more comprehensive school health program, in which nutrition is one of many components addressing the development of healthy behaviors in students.

Since children who go to school without breakfast do not perform as well as students who have eaten breakfast, many schools offer a breakfast program especially for students from low-income families. What schools serve in the cafeteria for breakfast and lunch and what they offer in vending machines as meals and snacks reveal the messages being communicated to students about what's appropriate and healthy to eat. Schools need to be sure that they are not sending students mixed messages about healthy food choices, with one message in the classroom and another in the cafeteria and vending machines.

School lunch programs can incorporate the principles of the Dietary Guidelines for Americans. The U.S. Department of Health and Human Services' *Healthy People 2000* recommends that we "increase to at least 90% the proportion of school lunch and breakfast services that are consistent with the nutritional principles in the Dietary Guidelines for Americans." To meet this objective, school lunches must provide choices that include low-fat foods, vegetables, fruits, and whole-grain products. High-fat foods, such as french fries and potato chips, should appear infrequently on the menu.

To help children learn to make choices, *Healthy People 2000* also recommends that schools offer "point-of-service" nutrition information in the school cafeteria. For example, some cafeteria-style restaurants now have an information card by each food listing its nutrient value and calories. Such information would have the added benefit of supporting children's learning experiences in the classroom, allowing them to practice the health knowledge and food selection skills introduced in the classroom. Educators are role models in the cafeteria, as well as in the classroom. When the school staff eat the food prepared at school, they send a positive message about that food. Even if teachers obtain their food in the cafeteria and then take it to the staff lounge, students will observe that adults are eating the same food as they are. This action provides an effective way to model food choices for students.

DIETING AND WEIGHT CONTROL
Body Image

There is a wide range of "normal" body shapes and sizes. This diversity of human body types is affected by both biological and cultural factors. For example, obesity tends to run in families. While obese people may have food and activity habits that foster their obesity, research also supports a conclusion that genetics plays an important role in body weight.

The ideal image of slenderness promoted by the mass media and various business interests sets many people up for unrealistic expectations. People—especially women—are led to believe that they can attain a certain body size and shape if they just buy or do the "right" things. This ideal ignores the basic reality of human diversity and perpetuates the stigma attached to those who vary from the ideal. It also furthers the fear of fat that has become endemic in American society.

This cultural ideal is very different from the ideal in many other societies. In some parts of the world where food is scarce, being fat is considered a sign of affluence and carries great prestige. In some countries, children and adults are often slim and athletic, but adults are expected to be heavy as a sign of maturity and status.

Weight and Health

At any one time, fifty million Americans are dieting to lose weight. Yet the relationship between weight and health has been debated for some time, and it still remains controversial. Nonetheless, some consistent trends have become apparent. Research shows that "yo-yo" dieting, the common cycle of repeatedly losing and gaining weight, may be as bad for people as weighing too much in the first place. Repeatedly, researchers have found that the body resists major weight change—loss *or* gain. An individual's normal range of weight is largely genetically determined. While diet and exercise play a definite role, they do so within limits set by heredity. Age also affects weight; between the ages of 20 and 55, Americans' median weight rises steadily—perhaps partly due to decreased physical activity.

In recognition of this age difference, in 1990 the US government began publishing recommended weight guidelines that give different ranges for older and younger adults. Women's "healthy weight" is near the lower end of each weight range, and men's "healthy weight" is at the higher end of the range.

A body shape and size that is "healthy" can be quite different from the thin ideal. Another way to determine whether your body weight is healthy is the waist-to-hip ratio. Research has consistently shown that the higher the ratio, the greater the risk of heart disease, especially among people who are overweight.

1. First, measure around your waist near your navel as you stand relaxed without pulling in your stomach.
2. Next, measure around your hips over the buttocks where hips are the largest.
3. Last, divide your waist measure by your hip measure.

The ratio should be less than .80 for women and .95 for men. Over these cutoff points, the risk of heart disease seems to increase. In addition, there is growing concern over the relationship between the amount of fat in the central abdominal cavity and the development of other serious health problems, such as hypertension (high blood pressure).

Dieting to Lose Weight

Traditional dieting—simply cutting calories to lose weight—has been shown not to work. Many dieters, frustrated by cycles of losing and then regaining weight, go from one fad diet or commercial diet program to another.

Fad diets, such as low carbohydrate diets or fasting, promise quick and easy weight loss without having to change eating habits. Despite their popularity and sales appeal, fad diets simply don't work. Not only do they fail, they can also cause health problems.

Americans now spend more than $3 billion a year on commercial diet companies' weight-loss programs. However, for most people, commercial weight-loss programs result in temporary weight loss, at best. The average dieter gained back almost half of the weight lost just 6 months after ending the program.

Healthy Ways to Control Weight

Since the likelihood is great that weight lost on a reducing diet will be gained back, anyone considering a diet should think seriously about whether losing weight is really necessary. Researchers now agree that increasing physical ac-

TABLE 12-1

Recommended Weight Guidelines

	Weight Without Clothes	
Height Without Shoes	**19-34 Years**	**35 Years and Over**
5'	97-128	108-138
5'1"	101-132	111-143
5'2"	104-137	115-148
5'3"	107-141	119-152
5'4"	111-146	122-157
5'5"	114-150	126-162
5'6"	118-155	130-167
5'7"	121-160	134-172
5'8"	125-164	138-178
5'9"	129-169	142-183
5'10"	132-174	146-188
5'11"	136-179	151-194
6'	140-184	155-199
6'1"	144-189	159-205
6'2"	148-195	164-210
6'3"	152-200	168-216
6'4"	156-205	173-222
6'5"	160-211	177-228
6'6"	164-216	182-234

tivity is critical to lasting weight loss and suggest that the approach most likely to succeed is a program that combines calorie reduction and aerobic exercise. Reducing the daily consumption of fats and increasing the consumption of foods high in dietary fiber, such as whole grains, fruits, and vegetables, can have an impact on weight as the increased fiber moves food through the body and the decreased fat results in less body fat. Regular exercise "burns off" fat and helps the body stay healthy.

EATING DISORDERS

Obsessive dieting can lead to eating disorders. Two eating disorders, bulimia and anorexia nervosa, have become increasingly common, especially in adolescent girls and young women. These conditions are extreme examples of the harm that is done by promoting an ideal of thinness and a fear of fat. Both conditions can have damaging effects on the body such as heart problems and can even cause death. Medical and psychological treatment are usually required to help the individual overcome the harmful eating patterns.

Bulimia is characterized by binge eating and then purging. Binges may last from a few minutes to several hours and then are followed by periods of self-induced purging by vomiting, use of laxatives, fasting, or vigorous exercise. A study of high school girls found that more than 10% used vomiting and nearly 5% used laxatives to lose weight.

Anorexia nervosa is self-induced starvation. Young people with this condition view themselves as much fatter than they really are and starve themselves to reduce body size. While those who are bulimic may appear normal in weight, girls who are anorexic are often skeleton-like in appearance. Social and psychological pressures contribute to both conditions. Some experts suggest that these conditions are related to a fear of growing up or a rebellion against standards set too high by others.

School counselors, the community hospital, or health services may give information and referrals to medical professionals and self-help groups.

SUMMARY

The body requires protein, fats, carbohydrates, vitamins, minerals, and water for health. The best way to obtain the necessary amounts of these nutrients is to eat a balanced diet choosing foods from each of the basic food groups: milk, cheese, and yogurt; meat, poultry, fish, dry beans, eggs, and nuts; fruits; vegetables; breads, cereals, pasta, and rice; and small amounts of fats, oils, and sweets. Within these groups, try to choose foods with high nutrient density most of the time.

As our knowledge about nutrition and health changes, the dietary recommendations nutritionists and health professionals make will also change. Because of this, it is important to be aware of what the current recommendations are and to continue to reexamine your eating habits. As a teacher, it will be even more important to

---

SYMPTOMS OF EATING DISORDERS

Eating disorders are often associated with one or more of the following symptoms:

- Abnormal weight loss
- Person appears to have a terminal disease
- Refusal to eat, except for tiny portions
- Binge-eating, often in secret
- Vomiting, often in secret
- Abuse of laxatives, diuretics, emetics, or diet pills
- Denial of hunger
- Excessive exercise
- Distorted body image, denies thinness, expresses concern over being "too fat"
- Preoccupation with food
- Absent or irregular menstruation in women
- Depression

be self-aware, since you will be modeling healthy food habits to students every day.

When dieting is taken to extremes or psychological problems accompany the desire to be thin, eating disorders can develop. Most common are anorexia nervosa and bulimia. If you suspect that you or someone you know has an eating disorder, it is critical to seek help. There are many treatment centers and medical professionals who specialize in these conditions.

In the section that follows are samples of classroom activities that can be used to help teach primary, intermediate, and middle school level students about nutrition.

REFERENCES

1. Berryman J, Breighner K: *Modeling healthy behavior*, Santa Cruz, Calif, 1993, ETR Associates.
2. Henderson A: *Healthy schools, healthy futures. The case for improving school environment*, Santa Cruz, Calif, 1993, ETR Associates.
3. Ikeda J, Naworski P: *Am I fat? Helping young children accept differences in body size*, Santa Cruz, Calif, 1992, ETR Associates.
4. Kane W: *Step by step to comprehensive school health*, Santa Cruz, Calif, 1993, ETR Associates.
5. Losing weight. What works. What doesn't. *Consumer Reports* 58(6): June 1993.
6. Nutrition and fitness: *Macmillan health encyclopedia*, vol 4, New York, 1993, Macmillan.
7. Nutrition and your health: dietary guidelines for Americans, ed 3, USDA USDHSS, Home Garden Bulletin no. 232, Washington, DC, 1990, US Government Printing Office.
8. Payne W, Hahn D: *Understanding your health*, ed 3, St. Louis, 1992, Mosby.
9. U.S. Department of Health and Human Services, Public Health Service: *Healthy People 2000: national health promotion and disease prevention objectives*, DHHS Publication No. (PHS)91-50212, Washington, DC, 1990.

LEARNING OPPORTUNITIES FOR NUTRITION

MATERIALS
Pictures of foods from magazines or food models
Food items: banana, grapes, pickle, apple

MATERIALS
Paper
Crayons

ACTIVITIES

1. Characteristics of Food
a. Show pictures of different foods (from magazines or food models) or actual foods to demonstrate taste (salty, sweet, sour), texture (rough, smooth, crunchy, slippery), smell (sweet, sour), and color.
b. Hold up three pictures of foods or food models of the same color (such as an apple, red jello, and a tomato). Ask "How are these foods the same?" (They are all red. "How are they different?" (They taste different: two are sweet, and one is not; one is crunchy; one is juicy.)
c. Ask the students to draw a picture of another food that is red (e.g., strawberries, pizza, cherries, watermelon, beets, or spaghetti sauce). Then have each student show the picture to the class and tell about the food. (It is crunchy; it is sweet; it is juicy; it smells sour.)

2. About Foods
Hand out the worksheet, *About Foods*. (Figure 12-2) Using crayons, students are to color the foods that are orange and circle the foods that are crunchy.

MATERIALS
Orange crayons
Worksheet: *About Foods*

3. **Three Dimensional Food Models**
   a. Have the students make three-dimensional food models from butcher paper stapled together and stuffed with newspaper. Make the food larger than life, perhaps as large as the students. An alternative is to have them make clay models of food. It may be helpful to put the students into groups for this activity. Have parents, older students, or teacher aides help out in each group.
   b. Display the stuffed food models around the room. Ask students who worked on the model to tell about their food.

MATERIALS
Butcher paper
Paints
Pencils
Staples
Scissors
Newspaper
Alternative: clay and paint

Evaluation: "Name That Food"
Play a simple game called "Name That Food." Begin by listing several characteristics of a food without naming the food. Continue describing the food until a student correctly guesses it. For example, "I am thinking of a food . . . it is red on the outside . . . it is crunchy . . . it is sweet . . . it is a fruit. . . . What is it?" (Apple.) Continue the game as time and the students' attention span permit.

FIGURE 12-2

Worksheet   Name _____

About Foods

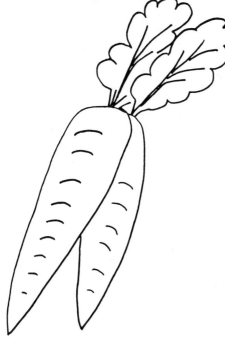

Directions:
1. Color all the orange foods.
2. Circle all the crunchy foods.

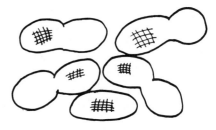

Peanuts

Carrots

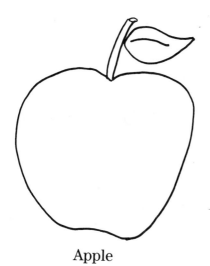

Apple

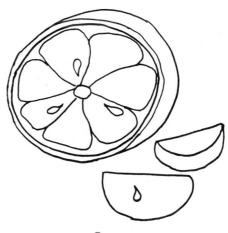

Orange

INTERMEDIATE LEVEL

OBJECTIVE: The student analyzes the nutritional value of food choices for meals and snacks.

LEVEL: Grades 4 to 6

INTEGRATION: Science, math

CONTENT GENERALIZATIONS: Fruits, vegetables, dairy foods, grain foods, and protein-rich foods should be eaten daily to provide adequate nutrition. Each of types of these food provides specific nutrients that are required to promote growth and maintain health. Children in grades 4 to 6 should eat three servings of dairy foods, two servings of protein-rich foods (also called meat), three servings of fruits and four servings of vegetables, and nine servings of bread and cereal (also called grain), daily for a nutritious diet. Certain foods are low in nutrient content. These are called *other* or *extra* foods and are usually high in sugar, fat, or both. These foods include cakes, candies, cookies, pies, salad dressings, mayonnaise, catsup, butter, margarine, jams, jellies, soda, and chips and should be consumed in moderation. A nutritious diet consists of a variety of foods selected from all of the food groups. Fruits, vegetables and whole-grain breads and cereal products also provide fiber.

VOCABULARY: Nutrients, protein, poultry, vitamins, minerals, carbohydrates

INITIATION: "Three-Day Food Diary"
Ask the students to keep a diary of all the foods they eat and drink, including meals and snacks. Begin the activity immediately by having the students write down everything they ate yesterday. That will be day 1 of the food diary. Today will be day 2, and tomorrow will be day 3. Tell the students they will be studying the foods they eat. Encourage them to eat normally and record all foods eaten including restaurant meals. Allow a little class time each day to fill in the food diary from the previous day.

ACTIVITIES
1. Types of Foods
Use food models or pictures of food to help discuss and identify various types of food. Hold a picture of a food up, and have the children identify the type of food (protein-rich dairy, fruit, vegetable, grain). Tell them that many foods we eat have more than one type of food in the same dish. Beef stew has protein foods and vegetables. Ask the students what types of food are represented in a cheese sandwich. (Milk and bread or grain.) Practice measuring dry food and water. Address the following questions in the discussion:

a. What are portions of foods or drinks that can be easily determined? (12 oz can of soda, 8 oz carton of milk, candy bar, apple, slice of bread, tablespoon of margarine)
b. What portions of foods or drinks are harder to figure out? (Pieces of meat, fish or chicken, food mixtures)
c. What are the different types of foods? (Milk, protein-rich vegetables, fruit, and bread and cereal or grain.)
d. What are some examples of milk foods? (Milk, cheese, cottage cheese, and yogurt.)
e. What are some examples of protein-rich foods? (Meats, fish, poultry, dried beans and peas, and nuts.)
f. What are some different forms of fruits and vegetables? (Juice, frozen, fresh, and canned.)
g. What are some examples of different kinds of grain foods? (Breads, cereals, rice, muffins, macaroni, pita bread, pasta, tortillas, and corn bread.)
h. How many servings of each type of food are needed for children your age? (Three milk foods, two protein-rich foods, 3 fruits, 4 vegetables, and nine grain foods.)

List their ideas on the board, then ask if they all agree that the listed foods do not fit into the food groups identified earlier.

MATERIALS
Worksheet: *Three-Day Food Diary* (3 copies per student) (Figure 12-3)

Measuring utensils for foods (liquid and dry measure), measuring spoons
Small ounce scale (postal scale) or balance
Dry food (example: cornflakes, macaroni), water (color with food coloring)
1 glass

2. Extra Foods

Ask the students if they can think of any foods that have not been mentioned. Explain that foods with a lot of sugar or fat do not have many of the nutrients needed for growth and health. Ask the children to help in making a list of extra foods, for example, cakes, candy, chips, butter, cookies, jams, soft drinks, margarine, catsup, jelly, mayonnaise, or salad dressing.

Explain that these foods should be eaten in moderation and should not be substituted for a food that is needed for a nutritious diet. Have the students make collages of extra foods using pictures from magazines. They can work alone or in groups. When all have finished, put the collages on a bulletin board.

MATERIALS

Food models or pictures of foods from magazines
Construction paper
Magazines
Glue
Scissors

3. How Well Did I Do?

Help students analyze their *Three-Day Food Diary* using the *Food Study Sheet*. Students should circle foods with a different-colored crayon to identify the type of food (including "extra" foods). Some foods should be circled with more than one color (for example, sandwiches, stews, pizza, and tacos). After the students have completed this, have them answer the following questions on a separate piece of paper.

a. How many days did you eat a nutritious diet?
b. Did you eat the minimum amounts of foods for each of the food groups? Which types of food were you low in?
c. Did you eat extra foods all 3 days?
d. What kind of foods do you need to eat more of?

MATERIALS

Worksheets: *Three-Day Food Diary* (completed earlier) (see Figure 12-3)
Student resource: *Food Study Sheet* (Figure 12-4)
Crayons: red, green, black, blue, brown, yellow (1 of each color per student)
Paper
Pencils

EVALUATION: "How Well Does Pat Eat?"

Have students analyze the worksheet, *How Well Does Pat Eat?* in the same way that they analyzed their own diets by circling the various types of food with crayons and answering the questions at the bottom of the page. Remind them that dishes which contain more than one type of food should be circled with more than one color. After students are finished, discuss the correct responses.

MATERIALS

Worksheet: *How Well Does Pat Eat?* (Figure 12-5)
Teacher resource: *How Well Does Pat Eat?* (Figure 12-6)
Crayons: red, green, black, blue, brown, yellow (1 of each color per student)

FIGURE 12-3

Worksheet   Name _____

Three-day Food Diary

DAY   1   2   3
(Circle one)

BREAKFAST	AMOUNT	SNACKS BETWEEN BREAKFAST AND LUNCH	AMOUNT
_____	_____	_____	_____
_____	_____	_____	_____
_____	_____	_____	_____
_____	_____	_____	_____
_____	_____	_____	_____
_____	_____	_____	_____
_____	_____		

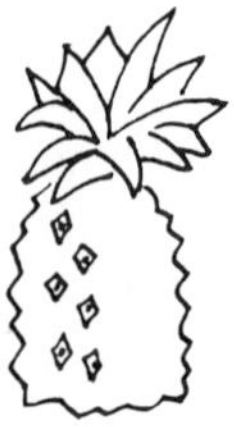

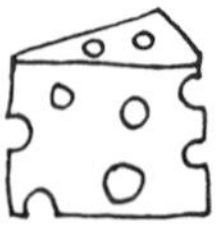

LUNCH	AMOUNT	SNACKS BETWEEN LUNCH AND DINNER (AFTER-SCHOOL SNACKS)	AMOUNT
_____	_____	_____	_____
_____	_____	_____	_____
_____	_____	_____	_____
_____	_____	_____	_____
_____	_____	_____	_____
_____	_____	_____	_____

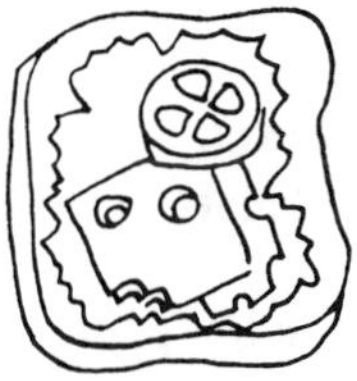

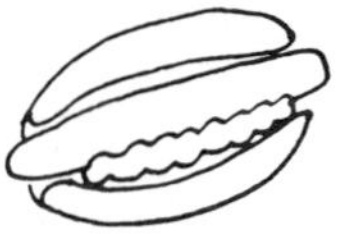

DINNER	AMOUNT	SNACKS AFTER DINNER	AMOUNT
_____	_____	_____	_____
_____	_____	_____	_____
_____	_____	_____	_____
_____	_____	_____	_____
_____	_____	_____	_____
_____	_____	_____	_____

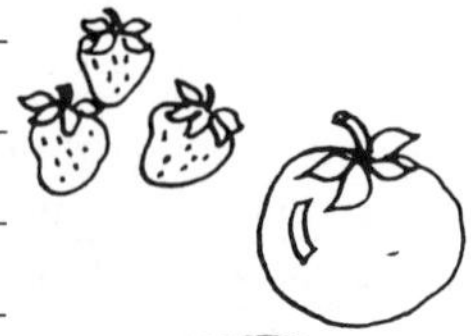

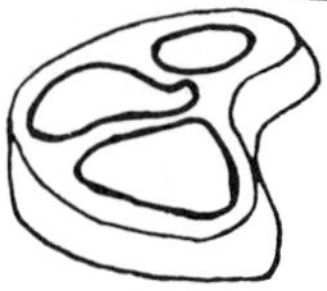

FIGURE 12-4

Student resource   Name _____

Food Study Sheet

TYPES OF FOOD	NUTRIENTS	PURPOSES	EXAMPLES OF FOOD

Fruits	Vitamin A
	Vitamin C
		Healthy gums
		Healthy skin
		Growth and
		  development
		Provides fiber to
		  prevent
		  constipation
			Apples
			Bananas
			Berries
			Strawberries
			Cantaloupe
			Grapefruit
			Oranges

Vegetables	Vitamin A
	Calcium
	Folic acid
	Iron
		Healthy skin
		Growth and
		  development
		Healthy bones
		Healthy teeth
		Healthy blood
		Provides fiber to
		  prevent
		  constipation
			Broccoli
			Carrots
			Celery
			Chinese pea pods
			Okra
			Greens
			Green beans

Milk	Calcium Phosphorus Riboflavin Protein Vitamin A Vitamin D (fortified)	Healthy bones Healthy teeth	Milk Nonfat milk Buttermilk Yogurt Cottage cheese Cheese

Grains	Carbohydrates
	B vitamins
	Iron
		Energy
		Provides fiber to
		  prevent
		  constipation
			Bread (whole wheat
			  or enriched)
			Cereal
			Pita
			Tortilla
			Matzo
			Rice
			Popcorn
			Pasta

TYPES OF FOOD	NUTRIENTS	PURPOSES	EXAMPLES OF FOOD
Proteins- Rich	Protein Iron Calcium B vitamins	Build body tissues Repair body tissues	Eggs Cheese and beans (legumes) Cereal and milk Poultry Meat Fish Nuts

FIGURE 12-5

Worksheet   Name _____

How Well Does Pat Eat?

Directions: Read the diet that Pat ate one day. He is an 11-year-old boy who
likes to play various sports. Did he get enough of the foods that he
needs? Circle all the different types of food eaten with different
colors to determine this. Then fill in the answers to the questions
at the bottom.

BREAKFAST

Bowl of cereal
Glass of milk
Glass of orange juice
Oatmeal muffin

SNACK BEFORE LUNCH

1 Apple

LUNCH

Hamburger on a bun
Catsup
Lettuce and tomato salad
Salad dressing
Glass of milk
Chocolate brownie

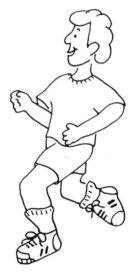

SNACK

1 piece of cheese pizza with tomato sauce
1 pear

DINNER

Fried chicken
Dish of carrots
Lettuce and tomato salad
Salad dressing
2 Dinner rolls
Piece of cake
Glass of milk

1. Did Pat have at least three
   servings of milk?_____

2. Did Pat have at least two servings
   of protein?_____

3. Did he have four to six servings of
   vegetables?_____

4. Did he have nine servings of
   grains?_____

5. Did he have three servings of
   fruit?_____

6. Did he eat any "extra" foods?_____

7. Did he substitute an "extra" food
   for a food needed in a food group?

   _____

FIGURE 12-6

Teacher resource   Name _____ **(Key)** _____

How Well Does Pat Eat?

Directions: Read the diet that Pat ate one day. He is an 11-year-old boy who likes to play various sports. Did he get enough of the foods that he needs? Circle all the different types of food eaten different colors to determine this. Then fill in the answers to the questions at the bottom.

BREAKFAST

B	Bowl of cereal
M	Glass of milk
F	Glass of orange juice
B	Oatmeal muffin

SNACK BEFORE LUNCH

F	1 Apple

LUNCH

Mt + 2 B	Hamburger on a bun
O	Catsup
V	Lettuce and tomato salad
O	Salad dressing
M	Glass of milk
O	Chocolate brownie

SNACK

M B V	1 piece of cheese pizza with tomato sauce
F	1 pear

DINNER

M	Fried chicken
V	Dish of carrots
V	Lettuce and tomato salad
O	Salad dressing
2 B	2 Dinner rolls

DINNER

O	Piece of cake
M	Glass of milk

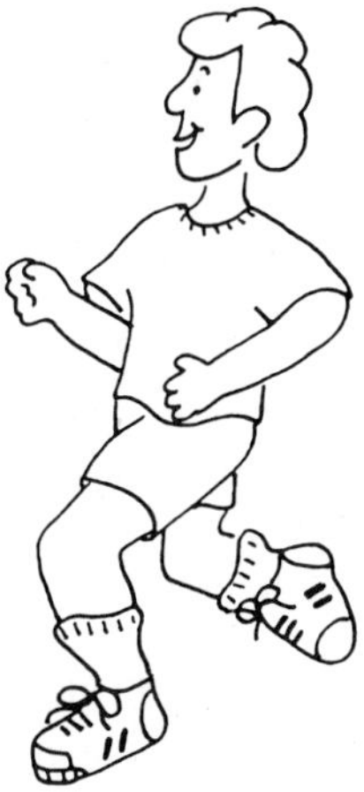

1. Did Pat have at least three servings of dairy? YES _____
2. Did Pat have at least two servings of protein? YES _____
3. Did he have four servings of vegetable? YES _____
4. Did he have three servings of fruit? YES _____
5. Did he have nine servings of grain? NO _____
6. Did he eat any "extra" foods? YES _____
7. Did he substitute an "extra" food for a food needed in a food group? NO _____

MINIMUM FOR CHILD SERVINGS

B = Breads and cereals	9
M = Milk	2-3
Mt = Meat and meat alternatives	2
V = Vegetable	4
F = Fruit	3
O = Other (high in fat, sugar)	_____

MIDDLE SCHOOL LEVEL

OBJECTIVE: The student explains the relationship between calorie intake, level of activity and body weight.

LEVEL: Grades 7 and 8

VOCABULARY: Calorie, balance, basal metabolism, energy

CONTENT GENERALIZATIONS: The amount of energy that foods provide is measured in terms of calories. Different foods have different caloric values, depending on the energy potential of that food. All foods provide calories. The body needs a certain amount of calories a day to function. Every activity of life from jogging to breathing requires energy. This energy is measured in calories. *Basal metabolism* refers to the minimum amount of energy required to maintain vital body functions, such as nerve, heart, kidney function and muscle tone. If an individual is balancing the calories eaten daily with the calories used daily, body weight will stay the same. If more calories are eaten than are used daily, weight will increase.

MATERIALS
Carrot (1 large, fresh)
Transparency: *What Is a Calorie?* (Figure 12-7)
Measuring tape
Food scale or balance (optional)

INITIATION: "What Is a Calorie?"
Hold up a large fresh carrot for the class to view. Ask "What are some ways to measure this carrot?" Students should be able to come up with various ways to measure the carrot, including weighing it and measuring its length, circumference, and diameter.

As each way to measure the carrot is suggested, ask a volunteer to actually measure the carrot and record the measurement on the board.

Suggest that there is one more measurement we have not yet done. We have not measured the food energy potential of the carrot. In other words, we have not determined the number of calories in the carrot.

Using the transparency, *What Is a Calorie?* explain that calories are a measure of energy. All foods have calories. The number of calories depends on how much energy it takes the body to burn up the food. Calories can be determined by the carbohydrate, fat and protein content of a food. A food's water, vitamin, and mineral content does not provide any calories. The term, *Kilocalorie*, can be substituted for Calorie. (Students should recognize the "kilo" prefix is metric for 1,000 or 1,000 calories = 1 Calorie or 1 Kilocalorie.

Tell the student that the average carrot has 35 Calories and have a student record the calorie measurement for the carrot on the board.

MATERIALS
Magazines
Scissors
Glue
Index cards (several per student)
Books: Several calorie equivalent books (purchased in drug stores or supermarkets)

ACTIVITIES
1. The Calories Are Right—A Game
To help students become more familiar with the caloric value of foods, have them work in small groups to make various flash cards. On the front of the card they should place a picture of a food. (Pictures can be cut from magazines or drawn.) On the back of the card they should write the number of Calories provided by that food. Students must look up the Calories in books. It is optimum to have one Calorie equivalent book per group, but one book can be shared by all the groups. Using the flash cards, play "The Calories Are Right" game. This game is similar to the television game, *The Price is Right;* however, instead of guessing the correct price of items, students

"bid" on the correct Calories of different foods. Ask for four or five volunteers to be contestants. Show a picture of a food to the class and the contestants. Ask for bids on the number of Calories from the contestants only. Contestants should write their bids on the board. Then the teacher can ask the rest of the class which bid they think is the closest answer without going over the correct Calorie amount. Reveal the correct answer, and declare a winner for that round. The winner of the round stays for the next round, and new contestants are chosen. Continue playing the game until everyone has had an opportunity to be a contestant. The contestant who has won the most rounds is the class winner.

2. A Balancing Act

Write the word *balance* on the board, and explain that the next activity is based on the concept of balance in calorie intake and expenditure. Tell the students, "Each person has individual calorie requirements, depending on his or her energy needs. During periods of growth, more calories usually are needed. Students your age often are active and require more calories. Your estimated calorie requirements are between 2400 and 2800 Calories per day. These numbers can be higher or lower depending on the individual and how active he or she is."

Hand out the worksheet, *A Balancing Act.* Use a transparency made from the worksheet. Read number 1 on the worksheet, and tell the students to complete the answer to item a. Ask for a volunteer to share his or her answer. Explain that our calorie needs are related directly to the amount of energy we use. When we eat more calories than we use, the body stores the excess as fat. When we eat fewer calories than we use, the body uses the stored fat for energy. Ask the students to answer item 1.b. on their worksheet, and then discuss it. Ask, "What will happen to Jose's weight?" (It

will stay the same.) Have the students finish the worksheet individually, then discuss numbers 2 and 3. Ask, "What will happen to Dennis' weight?" (It will increase.) "What about Sara's weight?" (It will decrease.)

Explain to the students that this is a gradual process, that over time a person who eats more calories than he or she uses will gain weight, and a person who eats less calories than those used will lose weight.

Ask students, "Why is excess body fat a problem?" Most may respond that it is physically unattractive. However, you may wish to point out that in some cultures, excess body fat is a sign of wealth because one has enough resources to be overnourished. However, obesity (excess body fat) is linked to diseases, such as diabetes mellitus, heart disease, high blood pressure, and certain cancers.

Divide students into boys and girls. Each group is given some large sheets of dark-colored construction paper. Ask the students to discuss with their group what they believe is the ideal body image for a young man and a young woman. When they reach a consensus, have them draw their ideal male and female images on the paper and cut silhouettes. This task should take no more than 15 minutes. Ask a spokesperson from each group to show their ideal silhouettes; compare images for male and female between groups. How similar are they? If different, ask what factors account for the differences. Ideal body images are strongly influenced by cultural expectations. This often leads to eating disorders and low self esteem for people of all ages. Ask, "What other individual characteristics determine self-image?"

MATERIALS

Worksheet and transparency: *A Balancing Act* (Figure 12-8)
Transparency pen

3. Burn Up Those Calories

Have the students consult the library or health texts to find out which activities burn more or less calories. They should list the activities they like, then find out the number of Calories burned per hour for each activity. Tell them to include watching television as an activity if it is something they do often in their leisure time.

Then have students complete the worksheet, *Burn Up Those Calories*. Students are to find or draw a picture of their favorite snack, then find out the Calorie equivalent for that snack and record it. They should figure out how long it will take to burn off that snack by participating in one of the activities they listed previously.

MATERIALS

Library resource books with Calorie Expenditure Charts for various activities
Worksheet: *Burn Up Those Calories* (Figure 12-9)

EVALUATION: "Dear Barry . . ."

Read the following story to the students, and have them respond in writing.

Barry is a good student. He spends most of his time after school doing homework. When he is done with his homework, he likes to watch television. He has noticed lately that he has gained some weight. It is not very much, but he is a little worried. He wonders why this is happening. Explain to Barry why this is happening, and offer a suggestion as to how he can avoid a further weight gain.

In the responses to the story, students should explain to Barry that he is probably eating more calories than he is using. They could suggest that Barry get involved in something more active than watching television after school.

FIGURE 12-7

Transparency master

What is a Calorie?

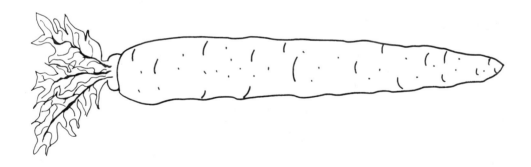

Calories are units of measure

8 INCHES: MEASURES THE LENGTH OF THIS CARROT

35 CALORIES: MEASURES THE AMOUNT OF HEAT ENERGY THIS FOOD CAN
                        PROVIDE

FIGURE 12-8

Worksheet   Name _____

A Balancing Act

1. Jose ate   During the day
   2400   +   he used 2400   =
   Calories.   Calories.

   a. Jose ate _____ Calories than
      he used.
      More   Less   The same

   b. In the box at the right, draw or
      write how this will affect his
      weight.

2. Dennis ate   During the day
   3000   +   he used 2000   =
   Calories.   Calories.

   a. Dennis ate _____ Calories than
      he used.
      More   Less   The same

   b. In the box at the right, draw or
      write how this will affect his
      weight.

3. Ana ate   During the day
   2000   +   she used 2800   =
   Calories   Calories.

   a. Ana ate _____ Calories than
      she used.
      More   Less   The same

   b. In the box at the right, draw or
      write how this will affect her
      weight.

FIGURE 12-9

Worksheet   Name _____

Burn Up Those Calories

Directions: 1. Find a picture of your favorite snack food and paste it in the box
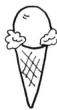
            below. (You may draw a picture of the food instead, if you like.)
        2. Look up the number of calories for that snack, and record it on the
            line under the box.
        3. Figure out how long it will take you to burn up that snack by
            participating in one of your favorite activities. (Find out information
            on how many calories are burned by different activities from books in
            the library or health texts.)

1. My favorite snack

2. _____ Calories

3. If I am _____, it will take me
          (Name of activity, e.g., jogging)

_____ minutes to use up the energy in the snack.

13 Disease Prevention and Control

When you finish this chapter, you should be able to:

- Differentiate among noninfectious, infectious and communicable diseases.
- Classify common modes of transmission for pathogens that cause disease in humans.
- Describe the most prevalant chronic, noninfectious diseases.
- Identify important lifestyle behaviors related to prevention of disease.
- Develop learning opportunities for elementary and middle school students in the area of disease prevention.

At the beginning of the twentieth century the leading causes of death in the United States were largely from diseases, such as pneumonia, influenza, and tuberculosis. With advances in medical science, we learned ways of preventing and controlling many diseases. These advances have increased life expectancy dramatically since 1900. Now more people die from cardiovascular diseases, cancer, and stroke.

Although these diseases generally affect people later in life, the chances of developing one of these conditions (and others, such as cirrhosis of the liver) are related to the lifestyle established early in life and to heredity. Even though the part that heredity plays has not been entirely determined, personal lifestyle choices involving good nutrition, exercise, avoidance of smoking, and good stress management can help prevent cardiovascular diseases. The development of cir-

rhosis of the liver is related to alcohol abuse, skin cancer to overexposure to the sun, and lung cancer to cigarette smoking. Hypertension, which is chronic high blood pressure, sometimes is controlled by lowering salt intake, not smoking, weight control, and regular aerobic exercise.

Studies on the relationship of lifestyle choices to the prevention of disease are continuing, and the information changes as new facts emerge. Most experts believe that the following factors contribute to longevity:

- Regular exercise (sustained aerobic exercise for at least 20 minutes, at least 3 times a week
- Good nutritional habits (a diet low in fats, sugar, and salt and high in fresh vegetables and fruits)
- Not smoking
- Regular use of safety belts

- Successful management of stress
- Abstinence or moderation in alcohol use
- Maintenance of a stable, normal weight

INFECTIOUS DISEASES

Microorganisms are minute living things that individually are too small to be seen with the naked eye. They are also sometimes called *germs* or *microbes*. Microorganisms are found almost everywhere. Most make important contributions by helping to maintain the balance of living organisms and chemicals in our environment. For instance, marine and freshwater microorganisms form the basis of the food chain in oceans, lakes, and rivers. Humans and many other animals depend on the bacteria in our intestines for digestion and synthesis of some vitamins, including some B vitamins for metabolism and vitamin K for blood clotting.

Only a minority of microorganisms are *pathogenic*, or disease-producing. Pathogenic microorganisms have special characteristics that allow them to invade the human body or produce toxins. *Infectious diseases* are illnesses caused by pathogenic microorganisms that invade and grow in the body.

One way of describing infectious diseases is by their mode of transmission. Any disease that spreads from one host or organism to another is called a *communicable* or *contagious disease*. Chickenpox, measles, genital herpes, and tuberculosis are examples. *Noncommunicable infectious diseases* are not spread from one host to another. These diseases are caused by microorganisms that normally live in the body and only occasionally cause disease, or by microorganisms that live outside the body and cause disease only when introduced into the body. An example is tetanus, which is introduced to the body through a wound.

Pathogens

Disease-causing organisms, or *pathogens*, that enter our bodies and resist our body immune system can flourish and produce illness or infection.

There are five major types of pathogens that cause infection in humans.

Bacteria are single-celled organisms that flourish in every environment. Important bacteria-caused diseases are typhoid fever, streptococcus and staphylococcus infections, tuberculosis, some sexually transmitted diseases, meningitis, and diphtheria.

Viruses are the smallest common pathogens. They are submicroscopic and difficult to study because they are not visible by regular light microscopes. Consequently there is still a great deal to learn about viruses. Some disorders that can be traced to viruses are the common cold, polio, viral hepatitis, smallpox, and AIDS. Researchers also believe that some cancers may be caused by viruses.

Protozoa are single-celled organisms larger than bacteria but not visible to the naked eye. Malaria is the best known disease caused by a protozoan.

Fungi are plantlike microorganisms that can live on the skin and cause disease. Athlete's foot and ringworm are caused by this pathogen.

Parasitic worms are not all microscopic but are important pathogens that cause significant infection. They are animals that live by obtaining the nutrients from a host, the organism that is infected with the worm. Tapeworms, pinworms, and roundworms are examples of parasitic worms.

Spread of Infection

For a disease to perpetuate itself, there must be a continual source of the disease pathogens. The source can be a living organism (human or animal) or an environment (soil, water) that provides a pathogen with adequate conditions for survival, multiplication and opportunities for transmission. These sources are called *reservoirs*.

The main living reservoir of human disease is the human body itself. Many people harbor pathogens and transmit them to others. People with obvious disease are transmitters. *Carriers* are people who act as reservoirs but have no outward evidence of disease. Some people have infections without having signs or symptoms of disease; others carry a disease during its symptom-free stages of incubation (before symptoms appear) or convalescence (recovery). Human carriers play an important role in the spread of diseases such as AIDS, diphtheria, typhoid fever, hepatitis, gonorrhea, amoebic dysentery, and streptococcal infections.

Both wild and domestic animals can be reservoirs of microorganisms that can cause human disease. People can become infected by direct contact with an animal. An example is rabies, which can be transmitted to humans by infected bats, skunks, dogs, cats, and foxes. Animals can be an indirect source of infection. This can occur if food or water is contaminated with animal wastes.

Infectious disease is spread by four routes: contact, a common vehicle, the airborne route, and vectors.

- **Contact** can be *direct* (through person-to-person contact, such as the common cold and sexually transmitted diseases), *indirect* (through a nonliving object, such as contaminated syringes that transmit HIV), or *droplet* (through saliva or mucous discharged into the air by sneezing, such as influenza).
- **Common vehicle** transmission means disease agents transmitted by an inanimate reservoir, such as food, water, drugs, or blood. Examples are food-borne salmonellosis (a type of "food poisoning") and water-borne shigellosis.
- **Airborne** transmission is infection by droplets or dust in the air that are inhaled. Q fever and histoplasmosis are transmitted this way.
- **Vectors** are animals that carry diseases from one host to another—such as the deer tick that transmits Lyme disease to humans.

Pathogens enter the body through a *portal of entry*, such as damaged mucous membranes or skin. For pathogens to cause disease in a population, they must also have a *portal of exit*—a way of leaving one host and moving on to the next. The most common portals of exit are the respiratory and gastrointestinal tracts. For example, respiratory infections often exit through the nose and mouth through coughing or sneezing. A healthy person becomes infected when they come in contact with the pathogen that is airborne in droplets.

Stages of Disease

A predictable sequence of events usually occurs when a person becomes infected and develops a disease. In order for disease to develop, there must be *predisposing factors*, conditions that make the body more susceptible to a disease. For example, inadequate nutrition and fatigue can be predisposing factors. Climate can also have an effect; during the winter there are more respiratory diseases, as people tend to stay indoors and have closer contact with one another.

Once a microorganism begins causing a disease, there are five steps that the disease course takes

1. *Period of incubation*—the time between actual infection with a pathogen and the first appearance of any signs or symptoms. This stage can vary in length from a few hours to a month or more, depending on the agent and the resistance of the host. A person can spread infection during this period.

2. *Prodromal period*—a short period of time following incubation in some diseases. Early, mild symptoms of the disease appear (such as a runny nose, watery eyes, and overall tiredness), the pathogen continues to multiply, and the host is now contagious. During this stage, hosts should stay away from others in order to protect them from infection.

3. *Period of illness*—also called the *acute* stage. This is the most uncomfortable stage, when all the signs and symptoms of the disease are seen. This is also the time when the likelihood of transmitting the disease is greatest. The body's defense mechanisms are marshalled, and the disease may be treated medically. Often,

these actions enable the body to overcome the illness.

4. *Period of decline*—the time when the signs and symptoms subside. The fever decreases, and the feeling of being ill diminishes.

5. *Period of convalescence*—the period when the person regains strength and the body returns to its pre-diseased state. This is also called recovery. It is important to know that people can spread infection during convalescence. For example, a person convalescing from typhoid fever or cholera can carry the pathogenic microorganism and infect others for months or even years.

Body Defenses Against Disease

The body has many natural defenses that help to protect from infection and disease. There are two general types of defenses —*mechanical* and *cellular.*

Mechanical defenses are "first line" defenses that physically separate the body from the external environment. Mechanical defenses include:

- *Skin:* Pathogens cannot enter the body through the skin unless a cut or opening is present. This is why it is important to keep sores and cuts clean.
- *Mucous membranes:* Mucous membranes are the tissues that line the openings of the body, the mouth, nose, and throat. Mucous is a sticky fluid that coats these body openings to trap dirt and pathogens.
- *Tears:* During every blink, tears wash the surface of the eyes to keep them clean. Tears contain chemicals that kill pathogens.
- *Hairs and cilia:* Tiny hairs and cilia in the nose filter the incoming air and shield against pathogens.
- *Ear wax:* Ear wax protects the ears by acting as a physical barrier to pathogens.

If the pathogens do get past these protective barriers, the body has a second line of defense: the cellular or *immune* system mentioned in Chapter 9. This complex system has two important components:

- *White blood cells:* These surround the pathogen and destroy it.
- *Antibodies:* Antibodies are substances that circulate in the bloodstream to help white blood cells identify and destroy pathogens.

Although we are born with the structural elements of immunity, our immune response must be "primed" to give us a state of *acquired immunity*. The development of acquired immunity can come about in several ways: naturally (by having disease), artificially (by vaccination), and passively (by receiving antibodies formed by others).

General Cleanliness Habits

In addition to the specific ways to prevent or control individual diseases described, there are some general cleanliness habits that can prevent infection and disease. Cleanliness habits are important because soap and water deter the growth of potentially harmful pathogens. General cleanliness habits for adults and children should include the following:

- Washing hands after using the bathroom and before eating
- Washing fruits and vegetables before eating them
- Washing cooking and eating utensils with hot, soapy water after each use
- Ensuring that hairbrushes, combs, towels, and toothbrushes are used by only one person and are washed regularly to help prevent the spread of disease
- Covering the nose and mouth when coughing or sneezing
- Immediately disposing of tissues after they are used
- Staying at home when ill to prevent transmitting the disease

NONINFECTIOUS DISEASES

The most important noninfectious diseases in the United States are the diseases often called *chronic diseases*. These are diseases that start slowly and develop over a period of years. (It should be remembered, though, that infectious diseases can also be chronic when they develop slowly and continue or recur for long periods of time—such as tuberculosis or leprosy.)

Chronic noninfectious diseases have varying causes. Some, such as diabetes, result from a metabolic defect, although they may be influenced by diet. Others, such as asthma, are frequently caused by allergies. Epilepsy is an electrical malfunction in the brain. Sometimes there is a hereditary predisposition to particular diseases.

Although biology, heredity, and environment contribute to diseases such as cancer, lung disorders, and cardiovascular disease, by far the leading cause is lifestyle. Because risk is linked to behavior, many diseases are preventable.

Cardiovascular Diseases

Cardiovascular diseases—diseases of the heart and blood vessels—account for nearly 50% of all deaths in the United States. Nearly one million people die of these diseases each year; this represents more deaths than result from all other causes combined. According to the American Heart Association, the five major forms of cardiovascular disease are coronary artery disease, hypertension, stroke, congenital heart disease, and rheumatic heart disease. A person may have one or several of these conditions at a time. Each condition can vary in severity, and all can cause damage to other body organs and body systems. The following information will describe the major forms of cardiovascular diseases: coronary artery disease, hypertension, and stroke.

Coronary Artery Disease   involves damage to the vessels that supply blood to the heart muscle. Most of this blood is supplied by the coronary arteries. Damage to these blood vessels can cause a reduction of blood (and oxygen and nutrients) to specific areas of the heart. The ultimate result is a heart attack.

In the development of most cases of heart disease, the major contributor is a condition called *atherosclerosis*, the buildup of fatty deposits called plaque on the inner walls of the arteries. The buildup reduces the blood supply to specific portions of the heart. When coronary arteries become narrowed, chest pain, or *angina pectoris*, may be felt. This usually occurs under stress or during strenuous exercise.

Some arteries can become so blocked that all blood flow is stopped. Heart muscle tissue begins to die when it lacks oxygen and nutrients. When this happens, there is a *myocardial infarction*, or heart attack. A heart attack can also result from a blood or fatty clot that blocks a coronary artery. Symptoms of a heart attack are uncomfortable pressure, squeezing, or pain in the center of the chest lasting two minutes or longer; pain spreading to the shoulders, neck or arms; and severe pain, dizziness, sweating, nausea or shortness of breath.

Elevated levels of serum cholesterol, a fatty substance manufactured in the liver and small intestine and needed for some body functions, are known to be associated with increased risk of atherosclerosis. About half of all Americans age 20 and older exceed the "borderline high" level of 200 mg/dl blood cholesterol, and about one in four adults has a "high" blood cholesterol level (240 mg/dl or greater).

Most people can reduce their serum cholesterol by making three dietary changes: eating less saturated fat; eating less dietary cholesterol; and lowering caloric intake. However, people's serum cholesterol will respond differently to these changes, and some will show no response. Other ways to reduce serum cholesterol are to exercise regularly and avoid smoking.

Hypertension refers to a consistently high blood pressure. Blood pressure is a measure of the force that your circulating blood exerts against the interior walls of your arteries and veins. Blood pressure is expressed as a fraction of *systolic pressure* (pressure when the heart contracts) over *diastolic pressure* (pressure when the heart relaxes). In general, concern over a young adult's blood pressure begins when there is a systolic reading of 140 or above and a diastolic pressure of 90 or above. More than 60 million American adults and children have hypertension. African Americans have a one-third greater

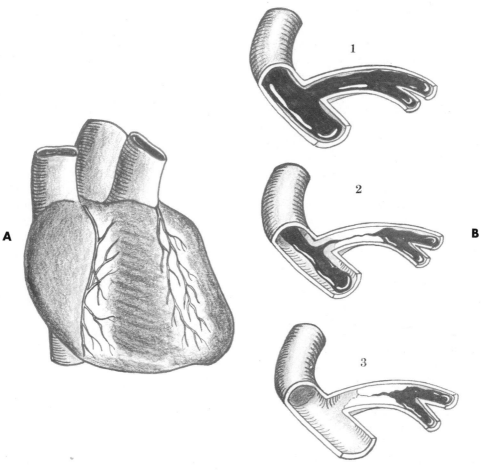

FIGURE 13-1
Progression from normal coronary arteries to arteries with atherosclerosis. A, The
heart showing right and left coronary arteries. **B,** The development of atherosclerosis: *1,* normal
blood flow; *2,* plaque build-up, restricted flow; *3,* completely blocked artery.

risk of developing hypertension than do white
Americans.

Many people with hypertension are unaware
of their condition. Uncontrolled hypertension is
dangerous, since it accelerates atherosclerosis,
requiring the heart to work much harder to pump
blood through narrowed vessels and causing
heart attack or heart failure. Hypertension also
accelerates *arteriosclerosis* (hardening of the arteries), making the vessel less elastic and more
susceptible to bursting.

To reduce hypertension, it is important to exercise regularly, reduce weight, decrease alcohol
use, and restrict the use of sodium or salt. Stress
reduction activities may also be helpful.

Strokes result from blood vessel damage in
the brain that often results from hypertension.
They are also called *cerebrovascular accidents.*
African Americans have a 60% greater risk of
stroke than white Americans, probably because
of the higher rate of hypertension among African
Americans.

Cardiovascular Risk Factors. A cardiovascular risk factor is a personal characteristic that increases the likelihood of developing some form of cardiovascular disease. There are some risk factors that a person can change and others that cannot be changed. Those that cannot be changed include heredity, sex, and age.

The major risk factors for most cardiovascular diseases are cigarette smoking, hypertension, high serum cholesterol, lack of exercise, and a family history of heart disease before age 60. Most health professionals agree that atherosclerosis and stroke are largely lifestyle diseases. Positive lifestyle changes can reduce a person's chances of developing certain cardiovascular diseases. Modifying exercise and eating habits, achieving optimal body weight, and stopping smoking can substantially reduce your risk.

Cancer

Cancer is the second leading cause of death for adults in the United States. It is a disease in which the mechanism that regulates normal cell behavior goes out of control. As a result there is uncontrolled growth of abnormal cells in the tissues and organs of the body. There are over 100 diseases included in the definition of cancer.

Cancer cells usually form a mass called a *tumor* in tissues and organs of the body. Some tumors are *benign,* or noncancerous, and do not spread to other tissues of the body. Others are *malignant,* or cancerous, and they invade or destroy surrounding tissue. Cancer spreads when some malignant tumor cells are shed and move into the lymphatic system or bloodstream, which carries them to other parts of the body. This process is called *metastasis.* Once a cancer has metastasized, it is much harder to treat, and the outlook for survival is less favorable.

The most common cancers in the United States are skin cancer, breast cancer, lung cancer, colorectal cancer, and prostate cancer.

Seven Warning Signs of Cancer. The American Cancer Society has identified seven key warning signs of cancer. These can alert an individual to possible cancerous growths:

1. *C*hange in bowel or bladder habits.
2. *A* sore that does not heal.
3. *U*nusual bleeding or discharge.
4. *T*hickening or lump in the breast or elsewhere.
5. *I*ndigestion or difficulty in swallowing.
6. *O*bvious change in a wart or mole.
7. *N*agging cough or hoarseness.

Other signs include rapid weight loss, persistent headaches along with visual or behavior changes, continuing abdominal pain, prolonged tiredness, and excessive or unexplained bruising. While these symptoms are not definite indicators of cancer, they should be checked by a physician if they persist for more than a few days.

Causes of Cancer. Cancer is thought to be caused by repeated or prolonged contact with cancer-causing agents called *carcinogens.* Suspected carcinogens include the tar in tobacco smoke, certain industrial chemicals, and ultraviolet radiation from the sun. Many years may pass between exposure to a carcinogen and evidence of disease. Heredity and possibly some bacterial and viral infections put some people at greater risk of developing cancer.

Treatment Methods. Treatment methods depend on the type of cancer and stage of the disease, but all aim to remove the abnormal cells as completely as possible. The earlier the cancer is identified, the better the chances for successful treatment.

Today almost half of all cancers can be cured completely through surgery, radiation therapy, or medications (chemotherapy). Combinations of treatments have also been effective. Currently there are some experimental methods being used to treat cancer, including the use of hormones and other biological agents to stimulate the body's immune system to attack malignant cells (*immunotherapy*).

Cancer Prevention. The key to prevention is to live in a way that reduces your exposure to risks. It is also important to be aware of the role of heredity. If cancer is prevalent in your family, you can act in ways that reduce your risk. For example, if you are a woman with a family history of breast cancer, it will be critical for you to carry out monthly breast self-examinations—which are recommended for all women but are especially necessary for you.

Other preventive measures include the following:

- Select your occupation carefully. Be aware of risks associated with certain jobs and avoid exposure to carcinogenic agents.
- Don't use tobacco products. About 30 percent of all cancer deaths are caused by cigarette smoking. Smoking is considered the number one preventable cause of death.
- Eat a healthy diet including foods high in fiber and low in saturated fats; avoid burning or overgrilling meat; and limit foods that are high in nitrites. Foods that are rich in Vitamins A and C (such as broccoli, spinach, carrots, peaches, and citrus fruits) may lower the risk of developing certain cancers.
- Control body weight. Obesity is related to a higher incidence of cancer of the uterus, ovary, and breast.
- Limit exposure to the sun and avoid unnecessary X rays.
- Drink alcohol moderately, if at all.

SUMMARY

In this chapter, we discussed the two major categories of disease—infectious and chronic, noninfectious. In the United States, most deaths are caused by the chronic, noninfectious diseases, especially cardiovascular diseases and cancer.

Infectious diseases are caused by pathogenic microorganisms that are harbored in living and nonliving "reservoirs" and can enter a "host" to cause disease. Infectious diseases that spread from one host to another are called communicable or contagious.

Five major types of pathogens cause disease in humans: bacteria, viruses, protozoa, fungi, and parasitic worms. Ways of spreading disease in a population are by contact, by common vehicle, by airborne transmission, and by vectors that carry diseases from one host to another.

Cardiovascular diseases and cancer are the two most significant chronic noninfectious diseases. While family history (genetics) plays a significant role in the development of these diseases, it is possible to alter one's lifestyle to reduce the risk of getting them and control some of their effects if they do develop.

REFERENCES

1. Communicable diseases. *Macmillan health encyclopedia*, vol 2, New York, 1993, Macmillan.
2. Hales D, Williams B: *An invitation to health.* Menlo Park, Calif, 1986, Benjamin/Cummings.
3. Lammers J: *I don't feel good. A guide to childhood complaints and diseases*, Santa Cruz, Calif, 1991, Network Publications.
4. Noncommunicable diseases and disorders. *Macmillan health encyclopedia*, vol 3, New York, 1993, Macmillan.
5. Payne W, Hahn D: *Understanding your health*, ed 3, St. Louis, 1992, Mosby.
6. Stang L, Miner K : *Disease and its prevention: health factors for teachers*, Santa Cruz, Calif, 1994, ETR Associates.
7. Tortora G, Funke B, Case C: *Microbiology. An introduction*, ed 7, Redwood City, Calif, 1991, Benjamin/Cummings.
8. U.S. Department of Health and Human Services, Public Health Service: *Healthy people 2000: National health promotion and disease prevention objectives*, DHHS Publication No. (PHS)91-50212, Washington, DC, 1990.

LEARNING OPPORTUNITIES FOR DISEASE PREVENTION AND CONTROL

PRIMARY LEVEL

OBJECTIVE: The student explains the difference between illness and wellness.

LEVEL: Kindergarten and grade 1

INTEGRATION: Reading, writing, language arts

VOCABULARY: Sick, ill, well, thermometer, fever, absent

CONTENT GENERALIZATIONS: Our degree of health may vary from day to day. Generally, when a person is ill, a disease, (severe or mild) is involved. The degree of illness or wellness usually affects the way we feel and the type of activities in which we can (or should) be involved. Most illnesses are accompanied by symptoms. If someone is ill, usually rest is recommended.

INITIATION: "Being Absent"
Read the following story, and follow up with the discussion questions.

BEING ABSENT

It was a beautiful Monday morning at school. When the school bell rang, Mrs. Owen opened the classroom door, and all the children in her first grade class filed in. Mary noticed that the place where her friend Judy sat was empty. When Mrs. Owen called the roll, Judy did not answer. Mrs. Owen said Judy was absent. Mary wondered where she was.

Ask the following discussion questions:
1. Why do you think Judy was absent? (She was ill.)

2. Have any of you been absent? Why?

3. What kind of illness did you have?

4. How did you feel when you were ill?

ACTIVITIES

1. Why Was Judy Absent?

a. Continue the story started in the initiation.

WHY WAS JUDY ABSENT?

On Sunday Judy felt fine. She went to the park with her dog Tippi and played fetch. She and Tippi ran all the way home. Later Sunday night Judy started to cough; she felt tired and did not want to play with Tippi. Her dad felt her forehead with his hand and said. "You feel warm; maybe you have a fever. I'll take your temperature." Sure enough, Judy's temperature was 101° Fahrenheit (F). She had a fever. So her dad put her to bed and said, "You are sick, and you need to rest to get well."

NOTE: Decide if the use of a Fahrenheit or centigrade thermometer is more appropriate for the students in your class.

The last time she had been sick, she had had to go to the doctor. She wondered if she would have to go again. On Monday morning Judy's fever was down to 99° F. Her mother said she should stay home from school until she was completely well again. On Tuesday, Judy's dad took her temperature again, and it was normal, so he said, "You can go to school today." Mary and Judy played as usual at school that day.

b. Discussion questions
  - Why was Judy at school Tuesday and not Monday? (She was ill on Monday.)
  - Was it a good idea for Judy to stay home from school on Monday? (She still had a fever.)

2. Who Should Stay Home?

Hand out and explain the worksheet *Who Should Stay Home?* (Maria is sneezing, feels tired, and has a fever; Donald feels good and full of energy and is happy.) Ask the children if they think either of the children should stay home from school. Have the students cut out the picture of the child who should stay home and paste that picture inside the house on the worksheet. Students then can take the worksheets home and explain them to their parents.

MATERIALS

Worksheet: *Who Should Stay Home?* (Figure 13-2)

Scissors

Paste or glue

3. Reading a Giant Thermometer

a. Show the children the *Giant Thermometer* (previously made from pattern.) Explain its purpose. Ask the children if anyone has ever had their temperature taken. Ask, "Has anyone ever had a fever? How did you know you had a fever?"

b. Place the *Giant Thermometer* on the bulletin board. Tell the children that this thermometer reads "normal." Then show various pictures of well children and explain that they probably have normal temperatures and are not sick. Ask the children to try to think of activities they like to do when they are well. Ask "Is it possible to do the things you like to do when you are sick? Why or why not?"

MATERIALS

Pattern: *Giant Thermometer* (teacher made) (Figure 13-3)

Pictures of well children having fun (skating, riding bicycles, playing games, etc.) from magazines or children's books

4. When We Are Well

Send a note home to parents explaining that their child is learning about illness and wellness. Ask the parents if they could send a photograph of their child to school. The photograph should be of the child when he or she was well and preferably doing something enjoyable. When the photographs are brought from home, have the children mount them on a piece of construction paper. Then put all the photographs on the bulletin board next to the *Giant Thermometer* with the title, "When We Are Well." This activity could be done with pictures cut from magazines or drawn by students if the teacher determines that photographs from home will be difficult to obtain.

MATERIALS

Letter to parents
Construction paper
Photographs of students from home, if possible

EVALUATION: "Who Is Well? Who Is Ill?"

Hand out the worksheet, *Who Is Well? Who Is Ill?* Ask the students to identify the child who looks ill and to explain how they can tell. Help them complete the words *ill* and *well* on the worksheets. They should color the well child and circle the ill child.

MATERIALS

Worksheet: *Who is Well? Who Is Ill?* (Figure 13-4)
Crayons

FIGURE 13-2

Worksheet

Name _____

Who Should Stay Home?

Maria is sneezing.
She feels tired.

Donald is smiling.
He feels good.

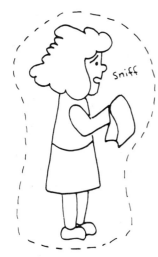

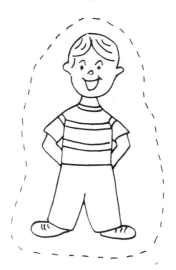

Cut out the picture of the
child who should stay home.

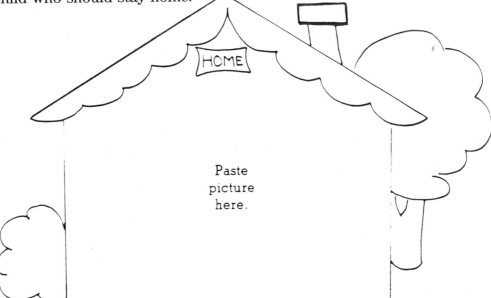

HOME

Paste
picture
here.

FIGURE 13-3

Pattern Name _____

Giant Thermometer

Directions:

1. Make a large thermometer out of white construction paper.

2. Mark the degrees in black.

3. Make a very large black line for 98.6° F (normal).

4. Make a long strip of construction paper, half red and half white.

5. Move it through the slits to demonstrate the way the thermometer works.

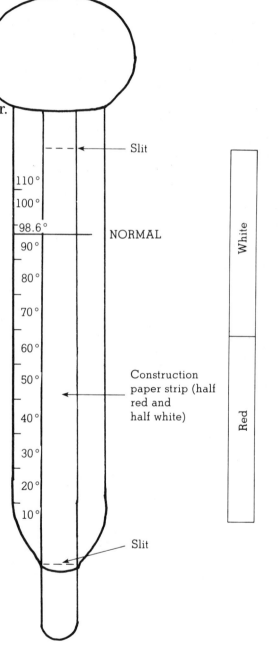

FIGURE 13-4

Worksheet

Name _____

Who Is Well? Who Is Ill?

Directions:
1. Circle the ill child.
2. Finish the words.
3. Color the well child.

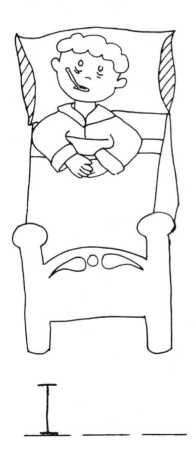

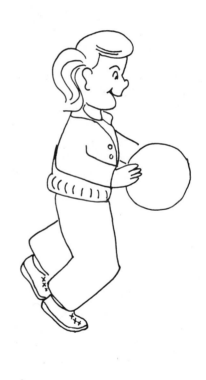

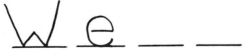

INTERMEDIATE LEVEL

OBJECTIVE: The student differentiates between control of infectious diseases and of noninfectious diseases.

LEVEL: Grades 4 to 6

INTEGRATION: Science, language arts, dictionary skills

VOCABULARY: Lifestyle, infectious, noninfectious, pathogens, heredity, environment

CONTENT GENERALIZATIONS: All women, men, and children are susceptible to both infectious diseases and noninfectious diseases. Infectious diseases are communicable diseases in which a person serves as a host to an invading pathogenic agent. Infectious diseases are best controlled by prevention. Preventive measures include immunizations, minimizing exposure to pathogenic agents, and isolation during the contagious stage. Examples of infectious diseases are colds, measles, influenza, sexually transmitted diseases, and rabies.

Noninfectious diseases are often diseases associated with lifestyle, environment, and heredity. Examples of noninfectious diseases are cardiovascular diseases, cancer, allergies, and arthritis.

INITIATION: "The Contagious "Handshake" Disease"

Ask every student in the class to stand and shake hands with five students. Allow them to move around the room quickly to do this. Encourage them to shake hands with both good friends and those whom they do not know particularly well. When the handshaking is done, everyone should sit down again.

Have two students who are seated in different parts of the room stand. (Try to choose students who are not easily embarrassed.)Then ask all the students who shook hands with these two students to stand. Tell the rest of the seated students that they should stand if they see someone standing with whom they shook hands. Eventually the entire class should be standing.

When all the students are standing, ask, "What if Mary and Joe (the names of the first two students) had a disease that could be transferred by a handshake?" (The entire class would have been exposed.) Explain that a disease that can be "caught" is called an infectious disease. Reassure students that Mary and Joe do not have a disease that is transferred by a handshake, but if they did, all students in the class would have been exposed. Write the word *infectious* on the blackboard and ask, "Who knows what this word means?" Through discussion with the students, reveal the meaning to be "catchable, transferable, and spreadable." Write descriptive words such as these under *infectious*. Similarly, write the word *noninfectious* on the blackboard, and ask for the meaning of this antonym. Terms such as "not catchable, not spreadable, and not transferable" should be suggested. List these words under *noninfectious*.

Inform the students that some diseases are infectious (transferable usually from person to person), whereas others are noninfectious and cannot be transferred from person to person.

ACTIVITIES

1. **What Kind of Disease?**
   a. Divide students into six groups. Hand each group one *What Kind of Disease Card*. Instruct the groups to do the following:
      ▪ Determine which of the diseases are infectious and which are noninfectious.
      ▪ Use health books, encyclopedias, or other references to find the information.
      ▪ For the diseases that are infectious, identify the way each is spread and controlled.
   b. On the board or on two large pieces of butcher paper, start two lists. Label one *infectious* and the other *noninfectious*. As the groups determine the category for the diseases on their card, they are to list them in the appropriate spot.

c. Ask a representative from each group to briefly explain the spread and control of the infectious diseases they studied.

MATERIALS

Teacher resource: *What Kind of Disease Cards* (a different card for each of the six groups) (Figure 13-5)
Reference materials: encyclopedias, health books, pamphlets, charts
Optional: butcher paper (two large pieces), felt pens

2. What are Infectious Diseases?

a. In a full group discussion and lecture, present these concepts. Infectious diseases can be spread through disease-causing microorganisms (pathogens) that can be transferred from person to person or animal to person. Each type of pathogen causes a particular type of disease. The spread of infectious diseases can be prevented through *immunizations* (vaccines). We do not have vaccines for all infectious diseases. (An example of an immunization is a vaccine for some types of measles.) A second preventive measure is *isolation* during the contagious stage (an example would be staying home from school when you have the chickenpox). A third way is *minimizing your exposure* (an example would be not going to your cousin's house when you know that he or she has been exposed to mumps and probably will be getting mumps). And finally, *taking care of yourself* and staying healthy is important. People who get enough sleep, eat the right foods, etc., are more able to resist the pathogens and resist getting a cold for instance.

b. Briefly review the four ways that infectious disease can be controlled, as discussed previously. Write them on the board if necessary. Have the students divide a piece of paper into four squares and draw a picture

that represents each of the ways to prevent the spread of infectious disease. Post the finished pictures on the bulletin board near the list of infectious diseases.

MATERIALS

Paper
Rulers
Crayons or felt pens

3. What Are Noninfectious Diseases?

a. Review the concept of infectious diseases and the definition of pathogens. Referring to the two lists of diseases, explain that noninfectious diseases cannot be transferred from person to person or animal to person. Through full group discussion, lecture, and use of the blackboard, present these concepts. Noninfectious diseases are not caused by pathogens. Noninfectious diseases result from how we live, the environment in which we live, and genetic weaknesses and resistances to disease that we inherit. An example of *heredity* is a person might be born with an inherited disease such as sickle cell anemia or hemophilia. Noninfectious diseases can be caused by *lifestyle*, or how one lives. A person who is overweight, gets little exercise, and smokes is more likely to suffer a heart attack. People who smoke or chew tobacco are more likely to develop oral and lung cancer. People cannot be immunized against noninfectious diseases. They cannot change their heredity; however, in some cases they can develop a healthful lifestyle to prevent or lower the risk of noninfectious diseases, and in other cases there are medical treatments available.

b. Discussion questions
   ▪ Why do immunizations not work against noninfectious diseases such as heart disease or emphysema? (There is no pathogen to isolate and make a vaccine.)

NOTE: There is current research regarding the possibility that viruses are related to cancer. Research eventually may produce vaccines for what are now viewed as noninfectious diseases as knowledge in medical science increases.

- How does lifestyle help prevent infectious, as well as noninfectious, diseases?
NOTE: AIDS is an excellent example of an infectious disease that is controlled by lifestyle choices. However, the example should only be used if students have had the opportunity to study this disease prior to this lesson.

4. What Do You Recommend?

Choose student volunteers to role play each of the following situations. Students may take turns being the patient with a disease and a physician who listens and discusses the problem. The student playing the patient should read the lines indicated, and the health educator should make up a response to the question.

SITUATION 1

Patient: I need help. What do you recommend? I just had a slight heart attack and recovered after being in the hospital for a month. I do not want another heart attack. *Can you tell me where I can get an immunization against a heart attack?*
Physician:

SITUATION 2

Patient: I am just about over my cold. I have had it for 3 days and feel much better. I cough and sneeze but only have a slight temperature. I am going back to work this afternoon. *Do you think this all right?*
Physician:

EVALUATION: "Preventing Disease"

Have each student complete the worksheet, *Preventing Disease.* Grade the worksheets, and return them to the students.

Suggest that the worksheets be taken home and shared with parents.

MATERIALS

Worksheet: *Preventing Disease* (p. Figure 13-6)

FIGURE 13-5

Teacher resource	Name ______________
What Kind of Disease Cards	
1. **Hepatitis (viral)** **Emphysema** **Mumps** **Measles (rubella)**	**4.** **Sickle cell anemia** **Rabies** **High blood pressure** **Cholera**
2. **Chickenpox** **Stroke** **Tetanus** **Heart attack**	**5.** **Rheumatic fever** **Influenza** **Mumps** **Diphtheria**
3. **Diphtheria** **Lung cancer** **Ringworm** **Influenza**	**6.** **Skin cancer** **Chickenpox** **Ringworm** **Emphysema**

FIGURE 13-6

Worksheet   Name _____

Preventing Disease

1. Molly has the chickenpox, an infectious disease. She has itchy spots all over
   her stomach and her face. Tell Molly one way the chickenpox might have
   been prevented.

2. Harry had a heart attack, a noninfectious disease. He is resting in bed, as
   recommended by the doctor. Tell Harry one way his heart attack might have
   been prevented.

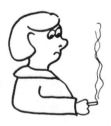

3. How are infectious diseases and noninfectious diseases different?

MIDDLE SCHOOL LEVEL

OBJECTIVE: The student analyzes the relationship of personal lifestyle choices to disease prevention.

LEVEL: Grades 6 to 8

VOCABULARY: Cardiovascular disease, hypertension, cancer, cirrhosis, lifestyle

CONTENT GENERALIZATIONS: People who get regular exercise, eat nutritious diets, avoid tobacco use, manage stress, and maintain an ideal weight increase their resistance to disease. It is also important to avoid contact with infectious diseases. All of these behaviors are lifestyle choices that each person must make individually. Some choices will contribute to health and help prevent disease, whereas others will increase the risks of developing a disease.

INITIATION: "Lifestyle Quiz"

Write the words *lifestyle choices* on the board, and ask the students what they mean. (The choices that we make regarding habits that affect our health.) Explain to students that habits established now can help prevent disease and prolong life. Hand out the worksheet, *Lifestyle Quiz*. Explain that this quiz is personal and will not be collected or graded. It is a way to look at current lifestyle choices to get an idea of the risk we have of contracting a disease as an adult.

MATERIALS

Worksheet: *Lifestyle Quiz* (Figure 13-7)

ACTIVITIES

1. Case Studies

Tell the students that they will be researching various diseases which are particularly affected by lifestyle choices. They are to do this research in groups and report their findings to the rest of the class. Each group will be given a case study about a person with a certain disease. The groups should do the following:

- Find out about the disease that affects the person in their case study.
- Identify the health habit choices of the person in their case study that may have contributed to the disease.
- Find out what, if any, treatment or changes in health habits can help this condition.
- List the various lifestyle choices that teenagers can make which could help to prevent this disease.

Hand out the worksheet, *Case Studies*, and allow class and library time to work on the reports. Tell the groups that they may want to prepare visual aids such as transparencies or posters for their reports. As each group presents a report, tell the rest of the class to record the health lifestyle choices discussed. When all the reports are finished, review the lists of choices accumulated, and summarize them on the board. They should include the following:

- Do not smoke or use other tobacco products.
- Get good nutrition (limit fatty foods, salt and sugar; eat more fresh fruits and vegetables).
- Get regular exercise.
- Control weight.
- Avoid overexposure to the sun.
- Do not use alcohol or other drugs.
- Learn how to manage stress.

2. Talking With Parents

Have the students rewrite the *Lifestyle Quiz* so that it is appropriate for adults. Suggest that they give it to their parents. (Giving the quiz to parents should be optional.)

MATERIALS

Worksheet: *Case Studies* (one case study per group) (Figure 13-8)

EVALUATION: "How's Your Lifestyle?"

Ask the students to analyze the lifestyle choices of two hypothetical teenagers in the worksheet, *How's Your Lifestyle?* Hand out a worksheet to each student, and explain the directions. They are to read about the lifestyles of each person and then determine if the choices are *excellent, average,* or *poor* for preventing disease later in life. Students also must explain why they think the lifestyle is excellent, average, or poor based on what they have learned about habits that promote or harm health.

MATERIALS

Worksheet: *How's Your Lifestyle?* (Figure 13-9)

FIGURE 13-7

Worksheet   Name _____

Lifestyle Quiz

Directions: In each of the areas below, circle the number that best describes your habits. Then total the number for each area, and find out what your scores mean on the next page.

CIGARETTE SMOKING

If you never smoke, enter a score of 10 and go on.

	ALWAYS	SOMETIMES	ALMOST NEVER
1. I avoid smoking cigarettes.	10	1	0

SMOKING SCORE _____

ALCOHOL AND DRUGS	ALWAYS	SOMETIMES	ALMOST NEVER
1. I avoid drinking alcoholic beverages.	4	1	0
2. I avoid using drugs (especially illegal drugs) as a way to handle problems	2	1	0
3. I do not drink alcohol or take other medicines.	2	1	0
4. I read the label and follow the directions on all medicines.	2	1	0

ALCOHOL AND DRUG SCORE _____

EATING HABITS	ALWAYS	SOMETIMES	ALMOST NEVER
1. I eat a variety of foods from each of the food groups.	4	1	0
2. I limit the amount of fatty foods I eat, such as butter, fat on meat, eggs, and shortening	2	1	0
3. I limit the amount of salt that I eat by not putting it on food at the table, not cooking with it, and not eating salty snacks.	2	1	0
4. I avoid eating too much sugar (especially candy and soft drinks).	2	1	0

EATING HABITS SCORE _____

EXERCISE AND FITNESS	ALWAYS	SOMETIMES	ALMOST NEVER
1. I maintain a desired weight and am not overweight or underweight.	3	1	0
2. I do hard exercise for 15 to 30 minutes at least three times a week (like running, swimming, or hard bicycle riding).	3	1	0
3. I do strength exercises for muscle tone for 15 to 30 minutes at least three times a week (like calisthenics, weight lifting, or yoga).	2	1	0
4. I use part of my leisure time for participating in sports activities.	2	1	0

EXERCISE AND FITNESS SCORE _____

Modified from Healthstyle: a self test, U.S. Public Health Service.

Continued.

FIGURE 13-7 cont'd

Worksheet   Name _____

Lifestyle Quiz

STRESS CONTROL	ALWAYS	SOMETIMES	ALMOST NEVER
1. I enjoy school or have a hobby I enjoy.	2	1	0
2. It is easy for me to relax and express my feelings.	2	1	0
3. I know what kind of situations make me feel stress.	2	1	0
4. I have close friends or relatives to talk to about my problems.	2	1	0
5. I belong to a club or have a group of friends that I enjoy.	2	1	0

STRESS CONTROL SCORE _____

SAFETY	ALWAYS	SOMETIMES	ALMOST NEVER
1. I wear a safety belt when riding in a car.	3	1	0
2. I avoid riding in cars with drivers who are under the influence of drugs or alcohol.	3	1	0
3. I obey traffic rules when riding a bicycle or walking.	2	1	0
4. I am careful when using potentially dangerous products or substances such as household cleansers, poisons, and electrical devices.	2	1	0

SAFETY SCORE _____

What your scores mean to YOU

Scores of 9 and 10
   Excellent. Your answers show that you are aware of the importance of this area to your health. More important, you are putting your knowledge to work for you by practicing good health habits. As long as you continue to do so, this area should not pose a serious health risk. It's likely that you are setting an example for your family and friends to follow. Since you got a very high test score on this part of the test, you may want to consider other areas where your scores indicate room for improvement.

Scores of 6 to 8
   Your health practices in this area are good, but there is room for improvement. Look again at the items you answered with a "Sometimes" or "Almost Never." What changes can you make to improve your score? Even a small change can often help you achieve better health.

Scores of 3 to 5
   Your health risks are showing! Would you like more information about the risks you are facing and about why it is important for you to change these behaviors? Perhaps you need help in deciding how to successfully make the changes you desire. In either case, help is available.

Scores of 0 to 2
   Obviously, you were concerned enough about your health to take the test, but your answers show that you may be taking serious and unnecessary risks with your health. Perhaps you are not aware of the risks and what to do about them. You can easily get the information and help you need to improve, if you wish. The next step is up to you.

FIGURE 13-8

Worksheet   Name _____

Case Studies

Lewis has just found out that he has hypertension.* He is 40 years old with a wife and two sons. He has a good job working in a bank. His boss does get on his nerves sometimes, and Lewis comes home in a bad mood. Lewis loves to eat steak and big batches of french fires with lots of salt. His wife fixes this meal often because it helps Lewis get out of his bad mood. Even though Lewis likes all kinds of sports, he spends more time watching them on television than actually participating. Therefore he has put on a few extra pounds in the last few years. He is really not certain what hypertension is and what he can do about it. Help Lewis out.

  1. Find out what hypertension is. What does this disease do to the body?
  2. What habits does Lewis have that may make the disease worse?
  3. What can be done about the disease (treatments and changes in habits)?
  4. What lifestyle choices can teenagers make that could help prevent this disease?
*Contact the American Heart Association for information on hypertension.

Jayne has skin cancer.* She is a very active woman of 38 years. She seems to be outdoors most of the time, both at work and at home. She loves to snow ski, garden, jog, and play tennis. Everyone is jealous of her wonderful year-round tan. She eats well, avoiding fatty and salty foods. She is also at her ideal weight. Jayne is a bit confused about why she has cancer. She lives such a healthy life. She would not think of smoking a cigarette, so why does she have cancer?

  1. Find out what skin cancer is. What does it do to the body?
  2. What life-style choices in Jayne's life could be the reason for her cancer?
  3. What can be done about the disease (treatments and changes in habits)?
  4. What lifestyle choices can teenagers make to help prevent this disease?
*Contact the American Cancer Society for information on skin cancer.

Harry has just suffered from a mild heart attack.* The physician said he needs to change some habits to prevent another attack. After all, he is only 42 years old with a daughter in junior high school. He has a good job as a stock broker. There is often a lot of pressure in the job, which is why he likes to come home and collapse in the chair with a drink, a cigarette, and some pretzels. Harry admits that he smokes too much, but it helps calm him down from his demanding job. He says he does not have time to exercise because of his job, his daughter, and his wife. The only free time he has is on Sundays, and then he likes to watch sports on television with the guys and eat chips, hamburgers, and beer.

  1. What is a heart attack? What happens to the body?
  2. What habits does Harry have that may have caused the heart attack?
  3. What can be done about someone who has a heart attack (treatments and changes in habits)?
  4. What choices in their lifestyles can teenagers make to prevent heart attacks?
*Contact the American Heart Association for information on heart attacks.

Continued.

FIGURE 13-8 cont'd

Case Studies

Shelia has emphysema.* She is 50 years old and has smoked cigarettes since she was 16. When she started smoking, it was very popular with her friends. She always thought she could quit whenever she really wanted to. Now her physician says she has to stop smoking cigarettes. Shelia is not certain she has the will-power to do it now. Cutting back to one pack a day has not seemed to help her gasping for air. It is still very difficult to breathe. She wonders, "Why bother to stop smoking all together?"

   1. What is emphysema? What does it do to the body?
   2. What habits does Shelia have that may be related to the disease?
   3. What can be done about the disease (treatments and changes in habits)?
   4. What choices can teenagers make in their lifestyle that can help prevent this disease?
*Contact the American Lung Association for information on emphysema.

Dennis has just been to the physician and found out that he has lung cancer.* He is 64 years old and is almost ready to retire. He has always been healthy—you have to be to work in construction. The only time he can even remember being sick was a few years ago when he had the flu. That is why he was never worried that he smokes two packs of cigarettes a day. His father smoked until he died of a heart attack at age 69. Dennis has always watched his weight and his diet. He does not eat salty foods and prefers fish and chicken to steak. He thinks the physician must be mistaken and that is too healthy to have cancer.

   1. What is lung cancer? What does it do to the body?
   2. What habits does Dennis have that may have caused the disease?
   3. What can be done about the disease (treatments and changes in habits)?
   4. What lifestyle choices can teenagers make to avoid getting lung cancer?
*Contact your local American Cancer Society for information on lung cancer.

Douglas has cirrhosis of the liver. He has always been a sociable guy. Everyone likes him. He usually stops by the local bar after work and has a few drinks with friends before going home. When he gets home, he has a few beers and watches television. Because he is single, he usually does not cook dinner for himself. He eats whatever he can find in the house. That often means hot dogs, potato chips, and beer. Sometimes he only has the beer. Douglas has never had a problem with his weight, even though he does not exercise. Why does he have cirrhosis of the liver?

   1. What is cirrhosis of the liver? What does it do to the body?
   2. What habits does Douglas have that may have caused the disease?
   3. What can be done about the disease (treatments or changes in behavior)?
   4. What lifestyle choices can teenagers make to prevent this disease?

FIGURE 13-9

Worksheet   Name _____

How's Your Lifestyle?

Directions: Read the following lifestyle choices for Mary and Steve. Decide if the
choices are excellent, average, or poor for preventing diseases later in
life. Explain why.

Mary is 16 years old. She is a good athlete and plays on several
school teams. She also jogs and rides her bicycle regularly with her
father. Sometimes she plays tennis with her mother. She enjoys being
active. Mary and her friends like to go to the movies and roller skating.
Once in a while some of her friends smoke cigarettes and drink. Mary
tried it one time, but did not like it, so she drinks cola instead of beer.

Mary watches what she eats. When she eats at home, she gets lots of
fresh fruits and vegetables, and her family has learned to enjoy foods
without adding salt. When she does out to eat with her friends, she does
eat fatty foods like french fries, hamburgers, and milkshakes.

How do you think Mary's lifestyle rates for preventing diseases later in
life? (Circle one)

        EXCELLENT   **AVERAGE**   **POOR**

Explain why:

Steve is 15 years old. He loves fried foods with lots of salt. He has
the menus of all the fast-food restaurants in town memorized! All his
friends hang out at the hamburger stand near school. Often they smoke
cigarettes and drink colas all afternoon. Steve usually meets his friends
there except during baseball season. Then he plays on the school team.
Baseball is really the only sport Steve is interested in. He is a good
catcher.

Steve likes to go to the movies too. Sometimes he and his friends sneak
beer into the theater. One time they got caught, and the theater manager
called their parents. Steve's mom was really mad, so he does not do it
much anymore.

How do you think Steve's life-style rates for preventing diseases later in
life? (Circle one)

        EXCELLENT   **AVERAGE**   **POOR**

Explain why:

14 Preventing STD and HIV: A Special Concern

When you finish this chapter, you should be able to:

- Define STD and HIV.
- Describe ways to prevent STD and HIV infection.
- Classify the behaviors most risky for the spread of HIV.
- Develop learning opportunities appropriate for elementary and middle school students.

STD and HIV are acronyms for crucial health concerns in this nation and the entire world. STD stands for *sexually transmitted disease.* STD is spread through sexual contact. HIV stands for the *human immunodeficiency virus,* which is transmitted sexually as are many other viruses and bacteria.

The most common STDs are chlamydia, gonorrhea, genital warts, herpes, syphilis, hepatitis B, and urinary and vaginal infections. Some are more easily treated than others. **ALL** are preventable. In fact the best way to avoid any health problem related to STD is to prevent contracting the infection.

SEXUALLY TRANSMITTED DISEASES

STDs, including HIV, are caused by various microorganisms that are spread through vaginal, anal, or oral intercourse. Anyone who is sexually active can contract STD and HIV regardless of race, sexual orientation, age, or gender. Some STDs are treatable; others are not.

The microorganisms, such as viruses and bacteria, that cause STDs are usually very fragile. They die easily when exposed to light and air. Furthermore, they usually need warm, dark, moist environments to grow and spread. The mucus linings of the vagina, penis, anus, and mouth are prime environments for these germs. Any break in the skin or damage to the mucous linings can allow the microbes to enter the body.

Each STD affects the body differently. In some cases, the infection is generally localized, affecting the genital areas and urinary tract. In others, like syphilis and AIDS, the microorganisms can spread into the blood and damage other parts of the body. In all cases, STD is serious. If not treated, STD can lead to long-lasting health problems, including sterility, nerve damage, and in the case of HIV/AIDS, death.

Signs and Symptoms

There are certain signs and symptoms that can mean you have an STD. Anyone who thinks they might have an STD needs to seek medical attention.

Following are some of the things to watch for:

- An unusual discharge from the anus, vagina, or penis
- Sores, blisters or bumps around the genitals or mouth
- Burning and pain during urination
- Swelling or redness in the throat
- Flulike feelings with fever chills and aches
- Swelling in the groin or around the genitals
- Pain in the pelvic area (for women)
- Burning and itching around the vagina (for women)
- Bleeding between menstrual periods for women
- Deep pelvic pain during intercourse for women

STD Prevention

There are two ways to help prevent STD infection. The surest way is to not have sexual intercourse, which is called *abstinence*. If abstinence is not the choice, then using a latex condom during every act of sexual intercourse provides a considerable degree of protection from STD infection including HIV. Using a contraceptive foam or jelly with nonoxynol-9 increases the protection. However, some people are allergic to nonoxynol-9. Only consistent use of condoms will provide protection. However, condoms only cover the penis. STD can be transmitted when body parts not protected by a condom make contact. Furthermore, condoms can break or slip off.

Couples thinking about engaging in sexual intercourse should talk about it. This is often difficult to do. But an important part of a relationship is open and honest communication. Unfortunately, not everyone is honest about their sexual histories. Talking about using protection against STD is essential.

HUMAN IMMUNODEFICIENCY VIRUS

As indicated, HIV is a virus. It is the virus that causes *acquired immunodeficiency syndrome* (AIDS). HIV attacks the immune system and damages the body's ability to fight off disease. A person who is infected with HIV will test HIV positive after undergoing special medical testing. People with HIV are said to have HIV infection or be HIV positive. An HIV-positive person's condition can range from healthy to very sick. However, people can live for many years (over 10 years) without showing any signs or symptoms. Currently, millions of people are believed to be infected with HIV and don't even know it.

AIDS

AIDS is the stage when an HIV-positive person's immune system no longer functions properly. When this happens, the body is vulnerable to many other diseases and infections. Many of these diseases are rarely seen when one's immune system is healthy. A diagnosis of AIDS is made when a person develops one or more specific conditions that indicate critical impairment of the immune system. These conditions include *Pneumocystis carinii* pneumonia (PCP) and Kaposi's sarcoma (KS). These are referred to as opportunistic diseases because a healthy immune system protects against infection. When one's immune system has been damaged by HIV, these rare infections have an opportunity to cause disease. Often HIV dementia and a wasting syndrome associated with HIV infection develop. To date, there is no vaccine to prevent HIV infection and no cure.

Symptoms of HIV

HIV can live in the body for many years without any symptoms. When symptoms do show up, they often are similar to those of minor illnesses or other infections. However, with HIV, the symptoms either don't go away or keep coming back. See your doctor if the following persist:

- Unexplained weight loss greater than ten pounds
- Recurring fever and/or night sweats
- Unexplained persistent tiredness
- Chronic diarrhea
- Swollen lymph glands
- Unexplained persistent dry cough
- White spots or unusual sores on the tongue or mouth

The only way to be certain of their significance is to be tested for HIV.

HIV Testing

HIV testing can indicate if a person has been infected with HIV by detecting the antibodies of such an infection. Since there is a possibility that false results can occur, a series of tests are performed on the same blood sample. Since it takes time to develop antibodies (usually about 3 months), a person recently exposed may have negative results. It is usually recommended that 2 tests approximately 6 months apart be taken. This assumes that no HIV-related risk behavior has occurred. Tests are widely available in public clinics, hospitals, doctor's offices, and many college campus clinics.

Other HIV Transmission

HIV can be tranmitted in other ways than through sexual contacts. HIV can get into the blood in other ways. Any needle use can be risky. Sharing needles for injection drugs, tattoos, ear piercing, or use of injectible steroids is high-risk behavior. This is why used needles are carefully disposed of in medical settings. Formerly, blood transfusions and use of blood products were a source of infection. However, today the risk of contracting HIV from receiving a blood transfusion or blood product is very low.

A mother infected with HIV can pass the virus on to the child either before birth or during birth. There are a few known cases in which HIV has been passed from mother to child through breast milk.

You don't get HIV from normal day-to-day contact between people. HIV is not transmitted through the air. You don't get it from the following:

- Touching, coughing, sneezing, or dry kissing
- Contact with toilet seats, eating utensils, water fountains, or telephones
- Hugging or touching
- Swimming pools, restrooms, or gyms
- Being close to other people, such as on a bus
- Mosquito or other insect bites
- Donating blood
- Tears or saliva

Figure 14-1 indicates the relative risk of various behaviors.

Protecting Yourself

You can protect yourself from STD and HIV by abstaining from sex. This is the only method that is truly effective all the time. You must, however, also avoid "dirty" needles.

If you are sexually active, condoms and contraceptive foam or jelly that contains nonoxynol 9 are very effective. However, condoms must be used *every single time* to reduce the risk of HIV. This method also prevents pregnancy. It is important to note, however, that some people are allergic to nonoxynol 9. Although no method can be 100% protective ("safe sex"), reducing the risk by practicing "safer sex" behaviors is possible.

Sex without the use of condoms is only safe if both partners are monogamous and are not infected. However, serial monogamy (only sexually involved with one person for a period of time such as in a relationship) is very risky. Many young people think that they are not at risk for STD, including HIV because they are monogamous when in a relationship. This is a myth. You must recognize that your partner may have been sexually active prior to "settling down" with you.

Don't use needles for injections unless for medical or dental use and under the supervision of a health-care worker. These people are trained to use hypodermic needles properly and with the least amount of risk. If you are unwilling to seek treatment for injection drug use, do not share

HIV Risk Behaviors

NO RISK	SOME RISK	RISKY

Massage
Receiving a
  blood transfu-
  sion today >>
Dry kissing
Abstaining
  from sex
Fantasizing
Masturbation
Hugging
Donating blood

Maintaining
  a lifetime,
  mutually
  monogamous
  relationship
  with an
  uninfected
  partner who
  does not use
  injection drugs
French kissing
Properly using
  condoms with
  nonoxynol-9
  or other
  spermicide
Mutual
  masturbation

Unprotected
  oral sex>>
<<Cleaning
  spilled blood
  without
  wearing
  gloves
<<Reusing a
  needle that
  has been
  cleaned with
  bleach

<<Breast-
  feeding by an
  infected mother
Intercourse
  using an oil-
  based lubri-
  cant and
  condom

Unprotected
  vaginal sex
Using the same
  condom twice
Anal sex

Sharing
  needles for
  anything,
  including
  injecting
  drugs, ear
  piercing,
  tattooing,
  and injecting
  steroids or
  vitamins
Reusing a
  needle that
  has been
  cleaned with
  water

<<This behavior could move slightly toward the left of the continuum.
>>This behavior could move slightly toward the right of the continuum.

Adapted from Collins JL, Britton PO: *Training educators in HIV prevention*, Santa Cruz, Calif, 1990, ETR Associates.

FIGURE 14-1
HIV Risk Behaviors.

needles. If you ignore the risk and do share needles, clean with bleach and water before use.

Treatment

Prevention is the only "vaccine" at this time. There is no cure for HIV infection. Although research is underway, a true cure is certainly many years away if it is ever possible. There are some treatments to slow down the progression of HIV infection that have been positive. And, some people are living much longer than expected with HIV infection. Responsible health practices have been thought to be very helpful in prolonging life.

A national AIDS hotline provides 24-hour,

confidential information, including referrals and educational materials. The hotline's toll-free numbers are 1-800-342-AIDS (English); 1-800-344-7432 (Spanish); 1-800-243-7889 (TDD/Deaf Access).

SUGGESTED READINGS

Barth R: *Reducing the risk: building skills to prevent pregnancy, STD and HIV*, ed 2, Santa Cruz, Calif, 1993, ETR Associates.

DeVault C, Strong B: *If you are a man . . . understanding STD*, Santa Cruz, Calif, 1993, ETR Associates.

Hiatt J: *STD facts*, Santa Cruz, Calif, 1989, ETR Associates.

Quackenbush M, Villarreal S: *Does AIDS hurt? Educating young children about AIDS*, ed 2, Santa Cruz, Calif, 1992, ETR Associates.

Quackenbush M, Clark K, Nelson M, eds: *The HIV Challenge: Prevention Education for Young People*, ed 2, Santa Cruz, Calif, 1994, ETR Associates.

LEARNING OPPORTUNITIES FOR PREVENTING STD AND HIV INFECTION

STD, including HIV infection naturally fall in the disease prevention and control content area. However, because of the seriousness and sensitivity of this topic, a separate chapter is provided.

Prevention of STD, including HIV infection, is critical, and instruction must start in elementary schools. Elementary teachers often question the reason for placement of this topic in the elementary curriculum. While most children are not at risk for HIV and other STDs, the fact is that some children do become infected. This fact necessitates that we assist children in preventing infection. It is important to remember with this topic that the information and learning opportunities must be developmentally relevant. It is, however, essential for teachers to be sensitive to the concerns of children and to be alert to the possibility of child abuse. Children who are sexually abused often will ask specific questions and may appear more knowledgeable than their peers.

It is not necessary to provide specific information if children are not developmentally ready for that information. Most of the learning opportunities for primary level children about STD, including HIV, will be embedded in lessons about disease. At this level, most often teachers need to be able to answer questions that come up about STD and HIV infection as a part of a general disease prevention lesson. HIV infection and STD can naturally be included when dealing with the concept that some diseases are infectious and some are not. *STD and HIV infection are infectious diseases that are very difficult to transmit, particularly for children.* This is an important point to make for young children.

When dealing with this topic, as well as other health topics, it is the role of the teacher to empower students with both information and skills to make decisions that keep them healthy. With increased media coverage and general openness about HIV infection and AIDS, it is safe to say that most children and adolescents in elementary school and middle school have some knowledge about STDs. However, it is also safe to say that the level and accuracy of their information is limited. Because of a variety of reasons, including children's limited amount of information, this topic is often scary. A general and important point to make for all students is that STD, including HIV, infection is easy to prevent.

The skills for prevention are far more important for their education than specific information about symptoms of diseases, treatments, or how they are spread. The **basic** behaviors that children and adolescents need to know about preventing HIV infection and STD are the following:

- Avoid all hypodermic needles, and tell a responsible adult if you see one
- Avoid contact with anyone else's blood
- Abstain from sexual activity

For younger children, the basic information is directly related to concepts about prevention of infectious disease in general. Children at the primary level learn the difference between sickness and illness, about germs (bacteria, viruses and other microorganisms), and that there are basic preventive measures for most diseases. These concepts lay the foundation for children understanding more specific information about preventing STD, including HIV, at an older age.

Specific lessons on HIV infection and AIDS are most appropriate at the intermediate level. At this level, students learn about the disease. In middle school, more emphasis is given to the value of abstinence as a means to prevent infection, as well as pregnancy. A school district must determine the appropriateness of lessons related to "safer sex." This may be an appropriate topic for some middle schools because of the prevalence of sexually active students. The appropriateness depends on the needs of the students in that community. If students in middle school are sexually active, lessons on safer sex are important. It is, however, a decision that must be made at the school board level. Teachers should not take it on themselves to teach about safer sex if it has not been approved by the board.

The following is a learning opportunity that serves as one example of how HIV can be addressed in the classroom. This lesson could be introduced at the intermediate level, but would also be appropriate at the middle school level. It must be reemphasized that even though this example is presented as appropriate for intermediate and middle school students, all lessons regarding HIV must be approved specifically by administrators in the school district. The learning objectives for children are the same as those for Chapter 13.

INTERMEDIATE LEVEL

OBJECTIVE: The student will be able to demonstrate how HIV infection (AIDS) affects the functioning of the immune system.*

LEVEL: Grades 4 to 6

VOCABULARY: AIDS, HIV virus, germs, immune

CONTENT GENERALIZATIONS: For this lesson, examples are woven into the description of the activities as is the style for the entire *Growing Healthy* Program referred to in Chapter 3.

INITIATION: "Germs, Germs, Germs"
Explain that germs are often the cause of disease. Tell students germs are so small that they can only be seen with powerful microscopes. Ask students to brainstorm ways that germs can enter the body. Tell them that a healthy immune system works to destroy all types of germs includ-

---

*Adapted from *AIDS and the immune system. A lesson for young people: Growing healthy: AIDS integration*, New York, 1988, National Center for Health Education

ing bacteria and viruses. Ask a student to tell what is meant when someone is "immune" to something. Help students to conclude that it means "protected" or "safe."

ACTIVITIES
1. Demonstration of the Immune System
  a. Hold the two ends of a 6 ft hose in one hand so the hose forms a circle, illustrating the skin as a barrier to keep germs out. As long as the skin remains uninjured, it holds the body's insides in and keeps the rest of the world safely out.
  b. Reveal the break in the hose and explain that when there is a break in the skin, germs can enter. Have students name ways that breaks occur (cuts, scratches, punctures, etc.). Review proper care for breaks in the skin. (Wash with soap and water to kill germs.)
  c. Lay the hose on a flat surface where it can be seen by students and roll the tennis balls and golf balls into the circle through the break in the hose (skin). These balls represent bacteria. The bacteria are large germs and are plentiful. Roll in the marbles, explaining that these represent viruses, very small germs.
  d. Tell them that our blood contains white blood cells that fight germs. One kind of white blood cell (phagocytes) moves through the blood and tissues to surround and eat germs. Use the sock puppet to demonstrate the action of the phagocytes (The sock puppet engulfs the marbles as a phagocyte engulfs germs.)
  e. Another kind of white blood cell produces chemicals, called antibodies, that destroy bacteria and viruses. Write "antibodies" on the chalkboard. These cells that produce antibodies are B-cells. Add B-cells to the circle.
  f. T-cells are another type of white blood cells that help fight germs. Some T-cells attack and destroy viruses. Other T-cells direct the battle. Add T-cells to the circle. Explain

that some T-cells serve as "command centers" for the body's battle against germs.

MATERIALS
6 foot hose
Tennis balls (3)
Golf balls (3)
Marbles (4)
Sock puppet (teacher-made)
Foam cut in "T" shape (3)
Foam cut in "B" shape (3)

g. Tell students that some of the antibodies stay in your blood and protect you in case you are exposed to the same disease again. That is immunity.

   Another way to get immunity for some diseases is by having a vaccine. We do not have vaccines for all diseases.

h. Conclude the demonstration by saying that the immune system works 24 hours a day in every part of the body to ensure good health.

2. **Discussion**
   a. Ask students what happens when the "command center" in a real battle involving soldiers is destroyed? Help students to conclude that germs could attack the white blood cells (in particular, the T-cells) that control the body's immune system; they could cripple the body's ability to fight off disease and infection.
   b. Ask if any students are aware of a new disease that results when the immune system is destroyed (AIDS). Explain that AIDS is a disease caused by a virus called HIV (the AIDS virus). Once HIV destroys the "command centers" (T-cells) of the immune system, the body cannot defend itself against infections. The person infected with HIV does not die of AIDS but of other diseases that the body can no longer fight off. Most often, people with AIDS die of a type of cancer or pneumonia. Many people are infected with HIV, and many people have died. It is a serious health problem.
   c. How do you get infected with HIV? Explain that HIV is very fragile. It dies in air and light. HIV can be passed on when infected body fluids enter another body. This can occur through sexual contact with a person who has the virus. Some babies have been infected with HIV because their mother had the virus in her blood when she was pregnant. Since we now know more about HIV and AIDS, women who want to have a baby can have a test to see if they are HIV infected before they get pregnant.
   d. Ask students if they have heard of any other ways that people can become infected with HIV. Write the words "IV drug use" on the board and explain that people who abuse drugs using needles to put the drugs directly into their veins are at great risk. Sharing a needle with a person who is infected with HIV risks exposure to the virus. Doctors and nurses are very careful when using hypodermic needles. Most of the time the needles used for giving shots or for giving blood are only used once and then disposed of. Students do not need to worry about needles used by doctors or nurses for medical reasons.
   e. Ask students if they have any ideas how to prevent the spread of HIV. Help them to conclude that avoiding sexual contact (sexual abstinence) is a sure way and the appropriate way for young people to avoid the virus. Avoiding the use of IV drugs is another preventive behavior. If they have any other specific questions about AIDS they should ask a trusted adult, a doctor, or call the local AIDS Hotline. Students can usually get the local Hotline number from the telephone directory or the directory operator.

EVALUATION: The Immune System Demonstration Revisited

Using the materials for the demonstration of the action of the immune system, have students take turns rolling the tennis balls, golf balls and marbles and explaining what each represents. Students then should use the sock puppet to demonstrate the action of the white blood cells. Students should "throw" in the foam "T" shapes and "B" shapes and explain their role in the func-tioning of the immune system. In the demonstration, students should explain how HIV destroys the immune system. As each student demonstrates, other students in the class should critique the demonstration.

MATERIALS

Sock puppet (teacher-made)

15 Injury Prevention and Safety

When you finish this chapter, you should be able to:

- Define injury prevention.
- Analyze situations for strategies for injury prevention.
- Explain guidelines for preventing injuries in a variety of settings and situations.
- Describe emergency and first-aid procedures.
- Develop learning opportunities for elementary and middle-school students in the area of injury prevention.

The major causes of death for children and adults have changed in the last 40 years. The ability to control disease, in particular infectious diseases such as polio, diphtheria, and pneumonia, has been a major factor. Injuries are a major public health problem. Although many infectious diseases are on the decline, injuries continue to threaten lives, particularly those of children and youth. In fact, injury is considered today's primary public health problem for Americans under the age of 40 years.

An important part of understanding injury prevention is related to the change in the terminology associated with this content area. The word *accident* is not used. An accident implies an unavoidable event. Many if not most injuries are the consequences of an event that was avoidable. The use of terms such as *injury control* and *injury prevention* rather than *accident prevention* helps clarify the potential for preventing these events. Injuries can be categorized as in-tentional (deliberate), such as in homicide and suicide, or unintentional (accidental), such as a fall or motor vehicle crashes. In both cases, prevention is the key to avoiding the injury event.

STRATEGIES FOR INJURY PREVENTION

Education/information and behavior change are key factors in injury prevention. People need to learn what behaviors are safer than others and choose to behave in a safe manner to prevent injuries. For example, one of the most important behaviors in the prevention of injury from motor vehicles crashes is the use of safety belts. Individuals need to know that safety belts work and how to properly use them. This is the education (information) part of injury prevention. The second and critical part of injury prevention relates to behavior. Individuals need to be motivated to use safety belts every time they get into a car. The motivation part of this prevention effort is different for every individual. Children who have been taught to use a safety belt and who see adults model similar behavior will most likely adopt this behavior easily. Others may find it difficult to adopt this habit.

Another important strategy to assist in preventing injuries is legislation (policy). Legislation and policy assist with the motivational aspect of injury prevention. It is a method for applying standards for expected behavior and an indication that consequences may apply. For example, many states have laws that require the use of safety belts. This is an example of legislation. However, systems for regulation and enforcement must be in place for laws to be effective. Traffic citations are used to encourage compliance with the law.

Prevention strategies are often most successful when used together. Another important strategy is technology. Significant engineering and technology advancements have occurred in the area of passenger restraints. Specifically, many motor vehicles have passive restraints. This means that they do not require an individual to take action or behave in a certain way. Air bags release on impact. Some safety belt chest straps are *automatically* in place when the door of the motor vehicle is closed. However, in most cases the lap belt still needs to be buckled for the passenger to be safe. The use of safety belts can save lives and prevent serious injury in a motor vehicle crash, but only about 60% of older children, adolescents, and adults use them consistently.

Technology has been an important injury prevention factor in many other areas as well. This is demonstrated in the development of protective equipment for recreation and sport, nonflammable materials for use in children's sleepwear, and smoke detectors.

Although education, laws and passive restraints help encourage the use of a product designed to promote safety, the modeling children observe will have the greatest impact on behavior.

Injury prevention strategies are complex and involve many aspects of society, including individuals, government, law enforcement, education, medical care, and emergency response mechanisms. Education and information are critical in influencing individual behavior.

SAFETY AT HOME

Many injuries occur in the home. Approximately 1 person in 10 is injured in the home each year. There are several ways to prevent injuries in the home. Knowing potential hazards and correcting them whenever possible help prevent injuries. The box lists common hazards in the home.

Most families should have a home safety plan that all family members know. Children as young as 3 or 4 years of age can learn the basics of injury prevention at home. In addition, they can be taught how to react in an emergency situation. It is particularly important for all family members to know how to react in case of fire. Following are steps to take in case of fire:

- Feel a door for heat before opening. If it does not feel warm, take a peek before opening.
- If there is smoke, crawl low and get out.
- If you are on fire—STOP, DROP, and ROLL.

Smoke detectors are lifesavers. Proper installation and regular checking are important steps

---

COMMON HOME HAZARDS

- Improper storage of poisonous or flammable chemicals, knives, and medicines
- Overloaded electrical outlets
- Open cupboard doors and drawers
- Improper storage of electrical appliances and tools
- Loose throw rugs (without rubberized backing)
- Poor lighting
- Clutter—particularly on steps
- Handles on pots and pans on the stove that protrude

to ensure continued effectiveness of this device. They assist in early warning of smoke and fire. Other important lifesavers are knowing two exits to every room and planning for the possibility of fire. Safety ladders should be available for exits from second and third floors.

One important aspect of fire safety is practice. Role playing what to do in case of a fire is invaluable. It clarifies and imprints actions to take, which is particularly vital for young children.

MOTOR VEHICLE AND PEDESTRIAN SAFETY

Motor vehicle occupant death rates peak from ages 16 to 19 years. Males are at the highest risk. Alcohol is an important contributor to traffic crashes that result in fatalities or serious injuries. It cannot be stressed enough how important the above the guidelines listed in the box are essential for preventing injury from crashes. The behavior choices, in particular the choice to wear a safety belt and not to operate a motor vehicle after drinking alcohol, significantly reduce the risk of injury or death due to traffic crashes.

Passengers have less control than drivers of behavior choices that can reduce the risk of injury. However, passengers can make personal decisions over the use of safety belts. In addition, passengers can and should refuse to ride in a car (or any other vehicle) driven by a driver who has been drinking.

RECREATIONAL SAFETY

Recreation is an important part of American life. From bicycling to aerobics and boating to hiking, recreation often involves activities that can put

---

TIPS FOR SAFE CYCLING

- Make sure your bicycle is in good working order—check the brakes and chain before riding.
- Use a light, reflective clothing, and reflectors on the bike, particularly in dim light or at night.
- ALWAYS wear a helmet.
- Follow all traffic laws.
- Avoid riding in rain or other bad weather conditions.
- Be aware of changes in the riding surface.

VEHICLE SAFETY FOR DRIVERS

- Know and follow traffic laws.
- Only operate vehicles that are in good working condition.
- Observe speed limits.
- ALWAYS wear safety belts, and require all passengers to wear appropriate restraints.
- NEVER drink alcohol and drive.
- Keep music or other noise to a reasonable level.
- Drive (or ride) defensively.
- Carry a first-aid kit.
- In bad weather, slow down and drive (ride) even more carefully.

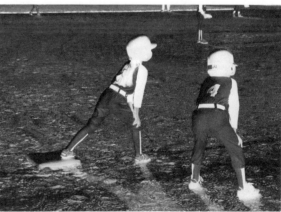

John Sabo

FIGURE 15-1
Safety in Sports.   Proper safety equipment is an important part of baseball. Note that both runner and base coach wear helmets.

TABLE 15-1

Preventing Sports/Activity Injuries

Sport/Activity	Common Site for Injury	Protective Strategy
Basketball	Knees, back, legs	Wear proper footwear
Baseball	Shoulder, elbows	Warm up, stretch, avoid muscle overuse
Ballet	Knees, feet, spine	Warm up, stretch, strengthen muscles
Biking	Skin (bruises, cuts), head	Bike on path or smooth surface, wear helmet, obey traffic laws
Gymnastics	Knees, back, shoulder	Warm up, stretch, strengthen muscles
Walking	Entire body (hit by car)	Wear reflective clothing at night, walk facing traffic, walk on sidewalk
Hockey	Knees, face, mouth	Warm up, wear protective gear
Running	Shin, foot, knee	Wear proper running shoes, run on a soft surface rather than pavement
Swimming/diving	Shoulders, broken neck, drowning	Warm up, check depth of water and current, do not swim alone, do not use drugs or alcohol

TABLE 15-2

First Aid

Specific Problem	What to Do
Asphyxiation	
Victim stops breathing and skin, lips, tongue, and fingernail beds turn bluish or gray.	Adult: Tip the head back with one hand on the forehead and the other lifting the lower jaw near the chin.
	Look, listen, and feel for breathing.
	If the victim is not breathing, place your mouth over the victim's mouth, pinch the nose, get a tight seal, and give 2 full breaths.
	Recheck the breathing; if the victim is still not breathing, give breaths once every 5 seconds for an adult, once every 4 seconds for a child, and once every 3 seconds for infants (do not exaggerate head tilt for babies).
Bleeding	
Victim bleeding severely can quickly go into shock and die within 1 or 2 minutes.	With the palm of your hand, apply firm, direct pressure to the wound with a clean dressing or pad.
	Elevate the body part if possible.
	Do not remove blood-soaked dressings; use additional layers, continue to apply pressure, and elevate the site.
Choking	
Accidental ingestion or inhalation of food or other objects causes suffocation that can quickly lead to death. There are over 3,000 deaths annually, mostly of infants, small children, and the elderly.	The Heimlich maneuver must be learned from a qualified instructor. The procedure varies somewhat for infants, children, adults, pregnant women, and obese persons.

TABLE 15-2—cont'd

First Aid

Specific Problem	What to Do
Hyperventilation Victim breathes too rapidly, often as the result of fear or anxiety. It may cause confusion, shortness of breath, dizziness, or fainting. Intentional hyperventilation before an underwater swim is especially dangerous because a swimmer may "pass out" in the water and drown.	Have the person relax and rest for a few minutes. Provide reassurance and a calming influence. Having the victim take a few breaths in a paper bag (not plastic) may be helpful. Do not permit swimmers to practice hyperventilation before attempting to swim.
Bee Stings Victims are not especially endangered except for persons who have developed an allergic hypersensitivity to a particular venom. Those who are not hypersensitive experience swelling, redness, and pain. Hypersensitive persons may develop extreme swelling, chest constriction, breathing difficulties, hives, and shock signs.	For nonsensitive persons, scrape the stinger from the skin and apply cool compresses or over-the-counter topical preparation for the insect bites. For sensitive persons, get professional help immediately. Scrape the stinger from the skin, position the person so that the bitten body part is below the level of the heart, help administer prescribed medication (if available), and apply cold compresses.
Poisoning Poisoning can often be prevented with adequate safety awareness. Children are frequent victims.	Call the poison control center immediately; follow the instructions provided. Keep syrup of ipecac on hand.
Shock A life-threatening depression of circulation, respiration, and temperature control is recognized by a victim's cool, clammy, pale skin; weak and rapid pulse; shallow breathing; weakness; nausea; and unconsciousness.	Provide psychological reassurance. Keep victim calm and in a comfortable, reclining position; loosen tight clothing. Prevent loss of body heat; cover the victim if necessary. Elevate legs 8 to 12 inches (if there are no head, neck, or back injuries or possible broken bones involving the hips or legs). Do not give food or fluids. Seek further emergency assistance.
Burns Burns can cause major tissue damage and lead to serious infection and shock.	For minor burns, immerse the area in cold water and then cover it with sterile dressings; do not apply butter or grease to burns. For major burns, seek help immediately, cover the affected area with large quantities of clean dressings or bandages, and do not try to clean the burned area or break blisters. For chemical burns, flood the area with running water.
Broken Bones Fractures are a common result of car accidents, falls, and recreational accidents.	Do not move the victim unless absolutely necessary to prevent further injury. Immobilize the affected area. Give care for shock while waiting for further emergency assistance.

individuals at risk for a variety of injuries. The same strategies apply for preventing injury in recreational situations as in any other situation. Education/information, behavior choices, laws, and technology are a part of injury prevention for recreational injuries.

Bicycling is a sport and a means of transportation for millions of people. Preadolescents are at the highest risk of injuries related to bicycles. Most deaths occur from collisions with motor vehicles and usually involve head injuries. Serious injuries that are not fatal are often the result of falls. The peak time for these injuries are the after-school hours of 3:00 to 7:00 P.M.

One important factor in saving lives and preventing serious injuries related to bicycles is the correct use of helmets. Technology has contributed greatly in the design of lightweight but sturdy helmets that protect the head, particularly in crashes with motor vehicles. Even so, less than 10% of the nation's 85 million bicycle riders use helmets. Helmets can prevent injuries (education/information) if used consistently. In some states, laws require helmet use for cyclists, particularly young cyclists. The strategies listed in the box can be effective in reducing the injuries related to cycling.

SPORTS AND SAFETY

Sports are the most frequent cause of nonfatal injuries that require medical attention. These injuries occur most often to males and females between the ages of 13 and 19 years. Physical contact is a major factor in sports-related injuries. Therefore there is a high rate of injuries in football and basketball. These injuries are usually trauma to the face, head, mouth, and eyes. Equipment such as mouth protectors and face guards have helped reduce injuries, particularly in football.

There are several important factors in the prevention of sports injuries. Qualified, trained coaches are important. Mandatory use of protective gear and maintenance of grounds help. However, an important part of preventing sports inju-

ries is education. You should know what the risks are for a sport and take action to prevent injury. Recommendations for some selected sports and activities are shown in Table 15-1, p. 372.

RESPONDING TO EMERGENCIES

Knowing what to do in an emergency is important. If someone is hurt, you must first make a decision about obtaining medical care. Many injuries, such as sports injuries, need attention but not emergency medical attention. In the case of a sports injury ask questions about how the injury occurred. Does it hurt? How much? Does it

---

SEVEN STEPS FOR ARTIFICIAL VENTILATION

1. **Tap and shout,** "Are you okay?" If no response, proceed to the next step.
2. **Check for a pulse** by placing two fingers (not the thumb) on the neck, just to the side of the trachea.
3. **Tilt the head,** with the chin pointing up. Place one hand under the head and gently lift. At the same time, push with the other hand on the victim's forehead. (This moves the tongue away from the back of the throat and opens the airway.)
4. Immediately place your cheek and ear close to the victim's mouth and nose. **Look** for the chest to rise and fall. **Listen** for air exchange. **Feel** for air blowing on your cheek.
5. For an adult, pinch the nostrils, take a deep breath, and blow into the mouth **two quick full breaths.** (For a baby, cover the nose and mouth with your mouth and give puffs of air.)
6. **Look, listen, and feel for air.** If there is still no breathing, proceed to the next step.
7. **Give 1 breath every 5 seconds** for an adult. To count each 5 seconds, blow, then say, "one thousand, two thousand, three thousand, four thousand." Blow, then continue the sequence. (Continue until help arrives or the victim starts breathing.)

TABLE 15-3

Epilepsy: Recognition and First Aid

Seizure Type	What It Looks Like	Often Mistaken For	What to Do	What Not to Do
Convulsive Generalized tonic-clonic, (grand mal)	Sudden cry, fall, rigidity, followed by muscle jerks, frothy saliva on lips, shallow breathing or temporarily suspended breathing, bluish skin, possible loss of bladder or bowel control, usually lasting 2-5 minutes; normal breathing then starting again; some confusion and/or fatigue possible, followed by return to full consciousness	Heart attack, stroke, unknown but lifethreatening emergency	Look for medical identification Protect the victim from nearby hazards Loosen the victim's tie or shirt collar Place a folded jacket under the head Turn victim on the side to keep the airway clear; reassure the victim when consciousness returns If single seizure lasts less than 10 minutes, ask the victim whether a hospital evaluation is wanted If multiple seizures occur or if one seizure lasts longer than 10 minutes, take the victim to the emergency room	Do not put any hard implement in the mouth Do not try to hold tongue; it cannot be swallowed Do not try to give liquids during or just after the seizure Do not use oxygen unless there are symptoms of a heart attack Do not use artificial respiration unless breathing is absent after muscle jerks subside or unless water has been inhaled Do not restrain
Nonconvulsive	Many different forms of seizures, ranging from temporary unawareness (petit mal) to brief, sudden, massive muscle jerks (myoclonic seizures)	Daydreaming, acting out, clumsiness, poor coordination, intoxication, random activity, mental illness	Usually no first aid is necessary other than to provide reassurance and emotional support; any nonconvulsive seizure that becomes convulsive should be managed as a convulsive seizure; medical evaluation is recommended	Do not shout at, restrain, expect verbal instructions to be obeyed, or grab a person having a nonconvulsive seizure (unless danger threatens)

hurt now more than when it happened? If the pain continues or increases, you should seek medical attention. You need to look at the injury. If there is obvious deformity, severe bleeding, or inability to move a body part, medical attention is necessary.

Although an injury is not severe enough to seek medical attention, it still needs attention. First, you should rest the injured part. Ice or cold treatment for approximately 20 minutes every few hours is often recommended. Elevation of an injured and swollen body part reduces the swelling. If an injury does not improve, you should seek medical attention.

FIRST AID

Specific procedures exist for first aid. Certification in first aid can be obtained from attending classes taught by instructors certified by the American Red Cross. This is an excellent way to prepare yourself for emergency situations. Tables 15-2 and 15-3 (pp. 372-373, 375) list general guidelines for emergency medical situations, but the information cannot substitute for a class on first aid.

VIOLENCE

Another area of injury is related to violence. Each year, more than 20,000 people die from and more than 2 million are victims of violent injury. Homicide and assault are a growing public health problem among adolescents and young adults.

Unfortunately, violence is often the first response of frustrated and emotionally stressed young people. It is portrayed in the media as a means to cope with conflict. This translates to youth as an effective mechanism for resolving conflict. The result is increased gang recruitment and warfare. Weapons are now common in many schools—from elementary to high schools.

The answers to violence prevention are complex. The underlying problems vary among communities. They must be addressed in a comprehensive way that integrates the efforts of all aspects of communities.

SUMMARY

Injury prevention presents a new way of thinking. Specific strategies help prevent both unintended and intended injuries. Many of the specifics of injury prevention rest in the knowledge (information) and behavior choices of individuals.

The following section of this chapter provides examples of learning opportunities that are appropriate for primary level, intermediate level, and middle-school students. In addition, you will find a listing of objectives that indicate the scope and sequence of content for this area.

SUGGESTED READINGS

Bike helmets: unused life savers, *Consumer Reports* May 1990.

Burton N: *Entering adulthood: understanding depression and suicide*, Santa Cruz, Calif, 1990, ETR Associates.

Hunter L, Lloyd-Kolkin D: *Entering adulthood: skills for injury prevention*, Santa Cruz, Calif, 1991, ETR Associates.

Kane W: *Safety is no accident: children's activities in injury prevention*, Santa Cruz, Calif, 1993, ETR Associates.

Payne W, Hahn D: *Understanding your health*, St Louis, 1992, Mosby.

Post J: *Into adolescence: stopping violence.* Santa Cruz, Calif, 1991, ETR Associates.

Prothrow-Stith D: *Violence prevention curriculum for adolescents*, Newton, Mass, 1987, Education Development Center.

Rivara FP: *Prevention of injuries to children and adolescents.* In Wallace HM and others, eds: *Principles and practices of student health*, vol I, Oakland, Calif, Third Party Press.

Sleet DA: *Injury prevention.* In Cortese P, Middleton K, eds: *The comprehensive school health challenge*, Santa Cruz, Calif, 1993, ETR Associates.

GENERAL STUDENT OBJECTIVES

Primary Level K-3

The student:
1. Explains the relationship between observing safety rules and preventing injuries.
2. Identifies potential hazards at home, school, and community.
3. Explains how to obtain help in an emergency.

Intermediate Level, 4/5-6

The student:
1. Evaluates actions of bicycle riders for their safety factor.
2. Demonstrates basic first aid procedures for stopped breathing.*
3. Identifies individual responsibilities for reducing hazards and preventing injuries.

Middle School Level 6/7-8

The student:
1. Develops a home safety program.*
2. Demonstrates standard first aid procedures appropriate in life threatening situations.
3. Explains how properly used protective equipment increases enjoyment and diminishes the possibility of injury when engaging in potentially risky activities.

*These objectives are illustrated by sample learning opportunities.

PRIMARY LEVEL

OBJECTIVE: The student illustrates basic first aid for minor injuries.

LEVEL: Grades 2 and 3

INTEGRATION: Writing, language arts, art

VOCABULARY: First aid, pressure, adhesive tape, adhesive bandage, wound, sterile pad

CONTENT GENERALIZATIONS: First aid is the immediate care given to an injured or suddenly ill person. Those who give first aid must be trained specifically to know what to do and what not to do. Basic first aid procedures include (1) wash wounds with soap and water; (2) apply direct pressure to stop bleeding; (3) treat minor burns with cool water; (4) always get help from an adult in an emergency situation or when an injury occurs; and (5) if a tooth is knocked out, save the tooth, and call the dentist immediately.

INITIATION: "First-Aid Box"
Show the students a box covered with white paper with a red cross on the sides and top. Ask the students what they think might be inside this box. (Students may recognize the first-aid symbol and guess items such as bandages, first aid cream, and adhesive tape.) Take out the items as they are guessed by students. Explain that the symbol on the box is recognized around the world. It means first aid to most people. First aid is the *first* help given to a person who is injured (hurt) or ill. It can be given to yourself or to another person but help always should be asked of an adult as quickly as possible.

MATERIALS

First-aid box (teacher-made)

Items to put in box: adhesive bandages, triangular bandages, sterile gauze pads, adhesive tape, first-aid cream

ACTIVITIES

1. Four Injuries

a. Following are four injury situations (stories). Use the same procedures for each story, and preferably do only one story a day.

b. An option is to ask for student volunteers to dramatize the story and demonstrate correct first aid procedures.

BRANDON AND THE COOKIE SHEET

Brandon could smell cookies baking in the oven. His mother was making his favorite kind—oatmeal with raisins! He ran into the kitchen and saw them in the oven. They looked done to him, and his mother was on the telephone. He got the pot holder out of the drawer and opened the oven. He did not realize how heavy the cookie sheet was. He dropped the cookie sheet and burned his arm.

Ask students, "What should be done?"

Brandon's mother ran into the kitchen. She saw that he had a minor burn on his arm. Immediately she lifted him up to the sink and ran *cool* water over the arm for a long time, which made Brandon's arm feel better. She looked at the arm very carefully and said, "Brandon, you are very lucky. There are no blisters. We don't have to go to the doctor."

Discussion Questions

- How did Brandon burn his arm? (He dropped a hot cookie sheet on his arm.)
- What did Brandon's mother do? (She ran cool water from the faucet over his arm.)
- What should Brandon do next time so he does not burn his arm? (Ask his mother or father for help when working in the kitchen.)

Hand out the worksheet, *Brandon and the Cookie Sheet*, and explain the directions. When the students are finished, allow them to tell about their pictures.

MATERIALS

Worksheet: *Brandon and the Cookie Sheet* (Figure 15-2)

JENNIFER AND THE ROLLER SKATES

Jennifer was at home alone while Grandma, with whom she lives, went to buy groceries for lunch. Grandma said she would be back in about 10 minutes. Jennifer slipped on her roller skates and took a spin on the sidewalk. She tripped over some gravel, fell, and scraped her knee. Her knee did not bleed, but it was scraped and had gravel and dirt on the surface. The scrape was about the size of a quarter.

Ask students, "What should be done?"

Jennifer took off her skates and went into the house. She washed the scrape and the surrounding skin with soap and warm water. She dried the scrape with a clean cloth and checked to make certain all the dirt and gravel was removed. Then she taped a sterile pad on the wound. When Grandma came home, Jennifer told her what had happened and how the wound had been cared for. Grandma said, "Why Jennifer, you could not have done any better!"

Discussion Questions

- How did Jennifer care for her scraped knee? (Cleaned it with soap and warm water, dried it, and applied a sterile pad.)
- If the scrape had been smaller, about the size of a dime, what could Jennifer have used instead of a sterile pad and adhesive tape? (Adhesive bandage.)
- Ask students to identify the items Jennifer used from the display.

Hand out the worksheet, *Jennifer and the Roller Skates*, and explain the directions. When the students are finished, allow them to tell about their pictures.

MATERIALS

Worksheet: *Jennifer and the Roller Skates* (Figure 15-3)

TIMMY AND THE SWING SET

Shirley saw Timmy, the little boy who lived next door, playing on the swing set in his front yard. The swing accidentally hit Timmy in the face, and his nose began to bleed. Frightened, Timmy yelled, "Help! My nose is bleeding!" and ran in circles while waving his arms.

Ask students, "What should be done?"

Shirley knew how to give Timmy immediate first aid for a nosebleed and went to help him. First, she told him to sit down quietly. Then she gently applied pressure to the nostril that was bleeding. When Timmy was sitting quietly, she showed him how to apply the pressure to his nose himself. Then she knocked on the front door to tell his dad what had happened. Timmy's dad sat with Timmy and told him to continue applying pressure as he leaned slightly forward. Timmy's Dad told Shirley, "Thank you for helping my son. You're a great neighbor who knew exactly what to do in this emergency." Timmy's nose stopped bleeding.

Discussion Questions

- What actions stopped Timmy's nose from bleeding? (Sitting down quietly, leaning slightly forward, and pinching the bleeding nostril.)
- How can you stop your nose from bleeding? (Same actions, and tell a parent or teacher.)

Hand out the worksheet, *Timmy and the Swing Set*, and explain the directions. When the students are finished, allow them to tell about the pictures.

MATERIALS

Worksheet: *Timmy and the Swing Set* (Figure 15-4)

MEI LING AND THE SOFTBALL

When Mei Ling was playing softball one Saturday, the ball hit her in the mouth and knocked out one of her new front teeth. It was *not* a loose "baby" tooth but a tight permanent tooth.

Ask students, "What should be done?"

Although Mei Ling was hurt, she knew exactly what to do. First, she found the tooth. She then wet a *clean* handkerchief at the drinking fountain and carefully wrapped the tooth in it. Mei Ling went home and told her mother, "My permanent tooth was knocked out. I wrapped it in this clean wet cloth." Mei Ling's mother replied, "You knew exactly what to do. I'll call our dentist right away. I hope Dr. Palmer will be able to put your tooth back." When Mei Ling and her mother arrived, Dr. Palmer said, "You have taken good care of this tooth! It was right to come see me right away because I will be able to put Mei Ling's tooth back. You have helped save Mei Ling's tooth through good first aid."

Discussion Questions

- How did Mei Ling and her mother help save Mei Ling's tooth? (Mei Ling found the tooth, placed it in a clean damp handkerchief, and told her mother right away; her mother brought Mei Ling and the tooth to the dentist right away.)
- It is best to wrap the tooth in a clean damp cloth. Mei Ling used her clean handkerchief. What else could have been used? (Clean damp paper towel, etc.)
- If no water, cloth, handkerchief, or paper towel had been available, what should Mei Ling have done? (She should have picked up the tooth with her hand and taken it home right away.)

Hand students the worksheet, *Mei Ling and the Softball*, and explain the directions. When they are finished, allow them to tell about their pictures.

MATERIALS

Worksheet: *Mei Ling and the Softball* (Figure 15-5)

2. **Minor Injuries Bulletin Board**

Help students make a class bulletin board chart of minor injuries that happen in and out of school over the period of 1 week. For each injury record the type of first aid administered. Discuss whether the first aid procedures administered for each injury were appropriate. If a minor injury occurs, allow the child to administer his or her own first aid with teacher supervision.

EVALUATION: "Randy and His Bicycle"

As Randy was riding his bicycle home from school, he made the turn into the driveway too sharply and skidded and fell. His elbow was bleeding and dirty. What should he do?

Have the students draw, demonstrate (act out), or write the proper first aid procedure for Randy's injury. (He should wash the wound with soap and water, cover the wound with a bandage, and tell an adult what happened.)

FIGURE 15-2

Worksheet   Name _____

Brandon and the Cookie Sheet

1. What happened to Brandon in the kitchen?

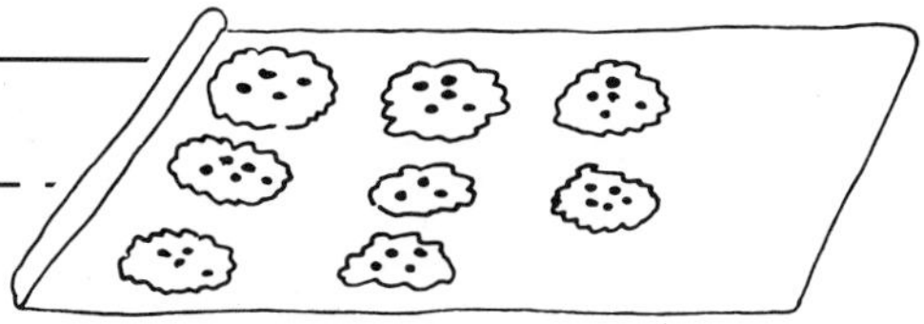

_____

– –

_____

_____

– – – – – – – – – – – – – – – – – – –

_____

2.   Draw or write what Brandon's mother did in the space below.

The correct first aid is . . .

FIGURE 15-3

Worksheet   Name _____

Jennifer and the Roller Skates

1. What happened to Jennifer when her grandmother went to the store?

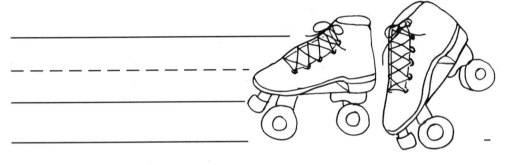

_____

— — — — — — — — — — — — — — — — —

_____

_____

— — — — — — — — — — — — — — — — — — — —

_____

2. Draw or write what Jennifer did in the space below.

The correct first aid is . . .

FIGURE 15-4

Worksheet   Name _____

Timmy and the Swing Set

1. What happened to Timmy in his backyard?

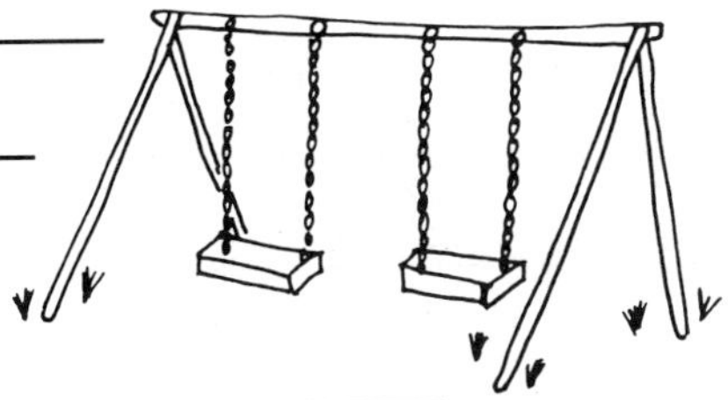

_____

— — — — — — — — — — — — — —

_____

_____

— — — — — — — — — — — — — — — — — — —

_____

2. Draw or write what Shirley did in the space below.

The correct first aid is . . .

FIGURE 15-5

Worksheet   Name _____

Mei Ling and the Softball

1. What happened to Mei Ling when she was playing softball?

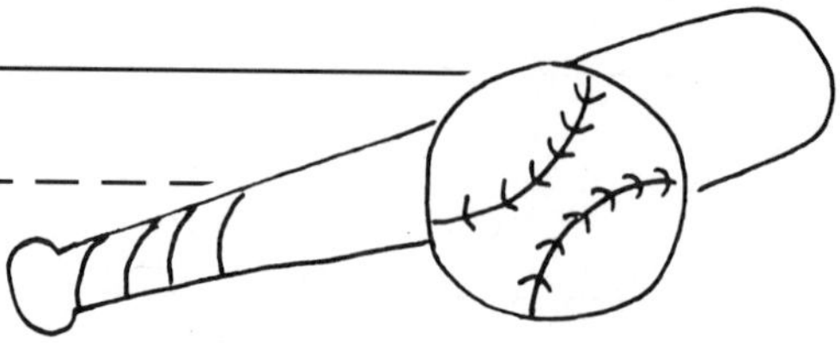

_____

_ _

_____

_____

_ _

_____

2. Draw or write what Mei Ling did in the space below.

The correct first aid is . . .

INTERMEDIATE LEVEL

OBJECTIVE: The student demonstrates basic first aid for stopped breathing.

LEVEL: Grades 4 to 6

INTEGRATION: Science

VOCABULARY: Lungs, inhale, exhale, artificial ventilation, mouth-to-mouth resuscitation

CONTENT GENERALIZATIONS: When normal breathing stops and too little oxygen is being taken into the lungs, the victim is in danger. If breathing is not restored, the victim may die within minutes. Artificial ventilation is the procedure for forcing air into the lungs of a person who has stopped breathing. Several specific steps should be followed and continued until help arrives.

NOTE: This lesson is a presentation of the most basic principles of artificial ventilation. Successful completion of these activities does not certify students in this procedure. The students should be aware that they should only administer this procedure in an emergency when no one else around can perform this life-saving technique. This procedure should not be confused with CPR, which involves chest compressions to start circulation, as well as mouth-to-mouth resuscitation. CPR should be taught only by a certified trainer. Contact the American Red Cross for guest speakers and other references.

INITIATION: "In and Out"
Ask the students to place their hands on their chest and feel it rise as they inhale and fall as they exhale. Hand out the worksheet, *In and Out.* Explain to students that, when we inhale, the diaphragm muscle moves down to allow more space in the chest for the lungs to expand. The dotted lines on the worksheet represent the general position of the diaphragm and the expansion of the lungs. When we exhale, the diaphragm pushes up on the lungs, decreasing the chest capacity and pushing air out of the lungs, which makes them smaller. This is represented by the solid lines on the worksheet. Have the students take a few big breaths and observe the increased size of their chest on inhalation and the decreased size during exhalation. Then the students should color their worksheets, using different colors to represent the lungs and diaphragm during inhalation and exhalation. The students also should label the basic parts of the respiratory system, including the trachea, bronchial tubes, lungs, alveoli (air sacks), and diaphragm. Put up a poster of the respiratory system or have them consult an encyclopedia to correctly label these parts.

MATERIALS
Worksheet and transparency: *In and Out* (Figure 15-6)
Poster: The Respiratory System
Encyclopedias
Resources
Guest speaker: school nurse or Red Cross volunteer to demonstrate artificial ventilation
Mannequin: Resusa Annie (American Red Cross)

ACTIVITIES

MATERIALS
Index cards (seven per student)
1. **Artificial Ventilation**
   Explain to students that breathing is called *respiration*. If a person is not breathing normally, another person can blow air into the nonbreathing person's lungs to try to keep him or her alive. This process is called *artificial ventilation*. Tell students that they will be learning and practicing the specific steps in this process. If possible, have a guest speaker demonstrate the following steps. The speaker may have access to a mannequin. (A mannequin should only be used by someone trained specifically in the use. There are certain health-related precautions that must be used.) If no mannequin is available, demonstrate the

procedure on a student. Do *not* blow into the student's mouth; blow to the side of the student's head. Tell the students that they will blow only to the side of their partner's head when practicing.

a. Write the following steps on the board:
- *Shout* and tap
- *Check* for pulse
- *Tilt* head to clear air passage
- *Look*, listen, and feel for air
- *Give four* quick breaths
- *Look*, listen, and feel for air
- *Give 1* breath every 5 seconds for an adult

b. Review these steps with the class, then demonstrate with a student volunteer. Blow air beside the head (not into the mouth) of the student.

c. Have students pair up, one being the victim and the other the rescuer. Lead students through each of the steps. Have students trade roles and repeat the process.

d. Inform students that to be certified to actually give artificial ventilation, young people and adults can take a class in basic first aid through the American Red Cross.

2. **Practice Mouth-to-Mouth Ventilation**

Organize the students into small groups of seven. In each group, one student describes the first step in administering artificial ventilation, then the person to the right states the following step and describes how it is done.

The process continues until each student has identified one of the seven steps. Students may take turns being first so that the cycle is repeated and reviewed seven times. *Optional:* Have the students make flash cards with the seven steps for artificial ventilation. They can quiz each other in pairs or in the groups.

3. **First Aid for Stopped Breathing**

Hand out the worksheet, *First Aid for Stopped Breathing*, and ask students to complete it individually. Go over the answers orally in class after everyone has finished.

MATERIALS

Worksheet: *First Aid for Stopped Breathing* (Figure 15-7)

EVALUATION: "Parent Letter"

Give the students a letter to take home to their parents. Explain that the letter informs parents of their learning the steps of artificial ventilation. Tell students to demonstrate these steps to their parents. Explain that the bottom half of the letter is to be returned after students have demonstrated the steps of artificial ventilation.

MATERIALS

Teacher resource: Sample Parent Letter (Figure 15-8)

FIGURE 15-6

Worksheet   Name _____

In and Out

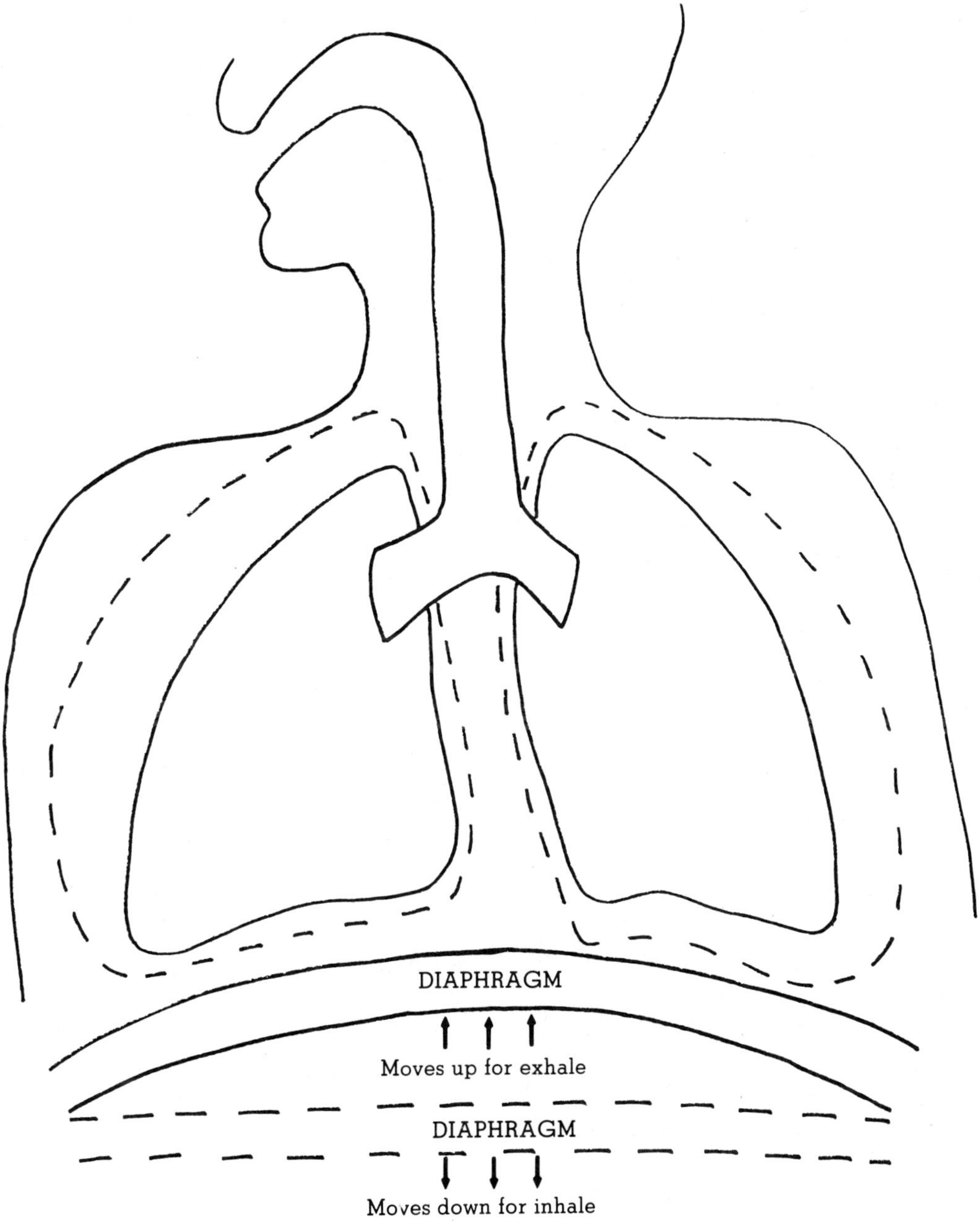

DIAPHRAGM

Moves up for exhale

DIAPHRAGM

Moves down for inhale

FIGURE 15-7

Worksheet   Name _____

First Aid for Stopped Breathing

Situation: You see a woman pull a man out of a lake. She says, "Can you
                  help me? This man is not breathing. Do you know artificial
                  ventilation?"

                  Can you help? Write the steps below in the correct order. (Hint:
                  The steps are at the bottom of the worksheet, but they are not in
                  order.)

                  STEPS FOR ARTIFICIAL VENTILATION

1. _____

2. _____

3. _____

4. _____

5. _____

6. _____

7. _____

- -

Use these steps for help in remembering, if needed. If you do not need to look
at these steps, all the better!

LOOK, LISTEN, AND FEEL FOR AIR

TILT HEAD

GIVE 1 BREATH EVERY 5 SECONDS

SHOUT AND TAP

GIVE FOUR QUICK BREATHS

LOOK, LISTEN, AND FEEL FOR AIR

CHECK FOR PULSE

FIGURE 15-8

Teacher resource   Name _____

Sample Parent Letter

Dear Parent:

 Your child _____ has been learning how to perform artificial ventilation during health class. To help him or her become more proficient, I have asked students to practice with their parents. These activities are limited. We did not learn how to perform CPR (cardiopulmonary resuscitation). If you or your child is interested in becoming certified in first-aid procedures, I suggest you contact the American Red Cross.

 As your child demonstrates the following steps, please check them off. Then return the bottom half of this sheet to me. Thank you for your cooperation.

           Sincerely,

         _____

           (Teacher)

- -

I have watched my son or daughter _____ demonstrate the following steps of artificial ventilation:

1. Shout and tap   _____

2. Check for pulse   _____

3. Tilt the head to clear the airway _____

4. Look, listen, and feel for air _____

5. Give 4 quick breaths   _____

6. Look, listen, and feel for air again _____

7. Give 1 breath every 5 seconds _____

         _____

          Signed (parent)

MIDDLE SCHOOL LEVEL

OBJECTIVE: The student develops a home safety program.

LEVEL: Grades 6 to 8

VOCABULARY: injury, hazard, emergency

CONTENT GENERALIZATIONS: Many injuries at home can be prevented if hazards are reduced and emergency plans have been made. Hazards exist in all rooms of the home. Correcting hazards can be a part of a home safety program. Reducing hazards and planning for possible emergencies make the home a safer place to live.

INITIATION: "A Hazard Looking for an Injury"

Using a great deal of dramatic flair, enter the classroom with a sign "A Hazard Looking for an Injury." Wear a large sloppy coat whose pockets are bulging with items that could be hazardous in the home, such as a plastic bag from the dry cleaners, a frayed electrical cord, a small throw rug without a rubberized backing, a bottle of cleaning fluid, or any other item that could be stuffed in the coat or put somewhere on your body. Dramatically pull out one item at a time, and tell a story about an injury that occurred related to the item. Make up the funny stories with nothing serious happening to the victims described. At the end of the "show" explain the reason we can laugh at these stories is because no one was really injured in these situations. This is not always the case.

Write the words *injury* and *hazard* on the board. Have the students look up these words and find out the difference between them (possibly for homework).

MATERIALS

Coat with lots of pockets
Items to represent hazards: Plastic dry-cleaning bag, frayed electrical cord, pot with handle, throw rug without rubberized backing, Sign: "A Hazard Looking for an Injury" (teacher-made)

ACTIVITIES

1. Home Safety Checklist

Hand out the worksheet, *Home Safety Checklist*. Explain that the students are to use it to check their home for hazards. Read through the *Home Safety Checklist* with the students. For each item on the checklist, ask why the situation described could be hazardous. Have them take the worksheet home and analyze their own home.

MATERIALS

Worksheet: *Home Safety Checklist* (Figure 15-9)

2. "Hazards" Pictures

Ask the students to take a picture of a hazard found in their own home. If a camera is not available, ask them to draw the hazard. Students then should correct the hazard and take or draw another picture of the situation. These pictures can be posted on a bulletin board, "Don't Let a Hazard Become an Injury." It may be necessary to rotate student pictures if several classes are involved in this activity.

MATERIALS

Camera and film for use by students in their own home (if available) or drawing paper and felt pens
Bulletin board: "Don't Let a Hazard Become an Injury"

3. In Case of Fire

Ask the students, "What is the purpose of fire drills at school?" (To practice the proper way to proceed if a fire occurs at school.) Ask them to describe the proper way to exit your classroom should a fire occur. Explain that it is important to be prepared for a possible fire at home as well.

Hand out the worksheet, *In Case of Fire*. Tell the students that this is a floor plan of a house. Using the transparency on the overhead projector, mark the normal exit route from the bedrooms to the outside. Ask the students, "What should be done if a fire in the hallway blocks an exit from the bedrooms?" (The door to the hallway should be closed, and a secondary exit should be taken. The family should have a prearranged meeting spot outside the home.) Ask students to locate a secondary exit route from each bedroom on their worksheet. Then discuss the routes and draw them on the transparency.

MATERIALS

Worksheet and transparency: *In Case of Fire* (Figure 15-10)
Overhead projector
Transparency pens (2 colors)

EVALUATION: "Be Prepared—First Aid at Home"

Ask the students to check at home for a first aid kit and a list of emergency numbers posted near the telephone. Hand out the worksheet, *Be Prepared*. Explain the assignment is to find out the emergency telephone numbers appropriate for their area and record them on the worksheet. Suggest that students look in the front pages of the telephone book for help in locating emergency numbers. The bottom part of the worksheet deals with the assembly of a first aid kit and the gathering of a few items that could be necessary in an emergency. Suggest that students work together with parents to gather items for the first aid kit and for possible emergencies. Set up a display of all the items indicated on the worksheet. Allow the students several weeks to complete this project. Tell them to get help from family members. It may be useful to discuss the problems students may be having in putting together first-aid kits for their homes. The discussions could be as a total class or in small groups. Encourage the students to help each other work out problems.

MATERIALS

Worksheet: *Be Prepared* (Figure 15-11)
Telephone book
Items for first-aid kit: bandages (several sizes and roller gauze), sterile pads (2×2 inches), antiseptic, adhesive tape, alcohol, tongue depressor, triangular bandages
Other items for emergency situations: flashlight with extra batteries, candles and matches, battery-operated radio, bottled water.

FIGURE 15-9

Worksheet   Name _____

Home Safety Checklist

Directions: Use the following list to check and correct hazards in your home. Do nothing on items that you have checked yes. Try to correct those where you have checked no.

STORAGE OF POISONOUS SUBSTANCES	YES	NO	CORRECTED
Medicines are out of reach of children.			
Labels are left on medicines and poisonous chemicals.			
Poisonous substances are always stored in original containers. (Do not put gasoline in a cola bottle for storage.)			
Household cleaners and chemicals are not stored on the same shelf as or a shelf above food.			
Kerosene, gasoline, and other flammable fluids are stored away from heat sources.			
PROPER USE AND STORAGE OF ELECTRICAL APPLIANCES			
All electrical cords are in good condition and not frayed.			
Electrical outlets are not overloaded.			
Extension cords are not under carpets, through doors, or over nails.			
Electrical appliances are used away from water.			
When not in use, electrical appliances and tools are stored neatly out of the reach of children.			
SAFETY AROUND THE HOUSE			
Hallways and stairs are well lit.			
Throw rugs have rubberized backing.			
Floors and steps are not cluttered.			
Water or grease on floors is quickly wiped up.			
Cupboard doors, closet doors, and drawers are kept closed.			
Stairways have handrails.			
Smoke detectors are in the home.			
SAFETY AROUND THE KITCHEN			
Pots and pans are used with handles not protruding from the stove.			
Curtains are not near the stove.			
The kitchen has a fire extinguisher.			
Knives are stored separately from other utensils and away from children.			
Matches are out of the reach of children			

FIGURE 15-10

Worksheet   Name _____

In Case of Fire

Directions: With the help of the teacher you will be locating the primary and
               secondary exit routes from the bedrooms of this house in case of fire.

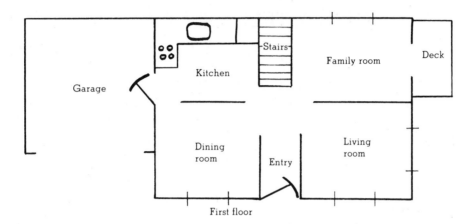

First floor

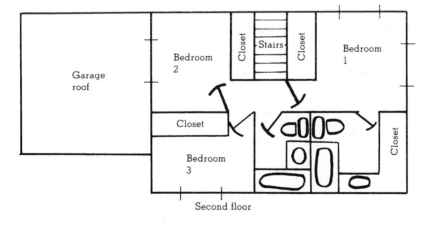

Second floor

FIGURE 15-11

Worksheet   Name _____

Be Prepared

Directions: Find the following emergency telephone numbers for your community.
Then cut along the dotted line and mount it on a 5 × 8 index card or a
piece of tagboard cut to the correct size. Place your sign near the
telephone in your home. If you have more than one telephone, make
other signs.

EMERGENCY TELEPHONE NUMBERS

Police _____

Fire _____

Ambulance _____

Poison control center _____

Work with your parents to assemble a first-aid kit for your home.

Include the following items. Check them off as you assemble the kit:

__ Bandages, several sizes   __ Tongue depressor

__ Sterile pad, 2 × 2 inches   __ Triangular bandage

__ Roller gauze   __ Optional items: flashlight, batteries,

__ Antiseptic   candles, matches, bottled water,

__ Adhesive tape   battery-operated radio

__ Alcohol

16 Consumer Health

When you finish this chapter, you should able to:

- Analyze methods of advertising approaches used to sell products that may have health benefits or hazards.
- Describe ways to enhance effective decision making before using health products and services.
- Identify criteria for selection of the variety of health-care providers and treatments.
- Explain methods used for consumer protection.
- Develop learning opportunities for elementary and middle-school students in the area of consumer health.

We are health consumers any time we buy or use a product for health reasons or use health-related services. We are also consumers of health-related information. It is often difficult to be discriminating in our choices. Advertisements may portray unhealthy products or services in a way that minimizes or denies the risk. Products that have no health value may be promoted as health-enhancing items. So many health products are on the market that it may be hard to tell which are effective. Being a knowledgable consumer of health products and services means learning to think critically about information we receive and to make decisions accordingly.

PRODUCTS AND ADVERTISING

Health-related products include over-the-counter and prescription medicines, toothpaste, shampoo, foods, vitamins, and first-aid products. Cosmetics and various hair and skin products are also often billed as health oriented. Many advertisements seek to promote a particular product by persuading consumers that the product is needed or desirable.

Advertising Approaches

We begin to encounter persuasion through advertising at a very young age, usually through commercials during children's television programs. These advertisements promote products that include vitamins, cereals, candies, and soft drinks. Even though parents do most of the purchasing, advertising directed toward children is very effective. Appeals to children's emotions and senses often include enticements such as, "It is fun to use or eat. It is tasty or smells good. It is popular to do. It is attractive." Claims that a particular product is healthful may also be used by advertisers. Finally, the packaging of foods and medications used by children is especially appealing. Games or toys are often included with a product as an enticement.

Early health instruction can make a difference in children's acceptance of advertising claims. Children can learn that the goal of advertising is sales, not health. They can also recognize the fact that advertised products are not necessarily useful.

Advertising on late afternoon or evening television, on radio, and in magazines is often directed at adolescents. Attractive people are portrayed enjoying life with a specific product; the advertisement conveys the idea that use of the product will somehow make life wonderful. Cigarette and smokeless tobacco advertisements often show young, active people having fun. People who use tobacco products and are terminally ill with lung cancer or disfigured by oral cancer are not used as models.

Another advertising approach is repetition. Constant repetition of the same message has an impact on the consumer, often in the form of a catch phrase or a visual image that people tend to remember. Consumers usually choose a product they have heard about over one they have not heard about, even when the message provides no real information.

Some other advertising approaches are the following:

- Use of testimonials and authority figures: Testimonials of "regular" people may also be used to show that people like the viewer have used a product successfully.
- Reference to scientific value with phrases such as *hospital tested* or *doctors recommend:* Actors may be pictured in white laboratory coats or in a setting that looks scientific or medical.
- Reference to widespread use of the product: This approach attempts to convince the consumer that "everyone" uses this product, so it must be effective.
- Appeal to the sense of superiority: This implies that consumers of this product are somehow better than other consumers.
- Instilling a sense of fear: This approach cautions consumers about potential consequences if they do not purchase a certain product (for example, insurance).

As some of these approaches indicate, advertising often makes use of symbols, and it presents a fictionalized version of social reality intended to persuade consumers to use a product. This approach can be effective for the general public and professionals. For example, the white laboratory coat has been used in television commercials and in advertisements in medical and nursing journals to symbolize scientific authority.

It is important to learn to look critically at advertisements, keeping in mind that the purpose is to sell a product or service. The negative aspects of the product or service will not be advertised. However, laws require cautionary statements to accompany some advertisements. Advertising appeals are usually more emotional than rational. Statements such as, "Nine out of ten doctors recommend" should be examined to see whether enough information is given in the advertisement to indicate that an actual study was conducted, who conducted it, how many doctors were involved, and whether they were physicians.

Many consumer health decisions are related to how people feel about themselves and what their background knowledge is on an issue. The desire for acceptance can lead young people in many directions. For those who have an *external locus of control*, decisions are more likely to be based on what others say or think; for those with an *internal locus of control*, decisions are more likely to be made independently, based on what the individual believes or thinks. Friends, parents, and advertisers can have a strong influence on a person's consumer decisions.

Personal Care Products

Personal care products include skin-care products, body-odor preparations, and hair-care preparations. Despite the array of products being marketed for skin care, soap and water may provide the lowest-cost and most effective skin care, especially when combined with a nutritious diet and a regular exercise program.

Two basic types of body-odor preparations are sold—antiperspirants and deodorants. Antiperspirants contain chemicals that reduce the amount of perspiration the body produces. Deodorants have chemicals that cover or mask odors. Perspiration is a normal body function that helps regulate temperature, rid the body of waste products, and keep the skin moist. When perspiration mixes with bacteria on the skin, odors usually result. Washing the areas of sweat production combined with the use of an antiperspirant or deodorant provides good hygiene.

The basic hair-care preparations are shampoos—with a basic soap substance that removes oil and dead cells from the hair and scalp—and conditioners—which replace some of the oils that shampoos wash out. Lanolin is often used as a conditioner in shampoos and conditioners. Hair-care preparations that contain proteins and vitamins are unnecessary. Advertisements may claim to "make healthy hair" or give hair "new life," but hair is "dead." (Hair shafts are composed of three layers of dead cells.)

Product Labeling

When purchasing health-related products, you should realize that many products contain valuable health information on the label. Packaged foods must have the ingredients listed from greatest to least according to the amount present. An ingredient list for cranberry juice cocktail may be water, cranberry juice, sugar, and vitamin C. This means that there is more added water than cranberry juice in the product, it has been fortified with extra vitamin C, and sugar was added.

Grocery shelves are filled with products that have labels making nutritional claims (1). In a sense, these also "advertise" a product to the consumer. The consumer's challenge is to get beyond the advertising to make wise decisions about which foods to purchase. A revised nutrient la-

Nutrition Facts

Serving Size 1/2 cup (114g)
Servings Per Container 4

Amount Per Serving

Calories 260   Calories from Fat 120

	% Daily Value*
Total Fat 13g	**20%**
Saturated Fat 5g	**25%**
Cholesterol 30mg	**10%**
Sodium 660 mg	**28%**
Total Carbohydrate 31g	**11%**
Dietary Fiber 0g	**0%**
Sugars 5g	
Protein 5g	

Vitamin A 4%	Vitamin C 2%
Calcium 15%	Iron 4%

*Percent Daily Values are based on a 2,000 calorie diet. Your daily values may be higher or lower depending on your calorie needs.

	Calories:	2000	2500
Total Fat	Less than	65g	80g
Sat. Fat	Less than	20g	25g
Cholesterol	Less than	300mg	300mg
Sodium	Less than	2,400mg	2,400mg
Total Carbohydrate		300g	375g
Dietary Fiber		25g	30g

Calories per gram:
Fat 9 • Carbohydrate 4 • Protein 4

FIGURE 16-1
New Nutrient Label

beling format (Figure 16-1) went into effect in 1993.

Drugs prescribed by a physician and provided by a pharmacist have detailed information sheets available that describe the drug. These pharmaceutical inserts provide valuable consumer information, including the drug's chemical formulation, its mode of action, and its contraindications—conditions that would prevent use of the drug. If asked, pharmacists will provide the insert for a consumer.

SELECTING HEALTH-CARE PROVIDERS

There are many reasons to consult a health-care provider. Most of us seek advice or care from a health-care provider only when we develop a specific problem. In these cases, we are seeking *diagnosis* and *treatment.*

Health providers may also offer *screening* for particular conditions or diseases. For example, blood tests are used to screen for high cholesterol. Sometimes these services are provided for large numbers of people at community locations such as shopping centers and schools. Community screening programs may not be as accurate as those performed by qualified medical laboratories, but it often identifies people who should seek further medical attention.

Another reason to use health-care providers is for *consultation.* Sometimes this means seeing a specialist for a problem. It can also mean obtaining a second opinion on a diagnosis or treatment plan when a person needs reassurance that these are appropriate.

Health-care providers can also help with strategies for *prevention.* Because many of the diseases of major concern today are not "curable," such as cardiovascular diseases and AIDS, prevention is critical to staying healthy.

Physicians

Physicians, or medical doctors, are trained and licensed to practice medicine. They diagnose and treat injuries and disease, prescribe medications, and perform surgery.

In the United States, there are two types of medical degrees—the doctor of medicine (MD), conferred at most medical schools, and the doctor of osteopathy (DO), conferred at osteopathic medical colleges. Although there were distinct differences in the two medical traditions, today the training is basically equivalent. MDs and DOs can become licensed to practice in any area of medicine. More than 90% of physicians are MDs.

Becoming a physician requires 4 years of college and 4 years of medical school; on graduation, the MD degree is conferred. Then 1 year of postgraduate training (internship) in a hospital is required. If the physician wants to practice in a specialty area, 2 to 6 more years of training (residency) are required and examinations taken in the specialty area. This allows a physician to be *board certified.* Before physicians can practice, they must also pass a state examination to be licensed to practice in a particular state.

Medical Specialists

Today, there are 23 main specialties. Three of these —*family practitioners, internists,* and *pediatricians*—are **primary care physicians;** the remainder are **specialists.**

Family Practitioners provide general care for people of all ages. *Internists* specialize in internal medicine and the diagnosis and nonsurgical treatment of diseases in adults. *Pediatricians* specialize in the care of children from birth through adolescence. They measure the physical and emotional development of their patients, identify health problems, and vaccinate children to prevent diseases such as polio.

Other specialists provide secondary care, or care for a specific problem that a primary care physician is not equipped to handle. A sample of some of these medical specialists are shown in Table 16-1.

TABLE 16-1

Sample Medical Specialists

Specialist	Condition or System
Allergist	Immune system
Cardiologist	Heart and blood vessels
Dermatologist	Skin
Neurologist	Nervous system
Obstetrician	Care for pregnant women and delivery of babies
Gynecologist	Female reproductive system
Ophthalmologist	Eyes diseases, visual problems
Urologist	Urinary tract, male reproductive system.

Choosing a Health-Care Provider

When choosing a doctor, dentist, or other health-care professional, you must consider many factors. For example, what are your attitudes about the provider's gender, age, or condition of the office? Did the provider answer your questions in a clear and complete manner? Did the provider seem to be genuinely interested in you? Does the provider make you feel comfortable? If you are dissatisfied, do you believe that your concerns are being addressed? What are the health provider's payment policies? Is the provider available on a 24-hour basis? If the answer to most of these questions is yes, you will probably be satisfied with the care provided.

Alternative Treatment Modes

A variety of other health-care practitioners offer services based on underlying philosophies that differ from that of "mainstream" medical practitioners in the United States and other Western countries. Mainstream medicine is *allopathic*, that is, relying on remedies often in the form of drugs. For example, physicians prescribe antibiotics to treat bacterial infections.

Many people turn to alternative types of treatment because they are dissatisfied with the emphasis on treatment and cures rather than prevention; others find certain alternative practices effective in relieving their symptoms or resolving their health problems. Some people prefer to use services provided by folk healers or "traditional practitioners" who may treat a variety of problems with methods not always recognized by mainstream medicine. For example, for Chinese Americans, the disorder of "heat imbalance" can be treated using traditional Chinese medicine. Many people use a combination of services depending on the nature of the problem and the options they perceive to be appropriate.

Acupuncture, an ancient Chinese practice of inserting fine-gauge needles at specific points on the body, is based on the theory that there are channels of energy, or meridians, running through the body and that specific points along the meridians correspond to individual organs. The needles are inserted and vibrated at these points to restore the organ to health. Acupuncture has been successful in relieving pain, as an anesthetic during surgery, and in treating depression and addictions. Some physicians work with acupuncturists or study acupuncture to provide a combined therapeutic approach to health problems.

Chiropractic is an approach to health care based on the theory that most health problems stem from the alignment of bones, especially those in the spinal column. Aligning or "adjusting" the spine is the major treatment used by chiropractors. This treatment method has been successful in relieving the pain of certain muscle and joint disorders, although there is no evidence that it is effective in treating diseases such as cancer and heart disease. In the past 20 years the length and quality of chiropractice education have been greatly enhanced. Medicare and many insurance companies now reimburse patients for chiropractic care.

Folk or *traditional medicine* is used by many ethnic groups in the United States, both at home and through traditional healers. In general, the treatments used are based on beliefs about the etiology—or causes—of disease. As mentioned previously, many ethnic groups describe conditions that may not be recognized by mainstream medicine. They may believe in etiologies of illness that are not accepted by mainstream health-care providers. Examples of such etiologies are wind and ghosts of the dead (traditional Navajo beliefs), the "evil eye" (some Latino populations, including Puerto Ricans and Mexican Americans), and supernatural causes such as "spirits" (Haitian Americans).

Self-Care

Taking more responsibility for our own health through prevention efforts or management of certain health conditions can often have a number of benefits: It can save on health care costs, it can be effective care for certain conditions, and it can result in more judicious use of community health-care facilities. Self-limiting illnesses, such as colds and flu, are acute problems that lend themselves to self-care. Chronic conditions such as asthma, diabetes, and hypertension are managed or monitored effectively with self-care, although acute episodes may require professional care.

The majority of illness episodes are treated outside mainstream medical facilities, either at home or by alternative healers. In dealing with chronic diseases, the patient and family ultimately become responsible for the care and management of the disease, as well as for health promotion activities. For many conditions, people consult family, friends, and others in their personal network to identify problems and recommend treatment.

Home preventive measures may also be taken, some routinely. For instance, many people take vitamins for this purpose, regardless of scientific evidence that they will be helpful. Herbal teas or tonics may be used for preventive purposes as well.

Health Insurance

Health insurance is a way of ensuring that medical expenses will be paid. Types of insurance include *basic health insurance*, which covers part of hospital, medical, and surgical expenses; *major medical insurance*, which pays for larger

medical expenses resulting from serious illness or injury; and *disability* insurance, which pays a reduced income to people who cannot work because of illness or injury.

In the United States, most people who have health insurance receive it as a work-related benefit. Currently, health-care coverage is a pressing national issue. Health-care costs have risen rapidly, and the cost of health insurance has become too great for many. Millions of Americans have no health insurance at all. The development of federal policies to reform the nation's health-care system and provide more affordable coverage for all people is now underway and should be closely watched by all health-care consumers.

SOURCES OF CONSUMER INFORMATION

Many organizations and agencies publish materials offering advice or information on health issues, products, and services. Several universities have begun publishing newsletters—for example, *The Harvard Medical School Health Letter* and *The Johns Hopkins Medical Letter: Health After 50*. Many health reference publications are on the market, including medical encyclopedias. Personal computer programs and videocassettes on health-related topics are also available.

Consumer Protection Agencies

Various nonprofit and governmental agencies produce information designed to help consumers recognize questionable products and services. Some of these, such as Consumers' Union, regularly evaluate products and services and publish the results.

A number of governmental agencies monitor laws that are designed to protect the consumer. Government enforcement agencies include the Food and Drug Administration (FDA), which requires all medical drugs, food additives, cosmetics, and other devices to pass tough tests to be certain that they are safe and effective. The Federal Trade Commission (FTC) monitors advertising misrepresentation, price fixing, and other unfair business practices. The U.S. Postal Service is responsible for protecting the public from mail fraud, including the sale and transportation of worthless or dangerous health remedies through the mail. The U.S. Department of Agriculture (USDA) ensures that food is safely processed. The Consumer Product Safety Commission (CPSC) enforces uniform safety standards for products in which injuries or illness could occur. An example of the importance of the CPSC is the enforcement of standards for children's sleepwear that require products to be flame retardant before they can be sold in the United States.

Voluntary Health Agencies

Agencies such as the American Heart Association and the American Cancer Society are voluntary health agencies. These and similar agencies focus on disseminating information that can be helpful for consumers or potential consumers of health-related products and services. On a local level, agencies such as these provide a valuable community service. For example, they may send speakers to public schools, support curriculum development, and distribute printed and visual materials.

AVOIDING MEDICAL FRAUD

When information about health is needed, it is important to be able to find an adviser who can provide accurate information. The first source of help for young adults in selecting health advisers is often their parents. School health personnel are qualified to provide certain health information and to refer students to appropriate health advisers. An appropriate health adviser is one who has the credentials for providing the health services needed. This usually means a degree from a college and a license to provide services. The credentials of particular physicians, dentists, and other health professionals can usually be verified by contacting the local medical society, dental society, or state licensing board.

Medical fraud, also called *health quackery*, is health care performed by unlicensed practitio-

ners or licensed practitioners in an unethical manner. Health quacks often prey on people with incurable diseases or chronic conditions for which there is no cure, such as arthritis, cancer, AIDS, diabetes, and multiple sclerosis. These patients are targets for quacks who promise quick, painless cures. These practitioners sometimes claim that the medical establishment does not use their special method because it wants the cure to be kept a "secret" so that physicians can make more money.

Medical fraud often does not hurt people directly, but when patients are in the care of a fraudulent practitioner, they are not getting the medical care they may need. Whenever seeking medical advice or care, people should investigate the qualifications and limitations of the individual involved. Most health professionals display their required licenses in a prominent place in an office, clinic, or pharmacy. If fraud is suspected, the Better Business Bureau, local medical society, or American Medical Association can be contacted.

BECOMING A SKILLED HEALTH-CARE CONSUMER

To become a skilled health-care consumer, you need to learn how to obtain valid and reliable information. Being able to think critically and evaluate the sources and nature of the information are also crucial.

To avoid medical fraud, you should not take advice from someone who (1) offers medical advice or treatment that is not available anywhere else; (2) discourages a second opinion from other medical personnel; (3) sells remedies door to door, through public lectures, or through advertisements in magazines or newspapers or on television; (4) uses testimonials, coupons, or guarantees; and (5) makes the service or product seem too good to be true. Common sense is often the best way to detect fraud. Ask yourself, "Is it really possible to lose 25 pounds in 2 weeks? Can creams and tonics really cause hair to grow on a bald head?"

SUMMARY

Becoming a skilled consumer of health-related products and services is not always easy. There are so many products on the market that it often is difficult to choose among them. Similarly, the array of services and service providers can also be confusing.

Consumers should be aware of advertising approaches and critically evaluate any advertising claims. They should keep in mind that the purpose of advertising is to sell a product or service. Many products have valuable information on their labels; understanding the labeled information helps consumers make good decisions about which products to buy. Professionals such as pharmacists can help with decisions about over-the-counter drugs and generic brands and provide information about drugs and their effects.

Consumers need to ask questions when choosing a medical provider. It is important to feel comfortable with your choice and to know that you can "shop around" if you are not satisfied.

Many people use alternative treatment modes such as acupuncture or chiropractic; some of these are now recognized as reimbursable by insurance companies. The use of personal networks and folk medicine is also widespread, and self-care can be effective in many cases.

Health insurance is a significant issue for all consumers of health care. You should be aware of the federal, state, and local decisions about health care.

Finally, consumers need to protect themselves against fraud and other risks. A number of government and nonprofit agencies offer help. However, consumers must protect themselves by becoming knowledgable and critical in evaluating the information they receive.

The following section provides suggested learning opportunities for students in elementary and middle schools to put into practice some of the principles and information presented in this chapter.

REFERENCES

1. Hisgen J: *Becoming a health-wise consumer*, Santa Cruz, Calif, 1990, ETR Associates.

SUGGESTED READINGS

Goffman E: *Gender advertisements*, Cambridge, Mass, 1979, Harvard University Press.

Harwood A: *Ethnicity and medical care*, Cambridge, Mass, 1981, Harvard University Press.

Health-care systems. Macmillan health encyclopedia, vol 9, New York, 1993, Macmillan Publishing.

Krantzler N: Media images of physicians and nurses in the United States, *Soc Sci Med* 22(9):933-952, 1986.

Payne W, Hahn D: *Understanding your health*, ed 3, St Louis, 1992, Mosby.

Zola I: Studying the decision to see a doctor: review, critique, corrective. *Adv Psychosomatic Med* 8:216-236, 1972.

LEARNING OPPORTUNITIES FOR CONSUMER HEALTH

PRIMARY LEVEL

OBJECTIVE: The student names people who help promote and protect health.

LEVEL: Kindergarten and grade 1

INTEGRATION: Art

VOCABULARY: MD, medical doctor, nurse, police officer

CONTENT GENERALIZATIONS: Many people promote *and* protect health. Some are health care workers, such as doctors, nurses, dentists, and hospital workers. Others in the community and school include fire fighters, police officers, crossing guards, custodians, school nurses, prin-principals, and teachers. Family members also help protect and promote the health of others.

INITIATION: "Health Helpers"

Read a story or book to the class about a health care worker, school worker, community worker, or family member who protects and promotes the health of others.

MATERIALS

Book or story

ACTIVITIES

1. "Who Am I"—Puppet Game

Use health puppets to play a game, "Who Am I?" Modify the patterns to make the puppets needed for your own version of the game.

  a. Hide the puppets behind a curtain while providing information regarding the role of each health helper, such as the following:

- I have a big light and a mirror so I can look inside your mouth at your teeth. I clean your teeth and tell you how to help your teeth stay healthy. Who am I? (Dentist or dental hygienist.)
- I keep the school clean, and I watch out for things around the school that might be unsafe. Who am I? (Custodian.)

  b. Have the students guess who each health helper is before bringing the puppet out from behind the curtain.

  c. Have the students use the puppets to put on a puppet show naming the health helpers in the show.

MATERIALS

Health helper puppets (teacher-made paper bag puppets using patterns *Health Helpers* (Figures 16-2 to 16-4)
puppet stage

2. Health Helper Pictures

Have the students color pictures of health helpers. When the pictures are done, have them show the pictures to the class, naming the helper displayed.

MATERIALS

Patterns: *Health Helpers* (see Figures 16-2 to 16-4)
Crayons
Resources
Guest speaker(s)

3. Health Helpers We See Every Day

Ask school health helpers, such as the custodian, cafeteria worker, crossing guard, or nurse to visit the class and tell about their job. Speakers may suggest ways students can help keep the school healthful.

EVALUATION: "Health Helper Collage"

Have the students help make a collage of health helpers from pictures in magazines, or have the class paint a mural of health helpers. Ask students to verbally name the health helpers in their work.

MATERIALS

Magazines
Glue
Poster paper (or butcher paper)
Poster paint

FIGURE 16-2

Pattern

Name _____

Health Helpers

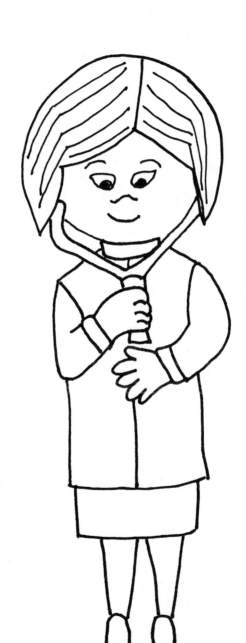

DOCTOR

FIGURE 16-3

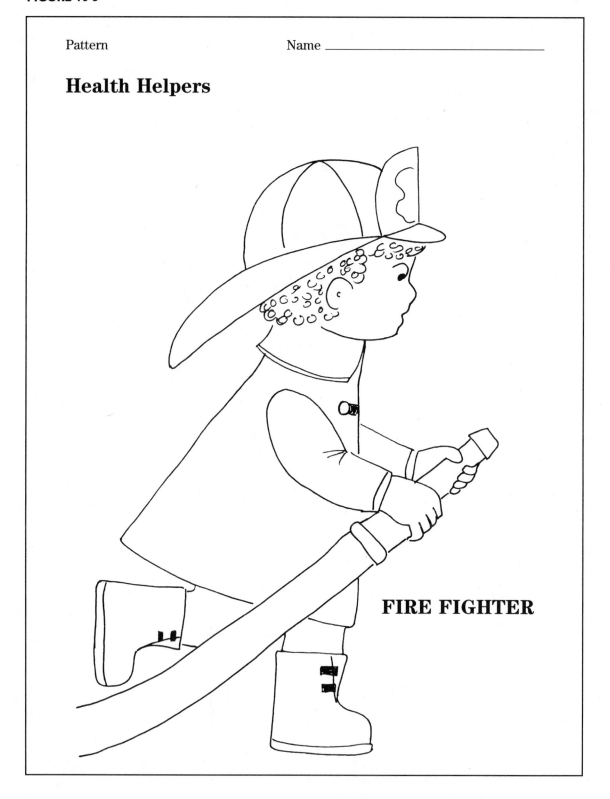

Pattern

Name _____

Health Helpers

FIRE FIGHTER

FIGURE 16-4

Pattern

Name _____

Health Helpers

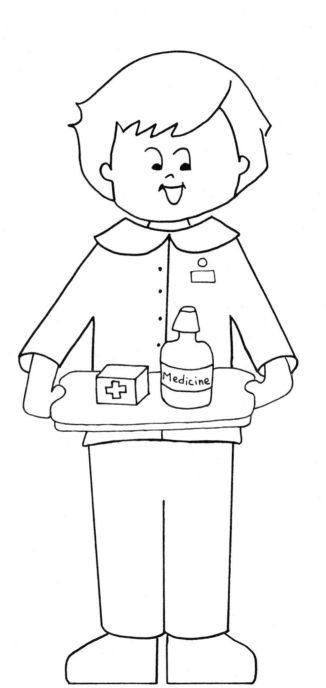

NURSE

INTERMEDIATE LEVEL

OBJECTIVE: The student describes appeals that promote the sale of foods and medications used by children.

LEVEL: Grades 4 to 6

VOCABULARY: Appeal, advertisement, claim, packaging

INTEGRATION: Reading, language arts, creative expression, scientific observation

MATERIALS
Teacher resource: *Advertisement Example* (Figure 16-5)
Shoe box
Construction paper
Felt pens
Red apple

CONTENT GENERALIZATIONS: Advertisements on television, radio, and billboards, and in magazines use various techniques to appeal to children. Food products, such as cereals or candy and gum, and medicines, such as children's vitamins, frequently have advertising aimed specifically at a child. Even if the child does not purchase the item personally, he or she often has an influence on the parent's purchase of various items. Appeals to children's emotions and senses often will include enticements, such as "It's fun to use or eat; it's tasty and smells good; it's popular to do; it's attractive." Powerful words and claims also may be used by advertisers. Finally, the packaging of foods and medications used by children is important. Often games and toys are included with a product as an enticement.

INITIATION: "Coming Soon—A Great Taste Treat"
A head of time, prepare a sign, advertisement, and package similar to the one in the *Advertisement Example.* Two days before the lesson, post

the sign "Coming Soon—A Great Taste Treat" on the bulletin board. The day before beginning the lesson, post the advertisement. Do not answer any questions about the signs. Tell students they will have to wait until they start the consumer health activities.

Write the word *advertising* on the board, and ask if anyone can tell what it means. Point to the signs on the bulletin board and the package, and explain that these are ways to advertise a product. Have students try to guess what it is. Then open the box, and display the product (a red apple). There may be some disappointment. Ask students what kind of product was expected. Use this opportunity to point out that often advertising gets us so excited about a product that we are disappointed when we try it because it is not what we expected.

Then ask students "What is the *purpose* of advertising?" (To get people to buy a product or service.) Tell them that it is important to remember this purpose whenever they see or hear an advertisement and that advertisers never point out the bad or useless aspects of a product.

MATERIALS
Five or six sheets of butcher paper
Felt pens or crayons

ACTIVITIES
1. **Commercials, Commercials, Commercials**
   a. Ask students if they pay much attention to commercials on television. (They will probably say *no.*) Ask them what kinds of products are usually advertised on television shows for children. (Cereals, candy, beverages, fast-food restaurants, cookies, gum, vitamins, toys.)
   b. Divide the students into groups of five or six. Give each group a large piece of newsprint or butcher paper and a felt pen or crayon. Explain that they are going to see which team can recall the most *brand* names for foods and drugs that are advertised on *children's* television programs. Allow students 5 minutes to work on their

lists. Then each group should post their list. Proclaim the "winner" and mention that we do remember products even though we *think* we are not paying attention to commercials.

c. Keep students in groups to continue more activities with their lists. Have the groups retrieve the lists that were posted and consider the following for each product:
- Is the product a food? If so mark an *F* after the product.
- Is the product a drug? If so mark a *D* after the product.
- Is the product high in sugar content? If so, circle the product.
- Put a large *A* next to the products that might be advertised on adult shows.

d. After this has been done for each product, ask the groups to make some generalizations about the types of products advertised on children's programs. If students need further direction, ask if the products advertised on children's television programs are the following:
- Mostly foods or mostly drugs
- Low or high in sugar content
- Seen more often on children's television shows or adult programs

e. If time allows, each group should report their findings (generalizations) to the class.

MATERIALS
Television commercials (3 or 4 recorded on videotape or cassette recorder)

2. Advertising Appeals
Explain to students that they will be focusing on products that are advertised to children, particularly foods and medications (such as vitamins).

a. Write the word *appeal* on the board, and explain that advertisers use various methods to try to make a product *appeal* to us so we will buy it. These methods are called advertising *appeals*.

- *Fun:* Commercials often make using a product look like fun. The people or characters are shown having lots of fun, or the commercial is funny (such as a cartoon). The result is that the product looks like it is fun to use.
- *Tasty:* Commercials often tell you how good the products taste. Remind students of their brainstorming activity in groups, and ask what kind of taste is advertised most often. (Sweet.)
- *Popular:* Commercials often make the product look like it is popular to use. People in commercials are portrayed as popular and attractive with lots of friends. In other words, *everybody* who is *anybody* uses this product.

b. Tell students that they are going to practice identifying these appeals with real commercials. Play three or four previously recorded commercials for the class. (Videotape is preferable, but cassette recordings of television commercials work just as well.) After each commercial ask students which appeals they observed. To give all students a chance to think about their answers, have them record their ideas on paper before calling on a volunteer to share his or her answer. **NOTE:** Because television advertising changes so frequently, it is not possible to provide examples of commercials using each appeal that still will be on television at the time of the lesson. The following are provided to give the teacher ideas.
- Trix cereal is a classic example of a commercial using appeals to *fun* and *taste*. The "silly" cartoon rabbit never gets the wonderful tasting Trix cereal.
- Dr. Pepper and Coca-Cola commercials have often used the *popular* appeal. Groups of attractive young adults convey the image that these beverages are used by the "in" crowd.

c. Refer back to the advertisement used in the initiation activity. Ask the students to identify the appeals used in this advertisement. (Taste and popularity.) Point out that another way to sell products is to use powerful words, or *power words*. Ask if anyone can identify a power word in the advertisement. Write the following power words on the board or on a sign hung on the bulletin board: wonderful, strong, great, super, new, exciting, and fun. Explain that these words often are used to attract attention to a product. Other power words also can be found in advertisements.

MATERIALS

Teacher resource: *Advertisement Example* (See Figure 16-5)

3. What's the Appeal?

a. As a homework assignment, hand out the worksheets, *What's the Appeal?* Students are to watch television commercials about foods or medications and look at children's magazines to complete their assignment. The two worksheets should be used while viewing four television commercials and two printed advertisements. (A separate sheet will be needed for each commercial and advertisement.) The printed advertisements can be found in children's magazines, comics, or the comic section of the weekend newspaper.

b. For each television commercial, the date, time of day observed, channel, and program are to be recorded. Explain that all scientific surveys involve gathering as much specific information as possible. The product being advertised must be listed, as well as a brief description of the advertisement. Then the advertising appeals observed should be listed, including any power words.

c. When the assignment is completed, put the students into their small groups to discuss their observations. What appeals were observed most often? What kind of products were observed most often? Were there many high-sugar foods? What power words were used most often? As time allows, the groups should report their findings to the class. Determine which appeal was observed most often by the entire class. Do the same for power words.

MATERIALS

Worksheet: *What's the Appeal? Television Commercials* (4 sheets per student) (Figure 16-6); *Printed Advertisements* (2 sheets per student) (Figure 16-7)

EVALUATION: "How Do They Sell That Product?"

Have the groups act out one of the commercials observed, without mentioning the product name. The class should guess the type of product (and specific brand if possible). Tell each student to describe on paper the methods used to sell this product. Advertising appeals and power words should be identified in their descriptions.

FIGURE 16-5

Teacher resource

Name _____

Advertisement Example

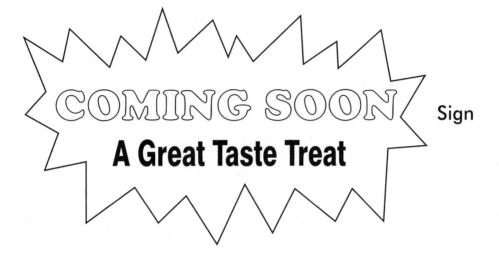

Sign

Try the **EXCITING** and **POPULAR** snack treat

RED & SWEET

Soooo Gooood   Yum Yum

<u>Great</u> any time of the day!

Advertisement

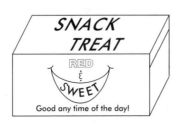

SNACK TREAT
RED & SWEET
Good any time of the day!

Package

FIGURE 16-6

Worksheet   Name _____

What's the Appeal?
Television Commercials

Directions: View four television commercials, and
analyze the methods used to sell a
product to children that is either food or
a drug. Use a separate sheet for each
commercial.

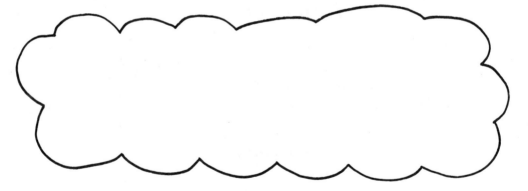

1. Product name_____

2. Television show where it was advertised_____

3. Date and time viewed_____

4. Channel_____

5. Brief description of what happens in the commercial:

6. Appeals used in the commercial_____
_____

7. Power words used in the commercial_____
_____

8. Is the product a FOOD or a MEDICATION?   (Circle one)

9. Is the product high in sugar?   YES   NO   (circle one)

FIGURE 16-7

Worksheet   Name _____

What's the Appeal?
Printed Advertisements

Directions: Find two printed advertisements in children's magazines, comics,
 or the comic section of the newspaper. Analyze the advertisement
              by answering the questions below. Complete a separate sheet for
              each advertisement.

1. Product name_____
2. Newspaper or magazine where it was found_____
3. Brief description of the advertisement (describe the picture or artwork)

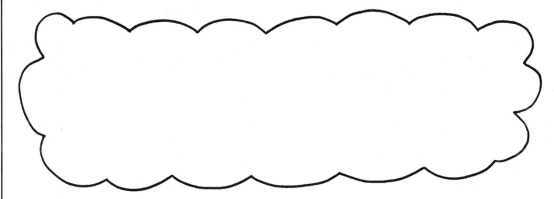

4. Appeals used in the advertisement_____
   _____
5. Power words used in the advertisement_____
   _____
6. Was the advertisement about a FOOD or a MEDICATION?   (Circle one)
7. Was the product high in sugar?   YES   NO   (Circle one)

MIDDLE SCHOOL LEVEL

OBJECTIVE: The student identifies criteria for the selection of an appropriate health adviser.

LEVEL: Grades 6 to 8

VOCABULARY: Advice, quackery, fraud, testimonials

CONTENT GENERALIZATIONS: The first source of help for the selection of health advisers is usually parents. Generally, select a health adviser who is trained to provide the information required and who is able and willing to refer you to another practitioner who may be more qualified to provide particular health services.

INITIATION: "Advice"
Write the word *advice* on the board. Ask the students to define the word. (A recommendation about what to do about a problem.)

Ask the students if they ever ask for advice from other people. Ask "Why do people need advice? Do we ever get bad advice? What might be some examples of bad advice?"

ACTIVITIES
1. What's Wrong Here?
Hand out the worksheet, *What's Wrong Here?* Review the directions with students. Explain that they are to read a story about someone who was seeking advice on a problem. Students are to write a short explanation of what each person did wrong in seeking advice. When they have finished the worksheets individually, ask them to share their responses with one or two others in the class. Then discuss the situations as a whole class. Ask the following questions:
- What is wrong with Peter asking his dentist to fix his car? (Peter has no idea if the dentist knows anything about cars. The dentist is not qualified to fix cars, only teeth.)

- What is wrong with Vicki asking her neighbor to fix her faucet? (Her neighbor is not qualified to fix plumbing. If he tries and something goes wrong, it may end up being a bigger problem.)
- What is wrong with Ken asking Bruce what to do about his cold and sore throat? (Bruce is not qualified to answer medical questions.)

After discussing each situation, ask the students "What is the most important factor to think about in seeking advice?" (Is the person qualified?) Remind the students that people may be qualified to give advice in some areas but not in others. For example, Peter's dentist certainly could give advice on care of the teeth but not on care of cars.

MATERIALS
Worksheet: *What's Wrong Here?* (Figure 16-8)

2. Criteria for Qualified Advisors
Ask the students if they have any idea how to choose someone to advise them on health matters. Ask "How do you know if a person is qualified?" After they have offered suggestions, explain that most people qualified to give health advice have been to school and have special training. Often the state requires that health professionals take a special test to get a license to practice in that state.

Write the following criteria on the board, and have the students copy it:
- Qualified health advisers have special training (for example, 8 to 15 years of schooling for medical doctors) and a license from the state.
- Qualified health advisers do not offer a secret cure that only they can provide; say that you do not need another adviser's opinion; sell products door-to-door, in magazines, or on television; use testimonials, coupons, or guarantees.

3. Reading the Fine Print

Have the students cut out advertisements from magazines about cures for problems such as baldness and obesity. Students should look for advertisements that seem too good to be true. Explain the importance of reading the fine print. Post them all on a bulletin board. From time to time during the activities on consumer health, ask for volunteers to share an advertisement they found particularly questionable.

EVALUATION: "Good Advice—Bad Advice"

Give each student a copy of the worksheet, *Good Advice—Bad Advice*. Tell them to circle *yes* if they think the advice will be from a qualified health adviser or *no* if they think the person may not be qualified.

After everyone has had a chance to circle their answers, go over each item in class. Ask for volunteers to share their responses and explain the reason for the choice.

MATERIALS

Worksheet: *Good Advice—Bad Advice*
(Figure 16–9)

FIGURE 16-8

Worksheet   Name _____

What's Wrong Here?

Directions: Below are several stories about people who needed advice. Read the
                story, then write an explanation about what the person did wrong in
                seeking advice on the problem.

1. Peter had car problems. Every time he started the car, black smoke
   would come out of the exhaust, and the car would make clunking
   noises. He had a problem, so he called his dentist. After all, his
   dentist was the smartest person he knew; certainly he could fix the
   car if Peter offered to pay him.

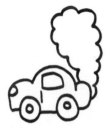

2. Vicki had a sink that dripped water from the faucet even when it was
   turned off. Her water bills were higher than normal, and the constant
   dripping noise was driving her crazy. She called her neighbor Sam. He
   was an accountant, but he had a few tools.

3. Ken was sneezing and coughing. He felt terrible. He asked his best
   friend Bruce what he should do about his cold and sore throat.
   Bruce's mother was a nurse, so certainly he would know what to do.

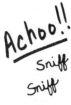

FIGURE 16-9

Worksheet   Name _____

Good Advice—Bad Advice

Directions: Circle yes if you think the person described is a qualified health adviser
and no if you think the person is not.

Would you take the advice of...

1. Someone with a diploma on the wall of her office who   YES   NO
   tells you she has a new cure for your sore throat that
   is still a secret and only available from her?

2. Someone who has been treating people in your family   YES   NO
   for many years and is licensed by your state to practice
   medicine?

3. Someone who is selling a diet remedy door to door?   YES   NO

4. Someone who has been practicing medicine in your   YES   NO
   community for a few months (The local medical
   society has never heard of him. He says that his license
   just has not been sent yet.)?

5. Someone who discourages you from getting a second   YES   NO
   opinion on your condition and thinks that you should
   just go ahead and get the surgery over with?

6. Someone who offers a quick, too-good-to-be-true cure   YES   NO
   for a health condition?

7. An actor who gives a testimonial on television about   YES   NO
   the health benefits of a certain product?

17 Drug Use Prevention

When you finish this chapter, you should be able to:

- Compare the short- and long-term effects of drug use among different categories of drugs.
- Describe the psychosocial factors of drug use.
- Identify types of treatment for drug use.
- Develop learning opportunities for primary, intermediate, and middle-school students in the area of drug use prevention.

DRUGS

Drugs change the physical and mental workings of the body. When used correctly, drugs can save lives, cure illness, prevent disease, and relieve pain. However, inappropriate use of drugs can lead to physical or psychological drug dependence or both. Any drug or medication has the potential of being useful or hazardous to health.

Medications

Medicines are drugs used to treat disease and the symptoms of disease. Medications are also used for treatments when injuries occur. Drugs used as medications can be obtained for use outside medical care settings. Some can be bought freely off the drugstore or market shelf (over the counter). Others can be purchased only with a prescription from a physican or dentist. Whether the drug is over the counter or prescription, you should read and follow the directions and pay at-

tention to any warnings that appear on the label. Medications are helpful and can save lives when used correctly but can be dangerous when used incorrectly.

Over-the-Counter Drugs

Over-the-counter drugs can be bought without a prescription—at food stores, drug stores, and many other places. There are over-the-counter drugs for headaches, allergies, colds, coughs, stomach aches, rashes, and certain infections. Recently more medications have been approved for use over the counter. A few examples include cortisone cream for treatment of rashes and insect bites and medication used to treat vaginal yeast infections.

Prescription Drugs

Physicians often treat illnesses with medication that can only be bought with a prescription.

These drugs are unsafe for self-medication and therefore must be filled by a pharmacist who is specially trained to prepare the prescription for individual use. It is particularly important to inform the pharmacist of other medications you are currently taking and to follow the directions carefully and fully. Many people believe that once they feel better, they can stop taking a course of medication. Unless otherwise indicated, most prescription medicines must be finished.

Psychoactive Drugs

Psychoactive drugs are drugs that interact with the central nervous system. These drugs alter an individual's mood, mental process, and behavior. Major forms and descriptions of common psychoactive drugs are described below.

Stimulants act on the central nervous system to increase pulse rate, blood pressure, strength of heart contractions, and muscle tension. Caffeine, amphetamines, methamphetamine ("ice"), cocaine/crack, and nicotine are examples of stimulant drugs.

Short-term effects are increased heart beat, blood pressure, and alertness and possible dizziness and a shaky feeling.

Long-term effects are mood changes, weight loss, depression, hallucinations, and brain, heart, and lung damage.

The use of **tobacco products** is considered to be related to more deaths than any other single health behavior. Tobacco contains a powerful drug called *nicotine*, a chemical often used as an insecticide. Nicotine is a "stimulant" drug and, when taken into the body, causes the circulatory and respiratory systems to speed up. Nicotine also causes the blood vessels to narrow so that the heart has to work harder to pump the blood through the body. Tobacco can be smoked in the form of cigarettes, cigars, and pipes or used in a smokeless form. Snuff and chewing tobacco are forms of smokeless tobacco.

Short-term effects are faster heartbeat, higher blood pressure, nausea, dizziness, bad breath, stained teeth, and relief of feelings of tensions.

Long-term effects are lung damage; cancer of the lung, mouth, and throat; high blood pressure; stomach ulcers; and loss of the sense of smell and taste.

Cocaine is a chemical made from the leaves of the coca plant. It is a powerful stimulant that usually comes in the form of a white powder. It is smoked (usually sprinkled on a cigarette or marijuana), snorted (breathed in through the nose), or injected with a needle. No matter which way it is used, it is very addictive.

Short-term effects are faster heart beat, higher blood pressure, higher body temperature, and the inability to sit still or sleep.

Long-term effects are permanent lung damage, ulcers in the nasal passages, personality changes and violent behavior, paranoia, and hallucinations.

Depressants are drugs that slow down the central nervous system. Alcohol is the most commonly used depressant drug. Others are tranquilizers and barbiturates. Effects of these drugs include lowering of inhibitions, sedation, and sleep; in higher doses, effects include coma and death.

Short-term effects are relaxed muscles, feelings of calmness or sleepiness, confusion, and slurred speech.

Long-term effects are chest infections, liver and brain damage associated with alcoholism, hallucinations, and possible death with an overdose.

Alcohol is a drug found in beer, wine, and liquor. It is a "depressant" drug that decreases the brain's ability to function and can cause dependency in certain individuals. Movement becomes slower, judgment and coordination are impaired, and the heart and respiratory systems slow. Use of alcohol with other drugs or while operating a car can be deadly.

Short-term effects are relaxation, loss of inhibitions, nausea, mood changes with possible feelings of violence or depression, and loss of muscle control (for example, staggering).

Long-term effects are permanent liver damage, permanent damage to the brain and heart, liver cancer, stomach ulcers, high blood pressure, and alcoholism.

Psychedelics and **hallucinogens** change the perceptions in some way. Peyote, psilocybin, LSD, PCP, and mescaline are examples of drugs in this group.

Short-term effects are faster heart beats, high blood pressure, hallucinations, and confusion (even panic).

Long-term effects are depression, memory loss, and other mental problems.

Narcotics provide pain relief and induce sleep. Examples of narcotics include opium, morphine, codeine, heroin, meperidine, and methadone.

Short-term effects are slower heartbeat, slower breathing, and nausea.

Long-term effects are lung damage, lower sex drive, constipation, and death with overdose.

Cannabis is a plant that is processed and sold as marijuana and hashish. The active ingredient in all cannabis products is THC (tetrahydrocannabinol). At low doses, THC produces effects similar to the depressant drugs. At higher levels, hallucinogenic effects are experienced, including sensory distortion and vivid hallucinations.

Short-term effects are feelings of calmness and relaxation, faster heart beat, slower reaction time, dry mouth and lips, and loss of the sense of time.

Long-term effects are heart and lung damage, lung cancer, inability to fight off colds and flus, memory loss, lower sperm count (for males), and disruption of the menstrual cycle (for women). Lung cancer may result from long-term smoking of marijuana.

Inhalants are chemicals that emit fumes. These fumes can be inhaled and cause a reaction in the body. There are numerous chemicals easily available for household use that are abused through inhalation. A few examples of these include glue, paint, hair spray, and household cleaners.

Short-term effects are dizziness, headaches, slurred speech, sneezing and bloody nose, nausea, and loss of control of bladder and bowels.

Long-term effects are permanent brain, lung, and kidney damage; fatigue; weakness of muscles; and possible death when used with alcohol or other depressants.

Steroids (anabolic steroids) are copies of the male hormone testosterone. Steroids assist in building up muscle and bone tissue in the body. They are used therapeutically to treat growth disorders.

Short-term effects are mood changes often resulting in feelings of depression or violence, acne, loss of hair, increased muscle growth, increased time to recover from injury, and lower sex drive.

Long-term effects are heart attacks, liver cancer, stopped growth in height, shrinking testicles, sterility (for males), and disruption of the menstrual cycle (for women).

PCP (phencycladine) is a chemical that is used as an animal tranquilizer.

Short-term effects are faster heartbeat, higher blood pressure, blurred eyesight, hallucinations, slurred speech, and slowed body movements and sense of time.

Long-term effects are permanent brain, heart, and lung damage; permanent speech problems, severe mental problems and fears, and memory loss.

DRUG MISUSE AND ABUSE

Drug misuse occurs when a drug is used in ways that can harm the body. Taking more medicine than the directions indicate and taking someone else's medicine are examples of drug misuse. Drug abuse occurs when drugs are used for purposes other than those for which they are intended. A person who abuses a drug risks becoming dependent on the drug and may suffer other ill effects.

LAWS REGULATING DRUGS AND USE

Many laws regulate the use of drugs. Federal, state, and local laws exist regarding drugs. Certain federal laws determine standards that drugs must pass to be legally sold in the United States.

WHAT ABOUT MY STUDENTS?

In the early years, content in this area should focus on safe behavior around unknown substances. Students in primary grades need to learn that drugs are medicines used only under the direction of a medical advisor or parent. Some people choose to use certain mood modifiers such as tobacco and alcohol. These substances should not be used by children. Because these kinds of mood modifiers can be harmful to health, many adults also choose to avoid these substances. Harmful substances may have special markings or special containers to help children identify them as dangerous. A skull and crossbones indicate that the contents are poisonous.

The Food and Drug Administration (FDA) sets these standards. The FDA also determines how drugs are sold legally. Some drugs are sold over the counter, which means that they can be purchased without a prescription. Others are prescription drugs and can be purchased only with a physician's order. Certain drugs are not usually taken for medical reasons. Some of these drugs are legal (such as alcohol and tobacco), and others are not (such as marijuana, cocaine, LSD, and PCP). State and local laws often regulate the sale of legal drugs, alcohol, and tobacco. Such laws regarding the age for purchasing these drugs, the penalty for drunk driving, hours when alcohol can be sold, and where a bar can be located, vary from state to state. Some countries do not allow the sale of alcohol. These are called *dry counties.*

Laws regulating the use of drugs are made for the sake of protection. In the case of prescription and over-the-counter drugs, the laws make drug companies prove that their drug is safe if used as directed. This means that drug companies must research their drugs carefully before they can sell them to the public or suggest that physicians prescribe the drugs. Thalidomide is an example of a drug that was thought safe and used in other countries. It was taken by many pregnant women in England and by some in the United States who got it while traveling or stationed abroad or was given by physicians who received the drug as samples and assumed that it was safe to distribute. The drug was later found to be the cause of severe birth defects. It had not been made legal to use in the United States because there was not enough research completed to meet the standards of the FDA.

Other drugs are thought to be unsafe and unhealthful and are not legal to use. However, controversy exists about whether some of these illegal drugs should be legalized. Marijuana has been shown to help cancer patients counteract the nausea of chemotherapy and is being prescribed for this purpose by physicians in some states. Some argue that marijuana is not as unsafe or unhealthful as the legal drugs alcohol and tobacco. Others argue that even if marijuana is not as harmful, it is not wise to legalize it and add to the problems caused by the use of alcohol and tobacco.

Laws concerning driving an automobile while under the influence of alcohol are meant to protect the innocent people who are involved in traffic incidents. Drunk drivers are responsible for approximately half the fatal automobile crashes in the United States. Many states have strict laws about driving while drinking or under the influence of alcohol.

Age requirements to legally buy cigarettes and alcohol exist because these drugs can be physically harmful. It is generally believed by society that the legal use of these drugs should be limited to adults who are better able to understand the consequences of their actions.

PSYCHOSOCIAL FACTORS AND DRUG USE

Many factors influence drug use or abuse, including family, culture, and religion. The beliefs and actions of friends and family members have a profound effect on personal use or abuse of drugs. Peers are particularly influential in the lives of adolescents, and adolescents often abuse drugs to be accepted by peers.

Modeling and media are important influences on drug use. Children act as they see adults act. If the adults around a child use alcohol, tobacco, or other drugs, a very strong use message is modeled. The old saying, "actions speak louder than words," is very appropriate when it comes to modeling drug use or nonuse. In addition to family members, teachers are strong models for children and adolescents.

The media (including movies and music videos) is a powerful modeling influence on almost everyone. The media defines beauty and sexuality, including femininity and masculinity, for many. When drug use is linked to these media images, strong messages supporting drug use occurs. Although tobacco has been banned from TV commercials for over 20 years, the image of the *Marlboro Man* as a handsome definition of masculinity lives on. Some believe that tobacco advertisements actually have more television than ever before with the advent of sponsored sports events. Sponsors get their names, logos, and even advertisements on almost anything. While watching a game on television, you may also be watching the donated scoreboard that bears the name of the sponsor. Professional athletes wear T-shirts, visors, shorts, and shoes and drive cars that sell various products. Some of these are for drugs—particularly tobacco and beer.

When *no use* policies and laws are enacted, the most powerful influence of all—*societal norms*—is exercised. If society values no use of a product, the behavior of individuals in society will follow. The example of the power of societal norms is most evident when it comes to cigarette smoking. In less than a generation, we have seen society model the nonuse message for cigarette smoking. It is no longer a right to light up anywhere. There are smoke-free restaurants, smoke-free workplaces, and smoke-free airline travel in the United States and many other countries. Laws and policies are important, but societal norms that support those policies and laws are driving the movement.

WHAT ABOUT MY STUDENTS AND PEER PRESSURE?

Children and adolescents should know what peer pressure is and that it is a normal part of growing up. Peer pressure is a part of adult life as well, although it is not as significant in influencing important adult decisions. Your students should understand that it is all right to be different and that if they are not interested in certain activities in which their friends are involved, perhaps they should find new friends.

Peer pressure is the most important factor contributing to adolescent use of drugs. Adolescents are very concerned about being accepted by group members. It is normal for adolescents to form groups of friends who dress similarly, are involved in the same activities, and explore new activities together. If these groups are involved in using drugs, there usually is a great deal of peer pressure for everyone to participate. Often this pressure is so great that adolescents will participate despite the wishes and values of their parents or themselves. In addition, knowing the health risks related to the abuse of drugs does not always act as a deterrent when peer pressure is involved.

Cultural and ethnic traditions are often a part of drug use. Attitudes about drug use vary among families and cultures. Teachers should become familiar with the cultural, ethnic, and economic diversity of their students. This will allow educators to better meet the needs of students. However, generalizations and assumptions cannot be made based on cultural and ethnic traditions.

When a person cannot stop using a drug, even though it causes serious problem, it is considered an addiction. There is a strong urge to use a drug that overpowers all other things. When this interferes with family, friends, jobs, school, money, or health, an individual is considered addicted to the drug. There are often legal indications of addiction. An addiction is considered a disease that can be treated.

When individuals depend on drugs to cope with feelings of fear, anxiety, and emotional pain, a drug dependency or addiction may be developing. Dependency may develop for persons who use drugs to escape pressures and problems in life. When drugs are used as coping mechanisms, the skills and emotional tools needed to become emotionally stable do not develop.

There are two basic types of addiction. Physically, drug addiction begins to occur when the brain "needs" the drug to feel normal. Without the drug, the individual can become sick. This is a physical addiction. When individuals learn that a drug makes them feel better in that it may cover up shyness, fear, anger, or other strong emotions, a psychological addiction can occur. Most often physical and psychological addictions appear together.

Many drugs are addictive, but some are more addictive than others. Nicotine (tobacco) is very addictive. A total of 9 out of 10 people who use tobacco get addicted. Other addictive drugs include cocaine, heroin, prescription narcotics such as pain pills, alcohol, LSD, PCP, and inhalants. Marijuana is also addictive. It stays in the body for a long time, resulting in fewer withdrawal symptoms, so people mistakenly think it is not addictive.

TREATMENT

Because the negative effects of many types of drug use are long-term, the health hazards related to the use of tobacco, alcohol, and other "social" drugs are often difficult to recognize. Often we use these drugs with no ill effects. Most of the physical diseases related to drugs take years to develop. In the case of tobacco and cardiovascular disease, the disease most often linked to cigarette smoking, 20 to 30 years may pass before any symptoms or problems appear. Cirrhosis of the liver, commonly linked to alcohol abuse, also takes years to develop. With chewing tobacco,

more problems related to the gums (including cancer) are being found.

Prevention of these conditions is more effective than treatment. Observation of immediate effects helps explain the risks. The effect of nicotine can be observed by testing pulse rate, blood pressure, and fine motor skills. A tobacco user will find it difficult to hold the hand as steady after using tobacco as before. Individuals who use smokeless tobacco can see changes in the soft tissues of the mouth in the area where the tobacco is "held." Staining of the teeth, recession of the gum tissue, and sensitivity to hot and cold are also signs of tobacco's effects.

Treatment for drug use will not be effective without personalization. This means that until individuals decide that they are at risk, they will not stop a habit or may be tempted to start. Many people cannot believe they have a drug problem even though it is clear to others. This is called *denial.* Denial is a major barrier to treatment and recovery.

Successful treatment consists of the following:

1. Stop using the drug and receive treatment for withdrawal if necessary.
2. Learn how the drug has become so important in your life.
3. Learn how to avoid using the drug again.

Types of Treatment

Treatment for drug abuse is difficult. Drug use affects not only the person who uses the drug but also the family and friends of that person. The basic approaches to drug abuse treatment are the following:

1. Detoxification—the supervised withdrawal from drug dependence.
2. Therapeutic communities—controlled environments in which drug abusers live and participate in counseling as they learn to develop drug-free lifestyles.
3. Outpatient drug-free programs—groups that emphasize various forms of counseling and support systems. Alcoholics Anonymous (AA) is an example of such an

organization. Other organizations have been formed to help persons with other drug-related problems (Narcotics Anonymous) and to help the families and friends of persons with drug dependencies (Al-anon and Alateen). Other groups, such as the American Cancer Society and the American Lung Association, offer programs for the cessation of tobacco use.

A WORD ABOUT ALCOHOL

Problem drinking and alcoholism among teenagers and young adults is becoming more prevalent in the United States and therefore demands particular attention. Anyone choosing to use alcohol must understand the concept of responsible drinking; if the decision is made to use alcohol, it should be used responsibly. That includes avoiding driving or riding a bicycle while under the influence, avoiding riding with a driver who has been drinking; being aware of alcohol habits, and not overdoing it. Drinking can be paced to allow the body time to metabolize the alcohol. It is always a good idea to eat food when consuming alcohol. Some people choose not to drink alcohol at all; their choice should be respected, and they should not be pushed into drinking.

HIV AND DRUGS

Because of the HIV epidemic, the issue of HIV and drug use must be addressed. The risk of HIV infection (infection with the virus that causes AIDS) is high with drug users. Those people particularly at risk are individuals using injection drugs (IV drugs). IV drug use is considered one of the most risky behaviors possible in the spread of HIV. The best choice is not to use IV drugs at all. If that is not your choice, you should *never* use a dirty needle.

SUMMARY

Drug use prevention is critical to the overall health of individuals and society. Teachers have a role to play, not only in teaching content and skills to refuse drugs but in modeling healthy behavior. The next section provides example learning opportunities for use at the primary level, intermediate level, and middle-school level.

SUGGESTED READINGS

Drugs, alcohol and tobacco. Macmillan health encyclopedia, vol 7, 1993, New York, Macmillan Publishing.

Evans D, Giarratano S: *Into adolescence: avoiding drugs*, Santa Cruz, Calif, 1990, ETR Associates.

Giarratano S, Evans D: *Entering adulthood: examining drugs and risks*, Santa Cruz, Calif, 1990, ETR Associates.

Henderson A: *Healthy schools, healthy futures: the case for improving school environment*, Santa Cruz, Calif, 1993, ETR Associates.

Payne W, Hahn D: *Understanding your health*, St Louis, 1992, Mosby.

Pruitt BE: *Alcohol and other drug use prevention education* In Cortese P, Middleton K, eds: *The comprehensive school health challenge*, Santa Cruz, Calif, 1994, ETR Associates.

Drug facts, Santa Cruz, Calif, 1990, ETR Associates.

Addiction facts, Santa Cruz, Calif, 1990, ETR Associates.

Villarreal SF, McKinney LE Quackenbush M: *Handle with care: helping children prenatally exposed to drugs and alcohol*, Santa Cruz, Calif, 1992, ETR Associates.

LEARNING OPPORTUNITIES FOR DRUG USE PREVENTION

GENERAL STUDENT OBJECTIVES

Primary Level K-3

The student:

1. Explains reasons for avoiding use of controlled drugs or unknown substances.
2. Explains reasons why many people avoid using any drugs including tobacco and alcohol.
3. Demonstrates effective ways of refusing offers of drugs*

Intermediate Level 4-5/6

The student:

1. Analyzes reasons why some people abuse drugs.
2. Explains why we have laws controlling use of drugs.*
3. Evaluates the effectiveness of problem solving skills in choosing alternatives to drug use.

Middle School Level 6/7-8

The student:

1. Predicts effects of drugs on physical, mental, and social functioning.
2. Analyzes factors motivating individuals to avoid or abuse drugs.
3. Interprets the significance of peer pressure on decisions regarding drug use.*

---

*These objectives are illustrated by sample learning opportunities.

PRIMARY LEVEL

OBJECTIVE: The student demonstrates effective ways of refusing offers of drugs.

LEVEL: Grades 2 to 3

INTEGRATION: Language arts

VOCABULARY: Refusals

CONTENT GENERALIZATIONS: Practicing the skills to refuse drugs in a classroom situation allows children the opportunity to deal with this situation in a "safe" environment. The skills learned in class can transfer to life situations.

Saying "no" in a way that is meaningful is a learned skill. Actually, all children know how to say "no." It is commonly a word heard by many a parent or teacher. However, to empower children to say no to drugs requires specific steps and practice. Body language that indicates that you mean no is important. Following are recommended for younger children:

- Look the person in the eye
- Say the word "no" with a voice that says you mean what you say
- Say why you mean "no"
- Offer an alternative (something else to do)
- Repeat the refusal over and over
- Walk away if necessary

INITIATION: "Do I Mean What I Say?"

Tell students to watch you carefully as you act out a situation. Set it up by telling the class that you were just offered a cigarette. (If you like, start with an offer of something other than a drug, such as a soda).

Using as much drama as you can, say no to the offer of the cigarette (soda). Using body language and your voice say "no" in an unconvincing way.

Ask students if they thought you really meant no. Most students this age will pick up the fact that you really didn't know what you wanted.

ACTIVITIES

1. Saying No and Meaning It

Conduct a discussion of the things that need to happen to communicate that you mean no. Use a poster that illustrates the big ideas. Keep it simple for students, but include the following in the discussion:

- Have eye contact
- Say no like you mean it and explain why
- Offer an alternative (something else to do)
- Walk away

MATERIALS

Poster: Say No! (teacher-made) (Figure 17-1)

1. Practice, Practice, Practice

a. Go to each child individually and offer a soda. Tell them to tell you no in a convincing way. After each offer, ask the rest of the class to critique the refusal. Review the steps on the poster during the critique.

b. Have students write a few sentences on "Why I don't want a cigarette."

c. Roleplay again by offering a cigarette. Have each child say why they don't want the cigarette. Critique again.

NOTE: for this exercise it is important for the teacher to make the offer and put light pressure on students. If you role play this with children making the offers, you will provide children practice in peer pressure to use drugs.

EVALUATION: "Can You Say No?" Individually have students demonstrate a refusal statement to your offer of drugs. Observe their ability to have eye contact, to say no in a convincing way, to say why they refuse, and to walk away.

FIGURE 17-1

Poster   Name _____

Say No!

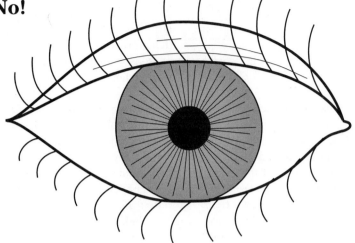

NO!

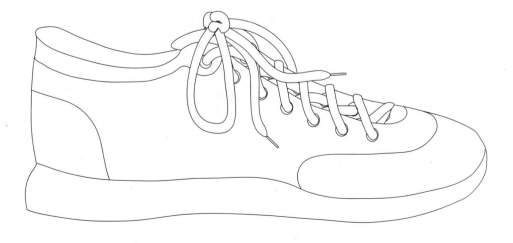

INTERMEDIATE LEVEL

OBJECTIVE: The student explains why we have laws controlling the use of drugs.

LEVEL: Grades 4 to 6

INTEGRATION: Language arts, media, social studies

VOCABULARY: Laws, legal, hazardous

CONTENT GENERALIZATIONS: There are many laws that regulate the sale and use of drugs. These laws exist for the protection of the health and safety of all of society. Legal drugs are those that have passed rigorous testing to prove their safety and usefulness. These include drugs prescribed by a physician and those sold over-the-counter in drug stores without a prescription. Two other drugs that are not used to treat diseases or to promote health are alcohol and tobacco, which are recreational drugs legal for use by adults. However, the sale and use of these drugs is controlled by state and local officials. In some places in the United States, the sale of alcohol is prohibited, and many cities and local communities have passed laws to regulate cigarette smoking in public places.

Other drugs are unsafe and unhealthful and are not legal to use at all. Experts believe that illegal drugs, such as marijuana, PCP, heroin, LSD, inhalants, cocaine, and crack are dangerous and that safe and responsible use is not possible. The use of legal and illegal drugs by young people is a serious problem in the United States.

MATERIALS
Chalkboard with 15 or so small pieces of chalk in tray

INITIATION: "Drugs and the Law—Where Do You Stand?"
Draw a line from one side of the board to the other. At one end of the line write the words, "More-Laws Larry" (or Lucy), and at the other end write "No-Laws Nelson" (or Nelli). Put a vertical line directly in the center of the long line.

Tell the students that the line represents all the attitudes about laws regulating drugs. The two mythical persons hold the *absolute* extreme attitudes on both ends. Explain to the students that you will be telling the class of these two persons' beliefs, and the students are to think of where their personal feelings are in relation to these two extremes.

Tell them, "More-Laws Larry thinks that all drugs should be available by prescription only. That includes aspirin, coffee, and cola drinks (because they contain caffeine). He thinks that alcohol and cigarettes should be totally against the law and that people caught with alcohol or cigarettes should be thrown in jail.

"No-Laws Nelson believes that there are already too many laws about drugs. People should be able to drink alcohol and smoke cigarettes whenever and wherever they please. There should be absolutely no age limits. In fact, he thinks kindergarten kids need to start drinking beer so they can learn how to hold their liquor. He thinks that all drugs should be legal and should be sold without a prescription, including marijuana, heroin, and crack."

Ask students to come to the board as a class and mark an X on the line where they think their beliefs lie regarding laws and drugs. Tell them that they cannot place their X on the center line. When the X's have been marked, ask, "Where do most people's beliefs about laws lie?" (Most will be around the center, but there will be a range.) Ask if they have observed a difference in people's attitudes about laws regulating drugs.

ACTIVITIES
1. And Now The News
Involve the entire class in a project designed to find out about the laws related to drugs in your local area, the reasons for these laws, and the viewpoints of different people in the community about the laws.

  a. Tell the class that they will be putting on a full-scale television show (or radio show if videotape equipment is not available). It will be a program called *Drugs and the Law*. Several committees (teams) will be formed to accomplish the task. Suggested committee organization and responsibilities are as outlined as follows. Write the team name on the board as each is explained.

- *Anchor host committee* (two cohosts) should provide leadership for the total production. They narrate the show and make certain all the teams are doing their jobs and will be on time for the taping.
- *Production committee* (three to five members) is responsible for the actual taping. They must plan the staging and background props and make suggestions for costuming.
- *Reporter teams* (several committees of four to six students, based on the number of drugs and related laws studied) must research the stories, write the stories, take appropriate pictures to enhance the stories, and appoint reporter(s) to read the story on the air.

b. **NOTE:** the anchor hosts are very important. These might be elected by the students. Explain that responsible persons are essential in these positions. Given the criteria, students probably will elect capable persons to the positions.

c. After the anchor hosts are identified, allow students to sign up for positions on the other teams. The various reporter teams possible include the following.
- Alcohol investigation team
- Cigarette investigation team
- Legal drugs investigation team (over-the-counter and prescription drugs)
- Illegal drugs investigation team (such as heroin, crack, inhalants, PCP, LSD, and marijuana)

d. Put a sign up sheet for students to list a first and second choice. Divide the students equally among the groups.

e. When the committees and teams have been identified, have them meet in groups and elect a leader. The leaders will be in close contact with the anchor hosts regarding progress.

f. Give each reporter team a worksheet that correlates with their team. Allow them to study the ideas on the sheet and plan their strategy for the investigation.

g. The responsibilities for the reporter teams will generally be the following.
- Identify the basic laws for that drug.
- Find out why there are laws about that drug.
- Find out how people in the community feel about the law and that drug.
- Write an interesting script that tells all these findings.
- Decide on a reporter(s) to be taped reading the script the team has written.
- Practice and rehearse the script, and time it. Change the script if it is too long or too short for the minutes assigned by the production team.

MATERIALS

Worksheets: *Investigating Alcohol/Investigating Cigarettes* (Figures 17-2 and 17-3); *Investigating Legal Drugs/Investigating Illegal Drugs* (Figures 17-4 and 17-5)

h. Have the production committee meet with the anchor host committee to plan the strategy for the production. They will have to plan the general format of the show, decide how much time will be given to the various reports, and plan and write an introduction and ending for the show. It also would be a good idea to set up deadline schedules, rehearsals, and trial tapings.

i. Give the students class time every day to meet with their teams. Circulate and troubleshoot. Also make certain the anchor hosts are meeting regularly with the other committee script writing. The production committee will have to prepare sets and become familiar with any equipment they may be using. Two to three weeks is approximately the amount of time needed to prepare for the taping.

j. Have the students rehearse the production and tape it with a cassette tape. Allow the class to listen to the tape and critique it. Have the teams modify the show based on the suggestions and rehearse again if desired.

MATERIALS
Cassette tape recorder and tape

2. Lights, Camera, Action

Have students put on the production. After viewing the show, ask various students questions such as:

a. Why are there laws about alcohol?
b. Why are some drugs legal to buy and others not?
c. Why are there age limits on certain drugs?
d. Why are there laws relating to drinking and driving?

MATERIALS
Videotape equipment
Video monitor

3. Parent Review

Invite parents to come to class and view the production. You may wish to have each team explain the part they played in the production process.

EVALUATION: "Why We Have Laws"

Have students write an essay titled, "Why We Have Laws About Drugs in [name of city or state]." Conduct a discussion of the reasons we have laws. The discussion should come from the reasons identified on their essays.

FIGURE 17-2

Worksheet   Name _____

Investigating Alcohol

Reporter   You are investigating three basic questions about alcohol. Find
information: several people in your community to interview. For each person
                   interviewed, get their exact name, age, and type of job. Try to find
                   different kinds of people to interview. The three areas you want to
                   find out about are the following:

1. What are the basic laws regarding alcohol?
    a. What are the age laws regarding the purchase of alcohol?
    b. When can alcohol be sold (days of week and hours)?
    c. Where can it be sold? Where can it be consumed (where can people drink
       it?)
    d. What are the laws regarding driving under the influence of alcohol?

2. Why do we have these various laws about alcohol?

3. How do people feel about the laws?
    a. Are the age limits too high? Too low?
    b. Should alcohol be available for purchase more hours in the day than it is
       now? Fewer hours?
    c. Are the laws about drinking and driving too strong? Not strong enough?

Interview people in your community about these and other questions. Decide as
a group who in the community should be interviewed. You may want to tape
your interview on a cassette tape and take photographs. (Make certain you get
permission to do this from the person being interviewed.) After the interviews
work as a group to write a script for the program. Remember your three basic
questions when writing the script. Decide on the readers for the script, practice,
and rehearse. Keep in mind the time allowed for your part of the program.
Check the time it takes your readers to read the script. Change the script if
necessary to fit the time allotted.

FIGURE 17-3

Worksheet   Name _____

Investigating Cigarettes

Reporter   You are investigating three basic questions about cigarettes. Find
information: several people in your community to interview. These should be
              different kinds of people with different kinds of jobs and different
              ages. For each person interviewed, get the exact name, age, and
              type of job. The three areas you want to find out about are the
              following:

1. What are the basic laws regarding cigarettes?
   a. What is the age limit for the sale of cigarettes?
   b. Where can they be sold?
   c. Are there laws about where you can and cannot smoke (that is, smoking
      and nonsmoking areas in public places)?

2. Why do we have laws about cigarettes?

3. How do people feel about the laws?
   a. Are the age limits too low? Too high?
   b. Should there be stronger laws about where they can be sold?
   c. Are the laws too strong about smoking and nonsmoking areas in public
      places? Not strong enough?

Interview people in your community about these and other questions. Decide as
a group who in the community should be interviewed. You may want to tape
your interview and take photographs. (Make certain you get permission to do
this from the person being interviewed.) After the interview work as a group to
write a script for the program. Remember your three basic questions when
writing the script. Decide on readers for the script, practice, and rehearse. Keep
in mind the time allowed for your part of the program. Check the time it takes
your readers to read the script. Change the script to fit the time allotted, if
necessary.

FIGURE 17-4

Worksheet   Name _____

Investigating Legal Drugs

Reporter   You are investigating three basic questions about legal drugs. Find
information: several people in your community who are familiar with these
                drugs. (Pharmacists, physicians, and nurses would be most
                helpful.) Get the exact name, age, and type of job for each person
                interviewed. The three areas you want to find out about are the
                following:

1. **What are the basic laws regarding legal drugs?**
   a. Who can buy over-the-counter drugs? Prescription drugs?
   b. Who can sell prescription drugs?
   c. Who can prescribe drugs?

2. **Why do we have laws regarding over-the-counter drugs and prescription drugs?**
   a. Why are certain drugs prescription drugs and others not?
   b. Why are some drugs that are legal in other countries not legal in the
       United States?

3. **How do people feel about the laws regulating legal drugs?**
   a. Are the laws too strong regarding prescription drugs? Should more drugs
       be available over the counter rather than by prescription?
   b. Should there be age limits on who can buy over-the-counter drugs?

Interview people in your community about these and other questions. Decide as
a group who in the community should be interviewed. You may want to tape
your interview on a cassette tape and take photographs. (Make certain you get
permission to do this from the person being interviewed.) After the interviews
work as a group to write a script for the program. Remember your three basic
questions when writing the script. Decide on readers for the script, practice,
and rehearse. Check the time it takes your readers to read the script. Change
the script if necessary to fit the time allowed.

FIGURE 17-5

Worksheet   Name _____

Investigating Illegal Drugs

Reporter information: You are investigating three basic questions about drugs that are illegal. Find several people in your community to interview. For each person interviewed, get their exact name, age, and type of job. These should be different kinds of people. You may want to start with someone on the police force in your community. The three areas that you want to find out about are the following:

1. What are the basic laws about illegal drugs?
   a. What drugs are illegal?
   b. Are there different laws regarding the sale and the possession of certain drugs?

2. Why do we have laws about these drugs? (Why are certain drugs legal to use and others not?)

3. How do people feel about the laws?
   a. Are the laws too harsh regarding illegal drugs? Too lenient?
   b. Should some of the drugs that are illegal be made legal? Should more drugs that are not legal be made illegal (for example, alcohol and cigarettes)?
   c. Should the penalties for using or possessing an illegal drug be stronger? Less harsh?

Interview people in your community about these and other questions. Decide as a group who in the community should be interviewed. You may want to tape your interview on a cassette tape and take photographs. (Make certain you get permission to do this from the person being interviewed.) After the interviews, work as a group to write a script for the program. Remember your three basic questions when writing the script. Decide on readers for the script, practice, and rehearse. Check the time it takes your reader to read the script. Change the script if necessary to fit the time allotted.

MIDDLE SCHOOL LEVEL

OBJECTIVE: The student interprets the significance of peer pressure on decisions to use drugs.

LEVEL: Grades 6 to 8

CONTENT GENERALIZATIONS: Peer pressure is considered the single most important factor contributing to adolescent use and abuse of drugs. Adolescents are very concerned about being accepted by group members. It is normal for adolescents to form groups of friends who dress similarly, are involved in the same activities, and explore new activities together. If these groups are involved in using drugs, there usually is a great deal of peer pressure for everyone to participate. Often this pressure is so great that adolescents will participate despite the wishes and values of their parents or themselves. Additionally, knowing the health risks related to the abuse of drugs does not necessarily act as a deterrent when peer pressure is involved.

It is helpful for adolescents to know what peer pressure is and that it is a normal part of growing up. In fact peer pressure is a part of adult life as well, although it is not as significant in influencing important adult decisions as for adolescents. Adolescents need help in understanding that it is all right to be different and that, if they are not interested in certain activities in which their friends are involved, perhaps they should find new friends.

VOCABULARY: Peer pressure

INITIATION: It's "In"
Find something to wear to class that will look strange to the students. It should be some mode of dress that is different from your normal attire. It should not be too bizarre, but it should be noticeable.

When the students remark on your new attire, and they will, tell them that this is the new "in" thing for teachers. Convince them that soon they will be seeing this type of attire on every teacher in the school. End your "act" by saying, "If any of the other teachers want to hang around with me, they're going to wear clothes like this." Then move immediately into activity 1.

MATERIALS
Unusual clothing that will cause students to remark on your appearance, such as:
Hat
New tie
Shoes

ACTIVITIES
1. Me and My Friends
Tell the students to just think "yes" or "no" answers to the following questions but not to answer aloud: "Are there certain kinds of clothes you and your friends wear? Are there certain activities that you and your friends like to do? Are there activities you have done that you probably would not have done unless your friends were there doing it too? Have you ever done something you wouldn't normally do, but one of your friends dared you to do it?" Ask them to raise their hands if they could answer yes to any of the questions. Tell the class as a whole, "Congratulations, you are all normal teenagers [or preteens]."

Hand out the worksheet, *Me and My Friends*, and ask the students to complete it as directed. The questions are similar to those previously asked in class, and students are to provide examples of activities influenced by their friends.
NOTE: Up to this point the discussions regarding peer pressure should have been general. The relationship of drug usage to peer pressure will be brought in gradually as it surfaces in discussions and on worksheets. The last item on the worksheet asks a simple yes or no question, "Do any of your friends smoke or drink?"

After the students have finished the worksheets, have them divide into groups to discuss their worksheets and to consider the question, "Are friends important in affecting the way you act and dress?" A representative from each group should share the group's ideas with the entire class at the end of the activity.

MATERIALS
Worksheet: *Me and My Friends* (Figure 17-6)

2. Survey Sheet—Peer Pressure Survey

Tell the students that they are to participate in a survey. Each student will use the worksheet, *Survey Sheet*, to ask an adult smoker some questions about when he or she started smoking. Explain to the students that the purpose of this survey is to find out if peer pressure was involved in that person's decision to start smoking. Review the questions on the *Survey Sheet*, and allow the students several days to complete the survey.

MATERIALS
Worksheet: *Survey Sheet* (Figure 17-7)

3. Tally Sheet—Peer Pressure Survey

Using butcher paper, make and post a large *Tally Sheet* for use in analyzing the data collected from the student surveys. As each student returns a completed survey, allow him or her to record the findings on the large class *Tally Sheet*. (One *Tally Sheet* could be used to collect data from several classes.)

MATERIALS
Teacher resource: *Tally Sheet* (Figure 17-8)
Butcher paper
Felt pens

4. Practice Saying "No"

Allow each student to practice "saying no" to peer pressure. Go around to each student in the class, and offer a cigarette to each. Tell them they must resist your pressure to smoke. Suggest that they give answers such as, "No thanks, I don't want lung cancer," "Are you kidding, those things are coffin nails," "No thanks, athletes don't smoke," or, "My mom would kill me, and I'm too young to die!" A more humorous response could be, "No thanks, I like clean breath and white teeth," or, "Are you kidding? I love to play tennis without breathing problems so I can get a natural high."

You may wish to repeat this activity several times during different class periods. It is important, however, that every student in the class has a chance to respond. Ham it up as the pressurer. **NOTE:** In this activity it is important that the teacher apply the pressure. Students should receive practice in *resisting* pressure, not *applying* pressure.

EVALUATION: "In My Opinion" Essay

Have the students write an essay describing their opinions on the question, "How important is peer pressure in the decision to smoke cigarettes or use drugs?" You may wish to provide students the option of taping their opinions on a cassette tape. In either case students should explain the reasons for their opinions.

FIGURE 17-6

Worksheet   Name _____

Me and My Friends

Directions: Read the questions below, and list what you do with or because of your
               friends.

1. What kind of clothes are "in" with your group of friends?

2. What do you like to do with your friends?

3. Do you have different friends at home than at school? If so, do you
   do different activities with these friends? List the activities you do.

4. Are there things you probably would not have done unless your
   friends were doing them also? List them.

5. Do any of your friends smoke cigarettes?   (Circle one)   YES NO
   Do any of your friends drink alcoholic beverages?
   (Circle one)   YES NO

FIGURE 17-7

Worksheet

Name _____

Survey Sheet

Directions: Use the questions on this worksheet to interview an adult about cigarette smoking. Ask a smoker when and why he or she started smoking cigarettes. The responses on your survey will be combined with the responses that other class members collect.

1. Name of adult smoker _____

2. Age of smoker   (Circle one)
   19 to 25 years, 26 to 35 years, 36 to 50 years, over 50 years

3. Questions

   a. How old were you when you first started smoking cigarettes? (Circle one)
      Under 10 years, 11 to 13 years, 14 to 16 years, 17 to 21 years, over 21 years

   b. Why did you start smoking?

   c. Did any of your friends smoke or start smoking at the same time you started?

   d. When you started smoking, did either of your parents smoke cigarettes? If the answer is yes, indicate whether it was the mother, father, or both.

   e. Did you know the health hazards of cigarette smoking before you started?

   f. Have you ever tried to quit smoking?

   g. Do you have any advice for young people who have not yet made the decision of whether to smoke or not?

FIGURE 17-8

Teacher resource   Name ______________________

Tally Sheet

Directions: Use a large sheet like the one shown here to tally the responses to the smoking survey. Several classes' responses could be recorded on one tally sheet posted in the classroom.

Age of smoker	19 to 25 years	26 to 35 years	36 to 50 years	Over 50 years
Age when started	Under 10 years	11 to 13 years	14 to 16 years	17 to 21 years
	Over 21			
Did friends smoke?	Yes	No		
Did parents smoke?	No	Yes, mother	Yes, father	Yes, both
Knew the hazards?	Yes	No		
Tried to quit?	Yes	No		

18 Environmental Health

When you finish this chapter, you should be able to:

- Explain the interrelationships among types of pollution and the ecosystem.
- Describe the causes and effects of the various types of pollution.
- Identify prevention and protection methods regarding environmental health.
- Develop learning opportunities for elementary and middle-school students in the area of environmental health.

The environment is a crucial factor in individual health. Everything in the environment, from the air we breathe to the number of persons inhabiting the earth, plays a role in our well-being. In this chapter, we will explore five types of environmental pollution—air, water, land, radiation, and noise pollution. Although we will be examining air, water, and land separately, in reality, they work together as part of a system. The *ecosystem* is the complex web linking animals, plants, air, water, and every other life form on earth. Any change in one part of the ecosystem affects other parts. Because of this, the earth's environment is a single system. When the environment in one part of the world is threatened, the rest of the world is also threatened.

Maintaining a clean and safe environment can enhance our lives physically, mentally, and socially. A clean environment decreases the spread of pathogenic microorganisms and lessens the chance of physical harm from potentially dangerous chemicals. A clean and safe environment is important for mental health. Many people believe that a pleasant natural environment helps reduce stress and stimulates the mind. Finally, relating to others is much easier in an environment in which the noise levels are tolerable.

AIR POLLUTION

Air pollution is a major problem in modern society. Although air pollution is usually a greater problem in metropolitan areas, pollutants contaminate air everywhere. These substances include gases and tiny particles that can harm human health and damage the environment. Some air pollution is caused by natural processes such as forest fires and volcanic eruptions. Of greatest concern is the pollution caused by human activity, especially the burning of fossil fuels—coal, oil, and natural gas.

Gaseous Pollutants

The most common gaseous pollutants are carbon dioxide, carbon monoxide, hydrocarbons, nitrogen oxides, sulphur oxides, and ozone. These chemical compounds are produced from a number of sources. The major source is the burning of fossil fuels in motor vehicles, power plants, and factories. Cigarette smoking, furnaces, gas ranges, certain construction materials, cleaning products, and home furnishings also release gaseous pollutants into the environment.

Greenhouse effect. Carbon dioxide is produced whenever fuels are burned. The major sources of carbon dioxide are industry, motor vehicle emissions, and electricity production. Many scientists believe that increasing levels of carbon dioxide may cause a *greenhouse effect* as part of a trend toward *global warming*—an increase in the earth's surface temperature. Carbon dioxide and other gases form a layer around the earth. As the earth is warmed by the sun, the heat radiates from the earth and becomes trapped by the layer of gases just as a greenhouse traps heat inside. A certain amount of greenhouse gases in the atmosphere is needed to make the earth warm, but activities such as the burning of fossil fuels are creating a gaseous layer that is too dense. Many scientists believe this increases the atmospheric temperature.

Since the beginning of the industrial revolution in the mid-1700s, the level of carbon dioxide in the atmosphere has increased 30%. Automobile use has been a major contributor of carbon dioxide to this process, as has tropical deforestation in Africa and South America (tropical forests naturally absorb carbon dioxide). With an increase of only a few degrees Fahrenheit, many scientists predict significant increases in violent storms, unbearable summer heat, and prolonged droughts. Another health concern of global warming is the spread of insects that can destroy crops or carry disease. Insects that could not survive colder temperatures can thrive in a warmer climate.

Acid rain. Some industrial processes—especially the burning of fossil fuels such as coal and oil—cause sulphur dioxide and nitrogen oxide emissions. As the particles travel through the air, they combine with water vapor to form sulphuric and nitric acids. Eventually the chemicals fall to earth as precipitation, or *acid rain*. When acid rain accumulates in lakes and rivers, it makes the water more acidic, damaging or killing aquatic life. It also damages crops and soil and may be associated with respiratory problems in humans. In the United States the leading producers of sulfur dioxide are Ohio, Pennsylvania, Indiana, Illinois, and New York. However, winds may carry the pollutants thousands of miles before they fall as dew, drizzle, fog, sleet, snow, or rain.

Damage to the Ozone Layer

Air pollution caused by the use of manufactured chemical compounds called *chlorofluorocarbons*, or *CFCs*, is depleting the earth's ozone layer. The ozone layer is a thin layer of a form of oxygen, consisting of three atoms of oxygen instead of the normal two, that occurs naturally in the earth's upper atmosphere. It is crucial to the survival of plant and animal life on earth. The ozone layer absorbs harmful ultraviolet (UV) radiation and prevents most of it from reaching the earth's surface. CFCs, a primary cause of ozone depletion, are used as coolants in air conditioners and refrigerators, solvents in the manufacture of electronic equipment, and foaming agents in insulation and food packaging. Until recently, CFCs were used as propellants in aerosol spray cans.

Ozone depletion is resulting in increasing levels of UV radiation on earth, posing significant danger to both plants and animals. The risks to humans include increased rates of skin cancer and cataracts, which can cause blindness. There may also be damaging genetic effects and diminished immune system capabilities.

Concern over the environmental effects of CFCs has led to efforts to sharply reduce their use by the end of this century. In 1978 the CFC freon gas was banned from use as a propellant in the United States, although it is still in use in other countries. Ways for consumers to help include avoiding the use of plastic foam packaging and insulation materials, using energy-efficient refrigerators, and having air conditioners serviced frequently. However, the extent of damage to the ozone layer now appears to be worse than initially anticipated, and the health risks are also greater. The Environmental Protection Agency (EPA) projects that more than 80 million additional cases of skin cancer will occur during the next 80 years because of the damage already done to the ozone layer (1).

Particulate Pollutants

Particulates are tiny particles of substances suspended in the air. As with gaseous pollutants, some particulate pollutants arise from natural processes, such as volcanic eruptions, but most are the result of human activities such as manufacturing, mining, and agriculture. Inhaling particulates can cause potentially fatal respiratory diseases—for example, *silicosis* from quartz dust and *asbestosis* and *lung cancer* from asbestos fibers. Other particulates of concern are soot, ashes, coal dust, and fragments of metals such as lead. These particulates can pollute the air indoors and outdoors.

Asbestos has been a major concern because its use is so widespread. In 1989 the EPA ordered the use of asbestos reduced by the year 1997. By this date, about 94% of all asbestos use will be eliminated. An estimated 27 million workers, many of whom will develop lung cancer and asbestosis, have been exposed to asbestos; to date, billions of dollars in damages have been assessed.

Chronic lead toxicity from the use of lead in various products is another serious health problem associated with particulate pollution. People who must live or work in areas with higher than acceptable levels of lead in the air may develop damage to hemoglobin, the gastrointestinal tract, and the central nervous system. Low-income minority children are most likely to be affected by lead toxicity. About 3 million children have dangerously high levels of lead in their blood.

Industry can lessen the release of particulates into the air by using smokestack scrubbing and emission control devices. People working in mining, industrial, and some textile occupations should wear face masks or other safety equipment to protect themselves from inhaling particulates at worksites. Government controls such as those established by the Clean Air acts have helped to reduce industrial particulates, but they are still a major source of air pollution.

WATER POLLUTION

Along with clean air, clean water is essential for sustaining life. In developing countries the most important health concern is the availability of clean and safe water. Many people in the United States take the abundance of clean water for granted. However, they are beginning to realize that our water resources must be protected to maintain the current standard of living. Waterways and resources can be polluted by sewer waste, garbage, and chemicals. Contaminated water transmits disease, thereby posing a great danger to animal life as well as to humans.

Water pollution is defined as any physical or chemical change in water that upsets the natural balance of aquatic life. As with air pollution, water pollution can be caused by natural processes and human activity. Surface and ground water can be polluted with minerals leeched from the soil, acids from decaying vegetation, and decaying animal products. Human pollutants can come from agricultural, urban, and industrial sources. Untreated human wastes are also a source of water pollution.

Polluted water can reduce the amount of water available for various needs, and it is associated with many human health problems. Water contaminated with sewage can cause diseases such as cholera and dysentery. If toxic substances enter sources of groundwater, streams, lakes, and oceans, they can enter the food chain and affect aquatic and human life.

Pathogenic Agents

Pathogens enter the water supply through human and animal wastes. In many parts of the world this type of water pollution is still common. In the United States and other developed countries, sewage treatment facilities remove disease-causing microorganisms from the water supply. However, pollution with pathogenic agents still occurs, for example, when sewage is flushed from boats. Animal wastes at feed lots and meat processing plants can enter and pollute the water supply.

Toxic Substances

In the United States, pollution from agricultural and industrial chemicals is a bigger problem than pathogenic microorganisms. These toxins are especially dangerous because they can enter the food chain. With each life form in the chain, their concentration per unit of weight increases; toxic chemicals become more concentrated as they move up the food chain. By the time humans eat the fish that have fed on contaminated lower life forms, the toxic chemicals can be highly concentrated. For example, mercury can accumulate in fish; when humans consume the contaminated fish regularly, the mercury can damage hemoglobin and central nervous system functioning and eventually cause death. Mercury poisoning can also cause mental retardation and physical deformities in children.

Pesticides used in American and Canadian agriculture are among the most toxic substances that can pollute water supplies. The *chlorinated hydrocarbons* such as DDT (now banned in the United States), chlordane, and Kepone, have been linked to cancer, birth defects, and reproductive system disorders. Drinking water contaminated with *polychlorinated biphenyls (PCBs)* has been associated with kidney and liver damage. These chemicals have been used extensively in transformers and electrical capacitors. In many parts of the United States, discarded electrical equipment has released PCBs into nearby water supplies. The extent of contamination and its related health effects are not fully known. The EPA ordered that all PCBs in electrical transformers be removed by 1990.

Approximately half of all Americans depend on groundwater beneath the surface of the earth for their drinking water (2). Groundwater is stored in aquifers, basins below the earth's surface made of sand, gravel, silt, and clay that absorb and store water. This water is obtained using wells. Common pollutants in groundwater are trichloroethylene (TCE), an industrial solvent and suspected human carcinogen, and vinyl chloride, a known human carcinogen. The EPA estimates that almost two thirds of rural Americans are drinking water contaminated with pesticides or other dangerous chemicals. The EPA has listed 700 compounds considered dangerous in drinking water and has rated the level of pollution as serious in 34 of the 50 states. If the quality of the drinking water in your home is in question, it can be tested. Your local water utility can give you more information about these tests.

Other Sources of Contamination

Oil spills can kill marine animals, fish, sea birds, and aquatic plants. Water damaged by oil spills must be treated by a variety of methods to restore it to a more normal state. These processes are costly and include vacuuming the oil and using detergents to break up oil slicks. Oil-eating bacteria can also be used to help clean up oil spills. The impact of oil spills on human health is not fully known.

Water Conservation

Water conservation is any action that is taken to avoid wasting water or to prevent it from becoming contaminated. All humans, animals, and plants need water to survive. Water makes up about two thirds of the human body. We need clean, fresh water for all kinds of uses—domestic, agricultural, and industrial. In the United States today, approximately 1500 gallons a day per person is used for recreation, cooling, food production, and industry.

Although fresh water is an abundant natural resource, it is not distributed evenly. In some areas, rainfall and water supplies are scarce, and in others they are plentiful. Some locations face serious water shortages. The pollution of many sources of water adds to the problem.

Water can be conserved by public and individual means. Many areas use *reservoirs* for their public water supply. These may be natural lakes or artificial bodies of water created by building dams on rivers or streams. *Groundwater*, the natural supply of water underground, is a source of water for some communities. Some groundwater comes from *aquifers*, large underground reservoirs. *Watersheds* are planned areas of vegetation that trap rainwater and allow it to soak into the ground, replenishing groundwater supplies. Preventing water pollution is another form of conservation.

Individuals can save thousands of gallons of water each year by following some simple conservation rules. The average household can save more than 30,000 gallons of water in a year by conserving water in the home. Some steps an individual and household can take to save water include the following:

- Do not let the water run while you are brushing your teeth or washing your face or hands.
- Install a low-flow shower head in your shower.
- Take a shower instead of a bath. (A shower can use about one third as much water as a bath if you use a low-flow shower head and keep the shower short.)
- Check faucets, toilets, and pipes for leaks. A leaky toilet can waste as much as 100 gallons of water a day.
- Water your yard only when it needs it.
- Run washing machines and dishwashers only with a full load.

LAND POLLUTION
Solid Waste

The greatest impact on our land comes from the products that we discard: solid waste and chemical waste. Solid waste is any kind of nonliquid refuse or trash. Types of solid waste are paper, food, glass, plastic, metal, junked automobiles, tires, appliances, furniture, and some agricultural and industrial wastes. During the past few decades the quantity of solid waste has greatly increased; in the United States, nearly a billion pounds of solid wastes are disposed of each day.

Most of this waste is generated by agriculture, mining, and industry rather than by individual households.

Solid waste disposal affects the environment and human health. The major methods of disposal include the following:

- *Open dumping:* Compaction and dumping of solid waste at a dump site. These actions are now discouraged or are illegal in many urban areas.
- *Ocean dumping:* Solid waste taken to offshore dump sites. Marine biologists worry that this practice changes the habitat of many marine plants and fish. Greater environmental awareness has led to the development of other, more controlled methods of solid waste disposal.
- *Sanitary landfills:* A more common method of disposal. Sanitary landfills are specially planned and supervised disposal sites where waste is disposed of in pits. Each day a layer of soil is pushed over the most recently dumped trash to encourage decomposition, reduce odors, and contain the material. Drawbacks are that harmful substances can seep into the ground and contaminate soil or water and that available space for these landfills is increasingly scarce.
- *Incineration:* Burning waste in specially designed furnaces. Materials are burned at very high temperatures, converting them to gases and leaving small amounts of residue that is usually disposed of in landfills. Incineration reduces the volume of waste and can be used to generate electricity or steam for heating. The disadvantage is that it can contribute to air pollution.

There are two ways to reduce solid waste—by reducing it at its source and by recycling. Manufacturers and consumers must make and buy products with reduced packaging or packaging that is reusable or biodegradable. *Biodegradable* products decompose naturally in the environment. *Recycling* involves converting disposable items into reusable materials. Some municipal areas have established curbside pickup of recycled materials, especially glass, aluminum, and newspaper. To be most effective, recycling requires planning, locating markets for recycled materials, establishing community or government support, and obtaining the active participation of individuals and households.

Chemical Waste

Disposal of hazardous chemicals is a serious problem. Because of the expense of detoxifying, recycling, and reusing toxic chemical products, chemical companies too often secretly and illegally bury their chemical wastes at dump sites. Because of this, the EPA is helping to fund the cleanup of approximately 1000 toxic waste disposal sites in the United States. Court decisions have also forced some companies to clean dump sites and pay fines.

Pesticides

Many hazardous pesticides such as DDT have been removed from the marketplace in the United States, and the EPA has established tighter controls over some less hazardous pesticides. Although farmers need to use effective methods of crop protection from insects and other pests, the effects pesticides can have on the entire ecosystem must be considered , and their use must be closely monitored.

The use of pesticides has increased the number of crops that can be grown. However, pesticides can leave a hazardous residue on plants eaten by humans. People exposed to greater amounts of pesticides can suffer serious health problems or even die from this exposure. In the United States, farmers and farm workers are at increased risk of pesticide-related health problems because of their daily exposure to pesticides.

Erosion

Erosion is another problem endangering our land. The soil needed to grow food is steadily eroding. Pesticides contribute to this erosion by permitting continuous cropping instead of crop rotation. An estimated 23 billion tons of soil are washed off the land each year worldwide. When the soil is eroded, vegetation disappears and the land dries out. When droughts occur, famine and starvation are the result.

RADIATION

Radiation includes several kinds of invisible energy, some occurring naturally in the environment and some created by humans. Usually the term is used to mean *ionizing radiation*, which produces electrically charged particles called *ions* in the molecules it strikes. Sources include cosmic rays, radioactivity, and x rays. *Nonionizing radiation*, the other major type, does not produce ions; examples of sources are microwaves and magnetic fields.

Although radiation has been important to the development of industrial and medical technology, there are health concerns with radiation exposure, especially exposure to ionizing radiation. Overexposure to ionizing radiation can cause cancer, damage to the immune system, and birth defects.

Radiation Exposure

Everyone is exposed to radiation from cosmic rays from the sun and universe. Natural radiation also comes from rocks and soil containing radioactive mineral deposits. These emit ionizing radiation as the radioactive material decays. A third source of ionizing radiation is *radon gas*, which is released from underlying rock formations and stone building materials.

Human activity has created other sources of ionizing radiation. Medical x-ray tests are a common source, and nuclear reactors also produce ionizing radiation. Nuclear radiation is potentially harmful if it leaks because of human error or equipment failure in operating the reactor. Reactors also produce nuclear wastes that require disposal, and no disposal methods are completely safe. In addition, the threat of mass exposure to ionizing radiation is a serious risk associated with the production of nuclear weapons.

Nonionizing radiation also comes from natural and artificial sources. A natural source is UV light from the sun. Most UV radiation is absorbed by the ozone layer in the atmosphere, although the depletion of this layer by air pollution is allowing more UV rays to reach the earth. The higher levels of UV radiation increase the risk of skin cancer and damage to the immune system.

Electromagnetic radiation is another type of nonionizing radiation. This type of radiation comes from appliances such as microwave ovens, televisions, and computer visual display terminals (VDTs). Some medical testing procedures, including ultrasound and magnetic resonance imaging (MRI), use equipment that emits nonionizing radiation. The magnetic fields around wires carrying electricity also emit this radiation. Scientists disagree about the health risks of exposure to electromagnetic radiation. Some studies have shown an association between exposure to high levels of electromagnetic radiation and birth defects or certain types of cancer, but a biological mechanism is unclear.

Radon is a colorless and odorless radioactive gas produced when uranium decays. It occurs naturally in certain soils, rocks, and groundwater and is emitted by building materials made from these soils or rocks. Radon is harmless in the open air but unsafe when it accumulates in enclosed spaces such as well-insulated buildings. Recent studies indicate that prolonged exposure can increase the risk of developing lung cancer. The combination of smoking and exposure to radon is especially lethal. Radon levels can be measured with a number of devices. If levels are high, some minor structural modifications can be made to the dwelling to reduce them.

Limiting exposure to radiation. You need to limit your exposure to potentially harmful radiation. Some steps you can take are to do the following:

- Limit the time spent in the sun.
- Use sun-block products to limit exposure to UV radiation.
- Limit exposure to x-ray tests only when

necessary. Pregnant women should not have x-ray examinations unless special precautions are taken.
- Reduce radon gas exposure in your home by sealing cracks in basement floors and walls and ensuring that basement and sump pump areas are vented to the outdoors.

NOISE POLLUTION

Noise pollution is any loud or annoying sound present in a person's environment. Prolonged exposure to noise affects health and may cause hearing loss. Noise loudness is measured using units called *decibels*. A soft whisper measures about 30 decibels, a lawn mower about 90 decibels, and a shotgun blast about 140 decibels. In general, the louder and higher the pitch, the more annoying and unpleasant the sound.

Noise is considered a physical and psychological stressor. Exposure to loud noise can cause increases in blood pressure, heart and respiration rates, cholesterol and hormone levels, and muscle tension. Prolonged exposure to noises of 85 decibels or more can cause hearing damage. Noise also produces emotional effects such as irritability and inability to concentrate. Some studies suggest a link between excessive noise in the workplace and rates of unintentional injury.

You can protect against the effects of noise by using earplugs or ear protectors when operating loud machinery and using sound-absorbing building materials. Some communities have adopted noise-reduction ordinances to control the noise level from machinery and other sources.

PROTECTING THE ENVIRONMENT

Protecting the environment requires that governments, industries, organizations, and individuals work together. Protecting the environment is a worldwide issue. We must "think globally and act locally."

Government

Nationally, the EPA was formed by the federal government to set standards and monitor and enforce regulations regarding the protection of the environment. The EPA has been partially responsible for the improvements in the nation's air and water in recent years. Another group formed by the U.S. government is the Council on Environmental Quality. The council makes recommendations about ways in which environmental problems should be handled. States and local governments also take measures to protect the environment by enacting laws that limit the amount of pollution from different sources.

Industries

Industries can help preserve the environment by adhering to the laws that regulate the amount of pollutants emitted as industrial by-products. They can experiment with ways to burn cleaner fuels and engage in and promote recycling of solid waste materials. Industries can also research methods to make wiser use of existing natural resources.

Organizations

In addition to the government and industry, other groups are trying to fight problems that affect the quality of the environment. Such groups include national citizens' organizations that provide education, lobbying, or actual clean-up work. The Sierra Club, National Wildlife Federation, Izaak Walton League, and the Audubon Society are groups that have raised money for research and management of pollution problems.

SUMMARY

The environment is a crucial factor in the health of individuals and communities. In this chapter, we discussed five major types of environmental pollution: air pollution, water pollution, land pollution, radiation, and noise. Although these components were considered separately, the air, wa-

---

INDIVIDUAL EFFORTS TO REDUCE POLLUTION

In reality, individuals must take steps to ensure the quality of the environment. Such practices include the following:
- Using soaps, paper products, and other materials that are biodegradable
- Using water sparingly
- Using electricity (lights and appliances) only when necessary
- Cutting down on use of disposable items
- Recycling materials
- Walking or bicycling for short trips
- Keeping cars, trucks, and motorcycles in good operating condition
- Promoting and supporting legislation that protects the environment.

---

ter, and land are interrelated and together make up our ecosystem.

Air pollution can be caused by gases or particulates in the atmosphere. Gaseous pollutants include carbon dioxide, which is thought to be responsible for the greenhouse effect as part of a dangerous trend toward global warming. Other industrial pollutants, sulphur dioxide and nitrogen oxides, are causing acid rain, which is harmful to all life. A third problem caused by air pollution is the depletion of the earth's ozone layer.

Particulate pollutants include asbestos and lead. Government controls have helped to reduce industrial emission of particulates, but they are still a major cause of pollution.

Clean water is basic to life. Without clean water, humans cannot survive. In many parts of the world, water polluted with human and animal wastes causes infection with pathogenic agents. In the United States the biggest problem is pollution from agricultural and industrial chemicals. Toxic substances contaminating water supplies include trace metals such as mercury, pesticides, and industrial solvents.

Water conservation practices should be

widely adopted. Individual households can save a great deal of water by following a few basic practices.

Land pollution includes solid waste, chemical waste, and pesticides. Erosion is another form of land pollution. Disposal of wastes has become a major problem. Recycling is one effective solution to the accumulation of massive quantities of waste.

Radiation occurs naturally and artificially in our environment. Exposure to radiation, particularly ionizing radiation, is a known health hazard and should be limited. Using sunblock and avoiding unnecessary x-ray examinations are other ways to avoid exposure to harmful radiation.

Excessive noise is also a type of pollution. Noise is a known physical and psychological stressor. It is important to protect the ears from excessive noise—noise exceeding 85 decibels.

In summary, protecting and conserving the environment is the responsibility of everyone—governments, industries, and individuals. Many organizations exist to work toward this aim.

In the section that follows, learning opportunities for primary, intermediate, and middle school level students offer ways to help students to think about these environmental issues.

REFERENCES

1. *Safety and environmental health: Macmillan health encyclopedia*, vol 8, New York, 1993, Macmillan Publishing.
2. Lloyd-Kolkin D: *Creating a healthy environment*, Santa Cruz, Calif, 1991, Network Publications.

SUGGESTED READINGS

Chiras D: *Environmental science: a framework for decision-making*, Menlo Park, 1985, Addison-Wesley.

Hunter L: *Caring for our planet and our health*, Santa Cruz, Calif, 1991, Network Publications.

Payne W, Hahn D: *Understanding your health*, St Louis, 1992, Mosby.

LEARNING OPPORTUNITIES FOR ENVIRONMENTAL HEALTH

GENERAL STUDENT OBJECTIVES

Primary Level K-3

The student:
1. Identifies the sources of environmental (air, land, and water) pollution.*
2. Names actions that conserve natural resources.
3. Describes way to work with others to help provide a healthful environment.

Intermediate Level 4-5/6

The student:
1. Explains how improving the environment can enhance physical, social, and mental health.
2. Identifies causes and preventives against environmental pollution.

Middle School Level 6/7-8

The student:
1. Analyze ways individuals and communities can promote a healthful and safe environment.
2. Evaluates the effects of community groups and agencies in improving and protecting the environment.*

*These objectives are illustrated by sample learning opportunities.

PRIMARY LEVEL

OBJECTIVE: The student identifies environmental (air, land, and water) pollution.

LEVEL: Kindergarten and grade 1

INTEGRATION: Reading readiness, writing readiness

VOCABULARY: Environment, pollution, land, water, air

CONTENT GENERALIZATIONS: The environment is the world around us, including land, water, and air. All living beings are dependent on a clean, usable, stable environment. When living quarters become dirty, contaminated, or unusable, they are polluted. Environmental pollution means the land, water, and air are dirty and unusable.

INITIATION: "Defining Environment"
Tell the students that they are going to learn a new long word today. It is a very important word. The new word is *environment*. Offer them the opportunity to say this new word individually and as a group. Applaud and praise their ability. Tell them that environment means *everything* in the world *around* us. This includes all the land, water, and air. Ask the students, "Are the land and all things on land a part of the environment?" "Are the air and all things in the air a part of the environment?" "Are the water and all things in the water a part of the environment?"

MATERIALS
Land pictures: empty fields, playgrounds, city buildings, houses, freeways
Air pictures: clear sky, clouded sky, stormy sky, sky with birds, sky with airplane
Water pictures: drinking fountain, river, lake, stream

Three shoe boxes, one labeled *land* with a picture of land; the second *water* with a picture of water; the third *air* with a picture of sky

ACTIVITIES

1. Air—Water—Land Learning Stations

Show some environmental pictures to the class. Initially, show all pictures of one type, emphasizing what each is, for example, "This is a picture of land, which is a part of the environment." Mix up the pictures, show them, and ask the students to tell whether they are part of the land environment, water environment, or air environment.

Rotate the students into learning stations in groups of four or five. They are to sort each picture into one of three appropriate boxes.

2. The Story of Diamond Lake

a. Inform the students that we want to keep our environment clean and healthful so that all the people, plants, and animals can live well in the environment. When the environment becomes dirty and unusable, we say it is polluted. Ask the students to listen to the following story about an environment that became polluted. The flannel board figures, *Goldie, Water, Trash*, are used during the presentation.

DIAMOND LAKE

Diamond Lake was so clean and beautiful that it sparkled. Many people and animals enjoyed Diamond Lake. Manuel and his family delighted in swimming at Diamond Lake each summer. Goldie Fish lived in the lake, which was clear and clean and filled with oxygen for her to breathe. Manuel and his family were careful not to throw trash in the lake so it would stay clean. But some people who came to Diamond Lake dumped their garbage into the lake. Diamond Lake became filled with old newspapers, soda cans, and dirty dishwater. Diamond Lake became a "polluted" lake. It no longer sparkled. Goldie Fish gasped for oxygen. Goldie's gills had to work very hard to get oxygen out of the polluted water. One summer Manuel and his family were very unhappy when they arrived at the lake. They could not go swimming because the water made their skin itch and hurt. Diamond Lake was dirty and polluted. Manuel said, "This is terrible! The lake is polluted, and we can no longer use it." Manuel was very sad. Goldie was very sad too.

b. **Discussion questions**
   - Why were Manuel and Goldie sad? (The lake was polluted.)
   - What happened to make the lake polluted? (People dumped garbage into the lake.)
   - What does "polluted water" mean? (The water is dirty and unusable.)
   - How can we keep lakes clean and unpolluted? (People must not throw garbage or other substances into lakes.)
   - Can Diamond Lake be saved? (Yes, with a great deal of work and help from many people, it is possible to restore Diamond Lake to its original beauty. It may take many years.)

MATERIALS

Flannel board figures: *Goldie, Water, Trash* (Figure 18-1)
Flannel board

3. Air and Land Pollution

Ask the students if they think that air and land can become polluted too. Ask them to speculate on what might cause the air to become polluted. Tell them to think about things that put smoke into the air. (Cars, airplanes, trucks, cigarettes, factories.) Use the same questioning for land pollution. Tell the students to think of things that might make the land and buildings messy and dirty. (Trash, litter, graffiti.)

Using the worksheet, *Air and Land*, help the students trace around the words *air* and *land*. For each picture on the worksheet ask, "Does this pollute the air or land?" After each picture is discussed, students should draw a check mark by pictures of things that pollute the air and an *X* by those which pollute the land. Ask the students if they have any ideas on how they can help keep the air and land from becoming polluted. (Do not litter, do not write graffiti on walls, and walk or ride a bicycle instead of riding in a car when possible.)

MATERIALS

Worksheet: *Air and Land* (Figure 18-2)
Pencils or crayons

EVALUATION: "Stop Pollution"

Hand each child a picture of the land, air, or water. Ask them to identify the type of environment and tell what might make that environment polluted. Also have the students tell how we might keep the environment from becoming polluted.

MATERIALS

Pictures of air, land, and water used earlier

FIGURE 18-1

Flannel board figures   Name _____

Goldie, Water, Trash

Use the pictures below to make flannel board figures for use with
the Diamond Lake story.

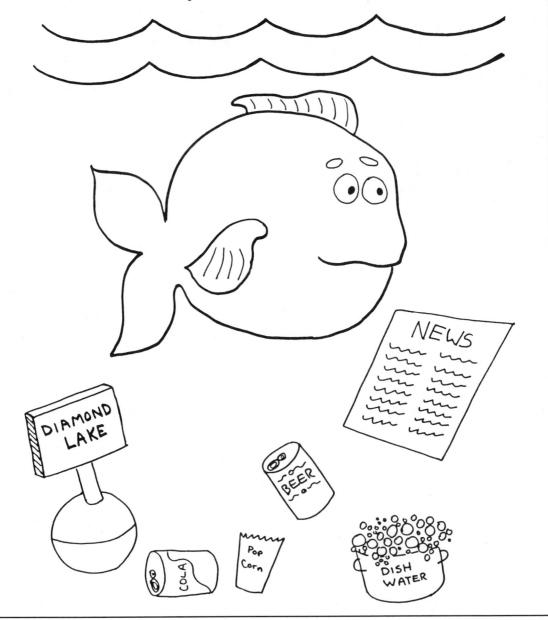

FIGURE 18-2

Worksheet   Name _____

Air and Land

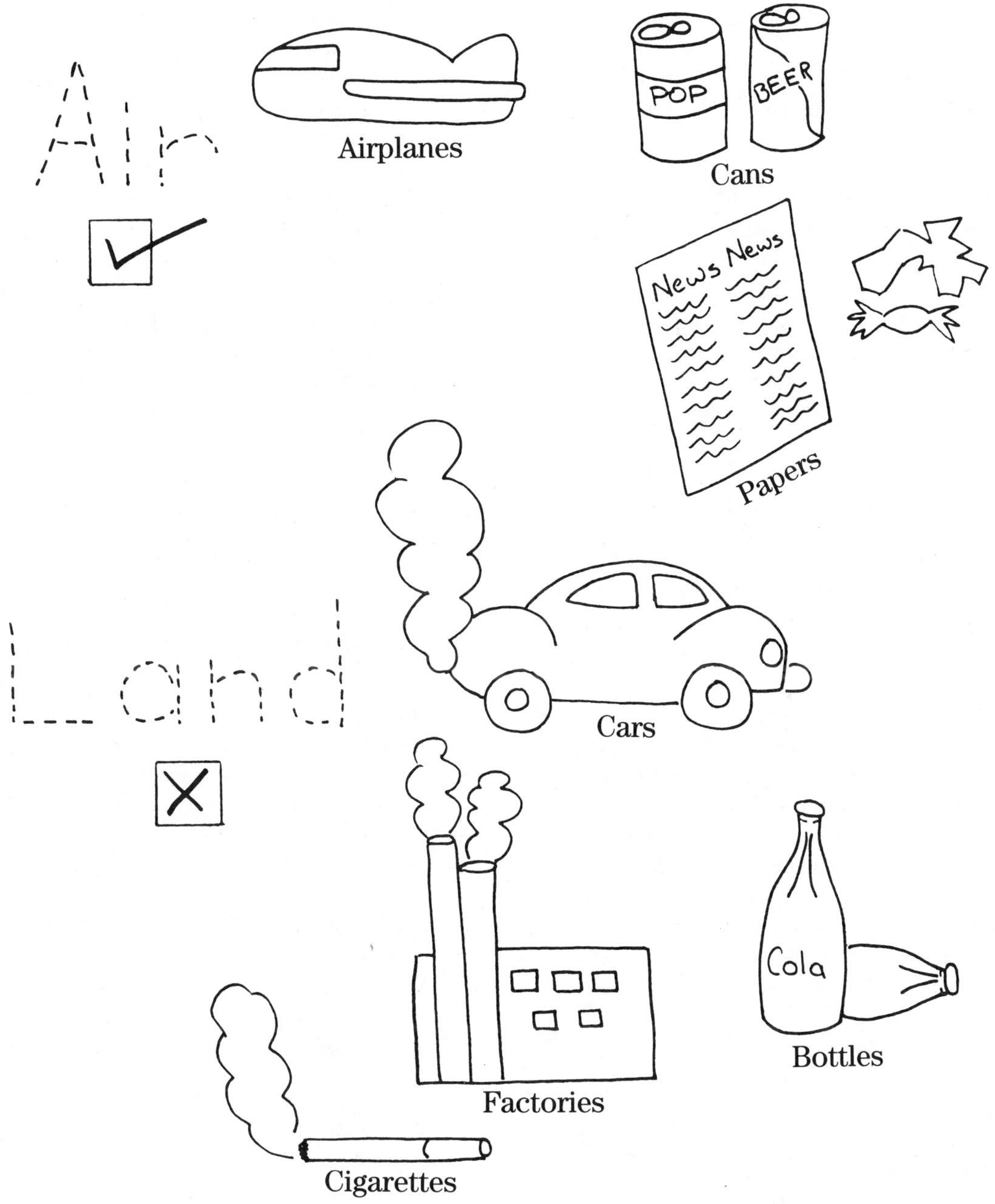

A̱i̱ṟ

☑

Airplanes

POP BEER

Cans

News News

Papers

Ḻa̱ṉḏ

☒

Cars

Factories

Bottles

Cola

Cigarettes

INTERMEDIATE LEVEL

OBJECTIVE: The student identifies causes of and ways to prevent environmental pollution.

LEVEL: Grades 4 to 6

INTEGRATION: Math, physical education, language arts, science, art

VOCABULARY: Environmental pollution, prevention, impact, cilia

CONTENT GENERALIZATIONS: People make an impact on their environment just by living in the world. Freeways, homes, factories, and office buildings noticeably modify the environment. An increase in the quality and comfort of life often is costly to the environment. Individuals can make choices in their daily lives that minimize personal contributions to environmental pollution.

There are several kinds of environmental pollution. Air pollution is caused largely by exhaust fumes from automobiles, airplanes, and factories. Walking or riding bicycles whenever possible is helpful in preventing air pollution. Water pollution often is caused by the use of water by industry and agriculture. Additionally, dumping trash and chemicals into lakes and streams will cause water pollution. Although industry causes much of the air and water pollution, individuals can help by doing their part to conserve water and not pollute water and air. Another kind of pollution is land pollution. This is caused by littering and the defacement of walls and other structures (graffiti). Individuals also can cause noise pollution. Being careful not to litter and to keep radios and stereos at a low level helps prevent these types of pollution.

INITIATION: How Much Water Do You Use In a Day?
Display a gallon jug of water. Ask the students to think about all the water they use daily. Tell them that we need clean water to live. Ask them if they can name some of the reasons we need clean water. (Washing, drinking, bathing, cooking.) Explain that the class is going to have a contest to see who can come closest to guessing the number of gallons of water that the average person uses every day. Pass out slips of paper for the students to use to make their guesses. Have a student volunteer collect the papers and arrange them in order from the highest number to the lowest number. Write the highest and lowest numbers guessed on the board. Then allow a student to open the envelope and read the correct answer (125 gallons). Compare the correct answer with the guesses made by class members. Declare the "winner."

Propose to the students that, if each one of us needs that much water every day, it must be important to make certain we keep our rivers, lakes, and oceans clean and pollution free. It also stands to reason that it is important not to waste water.

MATERIALS
Gallon jug of water
Slips of paper
Envelope containing the correct answer (125 gallons)

ACTIVITIES

1. Environmental Journal
Have the students begin an "Environmental Journal." Explain that this will be a notebook in which to keep papers, notes, worksheets, ideas, and feelings about the environment and pollution. The notebooks should be collected and read periodically to check progress and participation. Students should look through magazines to find a picture they like that represents the word *environment* for them. The picture should be glued on the front of a folded piece of paper to make their "Environmental Journal."

MATERIALS
Construction paper
Magazines
Scissors
Glue

a. The first item that students should place in the journal is a sheet of lined paper to keep definitions of words. They can begin by defining the following words.
   (1) Environment
   (2) Pollution
   (3) Impact
   (4) Litter
   (5) Wastes
   (6) Graffiti
b. The dictionary can be consulted for help, but the definitions should be written in the student's own words.

MATERIALS
Dictionaries

2. Environmental Health Survey

Tell the students they are going to take a personal survey to help them identify ways they contribute to environmental pollution. Explain that this survey is not for a grade. It is intended to provide information for personal use. The only way they will get an accurate idea about their personal impact on the environment is to be honest in answering the questions.

a. Hand out the worksheet, *Environmental Health Survey*, and allow the students to complete it. Provide help to students who need assistance in summation.
b. After all the students have completed their survey, tell them that a score of 50 is perfect; 45 to 49 is very good; 40 to 44 is good; 35 to 39 is fair; and below 35 is poor. Explain that these are all actions they can individually take to prevent or cause pollution.
c. Go over each statement on the survey orally with students. After each statement have the students write a letter to indicate the type of pollution they think it represents on the appropriate line. They should write an *A* for air pollution, *L* for land pollution, *W* for water pollution, *N* for noise pollution, and *C* for conservation. For each statement on the survey, ask students to

speculate what the impact might be if everyone did that particular activity.
d. Have the students put their surveys into their journal. If time allows, they can write a poem on the prevention of pollution for their journal.

MATERIALS
Worksheet: *Environmental Health Survey* (Figure 18-3)

3. Game: Stop That Pollutant

a. Conduct a short discussion on air pollution. Ask students to list various causes of air pollution. (This discussion should be brief.) Tell them that the next activity will help them identify causes of air pollution and demonstrate the way the body reacts to air pollutants (dirty particles in the air).
b. In preparation for this activity make three sets of signs from the patterns indicated in the margin. One set of signs will be needed for a third of the students in the class. Also make *dirty particle* labels. These are best done on pieces of masking tape. In the game a dirty particle label will be taped to a volleyball.
c. Take the students outside to a playing field or to a gymnasium to play a game called "Stop That Pollutant." Divide the students into three teams. One group is the *dirty particle team*, another is the *cilia team*, and the third is the *lungs team*. Give the students signs for their team to wear around their neck.
d. Briefly review the anatomy of the respiratory system. Explain that cilia are tiny hairlike projections in the bronchial tubes which sweep out dirty particles that are inhaled. But too much air pollution and cigarette smoking can damage the cilia.
e. Arrange the teams as in the illustration on p. 456. The cilia team lines up in two lines between the dirty particles team (throwers) and the lungs team (catchers). The rules are as follows:

- A member of the dirty particles team tapes a label on one volleyball and throws it.
- The dirty particle team members try to get the ball to the lungs team but must throw past the cilia team.
- Using one arm only, the cilia team members try to bat the ball back and keep it away from the lungs team.
- If the cilia team is successful, the dirty particles team must try again with that ball.
- If the ball gets past the cilia to the lungs, the member of the lungs team must take off and read the label on the ball. The label indicates the type of particle that has just gotten into the lungs (for example, car exhaust, cigarette smoke, factory waste, and fireplace smoke). After the type of pollutant is read, the lungs team should suggest a way that this type of pollution could be prevented.
- The object of the game is to see how many pollutants the dirty particles team can get into the lungs. The cilia and lungs teams are essentially on the same side. The cilia team tries to protect the lungs from the dirty particles, but once the ball gets past the cilia, a member of the lungs team *must* catch the ball.
- Have the teams trade roles.

MATERIALS
Teacher resource: *Game Directions: Stop That Pollutant* (Figure 18-4)
Patterns: *Game Signs for Stop That Pollutant* (Figure 18-5)

Masking tape
Construction paper
Crayons or felt pens
String
Game signs: "Lungs," "Cilia," and "Dirty Particles" (teacher made)
Volleyballs (3 to 5 balls)
Labels: "Dirty Particles" (30 labels, teacher made)

EVALUATION: "Environmental Mobile"
Give the students four tagboard circles. On one side of each circle they should glue or draw a picture representing a cause for each type of pollution (air, land, noise, and water). On the other side of each circle they should write a sentence about how that type of pollution could be prevented. Assess if students were able to identify a cause for each type of pollution.

Punch holes in the circles and suspend them from a hanger to make an environmental mobile. Others items that could be included on the mobile are poems about the environment and pictures of pleasant environments.

MATERIALS
Tagboard circles (4 per student, approximately 5 inches in diameter)
Crayons or felt pens
String
Hole punch
Hangers (1 per student)

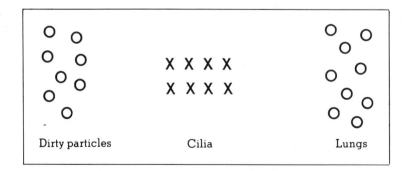

Dirty particles   Cilia   Lungs

FIGURE 18-3

Worksheet   Name _____

Environmental Health Survey

Directions: Read each question. Think carefully about whether you do what is described in the question. For each question, use the scale to describe how often you do the following:

Very often, circle 0
Often, circle 1
Sometimes, circle 3
Never, circle 5

	VERY OFTEN	OFTEN	SOME-TIMES	NEVER
1. I let the water run while brushing my teeth.	0	1	3	5
2. I spit chewing gum on the ground.	0	1	3	5
3. I use only one side of a piece of writing paper.	0	1	3	5
4. When walking, I drop food wrappers or paper on the side of the road.	0	1	3	5
5. I write words on walls.	0	1	3	5
6. I play my radio or stereo very loudly.	0	1	3	5
7. I chew tobacco and spit it on the ground.	0	1	3	5
8. When I am thirsty, I drink nonrecyclable canned or bottled soda pop.	0	1	3	5
9. I ask Mom or Dad to take me in the car when I could ride my bicycle or walk instead.	0	1	3	5
10. I throw usable toys or clothes in the trash when I no longer like them.	0	1	3	5

Now write the 10 numbers you circled and add them together.

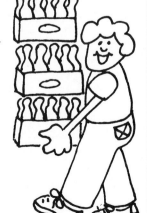

1. _____
2. _____
3. _____
4. _____
5. _____
6. _____
7. _____
8. _____
9. _____
10. _____
My score

FIGURE 18-4

Teacher resource

Game Directions:
Stop that Pollutant

1. Make signs on a tagboard for each team from sign patterns provided in this text. Each team will consist of a third of the students in the class. It may be useful to laminate the signs so that they may be used again.

2. Make labels titled "Dirty Particles." Use 1½- to 2-inch masking tape for the labels. Place a long section of tape onto a surface where the tape can be easily lifted off. Write the names of various air pollutants on the tape. Make about 30 labels using pollutant names over as necessary, such as the following:

Car exhaust	Factory smoke
Truck exhaust	Cigar smoke
Cigarette smoke	Fireplace smoke

3. Cut the labels from the long strip of tape, and mount them on a yardstick for easy access in the game.

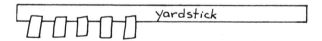

4. Organize the students outside or in a large gymnasium. Give each student a sign to wear indicating the team. Read the rules for the game as described in the activity section of this chapter. Trade off teams so that everyone has a chance to be on each team: lungs (catchers), cilia (one-handed defenders), and dirty particles (throwers).

FIGURE 18-5

Patterns

**Game Signs for
Stop that Pollutant**

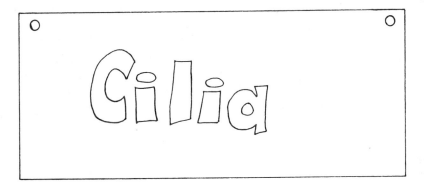

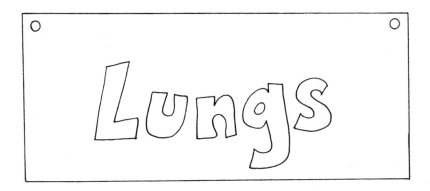

MIDDLE SCHOOL LEVEL

OBJECTIVE: The student evaluates the efforts of community groups and agencies in improving and protecting the environment.

LEVEL: Grades 6 to 8

VOCABULARY: Official agency, voluntary agency, community, environment

CONTENT GENERALIZATIONS: The individual is ultimately responsible for the health of the environment. For example, an individual can take personal responsibility for not polluting the air. However, if no one else in the community takes action to avoid pollution, the air still will be polluted. With environmental health concerns, in particular, it is necessary for people to work together to protect the environment. Several types of groups exist: official governmental agencies such as the public health department and the state environmental protection agency; voluntary agencies such as the American Lung Association; and special interest groups such as the Sierra Club, National Audubon Society, National Wildlife Federation, and American Camping Association. The individual can help protect the environment by participating in groups such as these and by following recommendations and laws designed to help the environment.

INITIATION: "Clean, Safe Water"
Display a large pitcher of water and paper cups. Ask if anyone wants a drink of water. Tell students that it is tap water and safe to drink. If there is a faucet in your classroom, fill the water pitcher in front of students to prove it is tap water.

After a few students have tasted the water, ask a few questions:
1. How does it taste?
2. Is it clean?
3. How do you know?
4. Can we trust the tap water to be safe in this city, state, or country?

5. Would you trust the tap water to be safe in other countries?

Explain to students that we often take for granted the clean water that comes out of the tap. In many places in the world, and sometimes even in the United States, the water that comes out of the tap is not safe to drink. The reason that we usually can trust our water is because we have groups of people in our community that work together to make certain our water is clean. (Typical groups in communities that do this are the public health department, water and power department, department of sanitation, and local ecology groups.)

MATERIALS
Water pitcher filled with tap water
Paper cups

ACTIVITIES
1. Mini-Lecture—Pollution
Write the words *land*, *air*, and *water* on the board. Ask the students to brainstorm actions that individuals can take to protect these valuable resources. This can be done in groups or as a full class. The students' list might include avoid littering, recycle glassware and aluminum, do not waste water, avoid polluting streams and lakes, walk or ride bicycles rather than use automobiles, and make certain all automobiles have proper equipment to filter exhaust fumes.

Explain to the students that it is important for individuals to do their part in protecting the environment; however, often certain problems must be solved by groups of people. It is also important that individuals support the work of community groups to protect the environment.
2. Protecting the Environment
Divide students into groups to do research on various groups that work to protect the environment. Hand out the worksheet, *Protecting the Environment*, and review the directions with students.

MATERIALS

Worksheet: *Protecting the Environment* (Figure 18-6)

a. Instruct each group to visit the library to identify an environmental issue (environmental concern in the community) they would like to study.

b. Once an issue has been identified, students should locate various groups that may be involved. The groups may be official (governmental), voluntary, or special interest.

c. The students should contact each group with a letter asking *specific* questions.

d. When the students get the correspondence back, they should prepare an oral report that describes the issue they have chosen and the work done by various groups in the community; they should evaluate how well the groups are doing in protecting the environment.

Encourage the students to use charts and other visual aids for their group presentation. Tell students that they may have to wait several weeks for a reply from the various agencies. If they do not hear from the agencies contacted, have them prepare a presentation without the letters.

NOTE: Review the issues chosen by groups and the lists of agencies that each plans to contact. It may be necessary to change the issues addressed to avoid sending too many letters to one agency.

3. Field Trip

Take a field trip to a local agency concerned with protecting the environment, such as one of the following.

- Water treatment plant
- Sanitation site
- Public health department
- State environmental protection agency

Contact the agency first, and ask for a guide who can explain the operation and the way that they work to protect the environment. Ask that the guide have suggestions for individuals that could make the agency's work easier. After the field trip ask the students to describe what that particular agency does to protect the environment. Also ask if they think the agency is doing a good job.

EVALUATION: "Certificate Of Appreciation"

List on the board all the agencies nominated by the class for a certificate of appreciation. Tell the students they must decide which agencies from the list should receive a certificate of appreciation from the class. For each agency a sentence or two describing why the award is deserved should be written by the group nominating it. Assess if students gave criteria for the nomination that demonstrates how the agency has helped to improve and protect the environment.

Have a committee of students tally the votes and determine which agencies will be awarded the certificate. Announce the winners to the class, and ask student volunteers to help in filling in and mailing the certificates.

MATERIALS

Teacher resource: *Certificate of Appreciation* (Figure 18-7)

FIGURE 18-6

Worksheet   Name _____

Protecting the Environment

Directions: In your groups you will be researching an environmental concern. You
                will be studying groups that are working to help the environment and try
                to figure out whether they are doing a good job of protecting the
                environment. As a group, follow the steps outlined below. Your group
                will be responsible for an oral presentation after you have done your
                research.

1. As a group, identify an environmental issue you would like to study.
   You may have to visit the library and talk to the librarian for help in
   this task.
   The environmental issue we will study is _____

2. Find out what groups are interested in the same environmental issue.
   Ask the librarian for help. Find out if the groups are governmental,
   voluntary, or special interest. You may have to look these words up in
   a dictionary first.
   The groups concerned with this issue are:

   _____   _____

   _____   _____

3. As a group, write a neat letter to each group identified in 2. Ask some
   specific questions such as the following: (1) What does your group do
   about (issue)? (2) What are some of the problems that your agency
   has dealing with (issue)? (3) Are there things that your agency would
   like to do about (issue) but for some reason cannot do at this time?
   (4) What can individuals in the community do about (issue)?

   All members in the group should sign the letter. Make certain that all
   words are spelled correctly and that you have indicated a return
   address. It might be a good idea to enclose a self-addressed stamped
   envelope.

4. When you have heard from all the agencies that you contacted,
   prepare an oral report that analyzes the effectiveness of the groups in
   protecting the environment. In other words, are they doing a good job
   or not?

   In your presentation you should have some visual aids prepared to
   add interest.

FIGURE 18-7

Teacher resource

Certificate of Appreciation

Directions: After the class has determined which agencies are doing a good job
protecting the environment, have a committee mail out certificates to
these agencies. An example is provided below.

CERTIFICATE OF APPRECIATION

The_____ class at _____ School

is awarding this special certificate of appreciation to

_____
  (Name of agency)

for outstanding efforts in protection of the environment in our community.

_____Signed_____
  (Date)   (Teacher)

Certificate of Appreciation Committee

_____   _____

_____   _____

_____   _____

19 Community Health

When you finish this chapter, you should be able to:

- Identify sources of health care within communities.
- Describe three roles and responsibilities of community health-care workers
- Compare private, public, and voluntary hospitals.
- List major voluntary health organizations that provide health education resources within communities.
- Explain how partnerships among health education agencies can benefit communities.
- Develop learning opportunities for elementary and middle school students in the area of community health.

M any health problems must be handled by the community as a whole. For any community health education program to be successful, the participation and cooperation of individuals within the community are necessary. Communication among health professionals, school staff, and elected officials is essential to identify health problems and determine possible solutions.

Not only these professionals must become involved; all citizens must accept responsibility and recognize that certain health problems cannot be solved without personal action. This action can take many forms, including volunteer work, financial donations to nonprofit health organizations, and political support of candidates concerned with the health problems of the community.

Today, experts agree that fostering healthy children is the shared responsibility of families, communities, and schools. As discussed in Chapter 13, in recent years behaviors have become the focus as the major causes of morbidity for Americans. The current threats to Americans' health are heart disease, cancer, sexually transmitted disease and unintended pregnancies, alcohol and other drug abuse, motor vehicle trauma, and suicide. In the past, youth were faced with the threat of infectious diseases such as smallpox, diphtheria, pertussis, and polio. Schools worked with the community to prevent these diseases by requiring students to be vaccinated and often by serving as sites for vaccination programs. Staff from schools and communities still work together to ensure that the school population is properly immunized, but helping to prepare students for a healthy future is more complex than just having proof of immunizations.

Because of this complexity, it has been observed that "The massive task of educating for awareness cannot be accomplished alone by the schools. Parents, the government and the private sector, the for-profit organizations and the not-for-profit organizations must all be drawn into the process" (1). Thus when we use the term *community health*, we refer to many health-related issues, including environmental concerns, prevention of communicable diseases, and education for healthy behavior.

In this chapter, we will briefly discuss some of the ways that a community can coordinate activities to promote health through services provided by various institutions and organizations. We will then explore potential career opportunities in the health field and examine the role that voluntary health agencies play within communities. Finally, we will look at current trends toward the development of comprehensive school health programs and community/school partnerships.

HEALTH-CARE FACILITIES

Most communities have a number of different types of health-care facilities, including hospitals, clinics, nursing homes, and rehabilitation centers. A recent development in many communities is the addition of private, 24-hour drop-in emergency and surgical centers.

Hospitals are categorized by their financial structure. They usually fall into one of three categories—private, public, or voluntary hospitals. *Private hospitals* (or proprietary hospitals) are profit-making institutions. They are not supported by tax funds and usually accept only patients who can pay all of their expenses. These hospitals tend to be relatively small and may provide limited services, specializing in the treatment of a few specific illnesses. They are often owned by a group of business investors, a large hospital corporation, or a group of physicians.

Public hospitals are hospitals that are mainly supported by taxes (publicly funded). They are run by federal, state, county, or city government agencies. For example, state mental hospitals, federal Veterans' Administration hospitals, and various military service hospitals are public hospitals. Large county or city hospitals are also public hospitals; these hospitals generally serve indigent population groups and may function as *teaching hospitals* for local medical schools. For example, medical students receive clinical experiences in teaching hospitals that are a valuable part of their education.

Voluntary hospitals are the most recognized type of hospital. They function as nonprofit institutions and usually offer a wider range of services than private or public hospitals or clinics. Many voluntary hospitals have expanded their scope of services to include specialized programs such as stress centers, cardiac rehabilitation centers, chemical dependence programs, and health education centers. These hospitals are supported by patient fees and contributions from the community.

Nursing homes and home care agencies are often private enterprises. Some nursing homes have begun to specialize in patient care, for example, in Alzheimer's disease. County departments of health and social services also offer health-related care for some low-income population groups.

Private drop-in emergency clinics and surgery centers are increasingly available for community use. These clinics have their own staff of physicians, nurses, and other health professionals. Some clinics specialize in meeting the health needs of certain segments of the population, such as women or older members of the community.

Many nonprofit agencies and organizations offer health care services to specific populations—for instance, minority groups (such as Latinos) or battered women. Planned Parenthood is an example of a nonprofit organization that provides educational materials and low cost health-care services for women. These clinics often operate on limited budgets; fund-raising efforts are necessary for maintaining their services.

CAREER OPPORTUNITIES

The health field offers a wide variety of career opportunities. Some examples of direct-care health workers are dentists, physicians, nurses, dental hygienists, dieticians, pharmacists, optometrists, physical therapists, and mental health counselors. Another category of health careers includes administrators of health institutions or other facilities. These jobs involve planning and administering the employees' services and policies of hospitals, clinics, voluntary health agencies, mental health facilities, nursing homes, and health departments.

Although direct-care health workers are also

a source of health information, education is the primary function of health educators. These individuals conduct community educational programs sponsored by hospitals, health departments, clinics, voluntary health agencies, and businesses and industries. School health educators are credentialed teachers of health in schools and universities.

Health research is essential, especially in the areas of disease prevention, and treatment. Researchers develop and test the safety and effectiveness of new drugs and medical devices. Individuals interested in laboratory sciences can find a career in the health field as well. Medical laboratory technicians and assistants perform tests to determine the presence and extent of a disease. Laboratory technicians need educational backgrounds in fields such as chemistry, human biology, and microbiology.

Those interested in health and food science may consider becoming a dietician or nutritionist. Others interested in health and journalism or art can become medical writers or illustrators. Careers in health field marketing usually involve the sale or promotion of new products or drugs to medical practitioners. As the demand for many kinds of health-care workers continues, individuals with an interest in science and health are likely to find a satisfying career. Exploring these career possibilities long before high-school graduation is a good idea.

VOLUNTARY HEALTH ORGANIZATIONS

Voluntary health organizations are agencies formed to deal with certain problems locally and nationally. They depend on donations of time and money from individuals in the community to function. Although there may be a few paid staff members, most of the work is performed by volunteers.

Voluntary health organizations exist because of an unmet need, and they frequently address problems that can be avoided with early preventive education. Some major voluntary health organizations are the American Red Cross, the American Cancer Society, the American Lung Association, and the American Heart Association. These agencies are extensively organized and have nationwide network of local chapters and volunteers.

A major focus of the work of voluntary health agencies is educational. Many of the organizations have developed printed and other educational materials and expertise in working with the media and policymakers. Some have also developed curriculum materials for students and in-service programs for teachers. In fact, many of these organizations now recognize that comprehensive school health education is one of the most effective ways to deliver their messages about preventing conditions such as heart disease, lung disease, and cancer.

COMMUNITY/SCHOOL PARTNERSHIPS

Involving families and the broader community as partners in planning a comprehensive school health program helps to ensure that the plan is responsive to family and community values and needs. Without the support of families and communities to reinforce the health messages presented in schools, a school-based health program cannot succeed. Students are quick to notice discrepancies between messages provided by different adults, as well as discrepancies between adults' messages and behavior. School health education programs are more likely to succeed when students receive consistent messages from their school, home, and community environments and when the behavior modeled by the adults in students' lives is also consistent with these messages.

Other programs for children and families also require a coordinated effort in the community. Services designed to help families with health-related problems are often not coordinated with related agencies. One organizational change being explored is a new type of collaborative effort in planning and delivering services, with a focus on prevention. Such partnerships can allow local agencies to pool their resources so that issues beyond the scope of one agency can be handled. These programs are usually offered in accessible neighborhood locations such as schools and clinics and are designed to address diverse cultural needs.

Although integrated services make sense to families, it is a major challenge for agencies and schools to create the necessary partnerships. Differences in professional training and vocabulary competition for sources of funding, agency organization, and legal guidelines make the integration of services difficult. Some of the ways a community can successfully work toward this goal are the following:

- Creating a "children's report card" to raise awareness about important health issues, highlight successes, and determine local needs
- Learning about each other's programs, service criteria, and funding restrictions
- Defining what a "partnership" means in terms of specific areas of collaboration
- Including formal and informal community leaders early in the process
- Viewing recipients as customers rather than clients
- Involving families in planning or evaluating services, often resulting in them feeling more responsibility for their own success
- Creating a community vision that has consistency and focus
- Reflecting local population diversity by designing services that are culturally and linguistically compatible
- Allowing adequate time for planning and development of integrated services
- Identifying local, state, and national barriers to collaboration and developing strategies for overcoming them (for example, confidentiality issues, job classification conflicts, and funding restrictions)
- Involving state and local elected officials because proposed changes may have political implications

PROMOTING HEALTHY PARTNERSHIPS

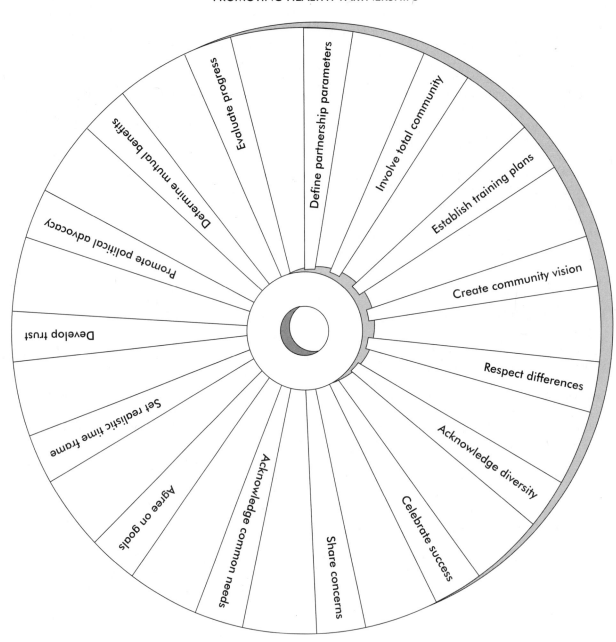

FIGURE 19-1
Promoting Healthy Partnerships

- Establishing evaluation methods and identifying meaningful outcome measures and ways of assessing cost savings
- Marketing the program and celebrating its successes as they occur

Currently, changes in professional training enable communities to achieve the goal of integrated services for children. For example, at many universities, teachers are educated in one school and social welfare workers in another. They have separate buildings and program requirements. These situations discourage student contact.

Similarly, credentials and licenses can create barriers. Professional conferences are exclusive rather than inclusive of other professionals. This situation is beginning to change as educators at universities recognize the contributions of other professional training programs.

SUMMARY

In this chapter, we have briefly considered some aspects of health from a community perspective. In every community, members must work together to solve certain problems. Career opportunities in the health-care field range from the provision of direct services to administrative and research-oriented job possibilities. Voluntary health agencies play an important health education role in communities, particularly in fighting specific problems or diseases.

Some new and innovative ways of working together to provide health education and services for families and children in communities are needed. Collaborative efforts between schools and community organizations are increasingly critical to fight the fragmentation of many types of services provided to students and their families. Although there are barriers to providing integrated services, these are often not as great as they initially appear, and the rewards are well worth the effort.

The next section of this chapter contains examples of learning opportunities for primary level, intermediate level, and middle-school students.

REFERENCES

1. Seffrin J: *Voluntary health organizations: the untapped resource.* In Cortese P, Middleton K, eds: *The comprehensive school health challenge*, vol 2, Santa Cruz, Calif, 1994, ETR Associates.

SUGGESTED READINGS

Berryman J, Breighner K: *Modeling healthy behavior*, Santa Cruz, Calif, 1993, ETR Associates.

Kane W: *Step by step to comprehensive school health.* Santa Cruz, Calif, 1993, ETR Associates.

Kirby D: Comprehensive school health and the larger community: issues and a possible scenario. *J School Health* 60(4):170, 1990.

Mason J: Forging working partnerships for school health education, *J School Health* 59(1):18, 1989.

Rice D: Ethics and equity in U.S. health care: the data, *Int J Health Services* 21(4):638, 1991.

Siri D: *Community/school partnerships.* In Cortese P, Middleton K, eds: *The comprehensive school health challenge*, vol 2, Santa Cruz, Calif, 1994, ETR Associates.

LEARNING OPPORTUNITIES FOR COMMUNITY HEALTH

GENERAL STUDENT OBJECTIVES

Primary Level K-3

The student:
1. Identifies familiar community health workers (health helpers)
2. Explains the function of various health workers in the community
3. Lists services provided by community health agencies and organizations*

Intermediate Level 4-5/6

The student:
1. Describes ways community members work together to solve health problems.
2. Identifies functions of interesting career opportunities in the health field*

Middle School Level 6/7-8

The student:
1. Describes community efforts to prevent and control disease.
2. Concludes that individual participation is essential if community health activities are to be successful.*

*These objectives are illustrated by sample learning activities.

PRIMARY LEVEL

OBJECTIVE: The student lists services provided by community health agencies and organizations.

LEVEL: Grades 2 and 3

INTEGRATION: Map skills, social studies, writing

VOCABULARY: Community, hospital, health department, sanitation department

CONTENT GENERALIZATIONS: A variety of health agencies and organizations exist in each community to safeguard the health of all people. There are many services needed and provided in communities. Agencies common in most communities include a hospital, health department, fire department, police department, sanitation department, and voluntary health agencies. Knowing where health services are available will en-

able citizens to take an active role in protecting the community's health.

INITIATION: "Health Worker" Play
Show pictures or teacher-made posters of community health workers, and discuss a main function of each. Review the functions to be certain that each child is familiar with each health worker. Then divide the class into small groups, and secretly assign each group a different health worker. Have each group or a member from each group act out the functions of their assigned health worker, and have classmates guess the health worker being represented. As each is identified, place a name card for the health worker on the left side of the bulletin board.

MATERIALS
Pictures of health workers or posters made from *Health Helpers* patterns (Figures 16-2, 16-3, and 16-4)
Name card for each health worker

ACTIVITIES

1. "Be a Wise Willy!" Bulletin Board Activity

a. One at a time, display large photographs of your community's health office building for each health worker you have studied. Use these pictures to complete the bulletin board display, *Be a Wise Willy!* For instance, show a picture of the local firehouse, doctors' building or hospital, police station, health department, and selected health agencies or organizations (such as the American Cancer Society and American Lung Association). For each photograph ask the following questions.

- How many of you have seen the building before?
- What is the name of the building?
- Which of the health workers works in this building?

b. If the students are unable to answer a question, provide clues or the information for them.

c. After the students identify a photograph and discuss it, mount it on the bulletin board display, *Be a Wise Willy!* Stretch pieces of large colorful yarn between the photographs and the names of the health workers in that building. There may be several strings attached to one card.

d. After discussing the bulletin board and allowing students to match the names with the photographs, explain that the yarn will be disconnected from the name cards and that students can come to the bulletin board during their free time and try to reattach the yarn to the correct photographs. To check their answers as they work independently, students can lift the index card beside each photograph and read the correct answer (name of health worker) for that photograph.

e. When a student has matched the items on the bulletin board correctly, he or she should write his or her name on the *Wise Willy* name card and detach the yarn pieces for the next student's use.

MATERIALS

Photographs of local community agencies (from the agencies' professional photographs or brochures or taken by the teacher)
Bulletin board display: *Be a Wise Willy!* (Figure 19-2)

2. Health Workers in My Community

a. Make a simple street map of your community similar to the sample worksheet provided here. If possible, it should include neighborhoods of all students in the class, school grounds, and downtown area. Using an overhead projector and a transparency of the handout, ask the students to point to the location of the school building, downtown area, their neighborhoods, and other familiar landmarks. Students should color significant points on the map (such as rivers, streets, and school).

b. Ask volunteers to identify the location of the community health buildings that are posted on the bulletin board. As students show the correct location, have one student write it on the transparency so that others can write it on their worksheets properly.

c. When all the worksheets are marked with the locations of the community health buildings, review the functions of each health worker.

MATERIALS

Worksheet and transparency: *Health Workers in My Community* (Figure 19-3)
Overhead projector
Transparency pen
Crayons

EVALUATION: "What Health Workers Do"

Divide the class into two teams. Have the first student from team A draw a slip of paper with the name of a health worker from a hat or bowl containing the names of all of them. The student is to name the function of the health worker drawn and use the transparency to show the location of the corresponding community building. If the student does this correctly, the team gets 1 point. Team B now gets a turn, then team A, and so on.

MATERIALS

Hat or bowl
Slips of paper with names of health workers
Transparency from worksheet: *Health Workers in My Community* (See Figure 19-3)
Overhead projector
Transparency pen

FIGURE 19-2

Bulletin board display

Name _____

Be a Wise Willy!

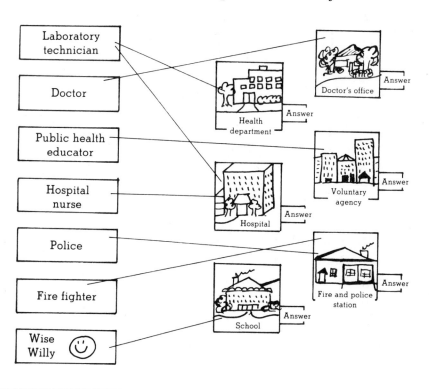

BE A WISE WILLY!

Know how to keep Toledo healthy!

Laboratory technician	
Doctor	
Public health educator	
Hospital nurse	
Police	
Fire fighter	
Wise Willy ☺	

Health department — Answer

Doctor's office — Answer

Voluntary agency — Answer

Hospital — Answer

Fire and police station — Answer

School — Answer

FIGURE 19-3

Worksheet   Name _____

Health Workers in My Community

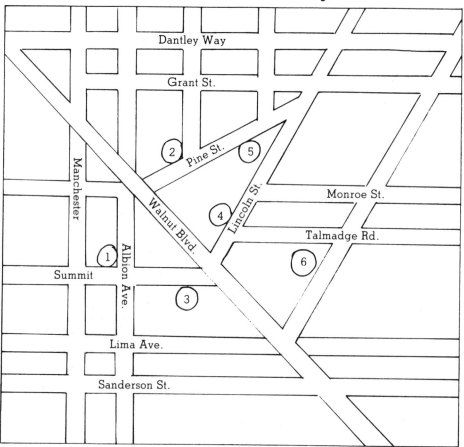

Key:

1. Fire department and police station
2. Health department
3. Health agency
4. Doctor's office
5. Owen School
6. Custer Hospital

INTERMEDIATE LEVEL

OBJECTIVE: The student identifies functions of interesting career opportunities in the health field.

LEVEL: Grades 4 to 6 (most appropriate for grade 4)

INTEGRATION: Dictionary skills, language arts, listening skills

VOCABULARY: Nurse, dentist, pharmacist, researcher, technician, physician

CONTENT GENERALIZATIONS: There are many career opportunities in the health field available to students, including dentist, dental hygienist, pharmacist, nurse (hospital, surgical, and school), laboratory technician, medical researcher, health educator (community, school, and industry), and physician. As the field of medicine expands, individuals who pursue a career in medicine are becoming more highly specialized. The types of physicians that children are most likely to see include pediatricians, allergists, family practitioners, otologists, internists, surgeons, and psychiatrists.

INITIATION: Health Careers That Interest Us
Conduct a brainstorming activity on the types of careers possible in the health field. Tell students to try to think of people who have helped them with their health. As ideas surface, write them on the board. If the students have difficulty, give clues such as the following:

1. What kind of people work at a dentist's office?
2. Who works in a hospital?
3. Is there someone here at school who helps you with your health?
4. What other kinds of doctors have you heard of?

When the brainstorming is finished, hand each student a strip of paper. Tell the students to print a health career on the paper that sounds interesting to them. They can copy the spelling off the board. They should print their name on the lower right corner of the paper. Mount the printed careers on a bulletin board entitled "Health Careers That Interest Us."

MATERIALS
Strips of paper (approximately 12 inches long)
Bulletin board sign: "Health Careers That Interest Us"

ACTIVITIES

1. Job Descriptions
a. Have students use encyclopedias to look up the career they printed on the slip of paper. They should write a paragraph about that job and draw a picture of a person in that career. Students may need out-of-class time to complete this assignment. When it is finished, they are to mount their paragraph and picture on the bulletin board.
b. Choose several career paragraphs to read aloud daily.

MATERIALS
Encyclopedias
Paper
Crayons, felt pens, or colored pencils

2. When Freddy Grows Up: A Play
Tell the students that a play will be presented because "Freddy" is trying to decide what he wants to be when he grows up. Choose two students to read the parts. Change the gender as necessary.

Option: Obtain two hand puppets and present the play as a puppet show. Or, have students present this play or puppet show to younger students in another class.

FREDDY WANTS A HEALTH CAREER

Freddy: Freddy: I feel great! I am only 10 years old, and I know what I want to be when I grow up [whistles, cheers, etc.].

Frieda: [Enters stage] Freddy, you are shouting and cheering. What happened? Did you win the softball game?

Freddy: Oh! Hello Frieda. No, it is better than that. I know exactly what I am going to be when I grow up.

Frieda: Last week you said you wanted to be a video game expert. Will that be your profession?

Freddy: Nope. Video games are for entertainment only.

Frieda: A ball player, then; you are a great pitcher.

Freddy: I pitched that idea too. I know exactly what I am going to be when I grow up. *Exactly.* [To student audience] can any of you guess what I am going to be?

Frieda: Now that everyone has guessed, tell us exactly what you want to be when you grow up.

Freddy: A doctor. D-O-C-T-O-R [waves card that says *doctor*].

Frieda: But exactly what kind of doctor?

Freddy: You know, a medical doctor, a physician [waves card that says *physician.*] A medical doctor is the same as a physician.

Frieda: Yes, that is true. But what *kind* of a physician?

Freddy: What do you mean?

Frieda: Well, my mom is a physician. She says that hardly any doctors take care of all the body parts—eyes, ears, feet—of all people, young and old. Doctors specialize in body parts or ages or diseases.

Freddy: Oh, doctors specialize in something. Then to know *exactly* what I am going to be I must know what *kind* of a doctor I am going to be.

Frieda: You have got the idea now. My mom is an ear doctor; she is an otologist [holds card that says *otologist*]. When people have trouble hearing, they see an otologist like my mom.

Freddy: An ear doctor is an otologist. Hmmm. No that is not for me. What other kinds of doctors are there?

Frieda: My brother goes to a dermatologist [holds up *dermatologist* card] because he sometimes has skin problems.

Freddy: That's a possibility. My sister goes to a dermatologist too.

Frieda: An allergist [holds *allergist* card] helps people who have allergies. People who break out in itchy bumps when they eat an orange or pet a cat see an allergy doctor—an allergist.

Freddy: Itchy bumps! That is not for me either. What else is there?

Frieda: The only other one I know of is a pediatrician [holds *pediatrician* card]. A pediatrician is a doctor who specializes in children. I am 10, and I go to a pediatrician.

Freddy: Let's look in the *Yellow Pages* of the telephone book to see what other kinds of physicians there are. There is one: psychiatrist [holds *psychiatrist* card]. A psychiatrist helps people with personal problems.

Frieda: Here is surgeon [holds *surgeon* card]. A surgeon operates to treat diseases or other problems.

Freddy: I found a family practitioner [holds *family practitioner* card]. They treat people of all ages.

Frieda: Internist [holds *internist* card]. An internist specializes in organs inside people, like your heart and lungs, but usually does not operate.

Freddy: That's it! I know *exactly* what I will be. I will be an internist, and treat people's heart, lungs, and other organs. Of course, I will tell them that if they keep healthy by playing baseball and sports and eating nutritious foods, they probably will not need an internist very often.

Frieda: [Asks students] Do you know the names of different types of physicians? See how many you can match to their job. Your teacher will give you a worksheet. You can ask your teacher for help.

Freddy and Frieda: Bye, good luck!

Ask the class, "If Freddy wants to have a health career when he grows up, what other jobs could he do other than being a physician?"

MATERIALS

Puppet stage (optional)

Two hand puppets that have the ability to grasp objects (optional)

Index cards with the following words printed (1 word on each card):

Doctor

Physician

Otologist

Dermatologist

Allergist

Pediatrician

Psychiatrist

Surgeon

Family practitioner

Internist

Telephone book

3. Different Kinds of Physicians

After the play, hand out the worksheet, *Different Kinds of Physicians*, for students to complete. Review the worksheet, and have students correct mistakes.

MATERIALS

Worksheet: *Different Kinds of Physicians* (Figure 19-4)

EVALUATION: "Who Does What?"

Have the students complete the worksheet, *Who Does What?*, individually and without assistance. Tell them that this worksheet is very similar to the one they already did on different kinds of physicians. However, this time there are other careers in addition to physicians on the worksheet.

MATERIALS

Worksheet: *Who Does What?* (Figure 19-5)

FIGURE 19-4

Worksheet   Name _____

Different Kinds of Physicians

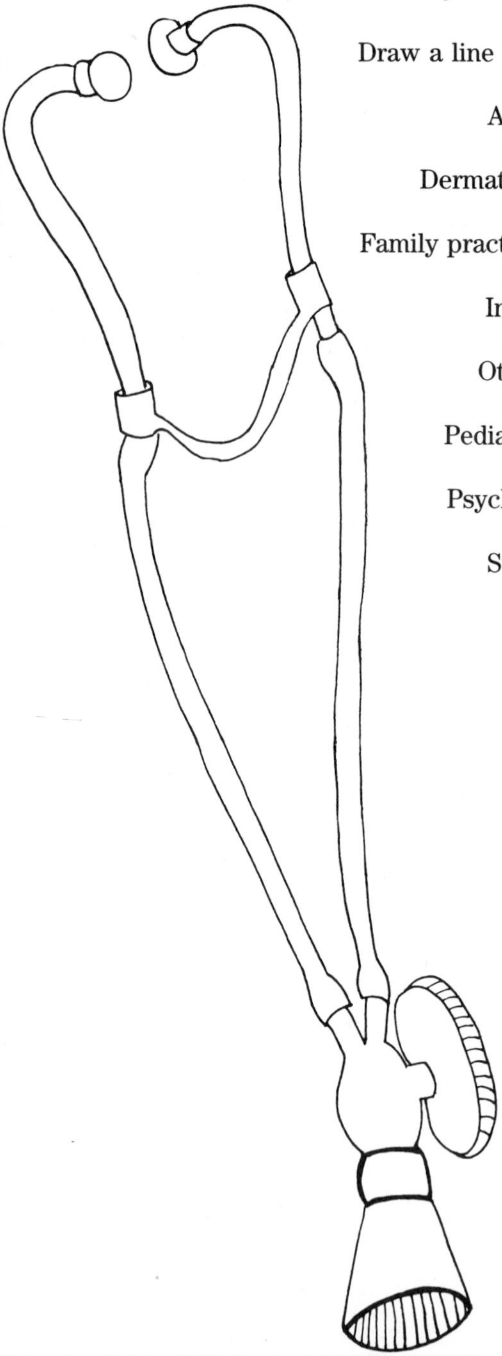

Draw a line from the type of physician to that person's job.

Allergist   Operates on internal organs

Dermatologist   Treats internal organs without
                     operating
Family practitioner
                     Treats people of all ages
Internist
                     Treats ear problems
Otologist
                     Treats itchy bumps from cats or other
Pediatrician   things

Psychiatrist   Treats skin problems

Surgeon   Treats mental problems

                     Treats children

FIGURE 19-5

Worksheet   Name _____

Who Does What?

Draw a line from the health career name to the sentence describing one of the
job responsibilities for that person.

School nurse   A person who teaches people about good health

Pharmacist   A person who helps children who are ill at school

Internist   A person who cleans your teeth

Dental hygienist   A physician who treats children

Surgical nurse   A person who assists a physician during operation

Pediatrician   A person who fills prescriptions written by physicians

Health educator   A physician who treats internal organs without operating

MIDDLE SCHOOL LEVEL

OBJECTIVE: The student concludes that individual participation is essential if community health activities are to be successful.

LEVEL: Grades 6 to 8

VOCABULARY: Volunteer, professions, organizations

CONTENT GENERALIZATIONS: Most communities have many organizations both public and private that are interested in the health of community members. The various types of organizations include voluntary health agencies (such as the American Cancer Society, American Lung Association, American Heart Association, and American Red Cross), official governmental organizations (such as the public health department and public hospitals), private industry (such as privately owned hospitals, local drug stores, private physicians, and other health professionals in private practice), professional organizations (such as local chapters of the American Medical Association [AMS], AMA Auxiliary, American Dental Association, and American Public Health Association), and service clubs (such as the Kiwanis, Rotary Club, and Lions Club). In most cases these organizations require individual voluntary participation to effectively carry out health activities in the community. Voluntary help and contributions are essential if these organizations are to accomplish their goals.

INITIATION: "Are You a Health Volunteer?"
Write the word *volunteer* on the board, and ask the students if they have ever volunteered to do something for an organization or for school. As students suggest activities, write or have a student write them on the board. Volunteer work they may have done includes collecting money for the American Red Cross or another organization; participating in a Walk-A-Thon or Bike-A-Thon for a voluntary agency, a club, or a cause; or participating in a recycling program with a club or the school.

Explain to students that in each case their voluntary help was probably very important. Often it takes many people working together to accomplish something. Voluntary participation is particularly important in community health activities. Many community health organizations would not be able to function without individual volunteers.

ACTIVITIES
1. Health Fair
Ask the students to help organize a health fair for the school. Explain that several health organizations will be invited to come to school and tell what they do for the health of the community and how they use volunteers. Booths or tables will be set up, and students can visit the different organization representatives to find out about their work.
2. Community Health Volunteers
Give each student a copy of the worksheet, *Community Health Volunteers*. Go over the worksheet with students to explain its use during the health fair. Students are to ask representatives from each organization a few questions about volunteer work. (It is a good idea to tell the representatives that students will be asking certain questions.) It may be helpful to rotate students around to the booths in small groups so that representatives can address these questions to several students at one time.

MATERIALS
Worksheet: *Community Health Volunteers* (Figure 19-6)

3. Health Volunteers Mural

After the health fair ask the students to participate in making a large wall chart entitled *Health Volunteers in Our Community*. Have students use their completed worksheets to make a chart of all the organizations and agencies that they surveyed at the health fair. Have small groups of students contact other agencies or organizations not at the fair to add to the wall chart. Groups should fill in the chart as they contact a new agency or organization about the use of volunteers. When the chart is finished, ask the students if they think individual participation in community health activities is important and why. Ask, "What would happen if no one volunteered to do things for the community? Are there any activities you may be interested in doing for the community?"

MATERIALS

Wall chart: *Health Volunteers in Our Community*
Butcher paper
Felt pens or crayons
Rulers
Worksheets: *Community Health Volunteers* (completed by students) (Figure 19-6); *Community Health Agencies and Organizations* (Figure 19-7)

EVALUATION: "Getting Involved"

Tell the students to imagine that a friend has just said, "My mom thinks I should go on a Walk-A-Thon for the March of Dimes—Birth Defects Foundation. It sure sounds like a dumb idea to me." Ask them to respond to their friend. In their response they should tell about individual participation in health activities in the community. These responses can be written or taped on a cassette recorder. Assess for student conclusions indicating the importance of individual participation in community efforts.

MATERIALS

Optional: Cassette recorder and tape

FIGURE 19-6

Worksheet   Name _____

Community Health Volunteers

Directions: Talk to various representatives from health agencies in your community. Use this worksheet to record your findings. For each agency, ask whether they use volunteers. If they do use volunteers, try to find out what kinds of jobs the volunteers do for the organization.

AGENCY OR ORGANIZATION	VOLUNTEERS		JOBS THAT VOLUNTEERS DO
1. _____	YES	NO	_____
2. _____	YES	NO	_____
3. _____	YES	NO	_____
4. _____	YES	NO	_____
5. _____	YES	NO	_____
6. _____	YES	NO	_____

FIGURE 19-7

Worksheet   Name _____

Community Health Agencies and Organizations

Directions: The following is a list of several agencies that may be in your
                community. Look in the telephone book for local chapters. Check off
                those located in your community.

- [ ] Al-Anon
- [ ] Alcoholics Anonymous
- [ ] Allergy Foundation of America
- [ ] American Association for Rehabilitation Therapy
- [ ] American Cancer Society
- [ ] American Diabetes Association, Inc.
- [ ] American Foundation for the Blind, Inc.
- [ ] American Geriatrics Society, Inc.
- [ ] American Hearing Society
- [ ] American Heart Association
- [ ] American Institute of Family Relations, Inc.
- [ ] American Lung Association
- [ ] American Parkinson Disease Association
- [ ] American Red Cross
- [ ] Arthritis Foundation
- [ ] Cystic Fibrosis Foundation
- [ ] Epilepsy Foundation
- [ ] Gray Panthers
- [ ] Leukemia Society
- [ ] March of Dimes—Birth Defects Foundation
- [ ] Medic Alert Foundation
- [ ] Muscular Dystrophy Association
- [ ] The Myasthenia Gravis Foundation, Inc.
- [ ] Association for Gifted Children
- [ ] Association for Mental Health
- [ ] Association for Retarded Children
- [ ] Child Safety Council
- [ ] Council on Aging
- [ ] Council on Alcoholism, Inc.
- [ ] Easter Seal Society for Crippled Children and Adults
- [ ] Hemophilia Foundation
- [ ] Kidney Foundation
- [ ] Multiple Sclerosis Society
- [ ] Society to Prevent Blindness
- [ ] Tay-Sachs and Allied Diseases Association, Inc.
- [ ] Planned Parenthood Federation
- [ ] Sickle Cell Disease Foundation of Greater New York
- [ ] United Cerebral Palsy Association, Inc.
- [ ] United Parkinson's Foundation

Joint Committee on Health Education Terminology

CONTEXTUAL DEFINITIONS

Health education takes place within the broad context of health. Certain health terms are defined to clarify how health education functions. These are the following:

Health: There are many definitions written for the word health. Examples are provided in Chapter 1.

Health promotion and disease prevention: Health promotion and disease prevention is the aggregate of all purposeful activities designed to improve personal and public health through a combination of strategies, including the competent implementation of behavioral change strategies, health education, health protection measures, risk factor detection, health enhancement, and health maintenance.

Healthy lifestyle: A healthy lifestyle is a set of health-enhancing behaviors shaped by internally consistent values, attitudes, beliefs, and external social and cultural forces.

Official health agency: An official health agency is a publicly supported governmental organization mandated by law and/or regulation for the protection and improvement of the health of the public.

Voluntary health organization: A voluntary health organization is a nonprofit association supported by contributions dedicated to conducting research and providing education and/or services related to particular health problems or concerns. (NOTE: Private voluntary organization (PVO) is used outside the United States to denote a voluntary health organization; in some countries and in connection with the United Nations,

nongovernmental organization (NGO) is used.)

Private health agency: A private health agency is a profit or nonprofit organization devoted to providing primary, secondary, and/or tertiary health services that may include health education.

PRIMARY HEALTH EDUCATION DEFINITIONS

Certain health education terms are generic and are defined here as follows:

Health education field: The health education field is the multidisciplinary practice concerned with designing, implementing, and evaluating educational programs that enable individuals, families, groups, organizations, and communities to play active roles in achieving, protecting, and sustaining health.

Health education process: The health education process is the continuum of learning enabling people, as individuals and members of social structures, to voluntarily make decisions, modify behaviors, and change social conditions in ways that are health enhancing.

Health education program: A health education program is a planned combination of activities developed with the involvement of specific populations and based on a needs assessment, sound principles of education, and periodic evaluation using a clear set of goals and objectives.

Health educator: A health educator is a practitioner who is professionally prepared in the field of health education, who demonstrates competence in both theory and practice, and who accepts responsibility to advance the aims of the health education profession. Examples of settings for health educators and the application of health education include but are not limited to the following:

- Schools
- Communities
- Post-secondary educational institutions
- Medical care institutions
- Voluntary health organizations
- Worksites (business and industry)
- Rehabilitation centers
- Professional associations
- Governmental agencies
- Public health agencies
- Environmental agencies
- Mental health agencies

Certified health education specialist (CHES): A certified health education specialist (CHES) is an individual who is credentialed as a result of demonstrating competency based on criteria established by the National Commission for Health Education Credentialing, Inc (NCHEC).

Health education coordinator: A health education coordinator is a professional health educator who is responsible for the management and coordination of all health education policies, activities, and resources within a particular setting or circumstance.

Health education administrator: A health education administrator is a professional health educator who has the authority and responsibility for the management and coordination of all health education policies, activities, and resources within a particular setting or circumstance.

Health information: Health information is the content of communications based on data derived from systematic and scientific methods as they relate to health issues, policies, programs, services, and other aspects of individual and public health, which can be used for informing various populations and in planning health education activities.

Health literacy: Health literacy is the capacity of an individual to obtain, interpret, and understand basic health information and services and the competence to use such information and services in ways that are health enhancing.

*Health advising:** Health advising is a process of informing and assisting individuals or groups in making decisions and solving problems related to health.

DEFINITIONS RELATED TO COMMUNITY SETTINGS

The terms that relate more specifically to community or public health education are defined as follows:

Community health education: Community health education is the application of a variety of methods that results in the education and mobilization of community members in actions for resolving health issues and problems affecting the community. These methods include but are not limited to group process, mass media, communication, community organization, organization development, strategic planning, skills training, legislation, policy making, and advocacy.

Community health educator: A community health educator is a practitioner who is professionally prepared in the field of community/public health education who demonstrates competence in the planning, implementation, and evaluation of a broad range of health-promoting or health-enhancing programs for community groups.

DEFINITIONS RELATED TO EDUCATIONAL SETTINGS

The terms that relate more specifically to school health education are defined as follows:

Comprehensive school health program: A comprehensive school health program is an organized set of policies, procedures, and activities

---

*The Committee believes that health counseling is a term that should be defined by the health counseling profession.

designed to protect and promote the health and well-being of students and staff. It has traditionally included health services, healthful school environment, and health education. It should also include but not be limited to guidance and counseling, physical education, food service, social work, psychological services, and employee health promotion.

School health education: School health education is one component of the comprehensive school health program that includes the development, delivery, and evaluation of a planned instructional program and other activities for students in preschool through grade 12, for parents, and for school staff and is designed to positively influence the health knowledge, attitudes, and skills of individuals.

School health services: School health services are that part of the school health program provided by physicians, nurses, dentists, health educators, allied health personnel, social workers, and teachers to appraise, protect, and promote the health of students and school personnel. These services are designed to ensure access to and appropriate use of primary health care services, prevent and control communicable disease, provide emergency care for injury or sudden illness, promote and provide optimal sanitary conditions in a safe school facility and environment, and provide concurrent learning opportunities conducive to the maintenance and promotion of individual and community health.

School health educator: A school health educator is a practitioner who is professionally prepared in the field of school health education, meets state teaching requirements, and demonstrates competence in the development, delivery, and evaluation of curricula for students and adults in the school setting that enhance health knowledge, attitudes, and problem-solving skills.

Comprehensive school health instruction: Comprehensive school health instruction refers to the development, delivery and evaluation of a planned curriculum, preschool through 12, with goals, objectives, content sequence, and specific classroom lessons that includes but is not limited to the following major content areas:

- Community health
- Consumer health
- Environmental health
- Family life
- Mental and emotional health
- Injury prevention and safety
- Nutrition
- Personal health
- Prevention and control of disease
- Substance use and abuse

Post-secondary health education program: A post-secondary health education program is a planned set of health education policies, procedures, activities, and services that are directed to students, faculty, and/or staff of colleges, universities, and other higher education institutions. This includes but is not limited to the following:

- General health courses for students
- Employee and student health promotion activities
- Health services
- Professional preparation of health educators and other professionals
- Self-help groups
- Student life

Governmental Agencies

Agency	Type of Materials	Health Topics	Levels
Environmental Protection Agency Forms and Publications Center Research Triangle Park, NC 27711 919/541-2111	Printed materials	Environmental health	General and adult
High Blood Pressure Information Center 1501 Wilson Blvd. Arlington, VA 22209 703/558-4880	Booklets	Disease prevention and control	General and adult
National Archives and Records Service General Services Administration National Audiovisual Center Washington, D.C. 20409 301/763-1896	Information lists Catalogues	Consumer health Drug use and abuse Environmental health Health careers Safety and first aid	General and adult
National Clearinghouse on Drug Abuse Information Room 10A56, Parklawn Building 5600 Fishers Lane Rockville, MD 20857 301/443-6500	Pamphlets Films	Drug use and abuse	General and adult
National Health Information Clearinghouse PO Box 1133 Washington, D.C. 20013 800/336-4797	Publications Pamphlets Information given over the telephone	Alcohol and smoking Consumer health Disease prevention and control Drug use and abuse Family life Mental health Physical fitness Personal health Safety	General and adult
National Heart, Lung and Blood Institute 9000 Rockville Pike National Institutes of Health Bldg. 31/4 A24 Bethesda, MD 20205 301/496-1051	Printed materials	Disease prevention and control Nutrition	General and adult

P, K through 3rd; I, 4th through 5th; M, 6th through 8th.

Agency	Type of Materials	Health Topics	Levels
National Highway Traffic Safety Administration U.S. Department of Transportation Washington, D.C. 20590 202/426-1828	Printed materials	Alcohol Safety	General and adult
National Institute on Alcohol Abuse and Alcohol- ism National Institutes of Mental Health 5600 Fishers Lane Rockville, MD 20857 301/468-2600	Pamphlets Reprints	Alcohol	General and adult
National Institute of Dental Research National Institutes of Health Bldg. 31/2 C34 Bethesda, MD 20205 301/496-4261	Pamphlets	Nutrition Personal health	M M General and adult
Office on Smoking and Health Room 1-10, Park Building 5600 Fishers Lane Rockville, MD 20857 301/443-1690	Technical information center	Smoking	General and adult
Public Documents Distribution Center Department 20 Pueblo, CO 81009	Pamphlets		General and adult
Public Health Service Environmental Health Service U.S. Department of Health, Education, and Welfare Rockville, MD 20857 301/881-1870	Pamphlets Reprints	Environmental health	General and adult
Superintendent of Documents U.S. Government Printing Office Washington, D.C. 20402 202/783-3238	Pamphlets Posters	Alcohol Community health Disease prevention and control Drug use and abuse Environmental health Growth and development Nutrition Personal health (dental) Safety and first aid Smoking	M I,M I,M I M P,I P,I,M I,M
U.S. Center for Health Promotion and Education Centers for Disease Control 1600 Clifton Atlanta, GA 30333 404/633-3311	Printed materials	General health education	General and adult
U.S. Office of Health Information and Health Promotion Hubert Humphrey Building 200 Independence Ave. S.W. Washington, D.C. 20201 202/655-4000	Printed materials	General health education	General and adult

Voluntary and Nonprofit Health Agencies

Agency	Type of Materials	Health Topics	Levels
Agency for Instructional Television 1111 W. 17th St. Bloomington, IN 47401 812/339-2203	Films Videocassettes	Mental and emotional health Safety Social health	General and adult
American Cancer Society, Inc. (national headquarters) Clyton Road Atlanta, GA 30030	Program packages: *Early Start to Good Health* (K-3), *Health Network* (4-6) Other instructional kits Films and guides Pamphlets Posters	Community health Consumer health Disease prevention and control Drugs, alcohol, and tobacco Family life Growth and development Mental and emotional health Nutrition Personal health	I, II, III III I,II,III I,II,III I,II,III I,II,III I,II,III II I,II,III
American Heart Association (national headquarters) The National Center 7320 Greenville Ave. Dallas, TX 75231 214/750-5300	Program packages: *Take Care of Your Heart; One Heart for Life* Brochures Pamphlets Films and filmstrips Cassettes Games Posters Photographic slides	Consumer health Disease prevention and control Drug use and abuse First aid Growth and development Nutrition Personal health	III III I,II III I,II,III I,II
American Lung Association (national headquarters) 1740 Broadway New York, NY 10019 212/245-8000	Program packages: *Lung Health Module* Films Literature and periodicals Posters Buttons and stickers Slides and cassettes	Community health Disease prevention and control Growth and development Environmental health	III I III
American Red Cross (national headquarters) 17th and E St. N.W. Washington, D.C. 20006 202/737-8300	Educational series on blood and circulatory system Films and filmstrips Pamphlets and leaflets Textbooks Posters	Community health Consumer health Family life Growth and development Mental and emotional health Personal health Safety and first aid	I III II,III I,II,III I III I,II,II

I, K through 3rd; *II*, 4th through 5th; *III*, 6th through 8th.-

Agency	Type of Materials	Health Topics	Levels
Arthritis Foundation (national headquarters) 3400 Peachtree Rd. N.E., Suite 1101 Atlanta, GA 30326 404/266-0795	Pamphlets Reprints	Disease prevention and control	I,II,III
Asthma and Allergy Foundation of America 1125 15th St. N.W., Suite 502 Washington, D.C. 20005	Pamphlets Films	Disease prevention and control Growth and development	General and adult
Cystic Fibrosis Foundation (national headquarters) 6000 Executive Blvd., Suite 309 Rockville, MD 20852 301/881-9130	Leaflets and pamphlets Films	Disease prevention and control Growth and development	General and adult
Epilepsy Foundation of America 4351 Garden City Dr. Landover, MD 20785 301/459-3700	Pamphlets Paperback books Films Cassettes Slides	Disease prevention and control	General and adult
Health Education Service, Inc. PO Box 7126 Albany, NY 12224 518/392-3951	Pamphlets Posters Videotapes	Family life Personal health (dental) Safety and first aid	III I II
March of Dimes—Birth Defects Foundation 1275 Mamaroneck Ave. PO Box 2000 White Plains, NY 10605 914/428-7100	Program packages: *Starting a Healthy Family* (Units I, II, III), *Preparenthood Education Program (PEP)* Films and filmstrips Pamphlets	Consumer health Disease prevention and control Drug use and abuse First aid Growth and development Nutrition Personal health	III III II III I,II,III II
Mental Health Materials Center PO Box 304 Bronxville, NY 10708 914/337-6596	Pamphlets Films	Family life Growth and development Mental and emotional health Personal health	General and adult
Muscular Dystrophy Association (national headquarters) 3561 E. Sunrise Dr. Tucson, AZ 85718 605/529-2000	Pamphlets Films	Disease prevention and control	I
National Association for Sickle Cell Disease, Inc. 3460 Wilshire Blvd., Suite 1012 Los Angeles, CA 90010 212/731-1166	Fact sheets Brochures	Disease prevention and control	II

Agency	Type of Materials	Health Topics	Levels
National Congress of Parents and Teachers (NCPT) 700 N. Rush St. Chicago, IL 60611 312/787-0977	Program package: *Alcohol Alley* Health education curricula Pamphlets	Consumer health Community health Disease prevention and control Drug use and abuse Environmental health Family life Growth and development Mental and emotional health Nutrition Personal health Safety and first aid	General and adult
National Council on Alcoholism and Drug Dependence 12 W. 21st St. New York, NY 10010 212/206-6770	Pamphlets Books	Alcohol	General and adult
National Easter Seal Society for Crippled Children and Adults 2023 W. Ogden Ave. Chicago, IL 60612 312/243-8400	Pamphlets	Dental health Disease prevention and control Growth and development Safety	General and adult
National Health Council 1730 M St. N.W., Suite 500 Washington, D.C. 20036 202/785-3913	Pamphlets	Health careers	General and adult
National Safety Council 425 N. Michigan Ave. Chicago, IL 60611 312/527-4800	Films Pamphlets Posters	Safety	General and adult
National Society to Prevent Blindness (NSPB) (national headquarters) 79 Madison Ave. New York, NY 10016 212/684-3505	Pamphlet Films Charts	Disease prevention and control Growth and development Safety and first aid	I I I
United Cerebral Palsy Association, Inc. (national headquarters) 7 Penn Plaza, Suite 804 New York, NY 10001 212/268-6655	Pamphlets	Disease prevention and control	General and adult
Wisconsin Clearinghouse for Alcohol and Other Drug Information 1954 E. Washington Ave. Madison, WI 53704-5271 608/263-2797	Pamphlets and booklets Fact sheets Posters	Drug use and abuse Family life Mental and emotional health Safety and first aid	III I,II,III II III

SOURCES OF FREE AND LOW-COST SPONSORED INSTRUCTIONAL AIDS FOR HEALTH TEACHING

The national organizations listed with asterisks have state or regional affiliates or offices. When this state or regional location is known, the teacher should first request materials or information from the nearest unit.

Abbott Laboratories
1 Abbott Park Rd.
Abbott Park, IL 60064
(708) 937-6100

Aetna Life and Casualty Companies
Public Relations and Advertising
151 Farmington Ave. DA06
Hartford, CT 06156
(203) 273-0123

*Al-Anon Family Group Headquarters
PO Box 862, Midtown Station
New York, NY 10018
(212) 302-7240

Allstate
Corporate Relations Department
Allstate Plaza
Northbrook, IL 60062
(312) 291-5000

American Alliance for Health, Physical
  Education, Recreation and Dance
1900 Association Dr.
Reston, VA 22091
(703) 476-3400

American Allergy Association
PO Box 7273
Menlo Park, CA 94026
(415) 322-1663

*American Automobile Association
Traffic Safety Department
1000 AAA Dr.
Heathrow, FL 32746-5063
(407) 444-7000

*American Dairy Association
6300 North River Rd.
Rosemont, IL 60018
(708) 696-1880

American Dairy Products Institute
130 North Franklin St.
Chicago, IL 60606
(312) 782-4888

American Dental Association
Bureau of Health Education and Audiovisual
  Services
211 East Chicago, Ave.
Chicago, IL 60611
(312) 440-2500

*American Diabetes Association
PO Box 25757
1660 Duke St.
Alexandria, VA 22314
(703) 549-1500

American Foundation for the Blind
15 West 16th St.
New York, NY 10011
(212) 620-2000

American Heart Association
7320 Greenville, Ave.
Dallas, TX 75231
(214) 373-6300

American Institute of Baking
Communications Department
1213 Bakers Way
Manhattan, KS 66502
(913) 537-4750

*American Lung Association
1740 Broadway
New York, NY 10019
(212) 315-8700

American Medical Association
515 N. State St.
Chicago, IL 60610
(312) 464-4818

American Social Health Association
PO Box 13827
Research Triangle Park, NC 27709
(919) 361-8400

Autism Society of America
8601 Georgia Ave., Suite 503
Silver Spring, MD 20910
(301) 565-0433

Children with Attention-Deficit Disorders
499 NW 70th Ave., Suite 308
Plantation, FL 33317
(305) 587-3700

The Hogg Foundation for Mental Health
University of Texas-Austin
Austin, TX 78713-7998
(512) 471-5041

Institute of Makers of Explosives
1120 19th St. NY, Suite 310
Washington, D.C. 20036
(202) 429-99280

Kellogg Company
PO Box 3599
Battle Creek, MI 49016
(616) 961-2006

Kemper Corporation
Long Grove, IL 60049
(708) 540-2000

Kemper Financial Services, Inc.
120 S. LaSalle St.
Chicago, IL 60603
(312) 781-1121

Kimberly-Clark Corporation
DFW Airport Station
PO Box 619100
Dallas, TX 75261
(214) 830-1200

Leukemia Society of America
733 3rd Ave.
New York, NY 10017
(212) 573-8484

Lever Brothers Company, Inc.
Lever House
390 Park Ave.
New York, NY 10022
(212) 688-6000

Mental Health Materials Center
PO Box 304
Bronxville, NY 10708
(914) 337-6596

Metropolitan Life Insurance Company
Health and Safety Education Division
One Madison Ave.
New York, NY 10019
(212) 578-2211

Millers' National Federation
600 Maryland Ave., SW, Suite 305 West Wing
Washington, D.C. 20024
(202) 484-2200

National Association for Hearing and Speech
   Action
10801 Rockville Pike
Rockville, MD 20852
(301) 897-8682

National Council on Family Relations
3989 Central Avenue, NE, Suite 550
St. Paul, MN 55421
(612) 781-9331

National Fire Protection Association
1 Batterymarch Park
PO Box 9101
Quincy, MA 02269-9101
(617) 770-3000

National Heart, Lung, and Blood Institute
Department of Health and Human Services
Bethesda, MD 20214
(301) 496-5161

Prudential Insurance Company of America
Public Relations and Advertising
Prudential Plaza
PO Box 36
Newark, NJ 07101
(201) 877-6000

Ralston Purina Company
Corporate Consumer Services
Public Relations
Checkerboard Square
St. Louis, MO 63164
(314) 982-1000

Rutgers Center of Alcohol Studies
Smithers Hall
Piscataway, NJ 08855-0969
(908) 932-2190

Schering-Plough Corporation
One Giralda Farms
Madison, NJ 07940
(201) 822-7000

Sex Information and Education Council of the
    United States
130 W. 42nd St., Suite 2500
New York, NY 10036
(212) 819-9770

Smithkline Pharmaceuticals Co.
1500 Spring Garden St.
PO Box 7929
Philadelphia, PA 19101
(215) 751-4000

State Farm Insurance Companies
Public Relations Department
One State Farm Plaza
Bloomington, IN 61761
(309) 766-2311

Sunkist Growers, Inc.
14130 Riverside Dr.
Sherman Oaks, CA 91423
(818) 986-4800

The Travelers Film Library
Travelers Ins. Co.
One Tower Square
Hartford, CT 06115
(203) 277-0111

Los Angeles Unified School District
Huntington Park High School
6020 Miles Avenue, Huntington Park, California 90255

LEONARD M. BRITTON
Superintendent of Schools
ANTONIO GARCIA
Principal

Dear Parent or Guardian:

You son/daughter is enrolled in a health education course at our school. This course covers such topics as drug and alcohol abuse, the importance of good nutrition, prevention of cancer and diabetes, prevention of AIDS and other sexually transmitted diseases, suicide prevention, first aid and CPR, family life, and sex education. The unit dealing with family life and sex education includes such topics as rape prevention, prevention of child abuse, ways to get along better with parents and brothers and sisters, and the importance of abstinence until marriage.

The units dealing with sexually transmitted diseases and family life and sex education will include one or more sessions in which the human reproductive organs may be described, illustrated, or discussed within the context of the study of human growth, maturation, and reproduction. Within the unit dealing with sexually transmitted diseases, sessions will be on the causes, symptoms, complications, and treatment.

The units dealing with family life and sex education and sexually transmitted diseases are optional, and the signed consent of a parent or guardian will be required for your son or daughter to receive this instruction. The *California Education Code* requires that instructional materials used in these classes be made available for you to inspect. In compliance with this requirement, a special display to provide you an opportunity to preview the materials will be presented in Room _____ on _____.

Please indicate on the tear-off below whether you wish your child to receive the optional instruction referred to above. Should you prefer that your child not receive this instruction, other assignments will be provided for him/her during the approximate 7-week period concerned.

Principal Antonio Garcia

- -tear-off -

To: Principal Antonio Garcia of Huntington Park High School

I do _____ do not _____ wish my son/daughter to receive the optional instruction dealing with family life and sex education being offered in the health course.

I do _____ do not _____ wish my son/daughter to receive the optional instruction on sexually transmitted diseases that will be offered in the health course.

Name of son or daughter _____

Signature of parent or guardian _____

Address _____ Date _____

An Analysis Checklist for Audiovisuals When Used as Educational Resources

Title _____

Distributor _____ Loan/Rental Terms _____

Media Type

___ 35 mm slides   ___ Videotape   ___ 16 mm film   ___ Film strip

___ Slide/tape   ___ Audiotape   ___ 8 mm film   ___ Other

EVALUATION INSTRUCTIONS

Listed below are general criteria to be used in analyzing and rating audiovisuals. Please read each element below each of the four dimensions listed: content, technical production, format, and characterization. Select one of the numbered descriptors that best describes your interpretation of how well each of the elements was used in the production. Place that number in the lined space to the right of each element. A space is provided for listing subtotals of each dimension and for circling the final overall rating. Please note the following example.

Example	Answer	Item code	
Are the facts and ideas worth stating? _____	3	3 = Excellent	I = Average
		2 = Good	0 = Poor

Content (based on proposed course or curriculum and the following additional criteria, is significance of content given primary importance?)

1. Are the facts and ideas worth stating? _____
2. Does the production indicate research practices of high standing? _____
3. Apparent usage of grammar/spelling _____
4. Accuracy of content _____
5. Viewer appeal _____
6. Writing style _____
7. Does audiovisual elicit or exude undue biases? _____

             TOTAL _____

Characterization (based on the following criteria, what was the overall quality and approach of announcers, cast, or crew?)

1. Voice quality _____
2. Fluency _____
3. Informative _____
4. Intimacy _____
5. Creativity _____
6. Interest _____
7. Terseness (concise, avoiding wordiness) _____

             TOTAL _____

Technical production (based on the following, are basic production elements used effectively in the audiovisual production?)

1. Unity _____
2. Center of interest _____
3. Variety _____
4. Cohesiveness _____
5. Conflict
6. Climax _____
7. Resolution of climax(es) _____
8. Pace _____
9. Warmth and emotion _____
10. Establishment of authoritativeness _____
11. Harmonious blending of all parts of the production? _____

TOTAL _____

Format: (based on the intended use of the audiovisual, do design elements do what they are set up to do?)

1. Use of special effects _____
2. Does film create proper mood? _____
3. Length of production _____
4. Volume levels of music, characters, special effects _____
5. How do audiovisual materials compare with similar A/V of this type? _____

TOTAL _____

Overall rating

Please circle the total number of points that indicates your total overall rating.

Excellent	75-99+
Good	50-74
Average	25-49
Poor	0-24

Health Education Software Evaluation Form

Title of program: _____ Version: _____

Distributor: _____ Copyright: _____

Address: _____ Cost: _____

Phone for technical support: _____ Serial # or site license agreement #: _____

    License restrictions: ☐ No copies allowed ☐ Backup copy only ☐ Multiple copies allowed

    ☐ Site license in effect

    Estimated operating time:_____

Hardware/software required:

Computer brand	☐IBM	☐Macintosh	☐Apple	☐Tandy ☐Other _____
Printer type	☐Laser	☐Dot-matrix	☐Letter quality	
Other	☐Mouse		☐Graphics required	☐Color monitor required

Amount of memory:_____

Version of DOS required:_____

Target population:

Age group:_____

Grade	☐Elementary	☐Middle	☐High school	☐Secondary ☐Adult
Ability	☐Advanced	☐Average	☐Low	☐Remedial
Grouping requirements	☐Individual	☐Pairs	☐Small group	

Accompanying instructional materials:

Continued.

Content evaluation:
☐Objectives stated clearly   ☐Content covers curricular needs
☐Content presented accurately   ☐Appropriate reading level
☐Free from stereotypes and bias   ☐Free from grammar/punctuation/spelling errors

Technical evaluation:
Check program features:
☐Graphics   ☐Music   ☐Time display
☐Color   ☐Voice   ☐Score display
☐Sound   ☐Windows   ☐Modem
☐Display screens legible   ☐Learner input errors handled effectively
☐Help screen available   ☐Can the rate of presentation be altered
☐Teacher can control or alter the content   ☐Reenter the program at last page of exit
☐Evidence the product has undergone revision ☐Level of skill is required for the instructor

Instructional evaluation:
☐Level of the learner assessed   ☐Branching based on individual needs
☐Record kept of learner progress   ☐Positive feedback provided to the learner
☐Learner practice or examples provided ☐Post-test provided
☐Personalization provided   ☐Instructions provided
☐Requisite skills stated

Documentation:
☐Documentation included   ☐Documentation easy to use
☐Results of pilot testing given in documentation ☐Suggestions of time allotments and use
☐On-screen documentation provided   of courseware provided
☐Technical support provided   ☐Instructor's manual provided
                                    ☐Student manual provided

Description of the program: Health content area(s):
                                   ☐Aging   ☐Exercise/fitness
                                   ☐Accidents   ☐Mental health
                                   ☐Community health   ☐Nutrition
                                   ☐Consumer health   ☐Personal health
                                   ☐Disease prevention ☐Sexuality
                                   ☐Environmental   ☐Substance abuse
                                   ☐Other _____

Reviewed by: _____ Date: _____

Glossary

affective domain relates to the values, beliefs, interests, attitudes, emotions, and feelings of individuals

affective objectives statements of teaching and learning purposes concerned with favorably influencing attitudes, values, or interests

AIDS (acquired immunodeficiency syndrome) an infection caused by a virus (HIV) transmitted through specific means, principally sexual intercourse, but also through sharing needles, syringes and other drug abuse paraphernalia, from an infected woman to her fetus or newborn infant, and by transfusion, specially in the case of hemophiliacs

anecdotal record a type of cumulative individual record that emphasizes episodes of behavior important in the character or personality

CAI Computer assisted instruction

child abuse any act of either commission or omission that endangers or hinders a child's physical or emotional growth and development

cognitive domain relates to the ability to deal with knowledge and factual information from an intellectual perspective

community health council cooperative body representative of all community health-interested organizations and agencies

competency ability to perform at some predetermined acceptable level of expertise, usually less than mastery

comprehensive school health program the planned coordinated provision of health services, a healthful environment, and health instruction for all children in a school, where each of the components complements and is integrated with the others in the total scope of the body of knowledge unique to health education

computer disk disk, also termed *floppy disk*, that stores information for later use or retrieval

concept an abstract idea or statement used as the focus of instruction relative to a broad area of subject matter

conceptual approach a curriculum organizational plan that employs generalizations or concepts as the framework of its scope

congenital a physical defect or abnormality existing at birth or before but not due to heredity, e.g., cerebral palsy, blindness or deafness of an infant whose mother suffered from measles (rubella) during her pregnancy

content the subject matter of health education; *see also* process

cooperative learning a teaching-learning strategy that focuses on team work, typically heterogeneous grouping of four students of various abilities, whose work is rewarded as a group, and dependent on the individual learning all its members

culminating activity a planned summarizing procedure or action providing a meaningful closure to a total learning experience

cumulative health folder a form used by school health service professionals to maintain records of screening tests, medical examinations, immunizations, illnesses or disabilities, anecdotal records of health-related behaviors that threaten a student's learning ability, and any other information relevant to the education and well-being of a schoolchild throughout his or her public school education

direct health teaching instruction given during regularly scheduled periods, having an organized, planned curriculum in equal status with all other basic studies

disease prevention deliberate actions planned and taken for the purpose of maintaining health, protecting against disease, early diagnosis and treatment of suspected disease, and rehabilitating disabled persons to the degree possible

elementary school usually refers to kindergarten to grade 6 or grade 8; in this text, refers to kindergarten to grade 8

enabling objectives subordinate objectives inferred as contributing to achievement of a general objective (see also instructional objectives)

evaluation a means of making informed decisions about the quality of a product or a performance; may be ongoing, or *formative*, as a means of determining total growth or change as a total outcome of some specified treatment or program; includes but is not limited to quantitative measurement

experiential teaching the provision of activities that are realistic, involve multiple senses, and require the learner to participate fully, affectively, physically, and cognitively; sometimes called hands-on learning (the student learns by doing)

face validity a quality of test design based on the fact that the items do match the subject matter of concern

footcandle the amount of light on a surface that can be seen at a distance of 1 foot from a lighted standard candle

follow-through procedures procedures used to check on the outcome of a referral of a child for further diagnosis or treatment of a health problem

free-response test one in which the student uses his or her own words to respond in writing to a relatively small number of questions

general objectives broad abstract statements expressing educational goals for several years; or to serve as guidelines for the more specific objectives of a given course of study

generalization a statement broadly representative of a class of subordinate ideas or data

handicapping conditions any condition that limits a child's mobility, strength, or well-being to the extent that special teaching may be required; includes mental retardation, speech impairment, visual impairment, hearing impairment, learning disability, emotional disturbance, orthopedic handicap, deaf-blindness, or health impairments associated with other conditions such as autism

health a quality of life involving dynamic interaction and interdependence of the physical, social, and mental and emotional dimensions of an individual's well-being

health attitudes relatively lasting clusters of feelings, beliefs, and behavior tendencies directed toward specific objects, persons, or situations related to health

health behavior actions customarily taken by an individual that have an impact on personal and community wellbeing

health belief a health-related statement or sense, declared or implied intellectually or emotionally, and accepted as being true by an individual or group; sometimes referred to as the conventional wisdom

health counseling procedures by which teachers, nurses, and physicians interpret a problem to students and their parents as a means of helping them find a solution

health education systematically organized activities designed to aid students in gaining the knowledge, skills, understanding, attitudes, and behavior patterns necessary for living healthfully; also health instruction, as a term used interchangeably in this book

health education goals long-range plans specified as the desired overall outcome of instruction

health guidance general assistance given by school personnel (such as nurses and teachers) to students and their parents to help them solve health problems that hinder a child's ability to learn

health habit a health practice that has become a routine activity

health knowledge authoritative concepts, generalizations, and supporting factual data deemed representative of the discipline of health education

health promotion any combination of health instruction and community organizations efforts supportive of individual or group behaviors conducive to improvement of their health status

health services all the efforts of the school to conserve, protect, and improve the health of the school population; includes appraisal of student health, prevention and control of disease, prevention or correction of physical defects, health guidance and supervision, and emergency care

healthful conducive to the maintenance or promotion of an individual's wellbeing

healthful school environment the quality of the physical, social, and emotional dimensions of a school; provided through procedures to maintain a safe and sanitary environment that promotes the health of both students and school personnel

healthy an optimum state or quality of life

hereditary a disease or tendency to certain diseases transmitted from parents to offspring, and carried by the genes, e.g., cystic fibrosis, sickle cell anemia, hemophilia

holistic health that state of being in which a person's body, mind, and spirit are in balance, functioning with utmost capacity or potential (high-level wellness), and in tune with natural and social environments, as well as with the cosmos (the spiritual environment)

hygiene personal health care, especially techniques and standards of grooming and cleanliness

incidental teaching ad lib attention to a health topic not scheduled or planned during a period of instruction but in response to current health problems or happenings of interest

infusion an alternative term used to describe the integration of health instruction or subject matter within other subject areas in the curriculum

initiating activity procedures to set the stage for what is to follow; may be done by recalling known related experiences, materials, or problems before entering into a new lesson

instructional objectives specific objectives serving as the focus of single lessons

integration in curriculum means by which a subject area is introduced and treated in a given educational situation so that subject areas are not treated separately, but logically as they relate to a broad unit of study

intermediate level in this text, grades 4 to 6

learning opportunity a situation in which relevant knowledge and activities are provided to stimulate the learner to become actively involved in the development of specified knowledge and skills.

liability responsibility for a tort or injury occurring on school grounds as legally determined by court action

life style decisions made and resulting actions taken by individuals that typically affect their health

mandates laws requiring that certain actions be carried out in prescribed ways

measurable objective one whose achievement can be assessed in the classroom by means of an evaluation procedure exactly matching the objective's expressed intent

measurement   quantitative description of student learning or progress; status determination

middle school   in many states a term currently used to designate grades 6 through 8, transitional between elementary school and preliminary to high school

mock-up   a simplified and clarified working model of part or all of a real device, for example, driver-training devices and the head and torso used in CPR practice

modem   a piece of equipment that enables the user to transfer copy from one computer to another, whatever the distance between the two may be; the term stands for *modulator-demodulator*

morbidity statistics   reported incidence of specified diseases and other health problems

need   (1) the degree to which the present condition of an individual differs from some acceptable norm (2) the natural urge to maintain a balance between internal drives and external conditions (physiological, psychological, and integrative needs) (3) felt needs: interests and concerns arising from intense desire to know about something or how to solve some problem

negligence   failure to do something that a reasonable person would do, or doing something that a reasonable and prudent person would not do

norms   average scores on a standardized test based on data obtained through its application to a population of students of a specified grade level or age

organizing elements   the range of subject areas or health topics considered to structure the body of knowledge of health education (body systems, health problems, content areas, topics, and generalizations or concepts).

organizing threads   continuing curriculum emphases, health concepts, values, and problem-solving skills that provide the basis for continuity and integration

permissive legislation   laws that establish the right to carry out a specified action, without requiring that it be done

primary level   the early elementary school years, specifically kindergarten to grade 3

problem-solving method   a logical process by means of which data are gathered and reasonable hypotheses are formulated and tested, until the best possible solution is discovered to a given health problem

process   all the cognitive operations applied in the use of the subject matter of health education; *see also* content

psychomotor objectives   those describing physical activities that can be practiced observably and demonstrated directly; for example, in health education, first aid techniques and toothbrushing skills

Public Law 94-142   legislation defining the rights of handicapped or disabled children to free public education in the least restrictive environment possible

reliability   the consistency and stability with which a test measures whatever it is measuring; an essential aspect of validity

resource persons   parents, health providers, and other concerned adults who voluntarily assist teachers and schools in the promotion of the school health program; may include health services, instruction, advisement, fund raising, and other appropriate activities

risk factors   characteristics or patterns of health behaviors that increase a person's risk of disease. These are either unmodifiable (e.g., age, sex) or modifiable, (e.g., cigarette smoking, overweight)

school health committee   a representative group of individuals drawn from school administration, faculty, staff, community, and students; a fact-finding, recommending, advisory body

school health education   instruction designed to improve health-related knowledge, attitudes, and behavior

scope   the entire range of organizing elements (subject matter categories) considered within health education curriculum plan

screening tests   preliminary appraisal techniques used by teachers or school nurses to identify children who appear to need diagnostic tests carried out by medical specialists

self care   the active involvement of lay persons on their own behalf in health promotion and disease prevention procedures or activities

semantic differential test   an instrument based on the scales developed by Osgood, Suci, and Tannenbaum* as a means of measuring attitudes toward specific concepts

sequence   a plan for the ordering of organizing elements either vertically (year to year) or horizontally (day to day and week to week) for any one course of study

Social Learning Theory (SLT)   the theory that every person exhibits a variety of behaviors that being reinforced by success recur when the stimulus is the same in later situations

software   a prepared set of instructions by which a microcomputers functions are activated and employed

standardized test   one whose validity and reliability have been established by means of careful statistical and other procedures; norms provided as well

---

*Osgood CE, Suci GJ, Tannenbaum PH: *The measurement of meaning,* Urbana, Ill, 1957, University of Illinois Press.

structured-answer test   an objectively scorable instrument by means of which the student indicates an answer to each item by checking or circling the best or correct choice among those alternatives offered

taxonomy of educational objectives   a scheme classifying educational objectives according to six levels of cognition, from lowest to highest in complexity, where the ability to demonstrate skill in each presupposes and depends on achievement of those preceding it in the hierarchy

teaching method   a process that involves the reasoned ordering or balancing of the elements of an educational function, that is, purposes, nature of the learner, materials of instruction, and total teaching and learning situation

teaching techniques   procedures or activities used by teachers for facilitating practice of instructional objectives, for example, field trips, role playing, lectures, and debates

tort law   civil liability laws governing torts (acts or failures to act by which a person injures another person or his or her property or reputation either directly or indirectly)

validity   the extent to which a test correlates with some criterion external to the test itself; that is, does it measure what it claims to measure?

values   preferences for ideas, things, or behaviors that are shared and transmitted within a community

Credits

Chapter 1

p. 13 (Figure 1-2). From Healthy People 2000, US Department of Health and Human Services, Public Health Service, 1990.

p. 20 (Figure 1-3). Health instruction responsibilities and competencies for elementary (k-6) classroom teachers. From *J Sch Health* 62(2):77, February 1992. Reprinted with permission. American School Health Association, Kent, Ohio.

Chapter 2

p. 27 (Figure 2-1). Adapted with permission from Edward B. Johns.

p. 29 (Figure 2-2). From Stone E: ACCESS: keystones for school health promotion, *J Sch Health* 60(7):298, September 1990. Reprinted with permission. American School Health Association, Kent, Ohio.

Chapter 3

p. 78 (Figure 3-1). Modified from School Health Education Study: *Health education: a conceptual approach to curriculum design*, St. Paul, 1967, 3M Education Press.

Chapter 5

p. 121 (Photograph). Copyright American Dental Association. Reprinted by permission.

Chapter 6

p. 160 (Box). Modified from Parker B: *Exec Educator* 3(8):24, 1980.

Chapter 7

p. 184 (Box). From Gilbert GG, Chairperson, Department of Health Education, University of Maryland.

Chapter 8

pp. 200-201 (Figure 8-1). Further information may be obtained by writing to the test author, Dr. Wanda Jubb, 2867 Greystone Lane, Atlanta, Georgia, 30341. Reprinted by permission.

Chapter 9

p. 218 (Figure 9-1), p. 219 (Figure 9-2), p. 221 (Figure 9-3) p. 222 (Figure 9-4), p. 223 (Figure 9-5), and p. 224 (Figure 9-6). From Payne W, Hahn D: *Understanding your health*, ed 3, St. Louis, 1992, Mosby–Year Book.

p. 225 (Figure 9-7). From Thibodeau G: *Structure and function of the body*, ed 9, St. Louis, 1992, Mosby–Year Book.

p. 227 (Figure 9-8) and p. 228 (Figure 9-9). From Payne W, Hahn D: *Understanding your health*, ed 3, St. Louis, 1992, Mosby–Year Book.

p. 229 (Figure 9-10). From Tate P, Seeley R, Stephens T: *Understanding the human body*, St. Louis, 1994, Mosby–Year Book.

p. 230 (Box). Copyright American Dental Association. Reprinted with permission.

p. 231 (Box). Helen Cease. Copyright American Dental Association. Reprinted with permission.

Chapter 11

p. 280 (Figure 11-1) and 281 (Figure 11-2). From Payne, W, Hahn D: *Understanding your health*, ed 3, St. Louis, 1992, Mosby–Year Book.

Chapter 12

p. 312 (Figure 12-1) and 313 (Box). US Department of Agriculture/US Department of Health and Human Services, 1992.

p. 316 (Table 12-1). From Payne W and Hahn D: *Understanding your health*, ed 3, St. Louis, 1992, Mosby–Year Book.

p. 317 (Box). Adapted from *National Anorexic Aid Society* Newsletter: 11:4, 1988.

Chapter 13

p. 339 (Figure 13-1). From Hockey RV: *Physical fitness: the pathway to healthful living*, ed 7, St. Louis, 1993, Mosby–Year Book.

Chapter 16

p. 397 (Figure 16-1). US Food and Drug Administration.

Chapter 19

p. 468 (Figure 19-1). Adapted from Siri D: *Community/school partnerships*. In Cortese P, Middletonk, eds: *The comprehensive school health challenge*, vol 2, Santa Cruz, Calif., 1994, ETR Associates.

Index